Baillière's Pharmacology and Drug Information for Nurses

Second Edition

UK Adaptation Team

From the Westminster Hospital, London

Frances Mary Wellington, SRN, RNT
Senior Nurse: Education
The Wolfson School of Nursing of Westminster

Denise Victoria Hoare, BSc(Hons), MPS
Staff Pharmacist, Drug Information
The Westminster Hospital

Jeremy Hyde, PhD, BPharm(Hons), MPS
Assistant General Manager, Charing Cross Hospital
Formerly Principal Pharmacist, The Westminster Hospital

Brigid Mary Knight, SRN, OND, DN(Lond), DipNEd(Lond)
Tutor
The Wolfson School of Nursing of Westminster

Dee Montague-Johnstone, RGN, RCNT, DipNEd(Lond)
Clinical Teacher
The Wolfson School of Nursing of Westminster

Diane Roberts, SRN, RSCN, RCNT
Clinical Teacher
The Wolfson School of Nursing of Westminster

The authors and publisher have exerted every effort to ensure that drug selection and dosage set forth in this text are in accord with current recommendations and practice at the time of publication. However, in view of ongoing research, changes in government regulations, and the constant flow of information relating to drug therapy and drug reactions, the reader is urged to check the package insert for each drug for any change in indications and dosage and for added warnings and precautions. This is particularly important when the recommended agent is a newly employed drug. Remember — drug names marked with a dagger (†) in the text are not currently available at NHS expense.

Baillière's Pharmacology and Drug Information for Nurses

Second Edition

Baillière Tindall London Philadelphia Toronto
Mexico City Rio de Janeiro Sydney Tokyo Hong Kong

Baillière Tindall
W. B. Saunders

33 The Avenue
Eastbourne, East Sussex BN21 3UN, England

West Washington Square
Philadelphia, PA 19105, USA

1 Goldthorne Avenue
Toronto, Ontario M8Z 5T9, Canada

Apartado 26370—Cedro 512
Mexico 4, DF Mexico

Rua Evaristo da Veiga 55, 20° andar
Rio de Janeiro—RJ, Brazil

ABP Australia Ltd, 44–50 Waterloo Road
North Ryde, NSW 2113, Australia

Ichibancho Central Building, 22–1 Ichibancho,
Chiyoda-ku, Tokyo 102, Japan

10/fl, Inter-Continental Plaza, 94 Granville Road,
Tsim Sha Tsui East, Kowloon, Hong Kong

Original Edition published under the aegis of the Society of Hospital pharmacists of Australia and published in 1985 by Holt-Saunders Pty Ltd, 9 Waltham Street, Artarmon, NSW 2064, Australia. Reprinted 1985.

This edition first published 1987.

Printed and bound in Great Britain by Mackays of Chatham Ltd

British Library Cataloguing in Publication Data

[Pharmacology and drug information for nurses]. Baillière's pharmacology and drug information for nurses.—2nd ed.
1. Pharmacology 2. Nursing
I. [Pharmacology and drug information for nurses] II. Title
615′.1′024613 RM300

ISBN 0-7020-1169-X

Contents

List of Tables

List of Figures

Preface

It has always been the duty of the nurse to administer drugs to patients, but that often simple act of drug administration carries with it a broader responsibility. The nurse must carry out this duty with accuracy and care and with an understanding of what benefits and hazards the drug may bring to the patient. The nurse will be required to give a degree of informed and responsible information when patients enquire about their drugs.

Pharmacists have been greatly involved in pharmacology lectures to nurses to prepare them for this duty. The original Australian book was written by a team of hospital pharmacists and other health professionals, with clinical experience at ward level and involvement in nurse education, in the belief that a new style of textbook in pharmacology for nurses was required. This British edition has been thoroughly adapted for use in the UK and the Republic of Ireland by nurse educators and pharmacists from the Westminster Hospital.

In addition to defining drug groups, drug action, uses, adverse reactions and precautions, this text has the following unique features:

1. The information has been directed towards the needs of the student nurse and practising nurse.
2. A section on nursing implications of drug uses is included in all chapters.
3. Learning objectives and self-evaluation questions are included.
4. The text reflects the availability of drugs under Limited List prescribing.

Of course, while comprehensive and practical in its coverage of drug information, it is not possible to provide full drug profiles in such a text.

The adaptation and originating teams are confident that this text will assist in bringing greater knowledge and understanding to the nurse's daily responsibility of drug administration and patient monitoring.

Virginia Richardson
Mary Wellington

Note
Drugs not available at NHS expense are marked in the text with a dagger (†).

Editorial Panel

Virginia E. Richardson BPharm, MSHP (Chairman, Editorial Panel)
Director of Pharmacy (Clinical Services)
Royal Prince Alfred Hospital
Sydney, NSW

Ross W. Holland EdD, PhD, MA, FSHP, FASCP, FAIPM, MACPP, MPS, PhC
Director, Pharmed Consultants
Registrar
Australian College of Pharmacy Practice

Editorial Advisory Panel

Joy B. Hobbes MPS, PhC, MSc, MAACB
Director of Pharmacy
Royal North Shore Hospital
Sydney, NSW

Rhondda Figgis Close DipEdStd, MPS, MSHP, PhC
Chief Pharmacist
The Nepean District Hospital
Penrith, NSW

Nursing Advisory Panel

Wendy Brockdorff SRN, DNE, MCN (NSW)
Nurse Educator
School of Nursing Studies
Royal Prince Alfred Hospital
Sydney, NSW

Jan Davis RN, RMRN Dip Neurosurgical and Neurological Nursing, BSc
Nurse Teacher
Nursing Education Centre
Prince Henry Hospital
Sydney, NSW

Marie Therese Eckert RN, RMN, Cardiothoracic Cert, CWM, BA DipEd (Nurs, SCAE), FCN (NSW)
Nurse Teacher
Nursing Education Centre
Prince Henry Hospital
Sydney, NSW

Jill O'Connor BSc (Hons), RN, Cardiac Nurs Cert, DipTertEd
Nurse Teacher
Nursing Education Centre
Prince Henry Hospital
Sydney, NSW

SECTION 1

Chapter 1
AN INTRODUCTION TO PHARMACOLOGY AND DRUG INFORMATION
Chapter 2
DRUG PROBLEMS
Chapter 3
DOSE CALCULATIONS
Chapter 4
TOXICOLOGY

1

AN INTRODUCTION TO PHARMACOLOGY AND DRUG INFORMATION

Rosalind T. Chate and Ross W. Holland

I firmly believe that if the whole Materia Medica, as now used, could be sunk to the bottom of the sea, it would be all the better for mankind — and all the worse for the fishes.

Oliver Wendell Holmes, American Physician, 1860.

DEFINITIONS

Pharmacology — is the study of the way in which drugs work in the body.

A drug — in the modern sense, is any substance which affects normal bodily function at the cellular level.

INTRODUCTION

In this chapter, three aspects of medication and its use will be considered. Firstly, there will be a brief overview of the historical use and effectiveness of drugs. Secondly, there will be a consideration of the administration of drugs within a hospital, with particular emphasis on the role of the nurse. The third and final section introduces some basic concepts with regard to the way in which drugs work and the dose forms by which they may be administered.

HISTORICAL PERSPECTIVES

Drugs, in one form or another, appear to predate civilisation. The Sumerians dwelling in the valleys of the Tigris and Euphrates Rivers 5000 years ago compounded medicines using asafoetida, thyme, cassis, myrtle, salt, saltpetre, and the roots, seeds and bark of the willow, fig, pear and date trees. Their prescriptions, written in cuneiform script on tablets of damp clay, were similar to this: the seed of the carpenter plant, gum resin of marhazi, thyme, pulverise and dissolve in beer, let the man drink.

It is reasonably presumed that their ancestors employed drugs and potions for many thousands of years prior to that time, perhaps up to 50 000 years ago.

Not only were many such remedies medicinally worthless, but druggists in ancient times compounded medications to effect what, to us, seem unlikely cures. An Egyptian remedy for blindness, for example, consisted of a mixture of pig's eyes, antimony, red ochre and honey. This was poured into the patient's ears! Another Egyptian remedy, for baldness, called for "... fat of lion, fat of hippopotamus, fat of crocodile, fat of cat, fat of serpent, fat of ibex ... ".

More recently, Bulleyn, a physician during the reign of King Henry VIII, described a potion that "kings and noblemen have used for their comfort" containing (among other items) "two drachms of white pearles, two little pieces of saphyre, emeralds, thin pieces of gold and silver". One must suspect that this cure provided more comfort to the physician than to the patient. With reliance on substances of little therapeutic worth and prescribing practices of such doubtful value, it is not surprising that Oliver Wendell Holmes felt constrained to make the comment quoted at the beginning of this chapter.

Many cures attributed to prescriptions such as these, where the patient survived in spite of the treatment, can be explained by the natural recovery of the patient from what may have been a self-limiting disease. They may also have been influenced by the ***placebo*** effect, where the patient's condition improves because they ***expect*** it to, rather than because of any direct action of the medication. (***Placebo*** means "I shall please".) It should be remembered that, even today, the aim of treatment is to assist the body's natural healing processes and that the placebo effect is as strong as ever.

However, not all remedies were without pharmacological justification. The Egyptians cured night blindness by taking the "liver of an ox, roasted and crushed". As night blindness is caused by a deficiency of Vitamin A, readily available in liver, this remedy may have been effective. Extract of pomegranate root, prescribed to eliminate roundworm, contains a potent vermifuge, so the results were probably satisfactory.

Indeed, many of today's drugs had their precursors in ancient times. Antibiotics, derived from moulds, are usually regarded as being a modern development in medication, yet the Chinese treated boils with mouldy bean curd around 2500 B.C., and other races applied mouldy cheese as a dressing for wounds. The Egyptians used the juice of poppy seeds, a crude form of opium. Morphine, a purified alkaloidal extract of opium, remains a potent and widely-used analgesic. The Greeks used extracts of willow bark to reduce fever. Aspirin, still one of the most effective drugs used to reduce fever, is closely related to that extract.

The sources of currently used drugs are diverse and include plants, animals, minerals, bacteria and synthetic substances. Of these, the majority are synthetic, that is, manufactured in the laboratory. Although the search for such products began with the industrial revolution and were made possible as a result of the advances in organic chemistry that occurred during the latter part of the 19th century, most of our modern drugs have been developed within the past fifty years. In contrast with earlier times, modern drug treatment is based on the measurable pharmacological activity of the substances used.

Pharmaceutical manufacturers have invested vast amounts of money in the research, development and production of new drugs. Before they are approved for general use, these substances must be subjected to extensive testing, first on animals and then on human volunteers. When trials have been successfully completed, approval to market the product must be sought from government health agencies. In the United Kingdom, this function is carried out by the Committee on the Safety of Medicines.

Having obtained approval to market a drug, the manufacturer must then submit each batch to strict quality control procedures to ensure uniformity of the purity, strength and, in some cases, the sterility of the product. In this way, the patient who has been stabilised on a drug can expect to obtain the same effect from every dose of that drug regardless of the batch from which it has been taken.

THE USE OF DRUGS

THE ROLE OF THE PRESCRIBER

The medical practitioner is responsible for diagnosis and initiation of therapy. Drugs must be ordered in the prescriber's own handwriting. If there is any doubt in reading or interpreting these orders by the nurse or the pharmacist, the medical practitioner must be contacted.

THE ROLE OF THE PHARMACIST

The pharmacist is legally responsible for the supply and distribution of drugs in accordance with the law and hospital policy. In addition, the pharmacist is responsible for the manufacture and preparation of a wide range of pharmaceutical products.

A third and most important role is that of resource person for drug information. In this role, the pharmacist acts as specialist consultant to the medical profession and is available to advise paramedical and nursing staff on all aspects of drug use and to counsel patients on the use of their medication.

THE ROLE OF THE NURSE

Because drugs have the power to help or harm a patient, their administration is one of the nurse's most important responsibilities. As the last link in the chain which makes the drug available to the patient, the nurse in the institutional setting in most cases assumes responsibility for administering the medication or for ensuring that it is taken by the patient.

Any nursing-care plan must incorporate drug therapy as an integral strand. It is the nurse who is best placed to assess a patient's needs and responses to treatment. Where a ward pharmacist is not available it is the nurse's responsibility to assess information the patient has, and needs to know, about the medication. The patient's physiological and psychosocial state should be assessed with regard to his ability to take drugs in the prescribed manner. For example, patients who have difficulty swallowing, who are vomiting or who have an aversion to a particular taste or to injections will be noted. Visual, hearing, intellectual or motor impairments that might interfere with a patient's ability to receive medication must be taken into account.

Establishment of a nursing plan in respect of drug therapy will take into account information gathered by observation of, and interviewing the patient or family, from other sources such as patient records and from appropriate professionals, particularly the pharmacist and medical officer. With regard to drug therapy, short-term goals might concentrate on patient cooperation in gaining maximum effect from drugs. Long-term goals will focus on patient and family education, the ability to self-medicate and compliance with therapy.

Such a plan will need to establish realistic goals and will involve drawing up schedules for drug administration taking into account the information gained from the assessment process, knowledge of drug actions, adverse effects, interactions, duration of effect and the prescription instructions. Planning should also take into account other activities in which the patient will be engaged. Time schedules need to take account of meals, rest periods and other treatments such as physiotherapy, and must be flexible enough to cope with unplanned events. Where strict time schedules are essential, these should be noted in the nursing plan.

Implementation of the nursing-care plan, with regard to drug therapy, requires that drug administration complies with five generally accepted principles: the right patient receives the right drug, in the right dose, by the right route at the right time.

The right patient

Before medication is given, the patient's identity should be checked using either the identity wrist band, or verbally. If the patient is incapable of verbal response, then some non-verbal response may be accepted, for example, nodding. If the patient is unable to identify himself or herself due to mental incompetence or unconsciousness, some other means of identification may be required. These practices vary from hospital to hospital. An infant should ***always*** be identified by its identity band.

The right drug

Drugs have both trade and generic (chemical) names. Any order using an unfamiliar trade name should be checked against the generic list and, if any doubt exists, the pharmacist should be consulted.

Before administering any drug, the label on the container should be double checked as follows: once, when the medication order has been read and the container is taken from the shelf; and then a second time as the container label is checked against the medication order. If the label is illegible, the container should be returned to the pharmacy and its contents not used. Should the contents be non-uniform, again the contents should not be used and the container returned to the pharmacy.

If the ***patient*** queries the drug, it should be checked again.

When giving the medication, the nurse should bear in mind the condition for which that drug has been ordered. This will help in learning drug names and their actions.

The right dose

Before administering any drug, the nurse should check the dosage. If any doubt arises, the nurse should consult the pharmacist or the prescriber before proceeding. Once again, if the ***patient*** queries the dose, it should be checked again. If, after checking with the pharmacist and/or prescriber, the nurse still has doubts about the dosage, she should refrain from administering it and inform both her nursing supervisor and the prescriber of her actions and her reasons. Particular attention should be paid to decimal points in a dosage and the difference between the abbreviations for milligrams (mg) and micrograms (mcg).

The dosage form provided by the manufacturer should not be divided unless it has been ascertained that it is appropriate to do so.

Some dosage forms are designed with a sustained release effect (for example, slow release potassium tablets — *Slow K, Micro K)*, so that various layers are designed to dissolve at different times. Other tablets are composed of a matrix which releases the drug gradually over a period of time. These tablets should never be cut or crushed as the structure of the releasing matrix could be destroyed, and the dosage delivered in an entirely different way to that which was intended.

Some tablets are given an enteric coating to protect them from destruction by gastric acid or to protect the gastric mucosa. Aspirin is often given in this form when it is to be taken in high dosage over a prolonged period.

As a general rule, a dosage form should *not* be altered — there is a good reason for it being the way it is. With toxic drugs, or for that matter with any drugs, the nurse should be alert to any adverse reactions which the patient may mention, for example, rashes or visual disturbances. It is the nurse to whom the patient is most likely to report any such signs, and the nurse is then in a unique position to convey these to the medical officer.

It is important to remember that the right dose for a robust middle-aged person is not necessarily the right dose for a person who is very young or very old. While most people are aware that the young require smaller doses, this fact is frequently forgotten when dealing with the elderly.

The nurse must be conversant with the drugs which her patients are receiving and their adverse effects, in order to evaluate their effectiveness.

The right route

Drugs may be administered by a number of different routes. Factors which determine the best route of administration include the patient's general condition, the rapidity of response required, the drug's chemical and physical properties, and the site of the desired action.

Drugs may be administered orally, parenterally, topically, rectally or by inhalation. A brief summary of each is listed below.

Oral

This is the preferred and most widely used route of administration as it is the most convenient, most economical and safest means of giving medication. Drugs may also be absorbed through the oral cavity *sublingually*, when the drug is held under the tongue until dissolved and absorbed, for example, glyceryl trinitrate tablets, and *buccally*, when the drug is held between the cheek and the gum until dissolved.

Parenteral

Drugs may be given parenterally (from the Greek *para* meaning "beside", *enteron* meaning "intestine", that is outside of the intestine or not via the alimentary tract) through a hollow needle by injection or by intravenous infusion.

Injections are used to insert small amounts of sterile liquid medicaments into the body via hypodermic syringe by various routes. These routes are termed *intramuscular* (injection into muscle), *intravenous* (injection into vein when necessary for the drug to enter the circulation rapidly), *subcutaneous* (injection just below the layers of skin), and *intradermal* (injections within the layers of skin).

Intravenous infusions are used when larger volumes of sterile fluids must be inserted into the circulation in order to supply electrolytes or drugs, or to replace fluid loss from tissue dehydration or depleted blood volume.

Topical

Topical medications include creams, ointments, lotions, liniments, sprays and paints, and may be used to lubricate, protect or to deliver a drug to a localised area, either on the skin or mucous membrane. Drugs which may be toxic if taken internally may sometimes be used effectively when applied to the skin.

Rectal

Medication may be delivered by the rectal route by enema or suppository. It may be for local effect (as in constipation or for haemorrhoids) or to deliver drugs for systemic effect in nausea when the stomach does not retain the drug; when medication smells or tastes objectionable; when the patient is unconscious; or to avoid irritation to the gastrointestinal tract.

Generally, suppositories are superior to enemas as a method of delivering drugs as retention is easier.

Inhalation
The respiratory tract has an enormous surface area of absorbing epithelium and so is useful for delivering drugs locally to the tract, for example, salbutamol *(Ventolin)* or beclomethasone *(Becotide, Becloforte)* sprays for asthma, or in an emergency situation (oxygen therapy).

Choice of route of administration

Both drug and patient factors are taken into account when deciding by which route to give a drug. The oral route is the most ancient method of drug administration and is also the safest, most economial and acceptable. The disadvantages are the necessity for patient cooperation, destruction of some drugs by digestive enzymes or inappropriate pH, formation of food-drug complexes which make it unavailable for absorption, and possible metabolism by the liver before the drug reaches the general circulation.

The advantages of the parenteral route are the lack of need for cooperation (for example, in an unconscious patient) and that absorption is usually more rapid and predictable than when a drug is given by mouth. The disadvantages of parenteral therapy include its increased cost and lesser safety over the oral route. It is essential to maintain strict asepsis to avoid infection, as both pain and infection (systemic and extravascular) may sometimes be caused.

The nurse should ascertain that a dose form is appropriate to the route available.

Although the medical officer prescribes the drug and route of administration, the nurse may question such an order when it seems inappropriate, for example, oral medication for a patient who is vomiting, or the parenteral route for a distressed person able to tolerate the drug orally.

The right area for injection should be chosen, avoiding trauma to the region where nerves run close to the skin. In the gluteal region, for example, the sciatic nerve runs down the inner aspect of the buttock, so injections should be made into the upper outer quadrant. To avoid the brachial vessels of the arm, injections should not be made below the V-point of, or behind, the deltoid muscle.

Special instructions regarding route of injection should be noted, for example, iron mixtures taken through a straw, IM iron injection through the Z administration technique.

The right time

It is important, especially with drugs whose efficacy depends on reaching and/or maintaining adequate blood levels, that drugs are given at the right time, in relation to time and to meals. If a drug should be taken before meals (*ante cibum* or a.c.) to obtain the required blood levels, it should be given about an hour before food. This applies to many of the antibiotics. Tetracycline, for example, is chelated (forming an insoluble compound) if given with milk or some foods, which effectively removes a large proportion of the drug before it can be absorbed. On the other hand, some drugs must be taken with or after food, either to avoid excessive irritation of the gut (for example, indomethacin) or to give higher blood levels (for example griseofulvin, which reaches much higher blood levels if given with fatty meal).

The medication should be charted *after it has been given* and the dose, the route, the time and by whom the drug was administered, recorded. If the patient refuses the drug, or if the medication is not administered, the reason should be noted and reported. The nurse must not assume that a drug has been taken when given to a patient but must check that it is so.

The recording of the administration of a controlled drug should also take place after the drug is given so that if the drug is dropped, broken or refused by the patient, the circumstances surrounding the reasons for the patient not receiving that particular dose can be documented. It is *not* acceptable practice to write up in advance that the drug has been given.

The nurse must also relate her knowledge of the patient's condition to the drug ordered and make a judgment as to the suitability of its administration at any given time, for example, giving an antihypertensive agent to a patient who is hypotensive, digoxin to a patient with a low apex beat, insulin to a diabetic with low blood sugar, waking a patient to give a sedative. In this respect, the nurse will need sound knowledge upon which to base her judgment.

When anyone administers medication, he or she is subjecting the patient to a potentially hazardous form of treatment. It is therefore essential that knowledge and commonsense form the basis for such actions. The kind of questions that should be asked include:

1. Is the drug being stored correctly (should it be refrigerated)?
2. Is the drug p.r.n. ("when necessary") sedation?
3. Is this the drug which the doctor intended for the patient's condition? If in doubt, communicate with the doctor.
4. Will this drug interact with some other drug or treatment the patient is receiving?
5. What are the possible or likely adverse reactions of this drug? Are any of these effects already present?
6. Are there any special precautions with this drug, for example, to be taken with plenty of water, injected deeply IM, or must not be intravenous (IV)?

Assessment of patient needs is especially important when administering drugs that are to be taken "when necessary" (*pro re nata* or p.r.n.). For example, careful consideration of potential causes, physical and physiological signs and the patient's own assessment are essential in adequately managing pain — a condition for which analgesics are frequently taken "when necessary". The nurse is often in a position to make recommendations to the prescriber based on such assessment.

LEGAL REQUIREMENTS

The nurse must be aware of and observe carefully the laws and institutional policy relating to drug use in the hospital. These include the patient's right to be informed and his or her right to refuse treatment.

The medication order

In Britain restricted substances and dangerous drugs must be ordered by a medical practitioner. This includes the majority of drugs ordered in a hospital.

The prescription or medication order *must* include, *in the prescriber's own handwriting*, the patient's name and identification number together with the name and strength of the drug, route of administration, dose and frequency, and the prescriber's signature. An order written by another person is *not valid*, even if signed by a medical practitioner.

Record of administration

The law requires that administration of controlled drugs be recorded in a separate drug register. In addition, hospital regulations may require that administration of other substances, such as sedatives and some analgesics, be similarly recorded. Also, it is general practice for all drug administration to be noted in the medication record or nursing notes. The nurse must be aware of and observe all such regulations.

Storage

For reasons of security and safety, some drugs must be stored separately in a locked cupboard. Once again, the nurse should observe the laws pertaining to drug storage.

INTERPRETATION OF ORDERS

Before administration of any drug, the nurse has to read and interpret the medical practioner's written orders. If the order is illegible or there is any doubt as to the prescriber's intention, it must be checked. In many cases the registered nurse will be able to read and interpret the order, but in some instances a pharmacist or the prescriber may have to be contacted. A list of the commonly used abbreviations and their meanings is included in Appendix A.

STORAGE

Three main factors must be considered in relation to the storage of drugs: temperature, position and expiry dates.

Temperature

Temperature is one of the most important factors governing the storage of drugs. Many drugs are thermolabile (destroyed or changed by heat) and must be kept within a specific temperature range. It is important that the temperature criteria are met if the drug is to have the efficacy and potency stated on the label. The main temperature requirements for drug storage are:

(a) ***In a cool place*** (defined by the *British Pharmacopoeia* as less than 15°C). Many drugs come into this group, for example, insulin (which has the added requirement that it must not be frozen).

(b) ***Refrigerated,*** some antibiotic syrups when dispensed and some antibiotic injections.

(c) Special temperature ranges: 2° to 10°C for most vaccines (for example, typhoid or measles vaccines) or *frozen,* for example, smallpox vaccine is stored below −5°C.

Expiry dates

Many drugs have an expiry date and must be used within the specified time. Loss of drugs due to expiry can be minimised by stock rotation, in which replacement stock is always placed at the rear of the shelf, thus ensuring that the older stock, which is moved forward, is used first.

Drugs stored incorrectly or for too long may lose or change their activity. Changes that should be noted include: colour changes in solids or liquids, clear solutions becoming cloudy, and moisture absorption by tablets.

Position

Drugs are toxic substances. It is therefore important that they be stored in a well-lit area, preferably at eye level and away from public access. They should be in locked cupboards or a locked drug trolley, particularly in a children's, psychiatric, or mental handicap ward. The law regarding storage of controlled drugs must be complied with.

GENERAL CONSIDERATION

Modern drugs tend to be more potent and more toxic than their predecessors, so a great deal of care and commonsense needs to be exercised when administering them. In the chain of events which leads to the patient receiving medication, the nurse usually administers the drug. It is therefore important that she or he sees that the patient not only receives the drug but actually takes it. As a general rule, medication should not be left on the bedside table for the patient to take later unless specifically directed by the prescriber.

When giving injections or intravenous solution, there are several points to remember. The injection or IV bottle or bag arrives at the ward with sterile contents. It is of little benefit to the patient if the manufacturer goes to the trouble of producing a sterile product only to have it contaminated at the point of administration. There is less likelihood of this happening if a little care is taken. The hands of the nurse who is giving the injection should *always* be washed, the ampoule should be checked for expiry dates, deterioration or damage, and the neck of the ampoule or entry site of the IV bottle or bag prepared with 70% alcohol.

Many ampoules when broken receive fragments of broken glass which are extremely difficult to see and can easily be drawn up through the needle. The injection of these particles may account for some of the phlebitis seen at IV injection sites. To avoid glass fragments, do not put the needle on the bottom of the ampoule or draw up the last portion of solution. All ampoules are manufactured with a small excess (called "overage") so there is no need to take the last few drops of solution. By this means it is hoped that the glass particles will be left behind. Sterile drawing-up plastic straws with built-in filters can be used to draw up solutions from ampoules. These are relatively inexpensive; while they do not remove bacteria, they certainly remove glass and particulate matter. When additives are being made into an IV solution, antimicrobial filters with pore size of 0.22 micron can be obtained. These will filter out not only particulate matter but also any bacteria which would otherwise be injected into the solution. They have the disadvantage of being expensive.

The charting of the medication both on the medication card and in the controlled drug book is a record of the patient having received the medication. *It should not be written up until after the patient has received and taken the medication.*

In Britain the cultural background of patients and nurses frequently differs. Recognition and acknowledgement of the influence of cultural differences on people's attitudes to drugs are important considerations as cultural differences may alter the usefulness of drug therapy for particular patients.

The results of drug therapy should be evaluated through direct and indirect observation for wanted and unwanted effects. Effects of drug/drug and drug/food interactions should be taken into account.

Discrepancies between the goals of care and the results should be critically examined. For example, it might be observed by the nurse or reported by the patient that symptoms are not relieved by a given drug within an appropriate time. The prescriber must be informed accordingly, and a decision must be made whether to alter the treatment.

THE RIGHTS OF THE PATIENT

At all times it must be remembered that the hospitalised patient has rights. These extend to the use of medication. Firstly, the patient has *the right to be informed* what the medication is for and what beneficial effects or adverse reactions might reasonably be expected from its use. In this regard prime responsibility rests with the prescriber, but it is sometimes the pharmacist and more often the nurse who performs this counselling function. To be effective, such counselling must be based on knowledge of pharmacology and therapeutics and be tempered with good judgment as to how much the patient needs to know.

The second is *the right to refuse.* Patients have the right to refuse medication. In the event of them so doing, the prescriber should be advised so that alternative treatment may be considered. Obviously there are cases where the patient is incompetent to make such decisions — when unconscious or perhaps mentally retarded — but this does not negate the general principle.

PATIENT EDUCATION

Educating the patient, family or other carers should be an essential part of any patient-management plan. The patient needs to know what benefits to expect from treatment, what adverse reactions are significant and should be referred to the medical practitioner. Compliance must be stressed. Injection techniques may need to be taught. When this has not been done by the prescriber or the pharmacist, nurses will often find themselves in the position of primary educator.

Before beginning to teach a patient about drugs, the following factors should be assessed:

(a) the patient's readiness to learn;
(b) the patient's ability to receive and use information effectively;
(c) the appropriate amount of information to be given to the patient;
(d) the patient's physical state, for example, motor and sensory functions;
(e) factors likely to interfere with learning such as fatigue, anxiety, fear, pain or social problems;
(f) other people to be included in the programme, for example, family, friends.

Time should be allowed for the education programme in the overall nursing plan. Information should be pitched at an appropriate level for the patient, using teaching aids, if available. Patients should be encouraged to participate by making some decisions themselves, and adequate time for evaluation and feedback should be allocated.

Long-term compliance with a drug regime may be dependent upon successful patient education. Every opportunity should be taken for co-operation between pharmacy staff and nursing staff in developing, implementing and evaluating such programmes.

THE ACTION OF DRUGS

Drugs act in a variety of ways. They may be given to maintain health, for example, thyroxine, insulin, vitamins; to relieve symptoms, for example, aspirin to relieve headaches; to reverse disease processes, for example digoxin in heart failure, antibiotics to fight infection; for prophylaxis (to prevent disease), for example Sabin vaccine to prevent poliomyelitis, cholera vaccine to prevent cholera; to change normal processes, for example, oral contraceptives; to aid in diagnosis, for example, barium meal for X-ray examination of the gastrointestinal tract or reagents to measure the sugar concentration in urine.

All drugs are individual entities and, as such, the action of each drug in the patient depends on its own pharmacodynamic properties (or biological and therapeutic effects), and pharmacokinetic properties (absorption, distribution, metabolism and excretion, or the way the individual patient utilises the drug). This means that the dose of the drugs needs to be tailored to the patient, especially with drugs where the therapeutic dose may be close to the toxic dose (for example phenytoin, digoxin), as no two people respond to a drug in an identical manner. This is highlighted by the fact that adverse reactions which appear in one patient do not necessarily appear in another who may have been given the same dose of the same drug.

The result of the drug activity depends on its interaction with tissue "receptors" at the site of action. Such an interaction gives the drug its characteristic effect. A receptor is difficult to define as a physical entity. It may be an area of cell membrane which results in the binding of a compound such as noradrenaline, or it could be an enzyme with which the drug combines to render it inactive.

ABSORPTION

Before a drug can exert its action, it must be absorbed. The lipid membrane of cells is selectively permeable to non-ionised drugs, and so drug presentation in this form aids its absorption.

There are several different mechanisms of absorption.

Passive diffusion

Lipid-soluble drugs are absorbed more rapidly than water-soluble drugs. When presented at the cell membrane in an aqueous solution, the non-polar lipid-soluble drug and polar substances with sufficient lipid solubility dissolve into the cellular membrane and pass through. Small water-soluble polar and non-polar substances pass through water channels in the membrane by a process called filtration. Passive diffusion requires no energy expenditure by the cell, and movement across the membrane depends on the concentration gradient. When the concentration is the same on both sides of the membrane, a steady state is reached.

Active transport

Active transport processes differ from passive processes in that they require energy and exhibit selectivity. A "carrier" transfers the substance across the membrane and then returns to repeat its work. Na^+, K^+ and amino acids are transported across the renal tubule in this way.

Many factors influence the rate of absorption. They can be related either to the drug or the person taking the drug.

Drug factors include the dose form (IM versus oral) and, if oral, such factors as disintegration time, rate of dissolution, particle size and the particular excipient (filling) or vehicle used in formulation can all influence the rate of absorption. These factors sometimes cause a problem when drug companies change the formulation of a particular product. It can have the effect of making the product more, or less, available (or bioavailable) with the result that patients previously stabilised on a particular dose of the drug have shown signs of over or under dosage. This problem has been experienced with *Lanoxin* tablets and *Epanutin* capsules.

Patient factors include surface area of epithelium to which the drug is exposed, for example that of gastrointestinal tract or alveolar epithelium. Patient factors in the gut include pH and presence and type of food. For example the calcium ions in milk combine with tetracycline, inactivating the drug. How long the drug takes to pass through the intestine (intestinal transit time) is another factor, as is the circulation at the absorption site.

DISTRIBUTION

After a drug is absorbed, it is transported to various parts of the body at a variable rate dependent upon cardiac output, regional blood flow and the physiochemical properties of the drug. Lipid-soluble drugs which readily cross cell membranes are distributed throughout the body, rapidly to highly perfused tissues such as heart, brain, liver and kidney, less promptly to muscle and more slowly into fat. Drugs which do not readily cross cell membranes are more restricted in their distribution and therefore more restricted in their potential sites of action.

Drugs may accumulate in tissues which then serve as a reservoir to prolong the effect of the drug. They can also become bound to plasma proteins, especially albumin, in a non-selective manner, which then acts in a similar way. Because of the competitiveness and non-selectivity of plasma-protein, binding problems can occur, for example, bilirubin encephalopathy in the newborn, caused when bilirubin is displaced by sulphonamides. Drug toxicity may occur when competition exists between two substances for the protein binding sites (for example, warfarin and glibenclamide).

METABOLISM

Many drugs must be transformed (metabolised) before they can be eliminated from the body. Drugs that are lipid soluble are not readily eliminated as they may be reabsorbed from the renal tubules after filtration. It is therefore necessary for the body to metabolise and transform them into more polar or ionised products which are not so readily reabsorbed. This biotransformation not only helps with the elimination of the drug but may inactivate it as well.

Many drugs are metabolised by the liver, and some can induce liver enzyme activity so that they actually increase the rate of their own metabolism as well as that of other drugs given concurrently. Unless monitored closely, this situation can be hazardous. For example, if a patient stabilised on a warfarin regime is given a barbiturate which is a microsomal-enzyme inducer, his anticoagulant level could be lowered. If the barbiturate causing the more rapid metabolism of the warfarin is then withdrawn, a far higher blood level of the anticoagulant occurs leading to the possibility of haemorrhage.

Knowledge of the way in which drugs are metabolised is thus very important.

EXCRETION

The body eliminates drugs either unchanged, as happens with polar compounds, or changed as metabolites, as with the non-polar or lipid-soluble drugs. These non-polar and lipid-soluble compounds are not readily eliminated unless they are first metabolised.

The chief organ of excretion is the kidney. Renal excretion involves three processes: glomerular filtration, active tubular secretion and passive tubular reabsorption. The amount of drug being filtered depends on the glomerular filtration rate. The proximal renal tubule adds to the glomerular filtrate by active secretion (as with, for example, penicillin). Reabsorption of non-ionised weak acids and bases takes place in the proximal and distal tubules. The rate of elimination of a drug by this route depends on the balance between these three processes.

Bile is the vehicle for many metabolites of drugs transformed in the liver. These metabolites may be excreted in the faeces or be reabsorbed into the blood and excreted by the kidney. Drugs can also be excreted by the sweat glands or in the saliva, in which they are usually swallowed and hence have the same fate as drugs taken orally. Excretion by these routes is not particularly important. Excretion of drugs in breast milk is important clinically in that basic compounds may be more concentrated in this fluid, thus subjecting an infant to unwanted effects of drugs taken by the mother.

DOSE FORMS

Drugs occur, or are prepared, in one or more of the three physical states, that is, solids, liquids and gases.

SOLID DOSE FORMS

Drugs in this group may be administered via any of four routes: oral, topical, rectal or vaginal.

Oral Forms

Oral forms are those taken by mouth. In most cases, it is preferable that the patient be given the oral form of the drug since it is the least costly dose form and the most convenient to administer. Oral forms include tablets, capsules and lozenges.

Tablets, which may be moulded or compressed come in a variety of shapes, sizes, colours and weights. Tablets may contain the pure drug, or be diluted with an inert substance to make up weight to produce a suitably sized tablet, or may contain two or more drugs for combined pharmacological effect. The tablet may be designed as a plain compressed tablet, a sublingual tablet (to be dissolved under the tongue), a buccal tablet (to be dissolved between cheek and gum), a sugar-coated tablet (to mask bad odour or taste), an enteric-coated tablet (to prevent disintegration in the stomach or preserve the tablet until it reaches the intestines), or a slow-release tablet (to release the drug over a prolonged period either by time-selective dissolving of layers, or slow release from a matrix).

Capsules are small oblong containers, usually made of gelatine, enclosing medicinal substances in the form of liquid, powder or pellets coated in such a way that they disintegrate at various predetermined rates so as to give a prolonged effect (for example, trifluoperazine sustained-release capsule or *Stelazine Spansule*).

Lozenges are solid doses of medicinal powders that act through slow disintegration in the mouth. They are useful when a local drug action in the mouth or throat is required.

Topical Forms

Topical forms of drugs are those used externally on the body and serve as protective agents for skin, or as vehicles for drugs.

The most important forms in this group are ointments and creams. Ointments tend to be greasy and therefore emollient, and stay on the skin for a long time. Creams are emulsions of oil in water (non-greasy "vanishing" creams, water being the external phase, for example, *Drapolene* cream) or water in oil (greasy, oil being the external phase, for example, zinc cream).

Suppositories

Suppositories are medicated masses made in a mould and designed to melt at body temperatures or to dissolve in body fluids (for example, glycerine suppositories). Suppositories are designed to deliver medication by the rectal route either for local effect or systemic absorption.

Pessaries

Pessaries are similar to suppositories but are designed for vaginal use.

LIQUID DOSE FORMS

There are three main groups of liquid drugs: solutions, suspensions and emulsions.

Solutions

Solutions are preparations of one or more drugs dissolved in a solvent, usually water. The main types are the following:

Syrups: concentrated solutions of sugar in water to which some medicinal substance may be added, such as syrup of Tolu.

Elixirs: clear, sweetened solutions containing alcohol and water, medication and flavouring, for example, elixir phenobarbitone.

Tinctures: alcoholic extracts of plants or chemical substances, for example, tincture of belladonna, tincture of iodine.

Injectables: solutions containing medication to be given via a syringe or an intravenous line.

Suspensions

Suspensions are preparations of finely divided powders suspended in a liquid and usually need shaking before use. They may be intended for either internal use (for example, penicillin suspension) or external use (for example, calamine lotion).

Emulsions
Emulsions are preparations containing either water globules suspended in oil by means of an emulsifying agent or (more usually) fat or oil globules suspended in water (for example, paraffin emulsion). As they are suspensions, they need shaking before use.

GASEOUS DOSE FORMS

The gaseous forms of drugs may be therapeutic or anaesthetic.

Therapeutic

Oxygen may be administered to alleviate hypoxia (lack of oxygen as found in cases of acute respiratory difficulty) or to counteract carbon-monoxide poisoning.

Carbon dioxide is used with oxygen to counteract respiratory depression, asphyxia and carbon-monoxide poisoning. In operative procedures it is used to increase speed of induction and recovery from anaesthesia.

Anaesthetic
Gaseous forms of drugs, for example, nitrous oxide or halothane, are used in operative procedures.

AEROSOL THERAPY

Any product depending on the power of liquefied or compressed gas to expel contents from the container is an aerosol. They may be solutions or powders.

Solutions
An aerosol solution is any liquid sprayed as a mist, for example, salbutamol *(Ventolin)* in a nebuliser.

Powders
An aerosol powder is any powder dispersed by a propellant.

2
DRUG PROBLEMS

Joy B. Hobbes

OBJECTIVES

At the conclusion of this chapter the student should be able to discuss:

1. the main factors predisposing to adverse drug reactions (ADR);
2. the fundamental mechanism of the allergic response;
3. the mechanisms of some of the clinically significant drug interactions;
4. the degrees of drug dependence, the type of drugs involved in drug abuse and the methods of treating drug abuse;
5. basic concepts of correct drug administration;
6. the importance of patient compliance in regard to drug therapy.

PREREQUISITE KNOWLEDGE

1. The physiology of the liver and its role in drug metabolism.
2. The physiology of the kidney and its role in drug elimination.
3. Documented toxic side effects of the drugs most frequently implicated in adverse drug reactions, for example, drugs with a low therapeutic index such as digitalis glycosides, cancer chemotherapeutic agents, antidiabetic drugs, oral anticoagulants.
4. The addictive properties of the narcotic analgesics and their toxic side effects.

DEFINITIONS

Drug — any substance given as therapy or for investigative purposes.
Adverse drug reaction (ADR) — any unintended or undesired effect of a drug administered in a therapeutic situation. The response may be a toxic reaction, either dose or non-dose related.
Side effect — a known response to drug administration within normal dose ranges. Because of its predictability, a side effect can be treated accordingly, if and when it arises, for example, tinnitus as a result of salicylate therapy, hypoglycaemia as a result of insulin therapy, severe

hypotension as a result of treatment with antihypertensives.

If the side effect is toxic and jeopardises the health of the patient, then the drug dosage must be modified or the drug withdrawn completely until the symptoms disappear.

Overdosage — a characteristic but excessive pharmacological effect of the drug caused by administration of a larger than usually recommended dose.

Hypersensitivity — a reaction not explained by the pharmacological effects of the drug, caused by altered reactivity of the patient and generally considered to be an allergic manifestation due to the suspected drug.

Idiosyncrasy — the reaction seen in a small number of patients who are abnormally sensitive to small doses of a drug.

Therapeutic index — a ratio of the lethal dose of a drug to the therapeutic dose. The closer these values, the greater the risk of toxicity. Cardiac glycosides, oral anticoagulants, oral antidiabetics and cancer chemotherapeutic agents are examples of drugs with a low therapeutic index.

In the past 20 years new and effective drugs have appeared on the market in increasing numbers. Examples of their success are the virtual eradication of many infections and advances in the control of cancer. Many naturally occurring drugs can be synthesised, in many instances improving the therapeutic value of the original material. Because of this recent and apparently continuing drug "explosion", it is extremely difficult for anyone concerned with drug therapy to be up-to-date with current literature on every new product. The manufacturer of a new drug must supply a product profile which clearly states therapeutic dosage levels, the common side effects of therapy, contraindications for use, toxicity of the drug and any other information relevant to its administration to humans.

The thalidomide disaster of the 1950s highlighted the absolute necessity for the proper evaluation of the safety of drugs administered to humans. In the United Kingdom doctors seeking advice and information on adverse reactions should contact The Medical Assessor, The Committee on Safety of Medicines, London. Marketing approval is withheld until the particular drug has been proven safe for therapeutic use in humans. Despite these stringent assessments, drugs still continue to cause problems in the community.

One reference claims that "1% to 3% of admissions to hospital for medical services are due to drug reactions". This figure excludes deliberate overdosage or drug abuse (*Merck Manual*, 13th Edition, p.1809). The reference continues, "among hospitalised patients, the incidence of mild to severe side effects may be as high as 10%".

The initial responsibility for correct drug therapy lies with the prescriber and the pharmacist who dispenses the prescribed drug. The ultimate responsibility for the administration of the correct drug to the patient rests with the nursing professional responsible for administering the prescribed drug to the patient.

This chapter aims to explain some of the problems that can arise as a result of drug use, whether correctly or incorrectly administered; the general abuse of drugs; the strict precautions which must be observed when administering drugs to a patient; the causes of adverse drug reactions and the mechanism of action for several types of drug interactions.

ADVERSE DRUG REACTIONS

An adverse drug reaction is any unintended or undesired effect due to a drug administered in a therapeutic situation. The response may be a toxic reaction, either dose or non-dose related.

FACTORS INFLUENCING THE INCIDENCE OF ADVERSE DRUG REACTIONS (ADRs)

1. The number of drugs per therapeutic regimen — the higher the number the greater the likelihood of an ADR.
2. Whether male or female. Women more than men are reported to take a greater number of prescribed and unprescribed "over-the-counter" drugs (*Boston Collaborative Survey* 1969).
3. Age. Both the elderly and neonates require modified dosage of the full adult dose due to reduced metabolic and detoxifying functions. Dosage in both cases is related to body weight and age.
4. The disease state itself can contribute to the incidence of an ADR. For example, nephrotoxicity during digoxin administration leads to accumulation of the drug and subsequent digoxin toxicity. In this instance the dose of digoxin should be reduced and digoxin blood levels continually monitored. Hypokalaemia in the presence of digoxin increases the sensitivity of cardiac muscle cells to the toxic effects of digoxin. Hepatic disease such as cirrhosis and hepatitis can lead to accumulation of any drug normally metabolised by the liver.
5. A history of allergic asthma or allergic reactions to drugs, food or clothing may indicate a predisposition to ADRs.
6. Treatment with cancer chemotherapeutic agents always leads to the onset of toxic side effects. In view of the serious nature of the disease, cancer chemotherapy is continued even though toxic symptoms are present.
7. Adverse drug reactions can occur as a result of increasing the dosage of a drug previously tolerated at a lower dose, varying the route of administration of a drug, or from different formulation characteristics of different brands of the same drug, leading to altered bioavailability of the drug.
8. Patient idiosyncrasy.
9. The immense array of drugs available on the market.
10. The similarity between brand names of drugs with different pharmacological actions may lead to error in administration. For example

Leukeran (cytotoxic drug); and *Lanoxin* (digitalis glycoside).

11. The easy availability of drugs, by prescription only or by purchase without a prescription, from a community pharmacy, and the possible complications from taking such products concurrently.

12. The lack of communication between physician and patient on the subject of correct use of drug therapy.

13. The increasing use by the community of illegally obtained drugs such as narcotics and hallucinogens, as well as tranquillisers and alcohol, and the potential dangers of combining any of these drug groups.

14. The genetic variation in the community, which influences the individual response to drug therapy.

CAUSES OF ADVERSE DRUG REACTIONS

Overdosage, accidental

1. Frequently occurs in the elderly who may forget that the daily dose of a drug has been taken already and repeat the dose.

2. The availability of several brands of the same generic drug form which leads to confusion on the patient's part, for example, frusemide, a potent diuretic, is known commercially as *Lasix, Aluzine, Dryptal* and *Frusid*.

3. Diseases which reduce metabolism of drugs by the liver or excretion of drugs by the kidney can lead to toxic blood levels of particular drugs, especially those with a low therapeutic index.

4. Emotional and mental disorders can lead to abuse of drugs used to treat such disease states, for example, barbiturates, antidepressants and tranquillisers.

Drug allergy (drug hypersensitivity)

Allergic reactions to drug therapy form the majority of adverse drug reactions and conform to a general pattern.

1. There is a delay in the establishment of the allergic state following initial exposure to the drug.

2. Once the allergic state has been established, the allergic reaction can be precipitated by minute amounts of the drug responsible.

3. The reaction occurs each time the drug is administered thereafter.

4. The reaction is not related to the anticipated pharmacological response.

5. The visible symptoms include skin lesions, sickness, bronchospasm and laryngeal oedema. The most common skin lesions are urticaria, exfoliative dermatitis, Stevens-Johnson syndrome, purpura and contact dermatitis. However, allergic reactions affect only a small percentage of patients, many of whom have a family history of allergic reactions involving mainly the skin, mucous membranes of the nose and bronchial smooth muscle. Such patients tend to react to foreign substances, whether food, clothing or drugs, which are harmless to the majority of the population.

A drug allergy may result in anaphylaxis.

Mechanism of allergic response

Allergic reactions, also referred to as hypersensitivity reactions, are due to an immunological response of the organism to a foreign substance called an *antigen*. Some of the antigens responsible for provoking an allergic response in humans are proteins, pollens, house dust, feathers, moulds, cereals and flour. Normally, antigens are molecules of high molecular weight.

NURSING IMPLICATIONS

A.K. SWONGER in *Nursing Pharmacology* (1978) suggests that 80% of adverse reactions are predictable and the remainder are avoidable. There has been some suggestion that the undesirable effects of a drug may be classified as iatrogenic disease or as adverse reactions. Whichever the perspective taken, it is possible to classify these reactions into five major groups: blood dyscrasia, hepatic toxicity, renal damage, dermatological effects and teratogenic effects.

As well as these syndromes, the consideration of drug problems involves the evaluation of the following adverse reactions and unpredictable responses:

drug allergy
hypersensitivity
idiosyncrasy
tolerance
accumulation
dependence
summation
synergism
antagonism
drug interaction

Based on the above discussion, the nursing process in drug problems must be implemented to gain a total perspective of the problem.

Assessment

This should be in the form of a nursing history which includes the following:

(a) previous medication history;
(b) habitual drug use or previous exposure to drugs or chemicals;
(c) prior adverse drug reactions or known allergies, hypersensitivities, or idiosyncratic reactions;
(d) past disease processes;
(e) current disease-related factors such as the presence of fever, or renal, hepatic or gastrointestinal pathology;
(f) present physiological conditions such as pregnancy or lactation;
(g) baseline vital signs;
(h) weight;
(i) blood screening parameters.

Management

This will vary depending on the nature of the adverse reaction. Close observation and immediate reporting of any abnormality is essential. In some cases it may be a situation of weighing the benefits and risks of a certain medication. Some options available in the management of drug problems follow.

Adverse reaction	***Management***
Hypersensitivity	Discontinuation of the drug.
Anaphylactic reaction	Immediate intervention with resuscitation measures.
Toxic extension	Possibly withhold medication until seen by a medical officer; possibly decrease the dose or discontinue the medication.
Tolerance	Possible increase of dose or change in therapy.
Interactions	Eliminate, or avoid, known interactions.

Evaluation

The most important aspects in the evaluation of ADRs is the observation and recognition of the type of reaction. It is also important to determine the significance of that reaction. Some side effects may present early in the course of administration and then disappear several days later. Others may be mild and cause the patient no discomfort. It is wise to suspect reactions to be associated with medications. It is also vital that any observed changes be documented and reported promptly to the appropriate people so that necessary management can be implemented effectively.

Note: The nurse should ensure that all details of adverse drug reactions are forwarded by the attending physician on the appropriate ADR form to The Medical Assessor, The Committee on Safety of Medicines, Market Towers, 1 Nine Elms Lane, London SW8 5NQ.

Drug molecules are usually of low molecular weight. In complexing with larger molecules such as proteins, a drug molecule may develop into a "hapten" which can act as a true antigen. The role of the antigen is to simulate the production of antibodies specific to the antigen, leading to an antigen-antibody reaction which may protect the organism from further invasive action by the antigen or cause noxious effects such as an allergic reaction, damaging the tissues in which the antigen-antibody reaction takes place.

As a result of this allergic reaction, certain pharmacological chemicals are released, including histamines, bradykinins and SRS-A (slow reacting substance of anaphylaxis) inducing the contraction of bronchial smooth muscle, dilation of blood vessels and increased permeability of capilliaries, which contribute to the visible symptoms outlined on page 26.

Antibodies are derived from the immunoglobulin molecules of the gammaglobulin fraction of serum. Five classes of immunoglobulins (Ig) are known: IgA, IgD, IgE, IgG and IgM. IgE antibodies have been implicated in the onset of the allergic response. Depending on the type of antigen-antibody reaction, allergic reactions have been divided into four basic categories.

TYPE 1 (anaphylactic reactions)

The onset of this reaction appears within minutes of the IV administration of a drug and is characterised by anaphylactic shock (even death) with acute urticaria, laryngeal oedema, acute asthma and hypotension. Anaphylaxis can also occur several hours after the oral administration of a drug.

Type 1 allergic diseases include allergic asthma, perennial allergic rhinitis, acute urticaria, and anaphylactic shock.

The drugs most commonly implicated in the onset of anaphylaxis are penicillins, dextrans, iodinated radiographic contrast media, IV anaesthetics and muscle relaxants.

TYPE 2 (cytotoxic reactions)

Cytotoxic reactions (implying cell destruction) are characterised by haemolysis of red blood cells. Examples of such reactions are haemolytic disease of the newborn, blood transfusion incompatibility, some haemolytic anaemias, purpura due to drug hypersensitivity, and agranulocytosis due to drugs.

Drugs implicated in this type of reaction are penicillins, cephalothin, quinidine, rifampicin (large doses, intermittent regime), methyldopa.

TYPE 3 (immune complex reactions)

Type 3 reactions are said to be rare and are characterised by fever, urticaria, arthralgia, thrombi, haemorrhages, nephritis and a chronic inflammatory state simulating rheumatoid arthritis.

Type 3 diseases include serum sickness, collagen diseases, systemic lupus erythematosus (SLE) and rheumatoid arthritis.

Drugs implicated include penicillins, streptomycin, thiouracils, rifampicin, sulphonamides, hydralazine, and INAH (isoniazid).

TYPE 4 (delayed hypersensitivity reactions)

Type 4 reactions are the most frequent. This reaction is not mediated by circulating antibodies but by special lymphocytes.

Type 4 diseases include contact dermatitis, graft rejection, auto-immune diseases and tuberculosis.

SYMPTOMS ASSOCIATED WITH ADVERSE DRUG REACTIONS

Symptoms associated with ADRs can be divided into three categories: life-threatening (as in anaphylactic reactions), severe, and irritating and uncomfortable.

Depending on the patient's condition and the severity of the reaction, a drug suspected of involvement in an ADR may or may not be withdrawn from therapy. The symptoms usually subside when the suspected drug is withdrawn. In the case of anaphylaxis the outcome may be fatal unless resuscitative equipment and appropriate drug therapy is on hand.

The following statistics from a major teaching hospital demonstrates the types of ADRs seen over a 12 month period at that hospital in descending order of frequency:

rash (unspecified)	21
rash (maculo-papular)	20
pruritus	20
rash (erythematous)	16
nausea	10
vomiting	9
bronchospasm	8
urticaria	8
agranulocytosis	7
fever	5
confusion	5

DETECTION OF THE CAUSATIVE DRUG IN AN ADVERSE DRUG REACTION

Many drugs in general use have common side effects such as nausea, vomiting, diarrhoea, rashes and pruritus. Therefore, in any given regimen of two or more drugs it is not always possible to state exactly which drug is implicated in the reaction, unless the patient undergoes rechallenge with the suspected drug. Because of the possible serious consequences of rechallenge, the severity of the symptoms and the patient's condition must be considered before embarking on this procedure.

Rechallenge is a means of detecting the drug responsible for the reaction. All therapy is withdrawn temporarily while the symptoms resolve. Then, one at a time, the drugs are reintroduced into the regimen. If the symptoms reappear on rechallenge with a particular drug, then proof of that drug as the causative agent is demonstrated.

Another method of detection is by intradermal testing. Four weeks after the reaction, 0.1 mL of a 1:1000 saline dilution of each drug is injected intradermally into the anterior surface of the forearm, using a tuberculin syringe and 26-gauge needle. The drug in the regimen is placed far enough away from the previous test area to avoid interference if a reaction is seen to occur. The forearm is observed for a half-hour for a positive weal and flare reaction. A positive reaction is regarded as one in which the weal exceeds 1.5 cm in diameter and persists a half-hour, thus implicating the specific drug as the cause of the reaction.

When a drug has been definitely implicated in an ADR, the patient's notes must be marked so that on future admissions that drug will not be administered. In the case of previous anaphylactic reactions, any patient so affected should wear a metal disc or carry a card stating that the patient is allergic to a particular drug.

The advancement of statistics on the incidence and type of reaction seen in hospitals and in the community depends on the reporting and recording of ADRs by cooperative prescribers. The prescriber fills out a special ADR form supplied to hospitals and local physicians, setting out the symptoms, dosage and drug therapy of the patient. This form is sent to The Committee on Safety of Medicines, Market Towers, 1 Nine Elms Lane, London SW8 5NQ where verification of all such reactions takes place. Data on ADRs can be of great benefit to prescribers when deciding which type of medication is most suitable for the patient. The completeness of information depends on the interest of the staff.

DRUG INTERACTIONS

When two or more drugs are administered concomitantly, a drug interaction may occur. The interaction is usually characterised by potentiation or antagonism of the effect of one of the drugs. Although theoretically possible, many drug interactions are not clinically significant because a combination of drugs may produce an interaction in one but not the majority of patients. This may be due to biological variability, patient idiosyncrasy or genetic factors. Some drug interactions are only of academic interest, having no adverse effect on the patient's well-being or on the drug regimen.

However, several drug groups have the potential to interact with other drugs, resulting in the potentiation of the pharmacological effects of the former. Drugs which may be potentiated include the following which have a low therapeutic index: the cardiac glycosides, oral hypoglycaemics, oral anticoagulants and cytotoxics. Interference with the pharmacokinetics of any of these drugs can lead to toxic blood levels. As in the case of drug reactions, the greater the number of drugs in a regimen, the greater the possibility of a drug interaction.

MECHANISMS OF DRUG INTERACTIONS

Because of the overwhelming number of possible drug interactions, only those of clinical significance will be discussed in regard to the mechanism of action. A single drug can react with another drug by a combination of physiological effects, so that more than one mechanism of action is possible at any one time. In this case the major component of the interaction is described.

Chemical incompatibility

Chemical incompatibility can occur during the preparation of any intravenous admixture. A precipitate is the usual sign of chemical incompatibility. However, the absence of a precipitate does not necessarily imply that the drug and its vehicle are compatible. An undetected microcrystalline precipitate is not clearly visible, yet the particles could occlude a vein. If in doubt, compatibility of drug and infusion fluid must *always be checked* with either the prescriber or pharmacy personnel *before* admixture is commenced.

Chemical incompatibility often occurs where two drugs are drawn up in the same syringe; this practice should be avoided. For example, penicillins are inactivated by aminoglycosides when mixed together in solution. Each drug should be drawn up separately and should be administered at different times if the potency of the penicillin is to be maintained for the requisite period of time.

Some chemical interactions are beneficial to the patient, for example the anticoagulant heparin (an acid) can be reversed by administering protamine (a base), the specific antidote for heparin overdosage.

Physical incompatibility

Sparingly soluble drugs precipitate out of solution when solubility is exceeded or the wrong vehicle is chosen for administration. For example, *Valium* is only slightly soluble in water and must be diluted according to the manufacturer's instructions.

Interference with gastrointestinal absorption

Interference with absorption from the gastrointestinal tract is another form of interaction leading to increased or decreased drug absorption.

Gastric emptying time and gut motility can be influenced by drugs; for example, metoclopramide accelerates gastric emptying rate which is important when considering digoxin. Digoxin is released upon dissolution of the tablet in the stomach and is absorbed across the small intestine. If the tablet does not dissolve completely because of the presence of metoclopramide, then the amount of digoxin available for absorption is reduced. If gastric emptying time is delayed, as with propantheline, an antispasmodic agent, the absorption of digoxin will be increased.

Chelating or binding of drugs in the intestinal lumen occurs frequently, with the formation of insoluble chelates which cannot be absorbed. Tetracyclines chelate with calcium (Ca^{2+}), magnesium (Mg^{2+}), and aluminium (Al^{3+}) all of which are components of antacids, and with iron (Fe^{2+}), resulting in low serum concentration of tetracycline if any of these ions is administered concurrently. Cholestyramine, a drug used to bind bile salts within the gastrointestinal lumen also binds other drugs, thus reducing their absorption; warfarin is one of the drugs so affected.

Plasma protein binding displacement

The free unbound drug in plasma is responsible for achieving the pharmacological effect. Binding sites on plasma proteins, especially albumin, can be occupied by any drug which has an affinity for such binding sites. Several drugs can occupy these sites on a competitive basis, those with the stronger binding potential displacing another drug already occupying those sites, thereby increasing the plasma level of the displaced drug. In the case of the drug groups with a low therapeutic index, an increased plasma concentration of unbound drug can be extremely dangerous; for example, the anticoagulant action of warfarin is potentiated by phenylbutazone, ethacrynic acid and the metabolites of chloral hydrate; the hypoglycaemic effect of tolbutamide and chlorpropamide is potentiated by phenylbutazone; and the effects of methotrexate are potentiated by salicylates and sulphonamides.

Modification of drug metabolism

Some drugs have the ability to stimulate metabolism of other drugs by the induction of hepatic microsomal enzyme activity. Barbiturates are well-known inducers of drug metabolism. When barbiturates are prescribed with oral anticoagulants, the dose of the latter will need to be increased to compensate for the increased rate of metabolism, but care must be taken to reduce the dose of the oral anticoagulant to the original level if the barbiturate therapy is withdrawn.

Inhibition of drug metabolism by inhibiting liver microsomal enzyme activity is another form of drug interaction which leads to prolonged action, accumulation and toxicity of the affected drug. For example:

1. Tolbutamide metabolism is inhibited by disulfiram and chloramphenicol.
2. Warfarin metabolism is inhibited by disulfiram.
3. Phenytoin metabolism is inhibited by disulfiram, chlorpromazine, prochlorperazine and diazepam.
4. The toxicity of mercaptopurine, a cytotoxic drug, is increased by allopurinol because mercaptopurine is metabolised by xanthine oxidase, an enzyme inhibited by allopurinol. Therefore the dose of mercaptopurine must be reduced to about 25% in the presence of allopurinol.
5. Acute ethanol intoxication slows the metabolism of warfarin and pentobarbitone.

Drugs which affect the same physiological system

Potentiation

The best example of this type of interaction is the potentiation of the depressant effect of hypnotics on the central nervous system (CNS) by other drugs which also depress the CNS, for example, alcohol, antihistamines, tranquillisers, narcotics, to name but a few. The combination of any two of these drugs could have serious consequences for anyone in charge of machinery.

Nephrotoxicity of cephaloridine and cephalothin is potentiated by frusemide.

Ototoxicity of aminoglycosides is increased by frusemide (high doses and injected rapidly IV) and ethacrynic acid.

Risk of bleeding is increased if oral anticoagulants and aspirin or other anti-inflammatory drugs are administered simultaneously, since all of these drugs affect platelet aggregation.

The anticoagulant effects of warfarin are potentiated by clofibrate.

Antagonism effect

Nalorphine and naloxone antagonise the respiratory depression induced by narcotics.

Vitamin K antagonises the haemorrhagic effects of the oral anticoagulants.

Thiazide diuretics, corticosteroids and oral contraceptives antagonise the effects of the oral hypoglycaemics.

Bacteriostatics such as tetracycline antagonise the bacterial effects of penicillins and cephalosporins.

Beneficial drug interactions

Drug interactions are beneficial in many instances, forming the basis of the emergency treatment of drug overdosage, for example, the use of British Anti-Lewisite (BAL) in cases of heavy metal poisoning, and the control with protamine of bleeding episodes due to heparin overdosage.

The effects of released physiological transmitters acting as agonists on various body receptors can be reversed with the specific antagonist synthesised for this purpose; for example, antihistamines antagonise the effects of released histamine; atropine enhances the effect of ß-adrenoreceptor stimulation.

Changes in urine pH alter the renal clearance of some drugs. Basic drugs are ionised in an acid urine, acidic drugs in an alkaline urine, and therefore are cleared more quickly in the urine. Advantage is taken of this concept in the renal clearance of poisons as an emergency procedure.

Competition between drugs

Competition between drugs for active renal tubular secretion results in the prolongation of action due to reduced renal clearance of one of the drugs; for example, probenecid competes in such a way with penicillins and cephalosporins, resulting in the reduced renal excretion of the latter two drug groups; salicylates and sulphonamides inhibit the excretion of methotrexate, a cytotoxic. In both examples, blood levels of the active agent can be maintained with smaller dosages of drug.

Changes in electrolyte balance

Changes in electrolyte balance also affect drug administration. Digoxin toxicity occurs when hypokalaemia is induced as a result of concurrent therapy with thiazide diuretics, carbenoxolone and amphotericin.

Food interactions

The importance of food in drug interactions cannot be overlooked. Monoamine oxidase inhibitors (MAOIs) such as phenelzine (*Nardil*), isocarboxazid (*Marplan*), iproniazid (*Marsilid*), tranylcypromine (*Parnate*, *Parstelin*) and foods rich in tyramine cause an acute hypertensive crisis or prolonged rise in blood pressure. The foods to avoid include avocados, matured cheese, spirits, wines, beer, pickled herrings, beef extracts and broad beans. Also, over-the-counter preparations containing pressor agents (found in cold remedies and nasal decongestants) can cause the same response with MAOIs. Knowledge of the interactions possible between groups of drugs given concurrently allows the prescriber to judge whether the patient will be at risk if certain drug groups are combined in a regimen. An understanding of the mechanism responsible for the drug interaction also allows the prescriber to modify the dosage of one or more of the drugs concerned in the interaction.

DRUG ABUSE

Drug abuse refers to the self-administration of a drug beyond the normal prescribed limits and hence covers the entire range of abnormal drug-taking, from the chronic abuse of aspirin and alcohol to addiction to narcotics. Recently "drug addiction" as a term has been replaced by "drug dependence" by the World Health Organization. Drugs which induce dependence have a common property — they modify the activity of the CNS in any of the following ways: they reduce anxiety and tension, cause feelings of elation, temporarily increase mental and physical ability, alter sensory perception and remove inhibitory controls.

Drug dependence can be divided into two components. ***Psychologic dependence*** describes mental reliance on a specific drug or drugs for the pleasure and/or comfort derived from ingesting it; such dependence can produce intense craving. ***Physical dependence*** defines a state of cellular adaptation to a drug which leads to the development of tolerance and a withdrawal syndrome.

The withdrawal syndrome is characterised by physiologic changes which occur when the abused drug is withdrawn abruptly, or when a specific antagonist to the drug is administered, as in narcotic overdosage. The symptoms of withdrawal due to the opiates include warm, moist, itchy skin; nausea and vomiting; restlessness; pinpoint pupils; running nose and eyes; yawning; chills; gooseflesh; rapid, irregular breathing; cramps and tremor. The severity of these symptoms differs according to the type of drug responsible, the dose level of the drug, and the period over which the drug was taken.

Tolerance describes the requirement for progressively larger doses of the drug to produce the original effect achieved at lower dose levels.

The drugs which cause dependence have varying components of physical and psychologic dependence, as shown in Table 1.

The drug-dependent personality is thought to be the product of several variables: personality, environment (home, social or work), the type of drug with abuse potential attractive to the person.

The ease of availability gives some drugs a greater potential for abuse by the public in general, for example, alcohol, cigarettes, aspirin compounds, night sedations, cough preparations and other non-prescription items which can be bought readily from the local pharmacy. In recent years, volatile industrial solvents have become popular with young people in whom partial tolerance develops with daily inhalation of the fumes.

Dependence varies according to the drug group abused and is divided into the following main groups:

1. Dependence of the opiate type.
2. Dependence of the barbiturate/alcohol type.
3. Dependence of the cannabis type.
4. Dependence of the cocaine type.
5. Dependence of the amphetamine type.
6. Dependence of the hallucinogen type.
7. Dependence of the volatile solvent type.
8. Dependence of the alcohol type.

Table 1
Commonly Used Substances with Potential for Dependence

Drug	Physical Dependence	Psychologic Dependence	Tolerance
CNS Depressants			
Opiates	++++	++++	+++
Synthetic narcotics	++++	++++	+++
Synthetic non-narcotic analgesics	+	+++	++
Barbiturates	+++	+++	++
Glutethimide	+++	+++	++
Methyprylon	+++	+++	++
Ethchlorvynol	+++	+++	++
Alcohol	+++	+++	+
Minor tranquillisers			
Meprobamate	+++	+++	++
Chlordiazepoxide	++	+++	++
Diazepam	++	+++	++
Stimulants			
Amphetamine	+	++++	++++
Methamphetamine	+	++++	++++
Cocaine	0	++++	0
Hallucinogens			
LSD	0	++	++
Mescaline, peyote	0	++	+
Marijuana			
(low-dose Δ.9 THC)	0	++	0
(high-dose Δ.9 THC)	0	++	+
DMT	0	++	0

(Reproduced from the *Merck Manual*, 13th edition, page 1506.)

Abbreviations:
LSD — Lysergic acid diethylamide
THC — tetrahydrocannabinol
DMT — dimethyltryptamine
0 — no effect
\+ — slight to ++++ marked effect

TREATMENT OF DRUG ABUSE

Depending on the type of drug abuse, treatment of withdrawal symptoms is based on two principles: replacement of the abused drug with a pharmacologically or physiologically equivalent drug, and gradual withdrawal of the equivalent drug.

Exceedingly higher doses than usual of the substitute drug may be necessary during the management of withdrawal symptoms of the abused drug. The period over which the substitute drug is withdrawn depends upon the patient's clinical state. In the past, sodium pentobarbitone, chloral hydrate and paraldehyde were used as substitutes in abuse of the alcohol/sedative type. Currently chlormethiazole *(Heminevrin)* is the drug of choice.

Heroin/opiate abuse is treated by the substitution of one narcotic by another. Methadone is the drug of choice for several reasons: it is active orally and therefore avoids the need for injection; it blocks the euphoric effect of heroin so that patients do not get a "high" on heroin if it is still being used; it is longer-acting than heroin or narcotics; and at high doses it blocks the patient's craving for heroin.

There are two methods of treatment. One method employs low doses of methadone (30 to 40 mg) followed by gradual withdrawal of this drug. The other relies on high doses of 120 mg (given daily in one dose) on which the patient is usually maintained. This second method is criticised on the grounds that the patient is still dependent on a narcotic.

Unfortunately, the success of either treatment is limited. Many addicts after detoxification return to their old haunts and associates, becoming involved again in the pattern of a life dependent on drugs. Many die young as a result of deliberate or accidental overdosage, of hepatitis, endocarditis, tetanus or other complications.

DRUG ADMINISTRATION ERRORS

A drug aministration error, apart from the administration of a wrong drug to a patient, includes other factors which modify or alter the intended drug therapy, for example, a missed drug dose; doubling the next dose to compensate for the missed one; administration of the correct drug at the wrong time, or administration of the correct drug by the wrong route.

In hospital the nurse is responsible for administering drug therapy to inpatients, and for ensuring that each patient receives what the prescriber intended. With such a responsibility, the nurse must be fully aware that a mistake in drug administration could have an adverse effect on the patient. In these days of litigation, a mistake could carry a heavy penalty.

All drug therapy in hospital is authorised by the prescriber in writing on a patient's treatment sheet and such a prescription must conform with Government regulations, for example, prescriptions should be written legibly and *signed* by the prescriber. The nurse must be conversant with these regulations and with individual hospital policy which sets down those drugs which can be administered by a nurse, those requiring supervision during administration, and nursing abbreviations used within the hospital.

If a drug administration error does occur, the nurse involved must contact the prescriber and senior nursing officials immediately the error is discovered, so that counter therapy can be initiated if necessary.

NURSING IMPLICATIONS

To reduce the incidence of administration errors, the following principles should be practised during the drug round.

1. Do not let your attention wander but concentrate entirely on the routine of the administration of drugs to patients.
2. Check the name on the treatment sheet with the patient's identification bracelet or in accordance with accepted hospital practice for patient identification.
3. Certain drug protocols require a complete understanding of the prescribed therapy, and the prescriber's instructions must be clearly stated. For example, corticosteroid therapy is never ceased abruptly but is withdrawn gradually, and some drugs used in cancer chemotherapy are administered at weekly intervals only. Before digoxin is administered the apex beat should be checked. A premedication check of urinalysis should be made before administering insulin. If *there is any doubt* as to the prescriber's intentions, check with him or her, or with the senior nursing staff or the ward pharmacist before proceeding with administration of the drug.
4. Be conversant with all the drugs used in your ward. Know the generic name, brand names, strength, indication and colour of each. Be aware of the confusion that can arise due to similar-looking or similar-sounding drug names, for example, clomiphene and clonidine; chlorambucil and *Chloromycetin;* disopyramide and dipyridamole; chlorpropamide and chlorpromazine. There are many others.
5. Check the label on the drug container with the treatment sheet at least three times during administration.
6. Check the calculations for toxic drugs such as *Lanoxin, Nepenthe* oral solution with senior nursing staff or the ward pharmacist. Inaccuracies are potentially fatal.
7. If a patient comments on the different colour or dose form of the drug check that the drug is as ordered.
8. If a dose has been missed, inform the physician and other nursing staff as soon as possible so that the missed dose can be safely compensated for.
9. See that the patient swallows any oral medication at the time of drug administration.
10. If a drug trolley is used, ensure that only drugs in use are kept in it and that the interior of the trolley is clear and uncluttered. Drugs will then be found quickly, with less chance of picking up the wrong container.
11. Never add drugs to any container issued by the pharmacy department.
12. Maintain all drug labels in a clear condition so that the label can be

read distinctly. If a drug container requires a new label, return it to the pharmacy department — do not relabel it yourself.

To summarise these basic concepts for correct drug administration:

- Check that the patient is the correct patient.
- Check that the drug is the correct drug and dose form.
- Check that the strength is the correct strength.
- Check that the time is the correct time for administration.
- Check that the route is the correct route.

COMPLIANCE

Compliance occurs when the drug regimen prescribed and administered in the hospital is followed. If such therapy must be continued after discharge from the hospital, it is important the patient understands and is capable of carrying out the prescribed therapy without supervision. Many disease states of a chronic nature require continuation of drug therapy, for example, the prophylactic use of *Intal* to reduce the incidence of asthma attacks; aspirin and associated analgesics and anti-flammatory agents to minimise the pain of rheumatoid arthritis; antihypertensives to control blood pressure in hypertension; continuing drug therapy is mandatory in order to overcome tuberculosis and to control diabetes. Once discharged, the patient must be relied upon to maintain adequate supplies of his prescribed medications and to take them at regular intervals.

Non-compliance can result from several factors involving the patient.

1. Inadequate understanding by the patient of what the drug is intended to achieve.
2. The patient not understanding the importance of adhering to the prescribed regimen in terms of prognosis.
3. Difficulty in obtaining the drug outside the hospital if the drug, by law, is restricted to the hospital only.
4. Cost of obtaining the drug outside the hospital.
5. Lack of interest in his condition by family or friends, who may be responsible for obtaining and/or administering medication.
6. Non acceptance of the condition or medication on the part of the patient.

Compliance in paediatric therapy depends on the full understanding and cooperation of the parents.

Senile and psychiatric patients often undergo multiple drug therapy, and therefore relatives must be fully aware of drug requirements for such patients.

Safe and effective drug therapy is only carried out when the patient or relative is fully informed of his medications and their use. To this end, the health team prior to the patient's discharge must ensure that the patient knows:

(a) the name and strength of the drug;
(b) the purpose for which the drug is to be taken;
(c) the amount of drug for a single dose;
(d) the total number of daily doses;
(e) the time the drug is to be taken, for example, in relation to meals;
(f) for how many days the drug regime is to be continued;
(g) the route of administration;

(h) any special directions required by the route of administration, for example, eye drops, suppositories;

(i) what action to take if a drug dose is missed, for example, especially digoxin, oral anticoagulant therapy.

As far as possible, much of this information appears on the label of the drug container supplied by the hospital's pharmacy department.

NURSING IMPLICATIONS

Basic counselling of the discharge patient should include such information as:

1. Instances when alcohol is contraindicated while taking certain drugs;
2. Special dietary precautions (for example, avoiding monoamine oxidase inhibitors with beef extracts, soft cheeses, chianti, broad beans);
3. What non-prescription drugs are contraindicated (for example, aspirin and analgesics with oral anticoagulant therapy);
4. Not to use complex machinery or drive cars in certain types of drug therapy;
5. What side effects to expect, and how to cope with them;
6. Correct storage conditions for the drug in use;
7. When to seek further medical advice.

SELF-EVALUATION TEST

1. Explain the importance of the disease state in regard to the onset of an adverse drug reaction.
2. List at least six other factors which influence the incidence of adverse drug reactions.
3. Explain the following terms: patient idiosyncrasy, therapeutic index, hypersensitivity reaction.
4. Which immunoglobulin has been implicated in the onset of allergic reactions?
5. Describe the symptoms of an anaphylactic reaction.
6. How many types of immunological reactions have so far been implicated in the allergic response?
7. Describe three ways in which the nurse can help in the detection of adverse drug reactions.
8. What features are common to all drugs which induce drug dependence?
9. What are the two components of drug dependence?
10. Explain the withdrawal syndrome.
11. Explain the basic principles of treatment of drug abuse.
12. Why is it important that a patient fully understands his or her drug therapy requirements?
13. Give some reasons for patient non-compliance.
14. State several ways in which the nurse can increase patient compliance with medication.
15. State the five basic concepts of correct drug interaction.
16. Describe six mechanisms of drug interaction.
17. What foods are contraindicated during therapy with MAOIs?
18. Name four drug groups involved in drug interactions.

3

DOSE CALCULATIONS

Ross W. Holland

OBJECTIVES

At the end of this chapter the student should be able to:

1. compute the doses required for solid-dose forms of medication (tablets, capsules) and liquid-dose forms (oral mixtures, injections);
2. compute the quantities required to make simple solutions, using both percentages and ratios
3. compute a dose based on body weight;
4. compute flow rates for intravenous infusions.

PREREQUISITE KNOWLEDGE

Simple arithmetic procedures up to and including the ability to:

1. multiply and divide in both decimals and fractions;
2. convert percentages to ratios and ratios to percentages;
3. resolve an equation with one unknown factor.

ARITHMETIC PRETEST

Students should work through the following exercises. Answers are given on page 48. If you are unable to successfully complete this pretest, review of the appropriate arithmetic principles should be undertaken before proceeding.

Conversion to fractions

1. $1\frac{3}{7} =$	**2.** $2\frac{2}{3} =$	**3.** $1\frac{4}{5} =$
4. $3\frac{1}{6} =$	**5.** $4\frac{1}{5} =$	**6.** $3\frac{3}{8} =$

Multiplying fractions

1. $\frac{1}{4} \times \frac{1}{3} =$	2. $\frac{3}{5} \times \frac{1}{2} =$	3. $\frac{1}{6} \times \frac{3}{4} =$
4. $1\frac{1}{5} \times \frac{5}{7} =$	5. $\frac{3}{2} \times \frac{4}{6} =$	6. $\frac{3}{8} \times \frac{2}{7} =$

Dividing fractions

1. $\frac{1}{5} \div \frac{1}{6} =$	2. $\frac{2}{3} \div \frac{4}{6} =$	3. $\frac{3}{8} \div \frac{1}{5} =$
4. $\frac{5}{7} \div \frac{3}{4} =$	5. $1\frac{2}{3} \div 1\frac{2}{3} =$	6. $1\frac{1}{4} \div \frac{1}{4} =$

Multiplying decimals

1. $1.6 \times 3.2 =$	2. $2.7 \times 1.75 =$	3. $6 \times 4.2 =$
4. $2.5 \times 1.7 =$	5. $16.8 \times 102 =$	6. $5.4 \times 30.5 =$

Dividing decimals

1. $16.4 \div 8 =$	2. $3.5 \div 0.7 =$	3. $6.5 \div 1.3 =$
4. $2.12 \div 0.424 =$	5. $7.5 \div 0.3 =$	6. $11.25 \div 3.75$

Converting ratios to percentages

1. 1 : 2 = %	2. 1 : 500 = %	3. 1 : 20 = %
4. 1 : 2000 = %	5. 1 : 5000 = %	6. 1 : 250 = %

Converting percentages to ratios

1. 1% = :	2. 20% = :	3. 5% = :
4. 0.02% = :	5. 1.5% = :	6. 0.45% = :

THE METRIC SYSTEM

The metric system is now used in all hospitals. It is simple, working in multiples of ten.

UNITS OF WEIGHT

1 kilogram (kg)	=	1000 grams (g)
1 gram (g)	=	1000 milligrams (mg)
1 milligram (mg)	=	1000 micrograms (mcg)

UNITS OF VOLUME

1 litre (L) = 1000 millilitres (mL)

Note: 1 litre of pure water under standard conditions weighs 1 kilogram. 1 millilitre of pure water under standard conditions weighs 1 gram. It is important to remember that the gram (g) corresponds in weight to the millilitre (mL), and the kilogram (kg) in weight to the litre (L). Only official abbreviations should be used. If possible, the terms "litre" and "microgram" should be written in full to avoid confusion.

EXPRESSING QUANTITIES AS DECIMALS

Quantities less than one unit are usually written in the next smaller unit. For example, half a gram is written as 500 mg rather than 0.5 g. If it is necessary to use the larger unit, a zero is *always* placed before the decimal, as shown above. To write .5 g could lead to confusion if the decimal point is indistinct. If 5 g of a drug were given in error for 0.5 g, the mistake could be fatal. Therefore, use whole numbers in the smaller unit whenever possible.

CONVERSION FROM GRAMS TO MILLIGRAMS AND VICE VERSA

We have already seen that 1 gram (g) = 1000 milligrams (mg). Therefore to convert grams to milligrams we multiply by 1000. For example:

$$2\text{ g} = (2 \times 1000)\text{ mg} = 2000\text{ mg}$$
$$2.165\text{ g} = (2.165 \times 1000)\text{ mg} = 2165\text{ mg}$$
$$1.23\text{ g} = (1.230 \times 1000)\text{ mg} = 1230\text{ mg}$$

In the last line it was helpful to write the 1.23 g as 1.230 g. We can then multiply by 1000 by moving the decimal point three places to the right. Conversely, when converting from milligrams to grams, we move the decimal point three places to the left. For example:

$$2060\text{ mg} = \frac{2060}{1000} = 2.06\text{ g}$$

Note that:

1. when the quantity is less than 1 gram (g), express it in milligrams;
2. as it is difficult to divide by decimals, for example 2.16, we can eliminate the decimal point by multiplying by $\frac{100}{100}$, which will not change the value.
   To divide by 2.16, we multiply by $\frac{1}{2.16}$
   $$\frac{1}{2.16} \times \frac{100}{100} = \frac{100}{216}$$, thus eliminating decimals.

DOSE CALCULATIONS

The quantity of a drug given, in terms of numbers of tablets or volume of a liquid, may be calculated in a number of ways. Any method of calculation that arrives at the correct answer is acceptable. However, only two will be presented here. They will be referred to as Method 1, which works from first principles, and Method 2, which involves the use of a formula.

Regardless of which method is used, it will be necessary *in all cases* to ensure that calculations are performed using the same *type of units* throughout, for example, milligrams, millilitres, percentage, ratio and so on. In many cases a conversion to similar units must be performed before the computation can begin. In addition, it will be necessary to specify the *type of units* to which your answer refers. An answer of six means little — it must specify the units: six tablets, six litres or whatever the appropriate unit happens to be.

CALCULATION FOR SOLID DOSE FORMS — TABLETS AND CAPSULES

Example How many tablets containing 62.5 micrograms of digoxin will be required to give a dose of 0.125 mg?

Method 1

Step 1 As the two doses are in different units, one in milligrams and the other in micrograms, one must be converted to the other.

$$0.125 \text{ mg} = (0.125 \times 1000) \text{ micrograms}$$
$$= 125 \text{ micrograms}$$

Step 2 If 1 tablet contains 62.5 micrograms and *X* tablets are required for a dose of 125 micrograms.

$$\text{then } X = \frac{125}{62.5} \times 1 \text{ tablet}$$
$$= 2 \text{ tablets}$$

Therefore, 2 tablets of digoxin 62.5 micrograms must be given for a 0.125 mg dose.

Method 2 This method involves the application of the following formula:

$$\text{quantity required} = \frac{\text{dose required}}{\text{dose available}} \times 1 \text{ (tablet, capsule)}$$

Step 1 As before, convert the dosages to similar units:

$$0.125 \text{ mg} = (0.125 \times 1000) \text{ micrograms}$$
$$= 125 \text{ micrograms}$$

Step 2 Substitute into the formula:

$$\frac{\text{dose required}}{\text{dose available}} = \frac{125 \text{ micrograms}}{62.5 \text{ micrograms}} \times 1 \text{ tablet}$$
$$= 2 \text{ tablets}$$

Therefore, 2 tablets of digoxin 62.5 micrograms must be given for a 0.125 mg dose.

Exercises

1. How many frusemide tablets 40 mg must be given for a 10 mg dose?
2. How many levodopa tablets 250 mg must be given for a 375 mg dose?

3. How many digoxin tablets 0.25 mg must be given for a dose of 125 micrograms?
4. How many haloperidol tablets 1.5 mg must be given for a 4.5 mg dose?

CALCULATIONS FOR LIQUID MEDICATION — MIXTURES AND INJECTIONS

Example 1 A dose of 75 mg of pethidine has been ordered. It is available in ampoules containing 100 mg in 2 millilitres. What volume must be administered?

Method 1 If 2 mL of solution contains 100 mg of pethidine, and X mL of solution contains 75 mg of pethidine.

$$\text{then } X = \frac{75}{100} \times \frac{2}{1} \text{ millilitres}$$

$$= \frac{150}{100} \text{ mL}$$

$$= 1.5 \text{ mL}$$

Therefore, 1.5 mL of pethidine injection 100 mg/2 mL would be required for a dose of 75 mg.

Method 2 Apply the formula:

$$\frac{\text{dose required}}{\text{dose available}} \times \text{volume of the dose available}$$

$$= \frac{75 \text{ mg}}{100 \text{ mg}} \times \frac{2}{1} \text{ mL}$$

$$= 1.5 \text{ mL}$$

Therefore, 1.5 mL of pethidine injection 100 mg/2 mL will be required for a dose of 75 mg.

Example 2 A dose of 150 mg of penicillin V suspension is ordered from a bottle labelled 125 mg/5 mL. What volume must be administered?

Method 1 If 5 mL of suspension contains 125 mg of penicillin V, and X mL of suspension contains 150 mg,

$$\text{then } X = \frac{150 \text{ mg}}{125 \text{ mg}} \times 5 \text{ mL}$$

$$= 6 \text{ mL}$$

Therefore, 6 mL of penicillin V suspension 125 mg/5 mL must be administered for a dose of 150 mg.
Note: The answer is a volume of suspension and is therefore expressed in millilitres.

Method 2 Apply the formula:

$$\text{dose required} = \frac{150 \text{ mg}}{125 \text{ mg}} \times 5 \text{ mL}$$
$$= 6 \text{ mL}$$

Therefore, 6 mL of penicillin V suspension 125 mg/5 mL must be given for a dose of 150 mg.

Exercises

1. A dose of 350 mg of potassium chloride has been ordered. A solution containing 1 g in 4 mL is available. What volume must be given?
2. A 100 mg dose of erythromycin has been ordered. Erythromycin suspension containing 125 mg/5 mL is available. How much must be given?
3. From ampoules containing atropine 0.6 mg/mL, what volume must be administered in order to give a 900 microgram dose?
4. A dose of 3 mg of chlorpheniramine has been ordered. Chlorpheniramine syrup containing 2 mg per 5 mL is available. How much must be given?

CALCULATIONS FOR EXTERNAL PREPARATIONS — ANTISEPTICS

Example 1 A 1 : 2000 solution of chlorhexidine is required and a 20% solution is available. How much of the 20% solution will be needed to make 2 litres of the 1 : 2000 solution?

Method 1

Step 1 As one strength is expressed as a ratio and the other as a percentage, one must be converted.

$$20\% = 20 \text{ parts per hundred}$$
$$= 20 : 100$$
$$= 1 : 5$$

Step 2 2000 mL of chlorhexidine requires *X* mL of chlorhexidine 1 : 5.

$$\text{therefore } X = \frac{1 : 2000}{1 : 5} \times 2000 \text{ mL}$$
$$= \frac{1}{2000} \times \frac{5}{1} \times \frac{2000}{1} \text{ mL}$$
$$= 5 \text{ mL}$$

Therefore, 5 mL of chlorhexidine 20% will be required to make 2 litres of a 1 : 2000 solution.

Method 2

Step 1 As above.

Step 2 Apply the formula:

$$\frac{\text{strength required}}{\text{strength available}} \times \text{quantity required}$$

$$= \frac{1:2000}{1:5} \times 2000 \text{ mL}$$

$$= \frac{1}{2000} \times \frac{5}{1} \times \frac{2000}{1} \text{ mL}$$

$$= 5 \text{ mL}$$

Therefore, 5 mL of 20% chlorhexidine solution will be required to make 2 litres of 1 : 2000 solution.

Exercises

1. How much *Eusol* 1 : 8 will be required to make 500 mL of a 1 : 20 solution?
2. How much *Savlon Concentrate* (100%) will be required to make 600 mL of a 5% solution?
3. How much *Hibitane* 5% will be required to make 1 litre of 1 : 1000 solution?
4. How much *Savlon* 1 : 2 will be required to make 1.5 litres of a 10% solution?

Example 2 A particular case which occurs only rarely in practice, but for which you should be prepared, is when a solid, such as powder or crystals, is to be dissolved. Consider the following.

Prepare 200 mL of a 0.5% solution of boracic acid (a powder) in water. Remember that for water, grams and millilitres are equivalent units in weight and volume respectively.

Method 1 200 mL of 0.5% solution requires X g of powder (100%)

$$X = \frac{0.5}{100} \times \frac{200}{1} \text{ grams}$$

$$= 1 \text{ g of boracic acid powder}$$

Therefore, 1 g of boracic acid powder will be required to make 200 mL of a 0.5% solution.

Method 2 Applying the formula from Example 1, we get:

$$\frac{\text{strength required}}{\text{strength available}} \times \text{quantity required}$$

$$= \frac{0.5\%}{100\%} \times 200 \text{ (g)}$$

$$= 1 \text{ g of boracic acid powder}$$

Note: As the answer is a quantity of boracic acid, a powder, the answer will be in units of weight, in this case grams.

Exercises

5. How much copper-sulphate crystals will be required to make 1 litre of a 1 : 2000 solution?
6. How much potassium-permanganate crystals will be required to make 2 litres of 1 : 5000 solution?

DILUTION OF INJECTIONS THAT ARE TO BE RECONSTITUTED

Some injections have to be reconstituted before use. That is, a diluent must be added to the powder. When the container specifies exact quantities and the final strength of the solution (for example, the final solution contains 100 mg/2 mL), there are no problems in calculating a fractional dose. Occasionally, however, no final strength is mentioned.

Consider the case of an antibiotic where you require a 125 mg dose. The antibiotic comes in a vial containing 250 mg to which you must add 2 mL of water for injection. The final volume will be a little over 2 mL because of the space occupied by the powder. The only way to administer a fractional dose will be to withdraw and measure the volume of the solution and to administer the correct fraction of that volume.

CALCULATION OF DOSES FROM BODY WEIGHT

Occasionally a dose may be expressed in the following form: give 1 mg/kg body weight. This requires the nursing staff to weigh the patient and give the appropriate dose based on that weight. If the patient weighed 75 kg, a simple calculation is all that is required to obtain the correct dose.

If 1 mg is to be given for 1 kg of body weight, and X mg is to be given for 75 kg body weight,

$$\text{then } X = \frac{75}{1} \times 1 \text{ mg}$$

$$= 75 \text{ mg}$$

A variation of this could be when the dose is expressed as follows: give 1 mg/kg/day in four divided doses. In this instance the total amount to be given per day would be calculated first, then divided into four equal doses and given at six-hour intervals.

CALCULATION OF INFUSION RATES USING DIFFERENT ADMINISTRATION SETS

Intravenous administration sets are calibrated to deliver a given number of drops per millilitre of solution. Current sets usually deliver 20 drops per millilitre or 60 drops/mL for the paediatric buretrol. Other sets are available, however, so the type in use must be known.

Because an intravenous order may be expressed as a volume to be given over a period of time (such as 500 mL over 4 hours), but the rate is roughly estimated by observing the flow in drops per minute, it is necessary to be able to calculate the conversion from drops per minute to millilitres per minute and vice versa using different administration sets.

Example 1 What flow rate is required to administer 500 mL of dextrose 5% in water over a period of 8 hours from a set delivering 15 drops per millilitre?

Step 1 Convert the hours to minutes.

$$\begin{aligned} 8 \text{ hours} &= 8 \times 60 \text{ minutes} \\ &= 480 \text{ minutes} \end{aligned}$$

Step 2 Calculate the required rate in millilitres per minute. If 500 mL are to be administered over 480 minutes, and *X* mL are to be administered over 1 minute,

$$\begin{aligned} \text{then } X &= \frac{500}{1} \times \frac{1}{480} \text{ mL} \\ &= 1 \text{ mL (approximately)} \end{aligned}$$

Step 3 Convert to a drop-rate per minute. Administration will be at the rate of 1 mL/minute (approximately). As the set delivers 15 drops/mL, the required rate will be 1 × 15 drops per minute or 15 drops/minute (approximately).

Note: As there are many possible sources of error in this procedure — variations due to different specific gravity of solutions, errors in observation, errors in calibration of the administration sets — answers to this type of question are approximations only. Decimal points need not be used as it would be impossible to observe 0.2 of a drop.

Example 2 Another situation that may arise is the need to administer a given amount of drug over a period of time. For example, at what rate must a solution containing 1000 mg of lignocaine in 500 mL of solution be given to a patient so as to receive 3 mg/minute from a set delivering 60 drops/millilitre?

Step 1 Calculate how much infusion solution contains 3 mg of lignocaine. If 500 mL of solution contains 1000 mg lignocaine, and *X* mL of solution contains 3 mg of lignocaine,

$$\begin{aligned} \text{then } X &= \frac{500 \text{ ml}}{1} \times \frac{3 \text{ mg}}{1000 \text{ mg}} \\ &= 1.5 \text{ mL} \end{aligned}$$

Thus, we need to give 1.5 mL each minute for a dose of 3 mg/minute. This must now be converted to a flow rate.

Step 2 Convert to a flow rate. If there are 60 drops in 1 mL, and there are X drops in 1.5 mL,

$$\text{then } X = \frac{60}{1} \times \frac{1.5}{1} \text{ drops}$$
$$= 90 \text{ drops}$$

Therefore, to administer lignocaine at 3 mg/minute from a solution containing 1000 mg/500 mL, using an administration set delivering 60 drops/mL, a flow rate of approximately 90 drops/minute must be maintained.

Exercises

1. What flow rate in drops/minute must be maintained using an administration set delivering 15 drops/mL to give 1 litre of normal saline by IV infusion over 12 hours?
2. How many drops/minute must be maintained to administer 50 mL of dextrose 10% over 1 hour using a paediatric set delivering 60 drops/mL?
3. What flow rate in drops/minute will be required to administer 1 mg/minute of aminophylline to a patient via a giving set calibrated to 15 drops/mL? The infusion solution has been prepared to contain 250 mg aminophylline in 500 mL.
4. Ampicillin has been ordered to be infused at a rate of 100 mg/hour via a set calibrated to 60 drops/mL. The infusion contains 500 mg of ampicillin per 500 mL. What flow rate will be required?

PAEDIATRIC DOSES

Correct doses are essential for the paediatric patient. It is, of course, the responsibility of the medical officer to precisely and unambiguously specify the dose required for a particular patient. If you wish to *roughly check* whether a paediatric dose is correct, several courses of action are available to you. Information concerning paediatric doses is available in the manufacturer's literature, in the *British National Formulary* and from the pharmacy department within your hospital. Alternatively, you may wish to convert a known adult dose by applying one of a number of formulae. Two such formulae are Clark's Rule and Young's Rule.

Clark's Rule

$$\text{Paediatric dose} = \frac{\text{weight of child in kilograms}}{70} \times \text{adult dose}$$

Young's Rule

$$\text{Paediatric dose} = \frac{\text{age}}{\text{age} + 12} \times \text{adult dose}$$

It must be stressed that these rules give rough estimations only. Any suspicion that a dose is incorrect should be checked with the pharmacist and referred back to the prescriber for verification or review.

ANSWERS TO SELF-EVALUATION PRETEST

Conversion to fractions

1. $\frac{10}{7}$	**2.** $\frac{8}{3}$	**3.** $\frac{9}{5}$
4. $\frac{19}{6}$	**5.** $\frac{21}{5}$	**6.** $\frac{27}{8}$

Multiplying fractions

1. $\frac{1}{12}$	**2.** $\frac{3}{10}$	**3.** $\frac{1}{8}$
4. $\frac{6}{7}$	**5.** 1	**6.** $\frac{3}{28}$

Dividing fractions

1. $1\frac{1}{5}$	**2.** 1	**3.** $1\frac{7}{8}$
4. $\frac{20}{21}$	**5.** 1	**6.** 5

Multiplying decimals

1. 5.12	**2.** 4.725	**3.** 25.2
4. 4.25	**5.** 1713.6	**6.** 164.7

Dividing decimals

1. 2.05	**2.** 5	**3.** 5
4. 5	**5.** 25	**6.** 3

Converting ratios to percentages

1. 50%	**2.** 0.2%	**3.** 5%
4. 0.05%	**5.** 0.02%	**6.** 0.4%

Converting percentages to ratios

1. 1 : 100	**2.** 1 : 5	**3.** 1 : 20
4. 1 : 5000	**5.** 15 : 1000	**6.** 45 : 10 000

ANSWERS TO EXERCISES

Calculations for solid dose forms

1. $\frac{1}{4}$ tablet	**2.** $1\frac{1}{2}$ tablets
3. $\frac{1}{2}$ tablet	**4.** 3 tablets

Calculations for liquid medications

1. 1.4 mL	**2.** 4 mL
3. 1.5 mL	**4.** 7.5 mL

Calculations for external preparations

1. 200 mL	**2.** 30 mL
3. 20 mL	**4.** 300 mL
5. 500 mg	**6.** 400 mg

Calculation of infusion rates

1. 21 drops/minute	**2.** 50 drops/minute
3. 30 drops/minute	**4.** 100 drops/minute

4
TOXICOLOGY

Andrew F. Petrie

OBJECTIVES

At the conclusion of this chapter, the reader should:

1. be able to list nine groups of substances with potential for causing human poisonings with examples from each group;
2. have an understanding of principles of management of poisoning, including initial therapy and exceptions to generalisations;
3. be able to list ten specific antidotes and describe their mode of action;
4. be able to list five routes of contact by which poisoning may occur with examples of substances toxic via these routes and their effects;
5. understand the concept of "range of toxicity";
6. understand the role of a Poisons Information Centre.

PREREQUISITE KNOWLEDGE

1. General human physiology.
2. Basic principles of chemistry.

In the sense of being a study of poisons and their effects on animals (including humans), toxicology predates recorded history. Poisons are mentioned on the Ebers papyrus, written about 1500 BC. They have figured prominently in Roman and Greek histories and on through the Middle Ages when, for example, the Borgias illustrated a working knowledge of the dosage and actions of poisons, if rather less interest and knowledge in how to treat their effects.

Paracelsus (1493-1541) could be regarded as the initiator of the modern approach to toxicology of identifying a particular toxin, the use of experimentation to examine responses to various chemicals in the therapeutic and toxic context and the potential involvement of environmental agents in toxicology. One statement attributed to Paracelsus provides an insight into both the breadth of the subject of toxicology and the relationship to pharmacology: "All substances are poisons; there is none which is not a poison. The right dose differentiates a poison and a remedy." This statement is both relevant and current.

While the intentional homicidal poisonings of the past have decreased as a major section of the study of toxicology, suicide attempts in adults are still a major problem, as are unintentional accidental poisonings in children — usually through experimentation in the developmental process of one to three year olds. Childhood poisoning as a form of child abuse and the neglect syndrome has also been well documented. In adults, industrial or agricultural accidents are significant causes of poisoning.

TYPES OF CONTACT

Having already expressed the large number of potentially poisonous substances, one should say that in particular situations contact through almost every portal of entry to the body may under the right circumstances, cause poisoning. Table 2 provides some illustration of the possible contacts with some representative toxins.

Table 2
Methods of Contact with Poisons

Type of Contact	Some Possible Effects	Example of Poison Active by This Route
Ingestion	Local in gastrointestinal tract Systemic poisoning	Overdose of medicines, some plants, petroleum distillates, pesticides
Topical - skin	Local irritation Absorption through skin to give systemic poisoning	Caustic soda (corrosive alkali) Organophosphate pesticides
Topical - eye	Local irritation	Acid and alkali, some plants, e.g. Meadow Saffron or Naked Ladies
	Specific effects on eye	Atropine
Inhalation	Irritation in upper and lower respiratory tract	Chlorine gas
	Absorption and systemic poisoning	Carbon monoxide (exhaust fumes)
Injection	Systemic	Overdose of therapeutic drugs Many cytotoxic drugs
	Local irritation, necrosis	

The type of contact which is significant and the extent of poisoning will depend on the substance concerned and its chemical properties.

Water-soluble substances, for example, are unlikely to be absorbed through the skin to produce systemic toxicity. However, if they are strongly acidic (for example, sulphuric acid) or alkaline (for example, caustic soda), they may react with the skin to cause a chemical burn. Some fat-soluble substances (for example, organophosphates like parathion and malathion) can be absorbed through the skin to produce systemic toxicity. A similar situation applies with ingestion where local irritation or absorption, or both, may occur depending on the chemical nature of the poison.

It should be noted that when a potential irritant like caustic soda has been swallowed there may be local burning in the mouth. However, the absence of burning in the mouth *cannot* be taken as indicative that there will not be serious burns in the oesophagus or stomach. In some cases the substance is swallowed quickly causing severe burns to the oesophagus but no effects in the mouth.

RANGE OF TOXICITY (Response and Dose)

The relevance of dose to toxicity can be well expressed by an example. Common salt (NaCl) in appropriate quantities is essential to life. We take it orally in our diet, and it is a standard ingredient of most intravenous infusion fluids. Normally the serum level of sodium will be in the range 130 to 150 mmol/litre. If this rises to 150-160 mmol/litre, CNS symptoms including convulsions will occur in approximately 10% of patients. Death is a frequent occurrence if levels exceed 185 mmol/litre. Two level dessertspoonfuls of sodium chloride (approximately 500 mmol of sodium) would, if retained and absorbed, raise the serum-sodium level of a two-year-old child by about 50 mmol/litre — a potentially lethal dose. Repeatedly, cases have been reported where children have died of salt overdose when it has been administered as an emetic. Salt should never be used for this purpose in children.

Ways of Expressing Toxicity

Unfortunately no simple relationship exists between the toxic dose of a substance and the therapeutic dose. For some substances, the toxic dose is close to the effective therapeutic dose (for example, cytotoxic drugs or tricyclic antidepressants). For other drugs, the therapeutic dose can be increased immensely before a toxic dose is reached (for example, penicillin).

Therapeutic index

This is the ratio of a toxic dose to effective dose. It gives an estimate of the relative safety of a drug in its normal usage. It is estimated as the ratio of LD 50 (lethal dose 50%) to ED 50 (effective dose in 50% of cases). As different effects may require different doses, a single drug may have a number of therapeutic indices. In practice a substance is usually referred to as having a "high" or "low" therapeutic index.

LD 50

This term is commonly used in toxicology literature. This is the dose which will kill 50% of an experimental population. For example, for the drug imipramine, an oral dose of 625 mg/kg given to a group of 100 rats would kill 50 of them. It is thus said to have an oral LD 50 (in rats) of 625 mg/kg. These data are helpful, but there is wide variation among species, as is shown in Table 3.

Table 3
Species Differences in LD 50 for Imipramine

LD 50 (oral, rats)	=	625 mg/kg
LD 50 (oral, mouse)	=	448 mg/kg
LD 50 (oral, dog)	=	100 mg/kg

Cases have been reported of children dying after ingestion of 15 mg/kg to 30 mg/kg. Hence, while animal data may be helpful, great caution must be exercised in using them to predict effects in humans.

ACUTE AND CHRONIC POISONING

Poisoning may be either acute (a single contact with a toxin) or chronic (repeated contacts with a toxin which is not, or is only poorly, excreted from the body, thus permitting a build-up over a period of time). The build-up of toxin or its effect may also be referred to as "cumulative". Often the symptoms of a chronic overdose differ from those of an acute overdose. As an example, a patient with acute lead poisoning (after ingestion of a soluble lead salt) may present with abdominal pain, vomiting, diarrhoea, metallic taste, black stools, oliguria, collapse or coma. A patient with chronic lead poisoning is more likely to present with a characteristic "lead line" on the gums and very non-specific symptoms of appetite loss, weight loss, constipation, vomiting, headache, weakness or loss of recently developed skills.

EPIDEMIOLOGY

During 1984 in Great Britain poisoning accounted for 6.8% of deaths due to accidents other than traffic accidents.

In childhood and adult poisonings, the most common substances involved are internal medications. Whereas barbiturates used to be the most common group ingested, these have been replaced with benzodiazepines (diazepam, oxazepam and so on). While the continued high incidence of sedative overdose is a source of great concern, there is some comfort in the greatly increased safety margin of benzodiazepines over barbiturates.

After medicines, common household items (cleaners, polishes, adhesives, insect repellants and so on) account for the biggest fraction of childhood poisonings.

Poisoning may be caused by substances from any of the following groups: internal medicines, external medicines, veterinary medicines, cosmetics, household and handyman products, pesticides, plants, animals and chemicals.

Details of an Individual Poisoning

In few cases will there be an accurate history of the quantity of substance swallowed, or even what the substance is. Adults who have attempted to take a suicidal dose of a substance are notorious for giving inaccurate histories of the quantity of substance ingested and may in fact be unconscious at the time of presentation. The history of a childhood poisoning will usually involve the patient (often too young to talk) having been found sitting amidst tablets or liquid spread across the floor. How much has been spilled and how much ingested cannot be accurately estimated. Children in the "at risk" age group (one to three years) cannot be relied on not to swallow something that tastes unpleasant. They may have ingested much more *or* much less than the mother thinks has been swallowed. At best, an educated guess can be made, based on the maximum that could have been swallowed. In some circumstances blood or urine assays may indicate the drug and quantity absorbed.

MANAGEMENT OF POISONING

In spite of the common association in people's minds between poisons and antidotes, *there are very few substances for which an antidote exists.*

The management of poisoning in the majority of cases involves two steps and occasionally a third: maintaining vital functions, removing contact between poison and the patient, and applying specific treatment (if appropriate). Some aspects are summarised in Table 4.

Table 4
Management of Poisoning

1. Maintain vital functions	Respiration, cardiovascular function, fluid and electrolyte maintenance, safeguard kidney function
2. Remove contact between poison and patient	If no contraindication, induce emesis; gastric lavage (rarely used in children); wash off skin or eye with water. Remove patient from gaseous poison. Speed excretion: catharsis, diuresis, dialysis Prevent absorption by adsorption onto activated charcoal
3. Apply specific treatment if appropriate	

EMESIS

Making a patient vomit an ingested poison is an early step in many poisonings, particularly in children. In general it should be carried out within about four hours of the ingestion and preferably earlier. In some cases delayed passage from stomach into the small intestine occurs, for example, with aspirin, atropine and its derivatives, tricyclic antidepressants and glutethimide. Where this happens, the induction of emesis later than four hours after an ingestion may be of value.

Emesis will not completely empty the stomach, and even with syrup of ipecac, as little as 30% of gastric contents will be removed, though often a greater volume may be achieved.

Contraindications to Emesis

There are four important cases where a patient should *not* be made to vomit. These are as follows.

1. The ingestion of corrosive substances (strong acids or alkalis, for example, caustic soda, drain cleaners, dishwashing machine detergent). In these cases there is possibility of perforation of the stomach or oesophagus and of further burning when the substance is vomited.
2. The ingestion of petroleum distillates (petrol, kerosene, fly spray, many polishes). These may be aspirated into the lungs causing a chemical pneumonitis. There are some exceptions to this generalisation if the potential risk from systemic poisoning is greater than that of aspiration. (Recent publications suggest there are some circumstances when emesis should be induced after petroleum distillate ingestion.)
3. The patient is unconscious (or likely to be unconscious by the time emesis occurs). There is a high danger of an unconscious patient aspirating vomitus into the lungs.
4. The patient is having a fit or convulsing.

Induction of Emesis

Over the years many substances including salt, mustard and copper sulphate have been used as emetics. Syrup of ipecacuanha or pharyngeal stimulation are probably the *only* methods which should be considered. Others are not effective in a high percentage of cases and may be toxic in their own right. Salt should never be used as an emetic in children.

Syrup of ipecacuanha (syrup of ipecac) is a preparation made from the root of the ipecacuanha plant. Over the years this has proved to be a safe and efficient emetic. Acting mainly on the CNS, it causes emesis in 95% of patients but normally takes between 15 and 30 minutes to work.

Syrup of ipecac

The *British National Formulary* (No. 10, 1985) lists the following dosage scale for syrup of ipecac:

Age	**Dose**
6-18 months	10 mL
Older children	15 mL
Adults	30 mL

The dose should be accompanied by a drink of water (approximately 100 mL for children and 200 mL for adults) and may be repeated once only if vomiting has not occurred within 20 minutes. In practice a 15 mL dose is usually effective in all paediatric patients. Note the contraindications to emesis listed previously.

Pharyngeal stimulation
This method is said to be largely ineffective but, if syrup of ipecac is not available, may be tried. For a child or baby, give 100 mL of water to drink, roll the child in a towel to restrict arms, place in "spanking position" (face down over the knees with head and shoulders sloping downwards), and with index finger, tickle the back of the tongue and throat. Continue giving water and tickling the throat until vomitus appears clear. For an adult, give 200 mL of water, lower the head of the patient between his knees and with the blunt end of a spoon handle, or the index finger, tickle the back of tongue or throat. Repeat giving water and tickling the throat until vomitus is clear.

Retain vomited matter
Vomitus should be saved and inspected for the presence of particles (for example, tablets) suggestive of the substance ingested to assist in confirmation of substance and quantity ingested. It may be necessary to have chemical analysis carried out for the same reason.

ADSORPTION

The process of adsorption involves using a chemical with a particularly large surface area (for example, activated charcoal) to adsorb other chemicals onto its surface. This is most frequently used to bind a toxic substance in the gastrointestinal tract and hence prevent the toxin passing into the blood stream. It may be used in other contexts, however. Specially prepared charcoal columns can be used in haemoperfusion (similar to dialysis) to remove toxins from the blood.

Adsorbents

Activated charcoal is the most frequently used adsorbent given orally. This substance has been specially prepared to increase its surface area and adsorbent properties. (Despite similar appearance, crushed burned toast is of no value as an adsorbent.) If it is being used in the same patient as ipecac syrup, activated charcoal needs to be given after the emetic has worked as it adsorbs ipecac.

Ideally a quantity of activated charcoal 5 to 10 times the amount of the ingested substance would be given. As the amount ingested is often not known, 500 mg/kg body weight (30 to 50g) is usually given as a slurry in water.

Activated charcoal must be kept in well-closed containers. Unless these are well sealed, the adsorptive power of the charcoal will be reduced as a result of substances in the atmosphere being adsorbed onto the charcoal. Some formulations for more palatable preparations have been published, but care must be taken in formulations of activated charcoal not to inactivate it.

Activated charcoal has been shown in humans or experimental animals to be of value in adsorbing the drugs listed in Table 5.

Fuller's Earth is also used as an adsorbent and is utilised in paraquat poisonings to minimise absorption into the blood stream.

Table 5
Drugs Adsorbed by Activated Charcoal

Analgesics	Hypnotics and Sedatives	Tranquillisers and Antidepressants	Others
Aspirin and sodium salicylate	Barbiturates, including barbitone	Chlorpromazine	Chloroquin
Salicylamide	Phenobarbitone	Imipramine	Chlorpheniramine
Dextropropoxyphene	Pentobarbitone	Nortriptyline	Ipecacuanha
Paracetamol	Quinalbarbitone		Isoniazid
Mefenamic acid	Glutethimide		Phenylpropanolamine
			Propantheline

CATHARSIS

Hastening the passage of gastrointestinal contents by administering a laxative is used to help remove unabsorbed poison from the body. The substances most commonly used are ***magnesium sulphate*** (Epsom salts) or ***mannitol 20% solution*** (500 mL orally for an adult).

NURSING IMPLICATIONS

Consideration of poisoning necessitates emphasis on aspects of first aid and hospitalisation.

Assessment

First-aid measures include the thorough assessment and identification of patient problems. Prompt intervention is imperative. These are, in essence, the "ABC" of first aid.

Management

1. Ensure cleared airways, adequate breathing and circulation.
2. Move the patient away from any toxic substance.
3. Remove toxic substance from the patient. For example, hosing or washing a substance from the body or removing contaminated clothing.
4. Manage convulsions if they occur.
5. Save any vomitus if possible.
6. Transport the patient to hospital as soon as possible. Certain information would assist in the management of the patient. Information should be noted and relayed to ambulance personnel or hospital staff.
   (a) Save bottle or container of substance.
   (b) Note the original purpose of the substance.
   (c) If known, the actual shape or form, colour, odour or texture of the substance.
   (d) Length of time of exposure to the poison or time since ingestion.
   (e) Any abnormal signs which have been observed, for example, fits, twitching, hallucinations or excited behaviour.

7. On arrival at hospital, careful assessment of any cardiovascular, respiratory or circulatory problems must be implemented. These may include cardiac arrhythmias or abnormal respiratory patterns.
8. Observation and assessment of any particular signs relevant to individual toxic substances should be noted. For example, carbon monoxide poisoning often results in a pinkish tinge in the lips and nail beds. Arsenic overdose often results in a garlicky smell to the breath. Assessment of consciousness level is essential. If possible identify the toxic substance. This will enable the appropriate antidote to be chosen. It will also enable the correct method of elimination to be implemented.

Elimination of poison

Depending on the type of poison or toxic substance and various contraindications, some of the following methods may be appropriate for elimination of the substance.

The most common are emesis and gastric lavage. Adsorbents (such as activated charcoal) and cathartics may be used for specific overdoses. Alkalization of the urine with intravenous sodium bicarbonate enhances the renal excretion of weak acids such as barbiturates and salicylates. Acidification of the urine enhances the renal excretion of weak bases such as amphetamines. Both of these processes may actually confound existing acidotic or alkalotic situations. Haemodialysis or peritoneal dialysis may augment the measures discussed, but the degree of usefulness depends on the special characteristics of the toxic substance.

Decontamination by removal of clothing and washing of the skin may be helpful in some gaseous or liquid exposures. Forced diuresis usually is helpful only in drugs which are totally excreted by the kidney. The usual diuretic is intravenous mannitol, 1 to 2 litres/hour. The problems associated with the use of mannitol are fluid overload and the induction of congestive cardiac failure and renal failure.

The management of such a patient involves supportive care.

SPECIFIC ANTIDOTES

Contrary to popular belief there are few poisons for which there are specific antidotes. However, when the few that do exist are used, they may be life saving. Table 6 lists the antidotes likely to be encountered and the substances for which they are antidotal.

INDIVIDUAL AGENTS

Acetylcysteine (*N*-acetylcysteine, *Parvolex* injection) used as antidote to paracetamol poisoning.

In part, the liver toxicity of paracetamol is due to a build-up of a toxic metabolite in excess of the ability of sulphydryl (-SH) containing enzymes to detoxify it. Acetylcysteine protects the liver from this metabolite and

Table 6
Antidotes for Specific Poisons

Antidote	Poison	Notes
Acetylcysteine	Paracetamol	IV, commence as soon as possible, not later than 10-12 hours after ingestion
Atropine	Organophosphate and carbamate insecticides	Large doses needed
Calcium (calcium gluconate, milk)	Fluoride	
Calcium disodium edetate (EDTA)	Lead	
Desferrioxamine	Iron poisoning	
Dicobalt EDTA	Cyanide	
Dimercaprol (BAL)	Heavy metals: mercury, arsenic	
Methionine	Paracetamol	Oral, commence as soon as possible, not later than 10-12 hours after ingestion
Naloxone	Narcotics, dextropropoxyphene	
Penicillamine	Copper, lead	
Physostigmine	Tricyclic antidepressants	Short duration of action
Pralidoxime (PAM)	Organophosphate pesticides	Do *not* use with carbamates, use early

is administered either orally or intravenously. Like all available paracetamol antidotes, it needs to be given as early as possible after the ingestion, certainly before 10 to 12 hours have elapsed. Orally, the usual dose is 140 mg/kg once, followed in four hours by 70 mg/kg every four hours for a total of 68 hours. For intravenous use, the dose is 150 mg/kg over 15 minutes followed by 50 mg/kg infused over four hours followed by 100 mg/kg over 16 hours, that is, a total of 300 mg/kg in 20 hours.

Atropine blocks the action of acetylcholine accumulated at nerve junctions and end plates in the parasympathetic nervous system (mainly affecting "muscarinic" receptors in smooth muscle, heart and exocrine glands).

It dries up excessive respiratory and other secretions, dilates pupils, causes flushing and reduces bradycardia. Unfortunately it has little effect on muscular weakness, including the respiratory muscles.

In cholinesterase-inhibitor poisoning, doses of atropine far in excess of usual are needed. For an adult, this may approximate 4mg to 8mg IV every 10 to 15 minutes.

Calcium (for example, as calcium gluconate, or milk in some mild cases) is used as an antidote to fluoride poisoning.

Most commonly, fluoride ingestion involves swallowing of low-dose tablets of sodium fluoride containing approximately 2mg. The potential lethal dose is much higher. While sodium fluoride is soluble (in water), calcium fluoride is insoluble and hence not absorbed from the stomach.

The route of administration needs to be adjusted to the particular situation.

Calcium disodium edetate (calcium EDTA or calcium disodium versonate) could theoretically be used to bind lead, iron, zinc, manganese, beryllium and copper, but the main practical use is with lead poisoning.

The drug is given by intravenous infusion or intramuscular injection, usually in courses lasting five days with a rest period between courses.

Renal toxicity and a febrile systemic reaction have been reported.

Desferrioxamine (*Desferal*) is used as an antidote for iron poisoning. Iron in the ferric (Fe^{3+}) state is absorbed onto desferrioxamine by the process of chelation to form a water-soluble complex which can be excreted in the urine (colouring urine red).

In treating iron poisoning, desferrioxamine is normally given by IV infusion at a rate not exceeding 15 mg/kg/hour. Oral administration to complex iron remaining in the stomach is controversial, some authorities feeling that this binds the iron in a non-toxic form, with others claiming that the effect is not beneficial. The bound complex is, to some extent, absorbed.

Allergic-type reactions have been recorded. Hypotension is probably the most significant effect.

Dicobalt EDTA (*Kelocyanor* or cobalt tetraracemate) is used as a cyanide antidote and has replaced sodium nitrate/sodium thiosulphate for this purpose.

Cyanide is toxic through inhibiting cellular respiration by blocking the enzyme cytochrome oxidase. Dicobalt EDTA is a chelating agent which forms a chemical complex with cyanide.

Dicobalt EDTA is given by IV injection. In adults, 300 mg (1 × 20 mL ampoule) is administered over one minute. This is followed by 50 mL of 50% dextrose injection. This may be repeated once if necessary. Vomiting is often caused, and anaphylactic reactions have been occasionally reported.

Dimercaprol (BAL; British Anti-Lewisite) is used as antidote for arsenic, mercury or gold.

Heavy metals such as these are toxic by combining with sulphydryl (-SH) containing enzymes within the cells. Dimercaprol contains two sulphydryls which bind preferentially to the metal, giving a water-soluble, reasonably stable compound that can be excreted in the urine.

Being supplied as an injection dissolved in an oil base, it must be given by intramuscular injection as the injection is painful. Dosage in severe poisoning commences at 3 to 5 mg/kg every four hours for two days, then reduces over a week.

Adverse reactions are common, depending on dosage, and can include anorexia, restlessness, elevated blood pressure, fever, tachycardia, convulsions and coma.

Methionine is used as an antidote to paracetamol poisoning.

See acetylcysteine for mode of action. Like the other paracetamol antidotes, methionine is a source of sulphydryl groups and either acts by these binding to paracetamol or by increasing liver production of glutathione (the enzyme which detoxifies paracetamol metabolites).

Normally methionine is given orally in a dose of 2.5 g every 4 hours for four doses only. Again, this should be commenced earlier than 10 to 12 hours after the ingestion to be effective.

Adverse reactions are rare. Methionine seems less prone to exacerbating liver damage than cysteamine if given late.

Naloxone *(Narcan)* is used as an antagonist to morphine and related drugs, pentazocine and dextropropoxyphene. (Nalorphine and levallorphan are also used as opiate antagonists but are ineffective against pentazocine).

Naloxone reverses the effects of these drugs, particularly respiratory depression, by competing with the narcotic for opioid receptor sites.

The drug may be given intravenously, intramuscularly or subcutaneously. It is not given orally because it is metabolised rapidly on first pass through the liver.

Most narcotic antagonists are capable of producing some opiate-like effects themselves. Naloxone does not do this. Care must be exercised in use with addicted patients, who may exhibit withdrawal symptoms.

Penicillamine *(Distamine, Pendramine)* is used to treat chronic lead poisoning (plumbism), acute lead overdose, and copper or mercury poisoning.

Penicillamine acts as a chelating agent, forming a soluble complex with these heavy metals.

Penicillamine is given orally. The following adverse effects have been described: skin rash, fever, leukopenia, thrombocytopenia, agranulocytosis and nephrotic syndrome.

Physostigmine is used in poisonings by tricyclic antidepressants (imipramine, amitriptyline and so on), atropine, hyoscine and propantheline.

Physostigmine acts as a parasympathomimetic by inhibiting the enzyme cholinesterase, that is, it acts similarly to an organophosphate pesticide. It crosses the blood-brain barrier and will reverse the coma of patients with these overdoses. They will quickly lapse back into unconsciousness. It is not recommended that repeated doses should be given to keep them conscious, but it is indicated for convulsions, severe hallucinations, hypertension and supraventricular arrhythmias.

Typical cholinesterase inhibitor symptoms may be expected if too much is given: tremor, increased peristalsis, pinpoint pupils, hypertension, vomiting, bronchial constriction, fainting, hypotension and bradycardia.

Pralidoxime (PAM) is used to treat organophosphate pesticide overdose. It is not normally used with carbamates, which are also cholinesterase inhibitors.

PAM combines with organophosphate, removing it from the receptor site of the cholinesterase enzyme, hence regenerating the enzyme. It thus acts differently from atropine, and the two drugs may be used in conjunction to treat organophosphate poisoning.

PAM is given by IV injection or infusion. The rate should not exceed 500 mg/minute. Normal adult dose is 1g repeated three times at eight to 12-hour intervals. There is little benefit in administering it more than 36 hours after a poisoning.

Doses significantly in excess of usual recommendations may result in PAM inhibiting cholinesterase itself. If given at a rate greater than 500 mg/minute, it can cause weakness, blurred vision, diplopia, headache, nausea and tachycardia.

SELF-EVALUATION TEST

1. List nine common groups of substances causing poisoning.
2. (a) List three initial steps in management of a poisoned patient.
   (b) Note exceptions to generalisations in 2(a).
3. List two poisons likely to cause serious, delayed-poisoning effects.
4. Which of the following should a Poisons Information Centre be contacted for?
   (a) Advice on ingredients of a substance swallowed by a patient.
   (b) Advice on how to manage a particular poisoning.
   (c) Advice about a plant poisoning.
5. List four poisons which have antidotes. Name the antidotes.
6. Which of the following are appropriate measures to induce vomiting in a two-year-old child?
   (a) syrup ipecacuanha
   (b) copper sulphate
   (c) salt
   (d) mustard
   (e) mechanical stimulation
7. The LD 50 of a drug "X" is said to be 700 mg/kg (oral, rats). The potential fatal dose in humans will be:
   (a) 700 mg/kg
   (b) 1 g/kg
   (c) 100 mg/kg
   (d) cannot tell from data.
8. If a patient presents having ingested mg/kg of the drug "X" referred to in the previous question, they should be:
   (a) Observed closely; are likely to have significant toxic effects.
   (b) Sent home at once; 700 mg/kg in rats doesn't mean it will harm humans.

Antidote	Poison	Nursing Implications
BAL (dimercaprol)	Mercury Arsenic Gold	***Assess:*** blood pressure, pulse rate, fits, consciousness. ***Administer:*** 2.5-3 mg/kg IM every four hours for two days then reduce over one week. ***Evaluate:*** therapeutic effect, adverse effects such as anorexia, restless behaviour, hypertension and tachycardia, fever, epilepsy and coma.
Naloxone	Narcotics Dextropropoxyphene	***Assess:*** narcotic addiction. ***Administer:*** IV, IM or SC. ***Evaluate:*** return of normal respiration; onset of withdrawal symptoms in addicted patients.
Penicillamine	Copper Lead Mercury	***Assess:*** blood pressure, pulse rate, blood screening, renal function, previous allergies. ***Administer:*** orally. ***Evaluate:*** therapeutic effect; adverse effects.
Physostigmine	Tricyclic antidepressants	***Assess:*** coma, epilepsy, hallucinations, blood pressure and cardiac status. ***Administer:*** until an anticholinesterase effect is reached. ***Evaluate:*** motor activity, GIT, irritability, pupil changes, hypertension, bradycardia, vomiting, bronchospasm, hypotension.
Pralidoxime (PAM)	Organophosphate pesticides	***Assess:*** current drug regime, concurrent use of atropine, blood pressure, consciousness. ***Administer:*** within 36 hours of ingestion; IV injection or infusion at a rate not greater than 500 mg/min; adult, 1 g every 8 h, to maximum of 3 g/24 h. ***Evaluate:*** therapeutic effect, adverse effects such as weakness, diplopia, headache, nausea and tachycardia.

Antidote	Poison	Nursing implications
Acetylcysteine	Paracetamol	***Assess:*** time since ingestion; pulmonary and liver fuction; renal function and blood sugar level. ***Administer:*** by intravenous infusion initially 150 mg/kg in 200 mL glucose IV infusion 5% over 15 minutes, followed by 50 mg/kg in 500 mL glucose IV infusion 5% over 4 hours and 100 mg/kg in 1000 mL glucose IV infusion 5% over 16 hours. ***Evaluate:*** therapeutic effect and liver function.
Methionine	Paracetamol	***Assess:*** as above; GIT for vomiting. ***Administer:*** within 10 to 12 hours of ingestion; orally 2.5 every four hours. ***Evaluate:*** therapeutic effect and liver function.
Atropine	Organophosphate Carbamate insecticides (Cholinesterase inhibitors)	***Assess:*** blood pressure, pulse rate, headache, confusion. GIT disturbances, profuse sweating, muscle twitching, convulsions. ***Administer:*** 4 to 8 mg IV 10 to 15 minutes to atropinisation, resulting in a rapid pulse (100 beats/min), dry skin, dilated pupils. ***Evaluate:*** therapeutic effect, which may only be partial.
Calcium EDTA	Fluoride Lead	***Assess:*** renal function and body temperature. ***Administer:*** IV or IM in courses consisting of five days as 50 to 75 mg/kg for adult; 1500 mg/m^2 of body surface for child; as IV solution, 2 g EDTA in 250 mL of normal saline slowly or every four hours in divided doses. ***Evaluate:*** for renal toxicity and hyperthermia.
Desferrioxamine	Iron poisoning	***Assess:*** blood pressure and pulse rate; pulmonary, GIT, renal and cerebral function; previous allergies. ***Administer:*** IV injection at a rate not exceeding 15 mg/kg/h, with a total dose of 80 mg/kg in 24 hours. ***Evaluate:*** therapeutic effect, allergic reaction, hypotension.
Dicobalt EDTA	Cyanide	***Assess:*** blood pressure, metabolic acidosis, cardiopulmonary function, previous allergies. ***Administer:*** 300 mg IV over 1 min; additional 300mg with oxygen and ventilation support. ***Evaluate:*** therapeutic effect, vomiting and anaphylactic reaction.

ROLE OF THE POISONS INFORMATION CENTRES

The United Kingdom and the Republic of Ireland are served by officially established Poisons Information Centres. These centres have been set up to provide up-to-date information on poisoning and provide a 24 hour service for medical practitioners.

Information can be provided on the extent of a particular problem, ingredients of ingested substances (under certain circumstances), and first aid or more detailed management of poisoning.

Table 8 lists the addresses and telephone numbers. In any situation where any doubt exists as to the management of a poisoning, the appropriate centre should be contacted for advice.

Table 8
Poisons Information Centres

City and Address	Telephone No.
London Poisons Information Service New Cross Hospital Avonley Road London SE14 5ER	01-635 9191
Edinburgh Poisons Information Service The Royal Infirmary Lauriston Place Edinburgh E3	031-229 2477
Belfast Poisons Information Service Royal Victoria Hospital Grosvenor Road Belfast B12 6BB	0232 240503
Dublin Poisons Information Service Jervis Street Hospital Dublin I	0001-745588
Cardiff Poisons Information Service Ambulance Headquarters Old Ty-Bronna Fairwater Road Fairwater, Cardiff CF5 3XP	0222 569200

SECTION 2

5
THE AUTONOMIC NERVOUS SYSTEM

William A. Thomson

OBJECTIVES

At the end of this chapter the reader should be able to:

1. describe the structure of the nervous system and the role of transmitter substances and receptors;
2. identify the actions of the sympathetic and parasympathetic nerve stimulation on major organs of the body;
3. identify and list drugs that interfere with nervous system function.

PREREQUISITE KNOWLEDGE

Anatomy of the nervous system.

STRUCTURE AND FUNCTION OF THE AUTONOMIC NERVOUS SYSTEM (ANS)

The following section on the autonomic nervous system is intended as a brief review of some aspects of the physiology of the ANS. For further information, physiology texts will give a more comprehensive description.

The ANS has been variously described as the vegetative, visceral or involuntary nervous system. Its major function is to regulate the internal environment of the body, for example, heart rate. Despite the name "involuntary nervous system", there is obvious interaction with and some modification of responses by the central nervous system. One such example is the effect of fear on heart rate.

STRUCTURE

The autonomic nervous system consists, peripherally, of two sets of fibres: input or afferent fibres and output or efferent fibres. Integration of the afferent and efferent fibres occurs in the central nervous system (CNS).

Afferent Fibres

Information is brought into the ANS via sensory afferent fibres, which obtain information from innervated organs and structures for processing in the CNS.

Central Autonomic Connections

Conversion of input information into output action occurs via efferent fibres at a number of levels, from the simple reflex arc in the spinal cord to the complex, which involves integration at various levels within the CNS and the subsequent outflow via efferent or motor fibres.

Peripheral (or efferent) ANS

The major divisions of the nervous systems are the sympathetic and parasympathetic nervous systems.

Sympathetic Nervous System

The preganglionic sympathetic nerve fibres leave the spinal cord from the thoracic and lumbar sections, synapse in ganglia adjacent to the spinal cord with postganglionic fibres, which then continue on to the innervated muscle or organ.

Parasympathetic Nervous System

The preganglionic parasympathetic nerve fibres leave the spinal cord from the midbrain, medulla and sacral portions of the central nervous system and synapse in ganglia situated either in or close to the innervated organ or muscle. Consequently the postganglionic parasympathetic nerve fibre is much shorter than the sympathetic postganglionic fibre.

DIFFERENCES BETWEEN SYMPATHETIC AND PARASYMPATHETIC NERVES

One of the major differences between the groups is the way in which sympathetic fibres ramify to a greater extent than parasympathetic fibres. This is exemplified by the fact that the ratio of sympathetic preganglionic fibres to postganglionic fibres may be as high as 1 : 20 whereas in the parasympathetic situation it is not unusual for the ratio to be 1: 1. This is aided in that the terminal ganglia are either in or very near to the organs being innervated, in contrast to the sympathetic system.

The ramification within the sympathetic nervous system will produce a more generalised discharge in contrast to the more discrete and localised effect of parasympathetic discharge.

TRANSMITTERS

There is evidence to show that, in order to transfer the information emanating from the CNS as an impulse to the effector organ, the synapse at the autonomic ganglion and the gap at the neuroeffector junction must be crossed with the aid of a chemical substance known as a transmitter. The two main transmitters involved are acetylcholine and noradrenaline.

These transmitters function in the following ways: ***Acetylcholine*** activates all autonomic ganglia, all parasympathetic neuroeffector junctions and some sympathetic neuroeffector junctions. On the other hand, ***noradrenaline*** activates most sympathetic neuroeffector junctions (see Figure 1).

The transmitter, after release from the nerve cell ending, is thought to work on a specific portion of the postjunctional cell called a receptor. After interaction with the receptor, the transmitter is either destroyed by an enzyme (cholinesterase in the case of acetylcholine or monoamine oxidase in the case of noradrenaline) or taken back up into the nerve ending. If this did not occur, then there would be no control to prevent the continual stimulation of the receptors.

FIGURE 1. LOCATION OF TRANSMITTERS.

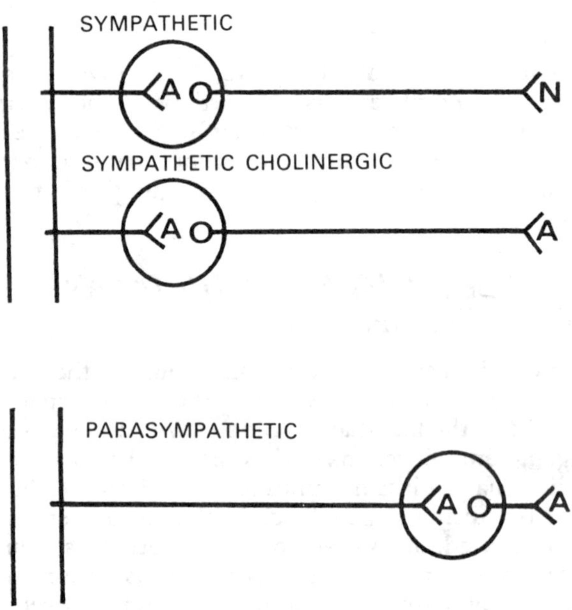

A—ACETYLCHOLINE
N—NORADRENALINE

RECEPTORS

Receptors are generally named after the transmitter which activates the receptor. Hence, *cholinergic receptors* are activated by acetylcholine and *noradrenergic receptors* by noradrenaline. Activation of the receptor by the transmitter leads to either initiation of depolarisation in the autonomic ganglion cells, resulting in the continuation of the impulse along the postganglion nerve fibre, or in the effector organ it may cause contraction or relaxation of smooth muscle. Not a great deal is known about the exact structure of receptors. However, it is thought that the structure allows for the specific combination with the transmitter.

An agent used to act on the receptor in a similar fashion to the transmitter is termed an *agonist;* the agent used to prevent the action of the transmitter at the receptor is an *antagonist.*

Cholinergic Receptors

Receptors which respond to acetylcholine or to drugs (cholinergics or cholinomimetics) which mimic the effect of acetylcholine are divided into nicotinic and muscarinic receptors. The muscarinic receptors will be the main parasympathetic nervous system receptors considered in this chapter. Drugs which stimulate muscarinic receptors and which mimic the effect of postganglionic parasympathetic nerve stimulation are called *parasympathomimetics.* Drugs which antagonise the effect of postganglionic parasympathetic nerve stimulation are called *parasympatholytics.*

* anticholinergics

Noradrenergic Receptors

Noradrenaline and drugs which mimic the effect of postganglionic sympathetic nerve stimulation are called *sympathomimetics.* The receptors on which these drugs produce their effect are called alpha receptors and beta receptors. The classification into alpha and beta receptors is basically determined on the varying agonist activities of sympathomimetic agents. Beta receptors are further divided into beta-1 and beta-2 receptors. Beta-2 receptors are found mainly in the lungs and beta-1 receptors in the heart. This difference in the location of beta receptors provides an opportunity to selectively stimulate certain groups of receptors without stimulating all beta receptors throughout the body.

ACTIONS OF SYMPATHETIC AND PARASYMPATHETIC NERVE STIMULATION

To gain an understanding of the various actions of drugs such as sympathomimetics, parasympathomimetics and other drugs which interplay with the ANS, it is necessary to have a basic understanding of some of the effects produced directly by the ANS. In many instances organs are innervated by both parasympathetic and sympathetic nerves, each producing an opposing effect, thereby offering a dual control system. A brief knowledge of their interplay is essential for understanding of the role of drug intervention in the ANS.

A summary of effects is shown in Table 9.

Table 9
Actions of Sympathetic and Parasympathetic Nerve Stimulation

Organ Innervated	Adrenergic receptor	Adrenergic responses	Cholinergic responses
Heart	Beta	Sinus tachycardia; force of contraction of atria and ventricles is increased	Sinus bradycardia; decreased AV conduction; decreased atrial contractility
Blood vessels			
Skin	Alpha	Vasoconstriction	Dilation
Skeletal muscle	Alpha	Vasoconstriction	Dilation
	Beta	Vasodilation	
Lungs	Beta	Smooth muscle relaxation, vasoconstriction	Smooth muscle contraction
Intestine			
Motility and tone	Alpha and Beta	Decreased	Increased
Sphincters	Alpha	Contraction	Relaxation
Secretion			Stimulation
Bladder			
Detrusor	Beta	Relaxation	Contraction
Trigone and sphincter	Alpha	Contraction	Relaxation
Salivary glands	Alpha	Sparse, thick secretion	Profuse, watery secretion
Eye			
Radial muscle (iris)	Alpha	Contraction (mydriasis)	Contraction (miosis)
Sphincter muscle (iris)		-	Contraction (near vision)
Ciliary muscle	Beta	Relaxation (far vision)	
Uterus	Alpha and Beta	Variable	Variable

DRUG INTERFERENCE WITH THE AUTONOMIC NERVOUS SYSTEM

Both the sympathetic and parasympathetic nervous systems contain several mechanisms by which drugs interfere with normal ANS functions. Several of these are common to both systems and include: drugs which mimic the effect of either sympathetic or parasympathetic stimulation; drugs which interfere with the enzymatic destruction of transmitters; and drugs which block the receptor to the transmitter.

DRUG INTERFERENCE WITH THE PARASYMPATHETIC SYSTEM

PARASYMPATHOMIMETICS

These are drugs which mimic the effect of parasympathetic nerve stimulation. Examples of these drugs and their usual strength, form and indications are shown in Table 10.

Table 10
Parasympathomimetics

Generic Name	Trade Name	Strength and Dose Form	Indication
Pilocarpine	*Isoptocarpine*	0.5 to 4%, eye drops	Glaucoma
Carbachol		0.25 mg, injection; SC	Postoperative intestinal atony
		2mg, tablets	Postoperative urinary retention
Bethanechol	*Myotonine Chloride*	10 mg or 25 mg, tablets	Postoperative urinary retention
		5 mg, injection; SC	Postoperative intestinal atony

Adverse Drug Reactions

The adverse reactions of parasympathomimetics include abdominal discomfort, salivation, flushing of the skin and sweating. Large doses will produce more pronounced parasympathetic effects.

Precautions

Parasympathomimetics are contraindicated in hyperthyroidism, pregnancy, peptic ulcer, bronchial asthma, bradycardia or hypotension, vasomotor instability, coronary artery disease, epilepsy and Parkinsonism. Their use is contraindicated following gastrointestinal or bladder surgery or obstruction, and in spastic gastrointestinal disturbances, acute inflammatory lesions of the gastrointestinal tract or in peritonitis.

The injectable form of this drug is intended for subcutaneous administration only. It should *never* be given intramuscularly or intravenously as violent symptoms due to severe cholinergic over-stimulation will occur.

ANTICHOLINESTERASE DRUGS

These are drugs which interfere with the enzyme responsible for the destruction of acetylcholine, that is, cholinesterase. Examples of these drugs and their usual strength, form and indications are shown in Table 11.

Table 11
Anticholinesterases

Generic Name	Trade Name	Strength and Dose Form	Indication
Physostigmine		0.5 %, eye drops	Glaucoma
Neostigmine	*Prostigmin*	15 mg, tablets 0.5 mg/mL, injection	Myasthenia gravis; antidote to curariform drugs; stimulants to bowel and bladder
Pyridostigmine bromide	*Mestinon*	60 mg, tablets; 1 mg/mL,	Myasthenia gravis
Edrophonium chloride	*Tensilon*	10 mg, injection	Diagnostic agent for myasthenia gravis
Distigmine bromide	*Ubretid*	5 mg, tablets; 0.5 mg/mL, injection	Stimulant to bowel and bladder movements

Adverse Drug Reactions

Adverse reactions to anticholinesterase drugs are due to excessive stimulation of cholinergic receptors and include: nausea, vomiting, abdominal pain, diarrhoea, salivation, sweating, lacrimation, miosis, bradycardia, hypotension, dyspnoea, urinary urgency and muscular twitching. These side effects can be controlled with atropine.

Precautions

These drugs should be used with caution in conditions where the potentiation of cholinergic effects is undesirable, for example, vagotonia, bronchial asthma, cardiac disease, peptic ulcer, epilepsy and Parkinsonism.

PARASYMPATHOLYTICS (ANTICHOLINERGICS)

These are drugs which block the receptor. Examples of these drugs are shown with usual strength, form and indications in Table 12.

Adverse Reactions

Adverse reactions to parasympatholytics include drying of salivary secretions, decreased sweating as well as mydriasis, blurred vision, tachycardia, urinary hesitancy and retention.

Table 12
Parasympatholytics (Anticholinergics)

Generic Name	Trade Name	Strength and Dose Form	Indication
Atropine sulphate		0.4 mg, injection 0.6 mg, injection 1.2 mg, injection 0.5% or 1%, eye drops	Preoperative medication; antidote for parasympathomimetics Ophthalmic examination
Atropine methonitrate	*Eumydrin*	0.6%, solution	Pyloric stenosis, intestinal, biliary colic
Hyoscine (scopolamine) hydrobromide		400 micrograms, injection	Preoperative medication usually combined with papaveretum
Hyoscine butyl bromide	*Buscopan*	10 mg, tablet 20 mg, injection	Spasm of gastrointestinal tract. By injection, for renal, biliary and gastrointestinal tract spasm
Dicyclomine hydrochloride	*Merbentyl*	10 mg, tablet	Gastrointestinal tract spasm
Propantheline bromide	*Pro-banthine*	15 mg, tablet	Gastrointestinal tract spasm
Ipratropium bromide	*Atrovent*	18 micrograms/ puff, inhaler	Asthma

Precautions

Use with caution in patients having severe cardiac disease and in elderly patients because of the possibility of urinary retention. These drugs must be avoided in patients with glaucoma, obstructive disease of the gastrointestinal tract or intestinal atony.

DRUG INTERFERENCE WITH THE SYMPATHETIC SYSTEM

SYMPATHOMIMETICS

These are drugs which mimic the effect of sympathetic nerve stimulation. Sympathomimetics vary in their ability to stimulate alpha, beta-1 and beta-2 receptors. Accordingly it is possible to use such agents as adrenaline, which stimulates both alpha and beta receptors, or salbutamol which preferentially stimulates beta-2 receptors. The degree of specificity of some of the agents enhances their therapeutic usefulness. Examples are shown in Table 13.

Although this is only a small group of the sympathomimetic drugs available, Table 13 does show the wide range of specificities encountered, thus providing clinicians with a variety of therapeutic solutions. For example, the drugs adrenaline, isoprenaline and salbutamol may all be used in the treatment of asthma. Adrenaline stimulates alpha, beta-1 and beta-2 sympathetic receptors and is therefore regarded as having the least specific action in the treatment of asthma. Isoprenaline is regarded as being more specific for the treatment of asthma as it stimulates only beta-1 and beta-2 sympathetic receptors. Salbutamol has the most specific effect of all three drugs because it stimulates only beta-2 sympathetic receptors.

Table 13
Sympathomimetics

Generic Name	**Trade Name**	**Receptor Stimulated**	**Strength and Dose Form**	**Indications**
Adrenaline tartrate		Alpha and Beta	1:1000, 1mL injection	Cardiac stimulant, asthma
Noradrenaline	*Levophed*	Alpha and Beta	2 mg/mL 0.2 mg/mL	Pressor agent
Methoxamine hydrochloride	*Vasoxine*	Alpha	20 mg/mL	Hypotension in anaesthesia
Isoprenaline hydrochloride	*Isuprel*	Beta 1 and Beta 2	0.2 mg/mL, injection	Cardiac stimulant, asthma
Dobutamine	*Dobutrex*	Beta 1	250 mg, injection	Cardiac failure
Salbutamol	*Ventolin*	Beta 2	100 microgram/puff inhaler; 0.5% respiratory solution; 500 microgram, injection	Asthma
Terbutaline	*Bricanyl*	Beta 2	250 microgram/puff inhaler; 1% respirator solution; 500 microgram, injection	Asthma

MONOAMINE OXIDASE INHIBITORS

These are drugs which interfere with the enzyme monoamine oxidase, which is partially responsible for the destruction of noradrenaline. See Table 14.

Table 14
Monoamine Oxidase Inhibitors

Generic Name	**Trade Name**	**Strength and Dose Form**	**Indication**
Phenelzine sulphate	*Nardil*	15 mg, tablet	Depression
Tranylcypromine sulphate	*Parnate*	10 mg, tablet	Depression

Adverse Drug Reactions

Adverse reactions seen include dizziness, palpitations, weakness, dry mouth and drowsiness.

Precautions

As these agents inhibit the action of one of the enzymes responsible for the destruction of noradrenaline, they can produce potentially serious interactions, on occasions life-threatening, with agents which either cause the release of more noradrenaline or the stimulation of adrenergic receptors directly. Therefore, concomitant administration of monoamine oxidase inhibitors with tricyclic antidepressants, anticold preparations (alpha-receptor stimulants) or foods containing tyramine should be avoided because of the risk of hypertensive crisis. If a hypertensive crisis occurs, phentolamine *(Rogitine)* in a dose of 5 mg to 10 mg should be used intravenously and may be repeated if necessary.

ALPHA-BLOCKING AND BETA-BLOCKING DRUGS

These drugs interfere with sympathetic transmission. Examples of *alpha-blocking drugs* are shown in Table 15.

Table 15
Alpha-blocking Drugs

Generic Name	Trade Name	Strength and Dose Form	Indication
Tolazoline hydrochloride	*Priscol*	25 mg, tablet	Peripheral vascular disease
Phenoxybenzamine hydrochloride	*Dibenyline*	10 mg, tablet	Peripheral vascular disease, hypertension
Phentolamine mesylate	*Rogitine*	10 mg, injection	Phaeochromocytoma, peripheral vascular disease

Adverse Drug Reactions

Adverse reactions to alpha-blocking drugs are mainly associated with vasodilation and include flushing, "goose-flesh", and a feeling of chilliness or warmth. Tachycardia may be experienced.

Precautions

Overdosage, particularly of the intravenous forms, may lead to hypotension which should be treated with noradrenaline infusion. Adrenaline should not be used.

Beta blocking drugs may be divided into drugs which block both beta-1 and beta-2 receptors and drugs which preferentially block beta-1 receptors, that is, cardioselective beta blockers. Examples of both types are shown in Table 16.

Table 16
Beta-blocking drugs

Generic Name	Trade Name	Strength and Dose Form	Indications
Non-selective beta-blocking drugs			
Propranolol	*Inderal*	1 mg, injection; 10 mg, 40 mg, 80 mg, 160 mg, tablets	Angina pectoris, hypertension cardiac arrhythmias
Pindolol	*Visken*	5 mg, 15 mg, tablets	Angina pectoris, hypertension, cardiac arrhythmias
Oxprenolol	*Trasicor*	2 mg, injection; 20 mg, 40 mg, 80 mg, tablets; 160 mg slow release tablet	Angina pectoris, hypertension, cardiac arrhythmias
Timolol	*Blocadren*	10 mg, tablet	Angina pectoris, hypertension, cardiac arrhythmias
Selective beta-blocking drugs			
Atenolol	*Tenormin*	50 mg, 100 mg, tablets	Angina pectoris, hypertension
Metoprolol	*Betaloc, Lopressor*	50 mg, 100 mg, tablets	Angina pectoris, hypertension

Adverse Reactions and Precautions

See Chapter 7, "Drugs Used in the Treatment of Cardiovascular Disease".

ADRENERGIC NEURONE-BLOCKING DRUGS

These are drugs which block the release of noradrenaline. Examples are shown in Table 17.

Table 17
Adrenergic Neurone-Blocking Drugs

Generic Name	Trade Name	Strength and Dose Form	Indication
Guanethidine monosulphate	*Ismelin*	10 mg, 25 mg, tablet	Hypertension
Bethanidine sulphate	*Esbatal*	10 mg, 50 mg, tablet	Hypertension
Debrisoquine sulphate	*Declinax*	10 mg, 20 mg, tablet	Hypertension

Adverse Drug Reactions

Adverse reactions to adrenergic neurone-blocking agents include postural hypotension, malaise, headache, sweating and failure of ejaculation. Fluid retention, depression, nocturia and frequency of micturition may occur also.

Precautions

Patients should be cautioned about sudden changes in posture, excessive exercise, or extremes of temperature which may precipitate hypotensive symptoms.

SELF-EVALUATION TEST

1. Describe briefly:
   (a) the structure of the autonomic nervous system;
   (b) the action of neural transmitters;
   (c) the role of cholinergic receptors;
   (d) the role of adrenergic receptors.
2. Define the following terms:
   (a) agonist;
   (b) antagonist;
   (c) parasympathomimetic;
   (d) anticholinergic.
3. What is the response to sympathetic stimulation of the following organs?
   (a) heart
   (b) lungs
   (c) uterus
4. What is the response to parasympathetic stimulation of the following organs?
   (a) intestine
   (b) blood vessels
   (c) heart
5. Give two examples of drugs that have the following actions:
   (a) parasympathomimetics;
   (b) anticholinesterases;
   (c) sympathomimetics;
   (d) beta-adrenergic blocking drugs;
   (e) alpha-adrenergic blocking drugs.

6

DRUGS USED IN THE TREATMENT OF RESPIRATORY DISEASES

Ross W. Holland and Vicky J. Grattan

OBJECTIVES

At the end of this chapter the reader should be able to:

1. classify drugs used in respiratory diseases according to their pharmacological action;
2. list adverse drug reactions of the substances used in treating respiratory conditions;
3. describe the correct method of administration of various inhalation therapies;
4. identify drugs with potential for over-use or abuse;
5. list nursing implications of the drugs used in respiratory diseases.

PREREQUISITE KNOWLEDGE

1. Anatomy of the respiratory system.
2. Physiology of the respiratory system, specifically the role of the autonomic nervous system in control of the lungs.
3. A working knowledge of the major respiratory diseases.
4. The role of the mast cell in allergy.

In this chapter the pharmacological treatment of two main areas of concern in respiratory diseases will be discussed in detail. These are the prevention and treatment of bronchoconstriction and the treatment of cough. The use of drugs in the treatment of respiratory infections will only briefly be covered, as a separate chapter considers in detail the use of anti-infective agents. Likewise, oncological drugs are considered elsewhere.

PREVENTION AND TREATMENT OF BRONCHOCONSTRICTION

Bronchoconstriction is the condition in which the airways, specifically the bronchioles, narrow. Such constriction may be muscular in origin or due to an inflammatory reaction. It may be caused by touch (for example, intubation or bronchoscopy), chemicals such as allergens or smoke, or cold, which compromises gas exchange and leads to breathing difficulties as seen in asthma and chronic obstructive airways diseases. Treatment is aimed at dilatation of the airways either by relaxation of the bronchiole musculature or reduction of the inflammatory processes.

BRONCHODILATING DRUGS

Three groups of drugs with a direct bronchodilating action are used clinically: beta-adrenergic agonists, anticholinergic drugs and xanthine derivatives.

Beta-Adrenergic Agonists

The muscle fibres surrounding the bronchioles are under the control of the sympathetic nervous system. The beta-2 receptor sites respond to adrenergic stimulation by relaxing the muscles, thereby leading to increased ventilation. The earliest substances used in this way, ***adrenaline***, ***isoprenaline*** (*Isuprel*) and ***ephedrine***, were fairly non-selective and had effects in many other areas of the body. Their cardiovascular actions, due to concurrent alpha and beta-1 receptor stimulation, led to tachycardia and palpitations. Combined with difficulty in breathing, these adverse reactions were not always reassuring to the patient.

Recent drugs are more specific to the beta-2 receptors in lung tissue and avoid the cardiac effects mentioned above except in very high doses or in hypertensive patients. Table 18 lists the most common of these drugs.

Table 18
Some of the Newer Adrenergic Agents Used as Bronchodilators

Generic Name	Trade Name
Orciprenaline	*Alupent*
Salbutamol	*Ventolin*
Terbutaline	*Bricanyl*
Fenoterol	*Berotec*

These drugs are available in a variety of forms including tablets, syrups and often injections for the acute attack, but the advent of metered aerosols, in which form they are all available, has led to marked advances in therapy. Aerosols are capable of delivering a small measured dose directly to the tissue involved, providing mucous plugs do not block access. This has two advantages: firstly, the dose is delivered directly to the affected area and secondly, the smaller dose required by this route reduces adverse reactions that may be seen when a larger dose is administered by another route. In addition, onset of action is more immediate, an important consideration for the patient suffering breathing difficulties.

The effect of all these newer substances, except fenoterol *(Berotec),* lasts about 6 to 8 hours, necessitating four doses a day. Fenoterol has a longer duration of action and requires only two or three doses per day. Increased dose or frequency rarely produces greater efficacy. Patients should therefore be discouraged from this course of action as no benefit is likely. Similarly, the use of different drugs within this group does not increase efficacy but may lead to adverse cardiac effects such as tachycardia and palpitations due to an additive action.

Another reason for therapeutic failure of aerosol treatment can be faulty administration technique, particularly with the very young and the elderly. Nursing staff should observe self-medication procedures and educate the patient if necessary. (See "Nursing Implications".)

Several of this class of drugs are also available for use in intermittent-positive-pressure-respiration (IPPR) machines. The nurse must carefully observe the dose and preparation procedures for each drug and correctly adjust the apparatus.

Anticholinergic Drugs

The role of the parasympathetic vagal pathways is to maintain a small amount of bronchial smooth-muscle tone within the airways. Bronchoconstriction may be superimposed by a reflex action in response to stimulation of the irritant receptors in the mucosal lining. This pathway is mediated by the chemical transmitter acetylcholine.

One way of interfering with this reflex is to use anticholinergic, atropine-like drugs such as ***ipratropium*** *(Atrovent).* Ipratropium is a clinically acceptable anticholinergic bronchodilator that acts by modifying the parasympathetic (vagal) effect of irritants on the bronchial smooth muscle. It is available in a metered aerosol form.

Anticholinergic side effects are unlikely to occur with this substance at therapeutic doses although in some cases there may be local dryness of the mouth or, if the substance enters the eyes due to inappropriate handling, a mild and reversible disturbance of accommodation may occur.

Xanthine Derivatives

Theophylline and ***aminophylline*** (a complex of theophylline and ethylenediamine) belong to the chemical class known as *xanthines.* These substances have a wide range of pharmacological activity as central-nervous and cardiac stimulants and in the relaxation of smooth muscle. This latter effect is put to use in the treatment of bronchospasm. They may therefore be used in the treatment of pulmonary emphysema, congestive heart failure, bronchial or cardiac asthma, status asthmaticus, Cheynes-Stokes respiration and bronchitis.

Theophylline is available in both tablet and liquid dose forms. Aminophylline, in addition, is available as suppositories and intramuscular and intravenous injections. (The intramuscular injection is very painful and therefore rarely used). A number of variations, such as choline theophyllinate, have been used from time to time.

The oral dose of aminophylline for an adult is 300 mg to 1200 mg per day in divided doses, and for theophylline, it is up to 900 mg per day, also in divided doses. Serum theophylline levels should be maintained within the therapeutic range of 10 to 20 mcg/mL. The use of controlled-release oral dose forms such as *Nuelin SR* and *Theo-Dur* provide a more constant rate of absorption with consequent smoother plasma levels than short-acting formulations. These dose forms are taken at 12-hour intervals and must be swallowed whole so as not to destroy the time-release delivery system.

The intravenous dose of aminophylline for an adult is 250 mg to 750 mg. It should be noted that aminophylline infusions are fairly unstable as a result of high pH, and the list of incompatibilities is long. Unless a pharmacist is consulted, no additives should be made to aminophylline infusions.

Adverse Drug Reactions

Nausea and vomiting are common adverse effects of the oral use of xanthines, and for this reason, administration with food is advisable. Alternatively, the rectal route may be used, although too frequent use of this route may lead to proctitis. Adverse effects particularly associated with rapid IV injection of aminophylline are headache, flushing, palpitation, dizziness, arrhythmias, tachycardia, hypotension and precordial pain. (See "Nursing Implications" for more detail.)

Combined Therapy

Because the three types of bronchodilators all have different mechanisms of action, they may be used in combination to advantage. Beta-2 adrenoreceptor agonists, whether given orally, IV or by inhalation, have an additive effect when given with the xanthine derivatives. Also, it is possible to achieve the same therapeutic effect with half doses of drugs from two different groups as with a full dose of one drug. This may sometimes, but not always, reduce side effects.

The anticholinergic ipratropium, when used in combination with a beta-agonist, produces a greater and more prolonged bronchodilatation than when a beta-agonist is used alone. The combination would appear to be synergistic, more than doubling the change in FEV_1 (forced expiratory volume in one second) produced by either.

CORTICOSTEROID THERAPY

An important use of corticosteroids is in the reduction of inflammation. This has been put to good effect in the treatment of various chest conditions. Bronchoconstriction may be caused, or at least complicated, by inflammatory processes. Reduction of these processes can lead to secondary bronchodilation and some reduction of associated pulmonary oedema.

In the acute attack, an IV dose of ***hydrocortisone sodium succinate,*** a soluble form of hydrocortisone, may be used. Alternatively, a course of ***prednisone***, ***prednisolone***, or ***betamethasone*** starting at a high dose (for example, 60 mg per day of prednisone) and reducing over a period of time, may be instituted. (Refer to Chapter 11, page 186 for the adverse effects of long-term high doses of these drugs and the effect of sudden cessation of steroid therapy.)

In many patients the long-term low dose use of corticosteroids has proved beneficial as a prophylactic measure. The introduction of ***beclomethasone*** *(Becloforte, Becotide)* in a metered aerosol has done much to improve the safety of this type of treatment. Small doses, 100 mcg, are delivered directly to the affected area. This not only increases efficacy but reduces the adverse systemic effects that may accompany long-term oral use. Patients should be told to gargle or drink fluids immediately after using beclomethasone to prevent the steroid remaining in the pharyngeal mucosa. Some recommend the prior use of an adrenergic bronchodilator to obtain better distribution of the steroid into the lungs.

OTHER PROPHYLACTIC MEASURES

Sodium cromoglycate *(Intal)*

Although asthma is in many cases mediated by an allergic reaction to pollens, dust-mite and the like, the condition responds poorly or not at all to antihistamines. This may be due to the fact that substances other than histamine are also released from damaged mast cells, for example, SRS-A, the slow release factor of anaphylaxis.

Sodium cromoglycate *(Intal)* blocks the release of histamine, SRS-A and other chemicals from sensitised mast cells after the formation of specific antigen-antibody complexes. It therefore has a prophylactic role in allergy-antibody complexes and is used in allergy-induced asthma. Sodium cromoglycate has no direct bronchodilator, antihistamine, anticholinergic or anti-inflammatory action. It is effective only as a prophylactic agent in patients with severe perennial bronchial asthma and has no role in the treatment of the acute attack. This substance is supplied in capsules but is administered by inhalation from a mechanical inhaler.

Adverse Drug Reactions

The most common adverse effect is irritation of the throat and trachea caused by inhalation of the dry powder, resulting in cough or bronchospasm. Caution should be used when decreasing the dose because asthmatic symptoms may recur.

NURSING IMPLICATIONS

Assessment

When drugs affecting the respiratory system are used, baseline observation of respiratory and cardiovascular parameters, colour, signs of hypoxia and hypercapnia should be documented. Nurses must know which drugs are used on a regular basis, for prophylaxis, and which are used for an acute attack of bronchoconstriction.

Administration

Oral preparations of xanthines in slow release forms, for example, *Nuelin S.R.* and *Theo-Dur*, are taken at 12-hour intervals and must be swallowed whole, so as not to destroy the time delivery system. Administration of oral xanthines with food is recommended, to reduce the incidence of nausea and vomiting. Diuresis should be expected with xanthine therapy.

Intravenous infusions of aminophylline should not be "caught up" if running too slowly. Cardiovascular effects may occur with too-rapid infusions. An infusion pump or microdrip giving set should be used, for maintenance of accurate flow rates. No drugs should be added to aminophylline infusions without first consulting the pharmacist or reliable literature because incompatibilities are extremely common. The dangers of rapid injection cannot be overemphasised, but care must be taken with all routes of administration. Deaths have been recorded in infants administered aminophylline by the rectal route.

From the previous discussion of adrenergic agents and of the use of corticosteroids in respiratory diseases, there can be seen a trend towards metered-aerosol therapy. It has the advantage of portability, reliability, the ability to deliver a measured dose and apparent ease of administration. However, frequent studies have reported poor response in up to 20% of patients using this form of therapy. In the majority of cases which occur with the very old and the very young, the problem has been traced to faulty administration techniques.

Instructions that should be given to the patient include:

1. Shake the container well and remove the cap.
2. Breathe out fully.
3. Place the inhaler in the mouth with the lips around the mouthpiece and tongue below the inhaler.
4. Tilt the head back slightly and breathe in deeply and slowly while fully depressing the top of the metered cannister.
5. Remove the inhaler from the mouth, and hold the breath for as long as is comfortable.
6. Slowly release the breath through pursed lips or the nose.
7. If two puffs have been ordered, wait one minute between puffs, and shake the container again before the second puff.
8. Clean the inhaler after every use.

Excessive inhalation of any aerosol should be avoided as it carries not only the potential hazard of overdose of the active ingredient but also the possibility of harm from the fluorocarbon propellants.

It is not uncommon for a patient with a respiratory disease that compromises breathing to be impatient for immediate relief from an acute attack. This often leads to too-frequent administration of a medication and a tendency to try a variety of drugs simultaneously. This can lead to additive adverse effects when similar drugs are taken together. Similarly, fear of an acute attack often leads to overuse of drugs in prophylactic regimes. Asthmatic patients in particular need to be aware of the purposes and limitations of the drugs they are using and counselled against excessive, unnecessary or unproductive use of the drugs at their disposal.

To reduce the incidence of oral candidiasis (thrush) the patient should be told to gargle or drink fluids immediately after using beclomethasone to prevent the steroid remaining in the pharyngeal mucosa. Improved dental hygiene also helps. In addition, these procedures should help to reduce the hoarseness, dry mouth and sore throat often associated with beclomethasone use. Some recommend the prior use of an adrenergic bronchodilator to obtain better distribution of the steroid into the lungs. This should be used 15 to 20 minutes before the administration of beclomethasone so that the bronchodilator may have maximal effect. When steroids are used prophylactically, the patient must be advised of the need for regular use. Use only when an attack occurs is not sufficient.

Sodium cromoglycate *(Intal)* is supplied in capsules but is administered by inhalation from a mechanical inhaler, usually four times a day for both children and adults. Patient education on proper use of the inhaler is particularly important to the therapeutic benefit of this agent. The main points are:

1. Patients must be advised that capsules are not to be taken orally as absorption does not occur by this route.
2. Load the inhaler with a capsule and pierce once, immediately before use.
3. Holding the inhaler away from the mouth, exhale and empty the air from the lungs as much as possible.
4. With the head tilted back and teeth apart, close the lips around the mouthpiece.
5. Inhale deeply and rapidly through the inhaler with a steady, even breath.
6. Remove the inhaler and hold the breath for a few seconds, then exhale slowly. (Do not exhale through the inhaler because moisture from the breath will interfere with proper function of the inhaler.)
7. Repeat several times until all the powder is inhaled. A light dusting of the powder remaining in the capsules is normal.

Nebuliser solutions: several of the beta-adrenergic agonists, such as salbutamol, are available for use in intermittent-positive-pressure breathing therapy or can be delivered as vapours with gases inhaled through nebulisers. The appropriate dose form must be selected, with careful attention being paid to the prescription for dose, diluent, gas (air or oxygen) and rate of delivery. The nurse must be familiar with the correct use and adjustment of each type of apparatus. Physiotherapists are appropriate resource personnel to be consulted about the operation of nebulisers and respirators. Particular care should be taken in the selection of the gas to vaporise solutions prescribed for patients with chronic hypercapnia, since oxygen may be contraindicated. If there is any doubt about the gas to be used, air is the safest alternative.

Evaluation

Nursing evaluation of bronchodilator therapy has several aspects:

(a) evaluation of clinical improvement of respiratory function;
(b) observation for adverse effects, particularly cardiovascular effects;
(c) evaluation of self-administration practices in order to prevent over-use of aerosols;
(d) evaluation of aerosol technique.

Demonstration of improved respiratory function may involve comparison of incentive spirometry and bedside lung-function testing (such as forced-expiratory volumes or peak-expiratory flow rates), before and after therapy. Nurses need to work closely with physiotherapists in evaluating the effects of bronchodilators and in motivating patients to use their drugs for maximum benefit.

Blood gases and serum aminophylline levels may be monitored.

Patient teaching

Again, nurses can reinforce the work of physiotherapists in educating patients about the nature of respiratory disease, the appropriate use of bronchodilators, and self-administration techniques.

The reason for therapeutic failure of aerosol and inhaler treatment can be faulty technique, particularly with the very young and the elderly. Patients must be taught correct techniques and must be observed during self-administration in order to evaluate the effectiveness of teaching. Placebo aerosols and inhalers are available for teaching purposes. Parents must be included when young children are taught. Patients must be cautioned about over-use and advised of the importance of following recommended doses. They must be able to distinguish between drugs intended for prophylactic use and those intended for the treatment of an acute attack.

THE TREATMENT OF COUGH

Cough is an important reflex for maintaining an open airway. As such, it should not be suppressed indiscriminately. There are two types of cough: the productive and the non-productive. Cough, when it expels secretions, exudates and foreign material (such as dust from the lungs) is productive and should be allowed to serve its purpose unless it is exhausting to the patient. The loose productive cough associated with asthma and bronchitis should not be suppressed. On the other hand, the dry, hacking, non-productive cough in which no sputum is expectorated should be made useful if possible by removing the source of irritation or loosening the secretions, or it should be stopped.

According to the condition, treatment should be aimed at:

1. removal of the source of irritation;
2. loosening the secretions to make the cough more productive;
3. cough suppression.

REMOVAL OF THE SOURCE OF IRRITATION

Where the cough arises due to irritation of the pharynx, use of demulcent substances such as ***syrups*** and ***glycerin*** which coat and thereby soothe the area can be made. A warm, moist atmosphere will often give relief when the cough arises from irritation below the pharynx, thus ***water inhalations*** with or without ***compound tincture of benzoin*** *(Friar's Balsam)* have a place.

If bacterial infection of the lungs is a causative or contributing factor, then appropriate anti-infective treatment should be instituted. Reference to the chapter on anti-infective agents will show a range of penicillins, erythromycins, tetracyclines and sulphonamides suitable for this purpose.

LOOSENING OF SECRETIONS TO MAKE THE COUGH MORE PRODUCTIVE

Expectorants

The theory behind the use of expectorants is that these substances stimulate cough and may have a direct or indirect action on bronchial secretory cells to produce a thin watery secretion. The efficacy of such agents has been questioned for some years, yet they continue to be used. Substances credited with this type of action include ***ammonium compounds, sodium citrate*** and older preparations such as ***ipecacuanha*** and ***squill.***

Mucolytic Agents

Mucolytic agents are substances that break down mucus. ***Acetylcysteine*** *(Fabrol)* acts by breaking down viscous sputum, but these breakdown substances have an unpleasant smell to which many object. It is administered via a respirator and acts within minutes. Bronchospasm may occur, so prior use of a bronchodilator is often recommended. In conjunction with physiotherapy this mode of treatment is effective, but it does nothing to prevent the formation of further mucus.

Bromhexine *(Bisolvon)* acts on the mucus at the formative stages in the glands and results in the formation of a thinner, watery, more mobile mucus which is easier to expectorate. However, it takes time to act – up to three or four weeks for full effect. Patients on this medication must be advised not to anticipate immediate action.

COUGH SUPPRESSION

In those cases where it is considered necessary to suppress cough arising in the lower respiratory tract, a range of substances is available. The major group comprises opium derivatives and acts by central nervous depression of the medullary cough centre. These include ***opium tincture, methadone, dihydrocodeinone, codeine, dihydrocodeine*** and ***pholcodine.*** The first three of these, although effective in the suppression of cough, have addictive properties. Their use is therefore restricted to the more urgent cases. Codeine and dihydrocodeine are effective but cause constipation and drowsiness. The potential for abuse also exists. Pholcodine, though less effective than other agents, has fewer adverse effects, nausea and drowsiness being the most common. It is widely used, particularly with children.

Two other antitussive agents with central nervous activity are ***dextromethorphan*** and ***diphenhydramine*** *(Benadryl).* Dextromethorphan, which is non-narcotic, is considered equipotent with codeine on a milligram-for-milligram basis as a cough suppressant, has no significant constipating effect and is not an analgesic. Diphenhydramine *(Benadryl)*, an antihistamine, has been shown to have antitussive properties. Twenty-five to 50 milligrams of diphenhydramine equals 15 milligrams of codeine as a cough suppressant, but sedation can be troublesome, and the drying and thickening effect on bronchial mucus can be counterproductive. Other antihistamines with less sedative effect have been used (chlorpheniramine, brompheniramine), but the problem of thickening mucus secretions remains.

Mixed Therapy

One of the problems in the treatment of cough is that there are usually concomitant symptoms, for example, nasal congestion, runny nose and fever. Many "cough mixtures" attempt to treat these associated symptoms as well and contain a range of chemical compounds with a variety of pharmacological actions. Not all combinations are rational. One such irrational combination would be a mixture containing both an expectorant to loosen mucus and an antihistamine which will thicken mucus. Similarly, compounds containing an expectorant and a systemic decongestant such as ephedrine or pseudoephedrine are considered suspect by some.

Nursing staff in some hospitals are authorised to give simple medication on a p.r.n. or "when necessary" basis. Before proceeding with treatment of a cough, it must be decided whether such action is in the patient's interest: should the cough be suppressed, or is an expectorant required? Combination products should be avoided. Other symptoms such as fever, headache or runny nose can be treated separately if necessary.

NURSING IMPLICATIONS

Assessment

The pattern of coughing, with regard to time of day, duration and frequency, should be determined. The effects of coughing on the patient should be observed, with particular attention to fatigue, colour and disturbance of rest and sleep. If the cough is productive, the characteristics of the sputum are significant, as is the patient's ability to remove secretions from the bronchial tree.

Nurses in some institutions are authorised to initiate treatment with medication for a cough, without a prescription from a medical officer. It is the responsibility of the nurse to be thoroughly conversant with local policy with regard to:

(a) the medications which can be administered;
(b) documentation;
(c) the number of doses that can be administered;
(d) method of administration;
(e) nursing evaluation of the treatment.

It is essential in such cases that nurses know the effects (both therapeutic and adverse) of the drugs administered and that a rigorous assessment of the cause of the cough is made.

Before proceeding with any p.r.n. or "when necessary" treatment of a cough, it must be decided whether such action is in the patient's interest to have the cough suppressed or whether an expectorant might be required.

Accompanying symptoms such as chest pain, fever, headache and runny nose should be documented and treated as they arise.

Administration

Combination medications, for example expectorants with antihistamines, should not be used unless specifically ordered by a medical practitioner.

Patients taking acetylcysteine *(Fabrol)* should be advised beforehand of the unpleasant smell associated with treatment.

Protection from burning must be afforded when water-vapour inhalers are used.

Evaluation

Changes in coughing pattern, sputum production and effects of cough suppression on ventilation must be observed and documented.

Patient teaching

Patients taking bromhexine *(Bisolvon)* should be advised that immediate results are not expected and to continue the treatment for one month before a final assessment of its efficacy is made. Correct administration of inhalation therapy should be taught if required. Patients must be warned about any sedative effects of cough medications.

ANTI-INFECTIVE THERAPY

Many respiratory conditions are either caused or complicated by infection. Anti-infective agents therefore play an important role in the treatment of such cases. ***Penicillin V*** or ***erythromycin*** are among the drugs of choice for upper-respiratory infections, while ***ampicillin, amoxycillin, the tetracyclines*** and ***sulphonamides*** are more widely used for lower-respiratory infections.

Reference should be made to Chapter 23 for a detailed discussion of the use of these and other anti-infective agents.

RESPIRATORY STIMULANTS

Respiratory stimulants are very rarely used in the treatment of barbiturate overdose and in pulmonary failure. Expert supervision is required. Use in these situations is usually short-term, while other measures, such as ventilation, are instituted. ***Aminophylline*** is the most common, being infused slowly intravenously. Adverse reactions to this drug have already been mentioned. Other central nervous stimulants that may be used are ***ethamivan*** *(Clairvan)*, ***doxapram hydrochloride*** *(Dopram)* and ***nikethamide.*** Restlessness and twitching, itching, vomiting and flushing may precede convulsions when these drugs are used in effective stimulant doses.

SELF-EVALUATION TEST

1. Place each of the following drugs into the appropriate pharmacological classification.

Drug	**Classification**
Salbutamol	Adrenergic bronchodilator
Beclomethasone	Xanthine derivative
Codeine	Corticosteroid
Squill	Mast cell stabiliser
Theophylline	Cough suppressant
Sodium cromoglycate	Cough expectorant
Aminophylline	Antihistamine with sedative properties
Fenoterol	Mucolytic agent
Prednisone	
Dextromethorphan	
Acetylcysteine	
Potassium iodide	
Diphenhydramine	
Bromhexine	
Terbutaline	

2. List the adverse reactions that may be experienced by a patient using the following drugs:
   (a) isoprenaline;
   (b) orciprenaline;
   (c) aminophylline;
   (d) codeine.
3. Describe the correct method of use of a:
   (a) metered aerosol inhalation;
   (b) spinhaler.
4. Name three drugs used in the treatment of asthma that tend to be overused by the patient.
5. Name two pharmacologically active cough suppressant agents that may be subject to abuse.
6. List the nursing implications associated with the use of drugs in the treatment of:
   (a) bronchospasm;
   (b) cough.

Summary — Drugs used in the Treatment of Respiratory Diseases

Drug Group	Drug Name	Use	Action	Adverse Reactions	Nursing Implications
BRONCHODILATORS					
Beta-adrenergic agonists	Orciprenaline Salbutamol Terbutaline Fenoterol	Bronchodilator in asthma and other airways diseases	Bronchiolar smooth-muscle relaxation	Increase in heart rate, anxiety, nervousness, palpitation, dizziness, headache, nausea and vomiting	
Anticholinergic	Ipratropium	Bronchodilator in asthma and other airways diseases	Bronchiolar smooth-muscle relaxation	Rare ADRs of anticholinergic nature; mainly dry mouth	
Xanthines	Theophylline Aminophylline	Bronchodilator in asthma and other airways diseases	Bronchiolar smooth-muscle relaxation	Oral: nausea and vomiting; rectal: proctitis; IV: headache, flushing, palpitation, dizziness, arrhythmias, tachycardia, hypotension, precordial pain	
STEROIDS					
Corticosteroids	Hydrocortisone Prednisone Prednisolone Betamethasone Dexamethasone Beclomethasone inhaler	Aids bronchodilation	Reduces inflammation in airways	See Chapter 11 on corticosteroids; ADR less common after inhalation therapy	***Assess:*** respiratory status, colour, level of consciousness; for chronic hypercapnia; cardiovascular status ***Administer:*** aerosols, inhalers and nebulizers – ensure correct technique used; IV aminophylline – microdrip giving set or infusion pump; do not add any drugs; do not "catch up" if behind time; oral – sustained release tablets must be swallowed whole, give every 12 hours. ***Evaluate:*** respiratory improvement by observation

					and spirometry; blood gases; serum aminophylline levels; for adverse effects ***Teach:*** correct technique with aerosols, inhalers; prophylactic and acute uses; dangers of over-use.
COUGH TREATMENT					
Expectorants	Guaiphenesin potassium iodide; ammonium compounds	Treatment of productive cough	Stimulate bronchial secretory cells	Nausea and vomiting; diarrhoea	
Mucolytics	Acetylcysteine	Mucolytic	Breakdown of viscous sputum	Nausea from unpleasant odour; bronchospasm; ADR rare; slow onset of action	***Assess:*** time, frequency and duration of cough; sputum characteristics; effects of cough – fatigue, sleep disturbance; chest pain, fever, headache, rhinorrhoea ***Administer:*** check local policies; suppressant or expectorant according to assessment; protect from burning during inhaler therapy ***Evaluate:*** change in cough pattern, sputum; sedative effects on ventilation ***Teach:*** results only after one month of bromhexine; inhalation method; sedative effects
	Bromhexine	Mucolytic	Causes production of watery mucus		
Cough suppressants	Dihydrocodeinone Dihydrocodeine Codeine Pholcodine	Cough suppression	Depression of medullary cough centre	Nausea, drowsiness, constipation	
	Dextromethorphan Diphenhydramine	Cough suppression	Depression of medullary cough centre	Sedation, thickening of mucus	
	Oxolamine	Cough suppression	Acts on lung receptors	Rare	

7

DRUGS USED IN THE TREATMENT OF CARDIOVASCULAR DISEASE

William A. Thomson, Ross W. Holland and Vicky J. Grattan

OBJECTIVES

At the end of this chapter the reader should be able to:

1. define the terms "oedema", "diuretic" and "antihypertensive agent";
2. name the main drugs used in the treatment of cardiovascular diseases and list important adverse reactions;
3. describe in general terms the mechanism of action of diuretics, antihypertensive agents, anti-arrhythmic drugs and those substances used in the treatment of congestive cardiac failure, angina and cardiac arrest;
4. identify the pharmacological activity of the various drugs mentioned;
5. list the nursing implications of the administration of these drugs.

PREREQUISITE KNOWLEDGE

1. Structure and function of the heart, the vascular system and the kidneys.
2. Physiology of these systems with particular emphasis on the role of the autonomic nervous system.
3. The principles of osmosis.
4. Diseases of the cardiovascular system.

DEFINITIONS

Cardiac failure — the failure of the heart to pump an amount of blood adequate to supply the metabolic needs of the body, and to maintain venous return.

Congestive cardiac failure — the occurrence of circulatory congestion due to decreased myocardial contractility. Cardiac output becomes insufficient to maintain blood flow to organs and tissue.

Oedema — the accumulation of excess fluid in the extracellular spaces of the body.
Diuretics — drugs which act within the kidneys to increase the production of urine. (They should not be confused with drugs that act on the bladder to increase micturition.)
Drug treatment of congestive cardiac failure — therapy aimed at increasing cardiac efficiency and reducing oedema, often with the aid of diuretics.

CONGESTIVE CARDIAC FAILURE (CCF)

For many centuries the leaves of the common foxglove *Digitalis purpurea* have been used in folk medicine as a cure for a variety of complaints. Only within the last 50 years has it been firmly established that the main value of digitalis — the chemical derived from the plant — lies in the treatment of congestive cardiac failure.

The leaves of *Digitalis lanata* contain a mixture of three natural glycosides (compounds which on hydrolysis yield a sugar and a non-sugar residue). They are widely found in plants and are crystalline, bitter and sometimes poisonous. One of those found in digitalis is ***digoxin,*** which is widely used. The main effect of digoxin is to increase the force of contraction of the heart muscle. That is, it has a positive *inotropic* action. Increase in the strength of the heart's contraction leads to increased cardiac output, decreased heart size, decreased venous pressure and consequent relief of oedema. In addition digoxin has a negative *chronotropic* effect in that it slows the heart rate. Digoxin also decreases conduction through the AV node which leads to protection of the ventricles from atrial tachyarrhythmia.

The dose must be accurately determined as there is only a small margin of safety before toxic effects become apparent. Digoxin is available in several dose forms including an injection which may be given for rapid digitalisation. (Digitalisation is the process of bringing a patient's blood concentration of digoxin to an effective level. This may be done by using loading doses of tablets or, more quickly, by using an injection.) Once an effective blood level has been achieved, a reduced maintenance dose is administered once or twice a day.

Tablets are available for oral administration in three strengths, 62.5 mcg, 125 mcg and 250 mcg. A paediatric elixir is also available.

Adverse Drug Reactions

The margin between therapeutic dose and toxic dose is narrow; consequently, the incidence of digitalis toxicity is high. The appearance of these toxic effects is not always predictable but may include: gastrointestinal disturbances (nausea, vomiting, anorexia, diarrhoea); cardiac arrhythmias, including sinus bradycardia, ectopic beats, bigeminy (coupled beats) and ventricular fibrillation; and fatigue, headache, mental confusion and blurred vision (these effects are less common).

Sensitivity to digoxin is increased by low potassium levels in the body, impaired renal function, advancing age, acute myocardial infarction, pulmonary heart disease accompanied by anorexia or recent cardiac surgery.

Treatment of Digoxin Toxicity

1. Withdraw the drug.
2. Correct hypokalaemia if present.
3. Use anti-arrhythmic drugs as indicated (for example, lignocaine).

NURSING IMPLICATIONS

Assessment

A baseline of cardiac function needs to be established, against which therapeutic effects and digoxin toxicity can be measured. Apex rate, peripheral pulse rate, rhythm and quality of the pulse wave, age, weight and electrolyte status should be recorded. If diuretics are used concurrently with digoxin, knowledge of the effects of those drugs on serum-potassium levels and the possibility of digoxin toxicity in hypokalaemia is essential. Other conditions predisposing to decreased potassium levels include gastrointestinal disturbances, stress and poor dietary intake.

Prior assessment of the patient's normal appetite will be useful in the early detection of toxicity. If recorded frequently, weight is a reliable indicator of fluid retention in the patient with congestive cardiac failure. The occurrence of dyspnoea, orthopnoea and crepitations should be noted.

Quinidine increases the serum level of digoxin, so the potential for toxicity increases when the drugs are used together, and digoxin doses need to be reduced accordingly.

Administration

As a general guide, digoxin is withheld when the heart rate, measured at the apex, is less than 60 beats per minute, counted over one full minute. However, since toxicity may be manifested by a range of arrhythmias, any change of rhythm and rate not in the therapeutic direction should be investigated.

If potassium levels fall below the normal limits, supplements will need to be prescribed to prevent toxicity.

Great care should be taken to administer the correct dose for individual patients, given the range of strengths, similarity of names of different preparations, and range of individual reactions to digoxin preparations. Particular care is essential when giving the drug to children.

Giving digoxin after meals will reduce local gastric irritation and allow for a more accurate assessment of the gastrointestinal signs of toxicity. Since daily doses are usually prescribed, administration at the same time each day is important in maintaining serum concentration.

Evaluation
The therapeutic effects of digoxin will be observed as decreased respiratory difficulty, peripheral oedema and tiredness; increased pulse volume and urinary output; and other signs of improved cardiac output, such as mental alertness and exercise tolerance. As congestion of the gastrointestinal blood vessels decreases, appetite should improve, and nausea should disappear. Where the underlying cause of heart failure cannot be removed, the improvement may be limited, and the need for drug treatment may become chronic.

Evaluation of toxicity is difficult because of the similarity of the features of congestive heart failure and those of digitalis toxicity. Continued gastrointestinal disturbances, apparent before digoxin treatment, may not indicate toxicity; but an initial improvement, followed by anorexia, nausea or vomiting, is more likely to be drug related. Visual disturbances, although rare, usually occur later. Although all new rhythm disturbances should be investigated, bradycardias and ventricular bigeminy are common in digitalis toxicity. Tachyarrhythmias may arise as a result of either heart failure or toxicity. Serum concentrations are useful in assessing toxicity, but observation of the patient's response to withdrawal of the drug is essential.

Patient teaching
Patients need to be taught to observe for signs of toxicity and the early signs of recurring congestive heart failure. They may need to be taught how to count peripheral pulse rates.

The distinction between brand names and generic names should be made, to avoid double-dosing when a patient leaves hospital with a prescription and still has tablets at home from a previous prescription.

OTHER DRUGS USED IN THE TREATMENT OF CCF

Diuretics play an important role in the treatment of oedema associated with heart failure. Refer to page 109 for a discussion of these substances.

ANTI-ARRHYTHMIC DRUGS

Disturbance of the normal rhythm of the heart is known as *arrhythmia*. This condition may be brought about by abnormal SA-node rhythm, ectopic foci generating premature beats or pacemaker shifts, circus movements or conduction blocks. Several drugs are available to correct this type of condition.

LIGNOCAINE

The local anaesthetic agent ***lignocaine*** (*Xylocard*) is particularly effective in controlling ventricular arrhythmias, such as those occurring during cardiac surgery or following acute myocardial infarction. This substance is available in injection form for both IM and IV use. Either a bolus dose or an infusion may be used when the IV route is chosen. There are several strengths and sizes available. The 100 mg/5 mL ampoule is used for bolus doses while the 1 g/5 mL is used to prepare infusion solutions, although the latter are now available ready prepared. Lignocaine is quick acting but short-lived in effect, the duration being about 20 minutes.

Adverse Drug Reactions

The most common adverse reactions associated with lignocaine therapy are paraesthesias, auditory difficulty, drowsiness, agitation, nausea, vomiting and muscle twitching. Major reactions include tonic-clonic seizures, hypotension, heart block and psychosis.

TOCAINIDE

Tocainide *(Tonocard)* is a derivative of lignocaine which is available in both oral and injectable dose forms. Like lignocaine, it acts by stabilising cell membranes so as to reduce the incidence of ectopic beats. Its major use is in treatment of ventricular arrhythmias. The injectable form may be administered intravenously as a slow injection or as an infusion in 50 to 100 mL of saline or glucose solution over 15 to 30 minutes. Doses must be individually adjusted. Orally, maintenance treatment is 1200 mg daily, divided into two or three doses.

Adverse Drug Reactions

The most common reactions are nausea, vomiting and anorexia, dizziness, tremor, confusion, nervousness and disorientation. More serious CNS and cardiovascular complications are rare at the normal dose range although overdosage usually results in signs of CNS toxicity.

Drug Interactions

Tocainide has been used with other oral antiarrhythmics and with beta-blocking agents without evidence of untoward effects. However concurrent use with lignocaine may lead to potentiation of CNS effects.

MEXILETINE

Mexiletine *(Mexitil)* is also related to lignocaine and is used for ventricular arrhythmias. The dose should be individualised, based on response and tolerance. Where initial therapy with the IV dose form is employed, changeover to the oral formulation following the manufacturer's guidelines is recommended as soon as the patient's condition warrants.

Adverse Drug Reactions

Side effects are relatively uncommon and are usually dose related. They include hypotension, bradycardia, drowsiness and confusion, nausea and vomiting and an unpleasant taste. Usually, they may be reversed by reducing the dose.

QUINIDINE

This substance is used for a wide range of atrial and ventricular arrhythmias. It decreases the excitability of the cardiac muscle and depresses conduction velocity and myocardial contractility. Quinidine is usually administered in the oral form. The most popular dose form is the sustained-release tablet, *Kinidin Durules,* which has the advantage of twice-daily dosage. However, the tablets must be swallowed whole to be effective.

Adverse Drug Reactions

The incidence of adverse effects is high — nausea, vomiting and diarrhoea being the most common. Hypersensitivity reactions include skin rash, haemolytic anaemia, thrombocytopenia or drug fever. Quinidine should be used with caution in heart block and digitalis intoxication.

Drug Interactions

Quinidine may potentiate the hypotensive effects of thiazide diuretics and hypertensive agents. Doses in excess of 500 mg per day potentiate the action of digoxin leading to digoxin toxicity. Care should be taken when these two drugs are taken together.

DISOPYRAMIDE

Although chemically dissimilar to other antiarrhythmics, ***disopyramide*** *(Rythmodan)* has a pharmacological action closely resembling quinidine. It is used for both atrial and ventricular arrhythmias and appears to be better tolerated than quinidine.

While an injectable form is available for intravenous use, the most common form is the oral capsule which is available in several strengths.

Adverse Drug Reactions

Among the more frequent adverse reactions are dry mouth, constipation, urinary hesitancy, blurred vision and dry nose. A long list of less common reactions have been reported, including death preceded by abdominal pain, in a few patients taking beta-blocking agents at the same time.

Drug Interactions

As with quinidine, caution should be exercised in patients taking disopyramide and digoxin concurrently.

PROCAINAMIDE

The action and use of procainamide *(Pronestyl)* is similar to that of quinidine, increasing the threshold to electric stimulation in both the atria and ventricles. Procainamide is most commonly used for the treatment of premature ventricular beats and ventricular tachycardia, although it may be used in atrial arrhythmias.

Procainamide is available in both injectable and oral forms. Administration by injection is via the intravenous route at a rate of 25-50 mg/ minute up to a total of about 1 gram. This should be carried out with ECG monitoring. The oral form is available in 250 mg tablets as *Pronestyl* and in slow release form as *Procainamide Durules* 500 mg.

Adverse Drug Reactions

These are the same as for quinidine, although there may be fewer central stimulant effects.

PHENYTOIN

The anticonvulsant agent phenytoin *(Epanutin)* is also effective in the treatment of ventricular arrhythmias, particularly those produced by overdoses of digoxin. Phenytoin depresses automaticity, which helps to control arrhythmias, and improves conduction leading to improved cardiac function.

Administration is by slow intravenous injection, no faster than 50 mg/ minute. If given too fast, bradycardia and severe hypotension may result. It should not be mixed with IV infusion solutions or other drugs as precipitation may occur.

Adverse Drug Reactions

Frequent adverse effects from short-term use include slurred speech, nystagmus, mental confusion and dizziness. These are usually dose-related. (For adverse reactions to long-term use, see Chapter 29.)

NURSING IMPLICATIONS

Assessment

Baseline assessment of vital signs and cardiac rhythm are essential. Neurological status should be documented in patients receiving lignocaine. Since antiarrhythmics are often given intravenously, a previous history of hypersensitivity is significant. Nurses caring for patients in the initial stages of treatment must be able to read and interpret electrocardiograms and be proficient in cardiopulmonary resuscitation techniques. Drug interactions have been observed between some antiarrhythmics and digoxin, so an accurate recent drug history is necessary.

Quinidine and procainamide solutions that have turned brown should not be used. Several strengths of lignocaine are available, for bolus injection and for slow infusion, so care must be taken to select the appropriate strength for the prescription. Lignocaine infusions are available in commercially prepared packs.

Administration

Closely regulated infusions will often be required, so infusion pumps are recommended. Continuous cardiac monitoring is advisable at the beginning of treatment.

Gastric irritation caused by quinidine can be reduced by giving tablets with food. Sustained-release tablets must be swallowed whole, not crushed.

Evaluation

The effects of this group of drugs on cardiac rhythm is most accurately evaluated by electrocardiographic monitoring. Patients with atrial flutter or fibrillation may have developed atrial thrombi, and embolisation may occur when atrial contraction is re-established. They should, therefore, be observed for signs of the life-threatening complications of arterial or pulmonary embolism.

Clinical signs of therapeutic action are related to improved cardiac output. Nurses need to be aware of the adverse reactions associated with the use of each drug.

Patient teaching

Patients should receive thorough instruction about doses and schedules. Families should be directed to cardiopulmonary resuscitation training programmes because of the possibility of cardiac emergencies.

ANGINA PECTORIS

Angina pectoris is a syndrome characterised by paroxysmal pain in the anterior chest. This pain occurs as a result of insufficient coronary blood flow leading to myocardial hypoxia. The pain varies greatly in severity. Typically starting over the precordium and upper sternum, it radiates to the left shoulder and may extend down the inner aspect of the arm to the fingers. In addition to pain, the patient suffers extreme apprehension and a feeling of impending death. Factors which predispose a patient towards angina include obesity, high serum-lipid levels, arrhythmias, hypertension, anaemia and hyperthyroidism. Acute attacks may be precipitated by emotional stress, heavy meals, sudden effort or exposure to cold.

Treatment in general is aimed at improving oxygen supply to the myocardium and decreasing the myocardial demand for oxygen.

THE ACUTE ATTACK

In many cases pain relief may be obtained by removing the cause of the attack. For example, angina of effort may be relieved by rest. Indeed the pain itself will often cause the sufferer to cease the activity immediately. In other situations rest alone may not provide either rapid or effective relief of pain, so that the use of drugs may become necessary.

Nitrites have long been the drugs of choice in the treatment of acute attacks of angina pectoris. ***Amyl nitrite,*** the first of these drugs, was administered by inhaling the contents of a small glass capsule which was crushed between the fingers. Due to its objectionable odour and the inconvenience of its method of administration, this drug is no longer in general use.

Glyceryl trinitrate 500 mcg and ***isosorbide dinitrate*** 5 mg *(Isordil)* are most frequently used to relieve the acute angina attack. Both are administered sublingually (under the tongue) and take effect within two minutes. The effect lasts about 20 minutes. Should pain relief not be readily obtained, the dose may be repeated within a few minutes to a maximum of three tablets. Many patients will notice a bitter taste or "sting" when taking glyceryl trinitrate.

The primary action of the nitrites is thought to be dilatation of the vascular smooth muscle. This reduces peripheral vascular resistance, and venous return to the heart is decreased. Thus myocardial oxygen demand is reduced. Nitrites may also improve the supply of oxygen to hypoxic areas by effecting a redistribution of coronary blood flow.

Potency of nitrites may be affected by heat, moisture and light. They should be stored in tightly closed, light-occluding containers (for example, in brown bottles) and kept in a cool, dry place. Expiry dates should be noted. The aerosol spray *(Coro-Nitro, Nitrolingual)* is another method of providing rapid relief, especially for those who cannot tolerate sublingual medication.

Adverse Drug Reactions

Flushing, together with severe or persistent headache, may occur with all nitrites or nitrates, particularly during the initial treatment. Hypotension may occur and can lead to episodes of dizziness, weakness and faintness. As the patient becomes accustomed to the drug, the headaches will tend to disappear. However, drug tolerance may develop so that the dose may have to be increased according to individual needs.

Drug Interactions

Alcohol accentuates vasodilation when combined with the nitrites and nitrates and may cause severe hypotension.

Glyceryl trinitrate *(Tridil)* is also available as a solution for preparation of an IV infusion. In this form it is used not only for the treatment of angina, but also to control blood pressure in perioperative hypertension, for controlled hypotension during neurological and orthopaedic surgery, and for congestive heart failure associated with myocardial infarction. Intravenous use is contraindicated in patients with anaemia, constricted pericarditis, increased intracranial pressure, hypotension, uncorrected hypovolaemia and sensitivity to organic nitrates.

Precautions

Tridil must be diluted with dextrose 5% or normal saline strictly in accordance with the manufacturer's instructions prior to use. *It is not for direct intravenous injection.*

Dose instructions must be followed with care as glyceryl trinitrate is absorbed into the PVC tubing on different giving sets at different rates. A change of giving set or infusion pump may therefore alter the dose required. Dilution and storage of IV solutions should be made only in glass parenteral-solution bottles or *suitable* plastic (i.e. non-PVC) containers.

Adverse Reactions

Overdosage may result in severe hypotension, transient headache and reflex tachycardia. Since the duration of action of glyceryl trinitrate is quite short, cessation of treatment and elevation of the legs is usually all that is required. Problems associated with drug tolerance, drug withdrawal and hypoxia have been reported.

Drug Interactions

Information on potential interactions with other drugs is poorly documented. However, caution should be observed in concomitant use of pancuronium, morphine, tricyclic antidepressants and anticholinergic agents. Alcohol should be avoided.

PREVENTION OF ANGINA PECTORIS

Long Acting Nitrates

Because of the effectiveness of short-acting nitrates in treating acute attacks of angina, it was logical that longer-acting compounds should be developed for prophylactic use. Although several have been developed, only ***isosorbide dinitrate*** 10 mg is used extensively. For maximum absorption, this drug is usually taken one hour before meals. Its effective time of action appears to be about two or three hours.

Glyceryl trinitrate is also available as long-acting preparations in the form of ointment *(Percutol)*, tablets *(Sustac* 2.6 mg, 6.4 mg, 10 mg) and impregnated dressings *(Transiderm Nitro)*. Their length of action varies: *Percutol* can be repeated every 3-4 hours as required, *Sustac* repeated every 6-8 hours, and *Transiderm Nitro* reapplied daily.

Adverse Drug Reactions

The adverse drug reactions for long-acting nitrates are the same as those listed for the short-acting compounds.

NURSING IMPLICATIONS

Assessment

The typical characteristics of angina pain must be distinguished from other types of chest pain. If angina is precipitated by particular activities, sublingual nitrates may be used to prevent pain, as well as to treat it. The duration of a particular episode of angina should be noted, since myocardial infarction can result from long periods of myocardial ischaemia. Distinction between the strengths and uses of isosorbide dinitrate is important.

Administration

Sublingual route

The time taken for glyceryl trinitrate or isosorbide dinitrate to relieve pain should be noted. Dosage may be repeated in a few minutes, up to a total of three tablets, if relief is not readily obtained. Patients commencing treatment should be advised that throbbing headaches, dizziness, fainting and/or slight palpitations may occur during the initial treatment. The patient should be resting in the recumbent position, without his legs dangling, to promote venous return. In order to avoid hypotension and faintness, he should not change position suddenly. When using isosorbide dinitrate *(Isordil)* the 5-mg tablet should be selected for sublingual administration during the acute attack. Many patients will notice a bitter taste or "sting" when taking glyceryl trinitrate.

Oral route

Isosorbide dinitrate 10 mg tablets, for prophylactic use, are given one hour before meals to promote absorption. The effective time of action appears to be about two or three hours.

Potency of nitrates may be affected by heat, moisture and light. Tablets should be stored in tightly closed, light-occluding containers (for example, in brown bottles) and kept in a cool, dry place. Expiry dates should be noted.

Topical route

Percutol is applied in ½-1 inch lengths using an Applirule and secured with a dressing; it is not rubbed in, and nurses should avoid direct skin contact with the ointment. Any convenient area of skin may be used. As the ointment is sticky, a less-hairy portion of the body is best. The chest, thigh or arm are often chosen. *Percutol* contains glyceryl trinitrate 2%. Its action lasts three to four hours, and the application may be repeated after this time. *Transiderm Nitro* should be applied to the lateral chest wall and reapplied every 24 hours, siting the new dressing on a different area of skin.

Intravenous route

This technique is currently employed only in the controlled environment of operating theatres or intensive care units. Glyceryl trinitrate solutions should be prepared in pharmacy whenever possible. Strict adherence to the manufacturer's instructions is essential at all times. Dosage and hence flow rates are critical and require constant monitoring. Use of polyethylene rather than PVC giving sets is recommended.

Evaluation

Relief from chest pain must be documented together with the time taken to achieve relief noted and the number of tablets required. The frequency of administration of nitrates can be a useful aid in the evaluation of angina. The occurrence of adverse effects and their acceptability to the patient should be noted. Failure of nitrates to relieve chest pain may indicate that myocardial infarction is occurring, and appropriate action must be taken. Recording of 12-lead electrocardiograms during chest pain and recovery may be used to document the effects of nitrates.

Patient teaching

Many patients self-administer nitrates, both in hospital and at home. It is therefore essential that they have adequate information about the drugs. Teaching should include:

(a) the correct method of sub-lingual administration;
(b) the need to carry nitrates at all times;

(c) the correct storage of tablets. They should not be kept in a metal box or in close contact with the body, and fresh supplies should be obtained regularly.
(d) the correct method of measurement and application of ointments.

Beta-blocking Agents

Beta-blocking agents are so named because they block the stimulation, by sympathetic nerve impulses, of beta-receptor sites at nerve endings. There are two main types of beta receptors: beta-1 receptors, which occur mainly in the myocardium, and beta-2 receptors, which are distributed through many organs, including the bronchi and blood vessels.

The most important clinical effects exerted on the heart by this group of drugs are reduced heart rate, reduction in the force of cardiac contraction, reduction of myocardial "irritability", and significant reduction in myocardial oxygen demand as a result of the previous effects. The reduction in heart rate and myocardial oxygen requirement makes these substances valuable in the control of angina pectoris. Those drugs which are cardio-selective are particularly useful. These are ***metoprolol*** (*Betaloc, Lopressor*) and ***atenolol*** (*Tenormin*). Other beta-blocking drugs are non-selective for cardiac tissue, acting on other systems in the body as well, and may in some cases lead to bronchoconstriction. Examples of this type are ***propranolol*** *(Inderal)*, ***oxprenolol*** *(Trasicor)* and ***pindolol*** *(Visken)*.

Adverse Drug Reactions

Beta-blocking drugs are becoming increasingly popular because they are well tolerated and have few adverse effects. Adverse effects may generally be avoided by gradual introduction of the drug. Reactions may include bradycardia and hypotension, nausea, vomiting, diarrhoea, lassitude and visual disturbances. More serious effects include severe nightmares and hallucinations, purpura or erythematous rashes and paraesthesias of the hands. Hypoglycaemia may be induced in the starving or ketotic diabetic.

Drug Interactions

Beta-blocking drugs may cause an altered reaction to stress. Prior to anaesthesia and surgery it may be necessary to withdraw them gradually, as there is a risk of myocardial infarction following sudden withdrawal. In emergency, when gradual withdrawal may not be practicable, the patient should be protected against vagal dominance by intravenous administration of atropine. Anaesthetic agents such as ether, cyclopropane and trichloroethylene should be avoided.

NURSING IMPLICATIONS

Assessment

Beta blockers are not usually given to patients with heart failure because they may be dependent upon sympathetic drive. Non-selective beta blockers should not be used for patients with asthma or any other form of bronchospasm. Baseline assessment should include heart rate, arterial blood pressure and respiratory status.

Administration

Several strengths of propranolol are available in tablet form, so care is needed to select the correct strength. There has been some controversy about the cessation of beta blockers for 48 hours before surgery, but it is generally considered wiser to continue them.

Evaluation

Regular monitoring of heart rate and arterial pressure is recommended. Patients must be observed for the first signs of congestive cardiac failure or bronchospasm.

Patient teaching

Since many patients will take beta blockers for long periods, they must know the signs of early cardiac failure and respiratory problems and must notify the medical practitioner if hypotension or bradycardia cause problems. They should be advised of the dangers of missing doses or stopping treatment suddenly, so a supply should always be at hand.

Calcium Antagonists

The calcium-channel blocking agents act by reducing the slow inward current of calcium ions across the cell membrane in cardiac muscle and in vascular smooth muscle. This reduction in calcium flow results in reduced contractility, heart rate and conductivity. The reduction in contraction of vascular smooth muscle, which causes both coronary and peripheral dilatation, is the basis for the drug's ability to decrease ventricular afterload and cardiac work and to prevent coronary vasospasm.

While it is becoming clear that these substances have a role as hypertensive agents and in the treatment of some arrhythmias, their main clinical use is in the treatment of angina.

Five calcium antagonists are available in Great Britain: ***verapamil*** *(Cordilox)*, ***nifedipine*** *(Adalat)*, ***lidoflazine*** *(Clinium)*, ***diltiazem*** *(Tildiem)* and ***nicardipine*** *(Cardene)*. All are available in oral dose form while verapamil is also available by injection. Although belonging to the same class of drugs, the chemical structures are different. This is reflected in their differing effects on the cardiovascular system. Nifedipine is preferred in the presence of congestive heart failure because of its afterload reducing effect. In CCF, verapamil should be avoided due to its negative inotropic effect, but diltiazem and nicardipine are much less likely to cause this problem.

Combination with beta-blocking agents may be beneficial, but caution is required with verapamil because of the additive negative inotropic effect.

Adverse Drug Reactions

Nifedipine frequently produces mild side effects as a result of its vasodilating action. Headache and congestion occur in about 6% of patients, with discontinuation of therapy necessary in only about 1%. Vomiting, nausea, hypotension and leg oedema are less common.

Verapamil generally has fewer reported reactions. There is a low incidence of headache, vertigo, nervousness, gastric discomfort, nausea, constipation and other non-specific symptoms. Serious adverse effects including hypotension, worsening heart failure, bradycardia and asystole have been reported with intravenous administration of verapamil, although the majority have occurred in patients receiving concomitant ß-adrenergic blockade.

Drug Interactions

Caution is required when using verapamil in digitalised patients as plasma digoxin concentrations may be increased.

NURSING IMPLICATIONS

Assessment

Cardiovascular status, including heart rate and arterial pressure, should be documented before therapy begins. Care should be taken to observe the patient closely when beta blockers are used concurrently.

Evaluation

Cardiovascular effects are similar to those of the beta blockers. Constipation caused by verapamil usually responds to dietary modification or stool softeners. Nifedipine may cause ankle oedema, requiring periodic elevation of the feet.

Patient teaching

Patients should be warned not to modify treatment without reference to their physician.

THE TREATMENT OF CARDIAC ARREST

Drugs used during cardiac arrest fall into three main groups: cardiac stimulants, anti-arrhythmic drugs and sodium bicarbonate. As the anti-arrhythmic drugs have already been described, they will not be included again.

CARDIAC STIMULANTS — ADRENERGICS

Reference to the chapter on the autonomic nervous sytem will show that control of the heart is a balance between the sympathetic (adrenergic) and the parasympathetic (cholinergic) systems. In general terms the adrenergic effects are to stimulate activity and the cholinergic effects are to slow activity. In the case of cardiac arrest, adrenergic drugs are used to stimulate the heart muscle to activity.

Adrenaline

Adrenaline stimulates the beta-1 receptors and:

1. stimulates the heart to spontaneous contraction;
2. in the case of ventricular fibrillation, increases myocardial tone prior to defibrillation;
3. increases conduction rate and velocity;
4. increases the perfusion developed by cardiac compression.

Adrenaline should be given early in the resuscitation effort and can be administered by the intracardiac route or intravenously. The IV route is preferred if it is immediately available. The usual dose is 500 mcg. Onset of action is immediate, reaching a peak in one to two minutes and lasting about five minutes. Adrenaline undergoes oxidative degradation (is broken down) by alkali, heat, air and light, therefore storage conditions are important, and it must not be mixed with aminophylline, phenytoin or sodium bicarbonate. It may also be incompatible with calcium salts.

Isoprenaline

Isoprenaline is similar in action to adrenaline, stimulating the myocardium to spontaneous contraction. Unlike adrenaline, it appears to be effective in the presence of acidosis. It is supplied as a 0.002% solution (0.2 mg/10 ml). The intracardiac dose is 20 mcg (0.1 mL) undiluted. By IV injection, the dose is 20 to 60 mcg initially, up to a total of 200 mcg. The infusion rate is usually about 5 mcg/min, adjusted to the patient's response.

As with adrenaline, isoprenaline is affected by alkalis and must therefore not be mixed with aminophylline, phenytoin or sodium bicarbonate. Isoprenaline and adrenaline should not be administered simultaneously but may be given alternately. In addition, the use of isoprenaline is hazardous in patients with digitalis intoxication, and in these cases extreme caution must be exercised.

Dobutamine

Dobutamine (*Dobutrex,* 250 mg injection) is a beta-1 selective adrenergic agonist. It is an inotropic agent whose primary activity results from stimulation of the beta receptors of the heart whilst producing mild chronotropic, hypertensive, arrhythmiogenic or vasodilator effects. The usual rate of infusion ranges from 2.5 to 10 mcg/kg/min. The patient's response ultimately determines the infusion rate.

Adverse Drug Reactions

The majority of adverse reactions are related to an extension of the pharmacological effects of dobutamine. Other reactions have included nausea, vomiting and headaches.

Dopamine

Dopamine *(Intropin)* stimulates alpha, beta and dopaminergic receptors. However, the serum concentration of the dopamine determines the receptor stimulated and the clinical effect seen. At low dosages (2 to 5 mcg/kg/min), dopaminergic receptors are stimulated, and renal and mesenteric vasodilation are seen. At dosages between 5 and 20 mcg/kg/min, the total peripheral resistance is relatively unchanged because of similar alpha and beta effects. However if the dose is greater than 20 mcg/kg/min, the predominating effect is vasoconstriction mediated via alpha-receptor stimulation.

Adverse Drug Reactions

Cardiovascular: ectopic beats, tachycardia, anginal pain, palpitation, hypotension and vasoconstriction.
Gastrointestinal: nausea, vomiting.
Central nervous system: headache.
Respiratory: dyspnoea.

Precautions

Dopamine should not be added to alkaline diluents as this will result in inactivation.

Patients taking monoamine oxidase inhibitors require a substantially reduced starting dose.

Care must be exercised in patients with peripheral vascular disease because of the danger of peripheral ischaemia and subsequent gangrene.

CARDIAC STIMULANTS — CALCIUM SALTS

Calcium chloride or ***calcium gluconate 10%*** may be given by IV injection (slowly) in the treatment of cardiac arrest. Its main actions are:

1. stimulation of the myocardium to spontaneous contraction; it is especially valuable where there is ECG evidence of coordinated electrical activity even though no pulse is palpable; it may stimulate such activity even when adrenaline has failed;

2. correction of myocardial calcium/potassium imbalance; this may be indicated where there has been some return of function of the ventricle, but myocardial contractions remain weak.

The adult dose of calcium gluconate is 1 g. Slow intravenous injection, 1 mL per minute, is essential.

Calcium gluconate should be administered with caution to digitalised patients. It must *not* be mixed with sodium-bicarbonate infusion as a precipitate will form immediately. Calcium gluconate is incompatible with adrenaline.

SODIUM BICARBONATE

Metabolic acidosis occurs rapidly following a cardiac arrest.

Sodium bicarbonate as an IV infusion solution of 8.4% (that is, 1 mmol/mL) is used to combat acidosis. It is important that this correction in base deficit be made early. The usual dose of 50 mmol may be repeated every eight to 10 minutes. Acid-base status should be determined as soon as possible to avoid overdose.

Precautions

1. Sodium bicarbonate solution is to be given by intravenous infusion only — never by any other route.
2. Calcium salts must not be added to sodium bicarbonate solutions as a precipitate will result. Many other drugs may be unstable in the pH range of the bicarbonate solution, including atropine, adrenaline, noradrenaline and isoprenaline. *It is therefore recommended that no drugs be mixed with sodium bicarbonate solution.*

NURSING IMPLICATIONS

Assessment

The duration of the cardiac arrest has significant bearing on the amounts of sodium bicarbonate required to correct acidosis, so the time of arrest must be noted. Monitoring of the ECG should be instituted as soon as possible, so that arrhythmias can be treated appropriately. Once circulation is re-established, frequent and regular checks of heart rate, arterial pressure and peripheral perfusion are required for the correct drug treatment to be prescribed.

Administration

Sodium bicarbonate solution should be prepared for infusion or bolus injection (from a pre-packed syringe) as soon as the equipment and sufficient personnel are available. If sodium bicarbonate is given through an intravenous line, it should be flushed with 5% dextrose solution or normal saline before other drugs are given into the same line in order to prevent interactions and precipitations.

An intravenous line should be established and other drugs prepared as required. The nurse must be thoroughly familiar with the location and lay out of the drug compartments of the resuscitation trolley. All medications must be carefully checked, clearly labelled and accurately recorded, even though speed is also essential. The time at which each dose is given should be documented.

When infusions (such as dopamine) are used, flow rates need to be accurately controlled, preferably by an infusion pump.

Evaluation
Constant observation of the ECG and clinical status of the patient provide the basis for evaluation of drug therapy in cardiac arrest. The record of the resuscitation procedure provides valuable information for evaluating performance and outcome.

DIURETICS

The volume of urine produced by the body is controlled by several factors. Although there are many mechanisms involved, the most important of these is related to the amount of sodium reabsorbed through the proximal portion of the renal tubule. Increased reabsorption of sodium leads to increased reabsorption of water, resulting in lessened urine formation. This appears to be largely an osmotic effect. Other factors, such as acid-base balance and the effects of aldosterone and anti-diuretic hormone, are also important but to a lesser extent.

FIGURE 2: DIAGRAMMATIC REPRESENTATION OF THE RENAL TUBULE SHOWING THE MAIN SITES OF ACTION OF VARIOUS CLASSES OF DIURETICS.

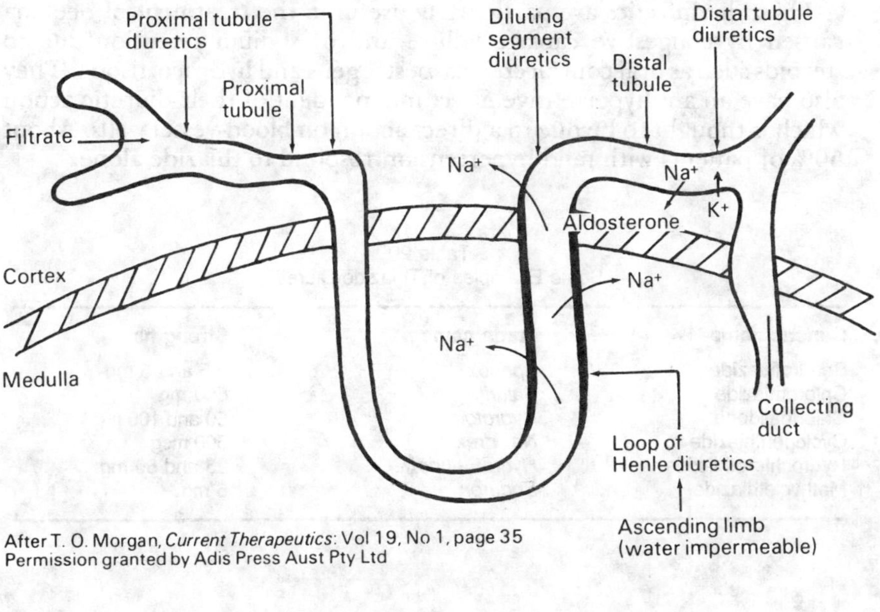

After T. O. Morgan, *Current Therapeutics*: Vol 19, No 1, page 35
Permission granted by Adis Press Aust Pty Ltd

In the normal situation these processes adjust themselves so that the renal excretion of sodium is equal to intake and oedema does not occur. If these renal adjustments fail, oedema will occur regardless of the nature of the primary disease which is usually cardiac, renal or hepatic in origin. Treatment is directed at both the primary cause of the condition and at the symptom, oedema.

Diuretics act within the kidney to increase production of urine, usually by blocking the reabsorption of sodium. Decreased reabsorption of sodium leads to decreased reabsorption of water, resulting in increased formation of urine. Figure 2 shows the main sites of diuretic action.

The diuretic effect of mercury has been known for centuries, but its systematic use did not start until the early 1920s with the introduction of mersalyl and mercaptomerin (*Thiomerin*). Both were highly effective drugs and toxic reactions were rare. Their use was limited because both had to be given by injection and were therefore inconvenient in chronic oedematous conditions.

Another group of drugs, now rarely used for generalised oedema, is that of the carbonic anhydrase inhibitors such as acetazolamide (*Diamox*). Experimentation with this group led to the development of the important thiazide diuretics.

THIAZIDE DIURETICS

This group of diuretics, of which ***chlorothiazide*** *(Saluric)* is the prototype, acts by inhibiting the reabsorption of sodium at the diluting segment of the ascending limb of the renal tubule (see Figure 2). Table 20 lists representatives of this class of diuretics, strengths available and some brand names. All thiazide diuretics may be taken orally.

Thiazide diuretics are particularly useful in the treatment of oedema caused by congestive cardiac failure and of sodium retention due to steroids such as oral contraceptives, oestrogens and hydrocortisone. They also have an antihypertensive effect independent of their diuretic action which is thought to be due to a direct action on blood-vessel walls. About 50% of patients with mild hypertension respond to thiazide alone.

Table 20
Some Examples of Thiazide Diuretics

Generic name	**Trade name**	**Strengths**
Bendrofluazide	*Aprinox*	2.5 and 5 mg
Chlorothiazide	*Saluric*	500 mg
Chlorthalidone*	*Hygroton*	50 and 100 mg
Cyclopenthiazide	*Navidrex*	500 mcg
Hydrochlorothiazide	*HydroSaluric*	25 and 50 mg
Methyclothiazide	*Enduron*	5 mg

Adverse Drug Reactions

This group of drugs may cause gastrointestinal irritation, dehydration if taken in excess, potassium depletion and an increase in plasma uric acid and glucose levels.

Gastrointestinal irritation may cause nausea, abdominal cramps or epigastric discomfort. The patient should be carefully observed for signs and symptoms of dehydration. Early in treatment, when diuresis is most profound and diet is likely to be restricted, weakness, paraesthesias and fatigue may occur due to potassium loss. Mild hypokalaemia is regarded as acceptable if the patient is not taking digoxin, and in the long term, less than 15% of patients require potassium supplements. However, in a patient taking digoxin, potassium levels must be maintained because hypokalaemia can induce digoxin toxicity.

Diuretics of this type cause elevation of plasma uric acid and glucose. Their effect may therefore cause or intensify gout or diabetes in susceptible or "borderline" patients. Rashes occur occasionally.

MORE POTENT DIURETICS — Frusemide and Bumetanide

Two diuretics act at the loop of Henle as well as at most proximal sites (see Figure 2). These two substances, ***frusemide*** *(Lasix)* and ***bumetanide*** *(Burinex)*, therefore have a more potent effect than the thiazides. They act more rapidly but for a shorter period of time (see Table 21). Frusemide is the more widely used. Special care must be taken to administer the correct dose. It is available in several strengths in both tablets and injection solution, a low-dose form for general use and a high-dose form for use in renal failure.

Table 21
Doses, Onset of Action and Duration Times of Some Diuretics

Generic name	**Dose range**	**Onset of action**	**Duration**
Amiloride	5-20 mg	2 hours	24 hours
Bendrofluazide	2.5-10 mg	2 hours	12-18 hours
Chlorothiazide	500 mg-2 g	2 hours	10 hours
Chlorthalidone	25-100 mg	2 hours	48 hours
Cyclopenthiazide	500 mcg-1.5 mg	2 hours	12 hours
Ethacrynic acid	100-400 mg	20 minutes	6 hours
Frusemide (low dose)	20-80 mg oral	15 minutes	4-6 hours
	20-100 mg IV	2 minutes	2 hours
Frusemide (high dose)	500 mg-2 g oral	15 minutes	4 hours
	250 mg-5 g IV	2 minutes	2 hours
Hydrochlorothiazide	25-200 mg	2 hours	12 hours
Mannitol	50–200 g IV	5 minutes	2 hours
Methyclothiazide	2.5–10 mg	2 hours	24 hours
Spironolactone	25–400 mg	24 hours	72 hours
Triamterene	100–250 mg	2 hours	10 hours

Adverse Drug Reactions

Both frusemide and bumetanide can cause elevated serum uric-acid levels, but the hyperglycaemic effect, while still present, is less than that of the thiazides. Transient deafness may result from both, and permanent deafness, although rare, has occurred with ethacrynic acid. The transient deafness related to the use of frusemide usually only presents a problem in the high-dose range, that is, over 500 mg orally or 250 mg by injection, but some incidences of hearing impairment have been reported with doses of 120 mg orally taken over a period of time.

Potassium loss with its associated symptoms of weakness and lassitude may be marked. Replacement potassium therapy is common with these two drugs.

POTASSIUM SUPPLEMENTS

To compensate for the loss of potassium caused by some diuretic agents, replacement therapy is often instituted. ***Potassium chloride*** is most often used and comes in several forms: a slow-release tablet *(Slow K)*, which must be swallowed whole, not crushed, in order to avoid damage to the stomach lining; effervescent tablets *(Sando K)* which must be dissolved in water; and liquid forms *(Kay-Cee-L)* which should be diluted in a glass of water or fruit juice before administration.

In acute cases of severe potassium depletion, the injectable form may be used.

"POTASSIUM-SPARING" DIURETICS

Not all diuretics have the potassium-depleting effect of those already mentioned. Several which act on the distal portion of the renal tubule (see Figure 2) have potassium-sparing effects. That is, potassium is retained by the body instead of being excreted.

One of these, ***spironolactone*** (*Aldactone*) is an aldosterone antagonist. Aldosterone normally causes sodium retention at the distal portion of the tubule. Spironolactone, by blocking the action of aldosterone, causes potassium retention, but loss of sodium with weak diuresis.

Two other drugs, ***amiloride*** (*Midamor*) and ***triamterene*** (*Dytac*), also retain potassium at the distal tubule but do so by a different mechanism. They have weak diuretic action and therefore are usually given for their potassium-sparing effects in combination with other more effective diuretics. Two such combination products, hydrochlorothiazide and amiloride (*Moduretic*), and hydrochlorothiazide and triamterene (*Dyazide*), are available. These combine the diuretic effect of one substance with the potassium-sparing effect of the other.

Adverse Drug Reactions

In using this group of drugs, care must be taken to avoid hyperkalaemia. This is only likely to occur if the patient is in renal failure or when supplementary potassium is being administered at the same time. Spironolactone may cause drowsiness, lethargy and, with prolonged use, gynaecomastia in males.

OSMOTIC DIURETICS

Mannitol, urea and ***glycerol*** are osmotically active substances that may be used as diuretics. Mannitol, usually given intravenously as a 10% to 20% infusion, is the most widely used. It exerts its effect at the tubule, inhibiting water reabsorption and hence increases urine formation. The chief use of this type of diuretic is in the reduction of cerebral oedema or intraocular pressure.

THE USE OF DIURETICS

As has already been noted, diuretics are used for the reduction of oedema, excess fluid being excreted as urine. The thiazide group have an additional action in the reduction of hypertension, either alone or in combination with other drugs with which they act synergistically (that is, the combined effect of the two drugs is greater than that expected from a simple additive effect). Diuretics may also be used in the treatment for some poisons. Drugs eliminated primarily via the kidneys may be removed from the body more quickly by means of "forced diuresis" when a diuretic (usually frusemide) and appropriate parenteral fluids and electrolytes are administered with a view to increasing elimination of the substance in urine.

NURSING IMPLICATIONS

Assessment

Baseline assessment should include cardiovascular status, degree of pulmonary and peripheral oedema, urinary output, weight and serum electrolytes. Diabetic patients taking thiazides may become hyperglycaemic, so blood-sugar levels should be assessed, even in the well-controlled diabetic. Thiazides and frusemide can also increase uric-acid levels, so patients with (or susceptible to) gout need to be identified as at risk. Hearing function should be assessed before beginning administration of frusemide, bumetanide or ethacrynic acid. Patients must be warned that urine output is expected to increase.

Administration

Diuretics are best taken in the early part of the day, for most people, because of the increase in urine output, the time of onset and the duration of action. If divided doses are prescribed, it is advisable to give the last dose during the early afternoon, rather than at night, unless the patient is catheterised.

If thiazide diuretics cause gastric irritation, they may be given with food.

If frusemide is given intravenously, the time of onset of action (two minutes) should be noted, and the patient warned, if he is not catheterised. A urine receptacle should be at hand.

When potassium supplements are given, the most appropriate dose form should be chosen. Some patients find the slow-release forms too large to swallow, and liquid forms may be more acceptable. Syrups are more palatable when diluted in water or fruit juice. For intragastric administration, liquid forms must be used. Intravenous potassium supplements are discussed in Chapter 34.

Evaluation

The degree of response to diuretics can be documented by recording fluid intake and output volumes, or more accurately by daily weight records. Fluid restrictions may need to be imposed at the same time as diuretics are given. Decreasing oedema and diminution in the other signs of heart failure are expected. However, patients should be observed for signs of dehydration if diuresis is excessive.

Potassium, uric acid and blood-glucose levels should be monitored frequently. Hyperkalaemia may occur when potassium-sparing diuretics are used; hypokalaemia may occur with other diuretics. The cardiac implications of potassium imbalance must be appreciated.

Hearing should be evaluated in patients taking ethacrynic acid.

Patients with prostatic hypertrophy must be observed for signs of urinary obstruction, especially after intravenous administration of diuretics.

Patient teaching

Patients must understand that increased urine output is the expected and desired effect of diuretics and that they need to determine the best time of day to take them, according to their daily routine. The importance of taking potassium supplements correctly should be emphasised. Signs of adverse reactions and failure of therapeutic action should be taught.

THE TREATMENT OF HYPERTENSION

Hypertension is a common disease in Britain. Figures show that in the order of 1.5% to 2% of people aged 40 or more have a diastolic blood pressure greater than 100 mmHg and a further 8% to 10% have a diastolic blood pressure in the range of 95 to 110 mmHg.

It has been shown that patients with diastolic blood pressures greater than 100 mmHg are at considerable risk from complications such as heart failure, cerebral haemorrhage or malignant hypertension. Even at lower diastolic blood pressures, the risk from one or more of these complications, although reduced, is significant. A study carried out in the 1970s among the mild-hypertensive category indicated that early treatment will significantly reduce the risk of associated complications of hypertension such as cardiovascular and renal damage.

Problems involved with the treatment of hypertension include lack of identification of the problem within the community. Patient-oriented problems are often complex and include poor understanding of the significance of treatment (which is reflected in poor compliance) and adverse drug reactions, which may predispose non-motivated patients to discontinue their therapy. This factor is particularly important as many patients have had little or no adverse effects from their hypertension in marked contrast to the potential adverse reactions from drug therapy. However, most patients can be adequately treated with careful drug and dosage selection. Combinations of antihypertensive drugs permit control of blood pressure with lower dosages and a subsequent reduction in side effects. The mechanisms by which drugs exert an antihypertensive effect are diverse and will be dealt with individually under each drug category.

Table 22
Some Antihypertensive Agents

Thiazide diuretics	
	Chlorothiazide *(Saluric)*
	Bendrofluazide *(Aprinox)*
	Cyclopenthiazide *(Navidrex)*
Drugs which reduce sympathetic outflow from the autonomic nervous system	
Centrally acting drugs	Clonidine *(Catapres)*
	Methyldopa *(Aldomet)*
Ganglion-blocking agents	Trimetaphan *(Arfonad)*
Adrenergic-neurone blocking agents	Guanethidine *(Ismelin)*
	Bethanidine *(Esbatal)*
	Debrisoquine *(Declinax)*
Drugs causing depletion of autonomic transmitter	Reserpine *(Serpasil)*
Drugs which block noradrenergic receptors	
(a) non-selective beta blockers	Propranolol *(Inderal)*
	Pindolol *(Visken)*
	Oxprenolol *(Trasicor)*
	Timolol *(Blocadren)*
(b) cardio-selective beta blockers	Metroprolol *(Betaloc, Lopressor)*
	Atenolol *(Tenormin)*
(c) alpha and beta receptor blockers	Labetalol *(Trandate)*
(d) postsynaptic alpha blockers	Prazosin *(Hypovase)*
Directly acting vasodilators	
	Hydralazine *(Apresoline)*
	Minoxidil *(Loniten)*
	Diazoxide *(Eudemine)*
	Sodium nitroprusside *(Nipride)*
Angiotensin-converting-enzyme inhibitors	
	Captopril *(Capoten)*
	Enalapril *(Innovace)*

THIAZIDE DIURETICS

Due to the high success rate of diuretics in the treatment of mild to moderate hypertension, their usage in the first line of treatment is widespread. They are also widely used in combination with other antihypertensive agents. (For details relating to the drugs used, dosage and adverse drug reactions, see the section on diuretics page 109).

DRUGS WHICH REDUCE SYMPATHETIC OUTFLOW FROM THE AUTONOMIC NERVOUS SYSTEM

Centrally Acting Drugs

Clonidine

The hypotensive action of clonidine (*Catapres* 100 and 300 mcg tablets) is produced mainly by its central effect of reducing sympathetic drive. Initially the dosage is 50-100 mcg 3 times daily, increasing every third day to a maximum daily dose of normally 1-2 mg.

Adverse Drug Reactions

Adverse reactions include dryness of mouth, sedation, constipation and fluid retention, all of which may necessitate the alteration of dosage. Rebound hypertension is a phenomenon associated with abrupt withdrawal of this drug, and patients should be advised accordingly not to alter their dosage or run out of medication.

Methyldopa

The main postulated mechanism of action of methyldopa (*Aldomet* 125 mg, 250 mg and 500 mg) in the CNS is due to its metabolism to alpha-methyl noradrenaline which then lowers arterial pressure by stimulation of central inhibitory alpha-adrenergic receptors. The recommended dosage range is between 500 mg and 3 g daily in divided doses.

Adverse Drug Reactions

Sedation, although transitory, is seen during initial treatment and usually when doses are increased. Other early reactions are headache and weakness. Symptoms of orthostatic hypotension, bradycardia, nasal stuffiness, mild dryness of mouth and gastrointestinal disturbances usually respond to reductions in dosage. Impotence in males has been reported.

Ganglion Blocking Agents

Agents like ***trimetaphan*** (*Arfonad*) act on the autonomic ganglia to prevent the transmitter acetylcholine from being able to stimulate the receptor on the postganglionic axon. The marked adverse reactions associated with these agents, including orthostatic hypotension and associated anticholinergic effects (blurred vision, dry mouth and urinary retention), tachycardia and respiratory depression make these agents unsuitable for most therapeutic situations, particularly with the wide variety of other agents available. Trimetaphan's use is limited to providing hypotension in surgery.

ADRENERGIC NEURONE-BLOCKING AGENTS

Adrenergic neurone-blocking agents prevent the release of noradrenaline from the postganglionic fibre, thereby reducing the number of noradrenergic receptors being stimulated. This reduction in the stimulation of noradrenergic receptors results in a subsequent reduction of blood pressure.

Guanethidine *(Ismelin,* 10 mg, 25 mg tablets), dosage 30 to 60 mg daily; in rare cases, 100 to 150 mg may be required. ***Bethanidine*** *(Esbatal,* 10 and 50 mg tablet), dosage 20 to 150 mg daily; the usual average daily dosage is 70 mg. ***Debrisoquine*** *(Declinax,* 10 mg, 20 mg tablets), dosage 20 to 120 mg daily.

Adverse Drug Reactions

Orthostatic hypotension is a major problem with adrenergic neurone-blocking drugs and is more commonly a problem in the morning when the patient rises. Diarrhoea is another commonly encountered adverse reaction with guanethidine. Sexual impotence occurs only occasionally with guanethidine. The extent and severity of adverse reactions associated with this group of drugs has, in general, led to a reduction in their usage, particularly with the advent of newer types of drugs with lesser adverse effects.

DRUGS CAUSING DEPLETION OF AUTONOMIC TRANSMITTER

Reserpine *(Serpasil,* 250 mcg tablet)
The mechanism of action of reserpine is by the depletion of noradrenaline from postganglionic neurones. Dosage is 0.25 to 1.0 mg daily in divided doses.

Adverse Drug Reactions

Mental depression occurs at high doses. Nasal stuffiness, lethargy and apathy, gain in weight and diarrhoea also occur. Special care should be taken in general anaesthesia to avoid hypotension. Long-term use has been associated with the promotion of breast cancer.

DRUGS WHICH BLOCK NORADRENERGIC RECEPTORS — BETA-BLOCKING DRUGS

Non-selective beta-blocking drugs will block both beta-1 and beta-2 receptors. Cardioselective beta-blockers will only block beta-1 receptors. Cardioselective beta-blocking drugs represent an advantage in that they will not significantly block beta-2 receptors responsible for bronchodilation in the lung. Despite their selectivity, they are still not recommended for asthmatics because of the likelihood of precipitation of asthma when administered in high doses.

When discontinuing beta-blocking agents, care should be taken to reduce the dosage gradually, for example, over seven to 10 days, particularly in the case of ischaemic heart disease, as an abrupt withdrawal may result in an acute deterioration of the patient's condition.

Care must be exercised in patients undergoing surgery due to the possibilities of interactions between anaesthetic agents and beta-blocking agents. However, the use of atropine is usually sufficient to overcome any cardiac problems and withdrawal of beta-blockers is generally unnecessary.

The mechanism of beta-blockers in hypertension is complex and not completely understood. Some of the possible actions include a central mode of action, reduction in cardiac output and peripheral effects.

Non selective beta blockers
Propranolol *(Inderal,* 10, 40, 80, 160 mg tablets)
Dosage is 160 to 320 mg daily. In a few cases, as much as 1 g per day is necessary to control blood pressure.
Pindolol *(Visken,* 5 mg, 15 mg tablets)
Dosage is 15 to 45 mg daily in divided doses.
Oxprenolol *(Trasicor,* 20 mg, 40 mg, 80 mg, 160 mg tablets)
Dosage is 120 to 480 mg daily in divided doses.
Timolol *(Blocadren,* 10 mg tablet)
Dosage is 20 to 60 mg daily. The majority of patients respond to 30 mg.

Adverse Drug Reactions

Patients with a history of asthma or obstructive airways disease should not receive beta-blockers because of the possiblity of bronchospasm. Similarly these drugs should be avoided in patients with bradycardia or atrioventricular conduction disturbances.

Central nervous system reactions include hallucinations, bizarre dreams, nightmares, insomnia and depression, especially with propranolol and pindolol. Other adverse reactions include gastrointestinal effects such as nausea and diarrhoea, lethargy, tiredness, mild depression and various skin reactions.

Cardio-selective beta blockers
These drugs essentially block beta receptors in the heart (beta-1) resulting in a greater specificity of action compared with non-selective beta blockers. Despite this specificity of action, their use in patients with asthma or obstructive airways disease is not recommended because of the possibility of bronchospasm.

Metoprolol *(Betaloc, Lopressor,* 50 mg, 100 mg tablets)
Dosage is 100 to 200 mg twice daily.

Adverse Drug Reactions

Effects reported include bronchospasm, cardiac failure, muscular cramps, weakness, oedema, prolongation of AV conduction time, insomnia, lethargy, increased dreaming and a positive anti-nuclear factor (ANF). Other effects include ocular and skin reactions.

Atenolol *(Tenormin,* 50 mg, 100 mg tablets)
Dosage is 100 mg daily and controls a majority of patients.

Adverse Drug Reactions

These include bradycardia, coldness of the extremities and muscular weakness. Sleep disturbances are rare. Dizziness and skin rashes have been reported.

Alpha and beta receptor blockers
Labetalol *(Trandate,* 100 mg, 200 mg, 400 mg tablets)
Labetalol is the only example of a drug used clinically for alpha and beta blockade. The mechanism of action of labetalol in lowering blood pressure is to reduce peripheral resistance by blocking alpha receptors. The beta blockade blocks reflex increases in heart rate caused by peripheral vasodilation. Dosage is 200 to 2400 mg daily.

Adverse Drug Reactions

Headache, gastrointestinal tract disturbances, dizziness, lassitude, lethargy, tiredness and malaise have been reported. Bronchospasm may occur in susceptible individuals.

Postsynaptic alpha blocker
Prazosin *(Hypovase,* 0.5 mg, 1 mg, 2 mg, 5 mg tablets)
Prazosin, although often classified as a vasodilator, actually allows vasodilation to occur by blocking postsynaptic alpha receptors. Dosage therapy must be initiated slowly to prevent the possibility of sudden loss of consciousness. Initial doses are usually 500 mcg three times daily, increasing gradually to maintenance doses of between 3 mg and 20 mg in divided doses.

Adverse Drug Reactions

Postural dizziness, drowsiness, palpitations, urinary frequency and diaphoresis have been reported.

DIRECTLY ACTING VASODILATORS

The mechanism of action of this group of drugs is to produce vasodilation resulting in a drop in blood pressure. The actual mechanism by which these drugs produce this effect differs.

Hydralazine *(Apresoline,* 25 mg, 50 mg tablets)
The dosage for initial therapy is 25 mg to 50 mg daily with doses being raised to 100 mg daily, according to individual response. In causing vasodilation, hydralazine usually causes a reflex tachycardia and hence is often combined with beta-blocking drugs to overcome this problem.

Adverse Drug Reactions

Tachycardia, vomiting, headache, localised oedema, skin rashes and urticaria have been reported. Doses in excess of 200 mg per day have, in some cases, been associated with a clinical picture resembling acute systemic lupus erythematosus.

Minoxidil *(Loniten,* 2.5 mg, 5 mg, 10 mg tablets)
Minoxidil is a potent orally active vasodilator agent which acts on peripheral arteriolar smooth musculature, reducing peripheral vascular resistance and arterial blood pressure. The recommended dosage regimen is to initiate therapy with 5 mg per day. Increments of 5 mg to 10 mg are then made at three-day intervals until 50 mg/day is reached.

Adverse Drug Reactions

Cardiovascular reactions include pericarditis, pericardial effusions, salt and water retention, peripheral oedema, reflex tachycardia, arrhythmias and hypotension. Dermatological reactions include hypertrichosis in between 50% and 70% of patients, skin rashes and pruritus. Respiratory reactions include dyspnoea and bronchospasm.

Diazoxide (*Eudemine* 300 mg/20 mL IV injection)
Diazoxide is a potent vasodilating agent structurally related to the thiazide diuretics. It is, however, devoid of a diuretic action. Diazoxide produces a reduction in blood pressure by a direct effect on arteriolar smooth muscle. This fall in peripheral resistance is offset to a small extent by an increase in heart rate and cardiac output. Dosage is given as a rapid intravenous injection of 300 mg for adults. In children a dose of 5 mg/kg is usually used.

Adverse Drug Reactions

Hypotension has occasionally been observed. Gastrointestinal upsets include nausea, vomiting and abdominal discomfort. Transient hyperglycaemia and the retention of sodium and water occur frequently but rarely require treatment.

Sodium nitroprusside (*Nipride,* vial 50 mg)
Sodium nitroprusside is a powerful dilator of both arterioles and venules. However, its action only lasts for one or two minutes and the drug must be administered by constant intravenous infusion. On discontinuing the infusion, blood pressure returns to pretreatment levels within two to three minutes. The drug is light-sensitive, and intravenous bottles containing sodium nitroprusside should be wrapped to protect the drug from degradation. Dosage is dependent on response, but initial dose would be 100 mg/L in 5% dextrose in water at a rate of 20 microdrops per minute.

Adverse Drug Reactions

These include sweating, muscular twitching, nausea, anxiety and apprehension which are generally related to a rapid reduction in blood pressure and can be overcome by reducing the administration rate. If administration continues for more than 72 hours, thiocyanate (a metabolite) toxicity may become apparent, manifested by delirium and psychosis.

ANGIOTENSIN CONVERTING ENZYME INHIBITORS

Captopril (*Capoten,* 12.5 mg, 25 mg, 50 mg tablets)
Although the exact mechanism of action of captopril is not fully understood, it is thought to lower blood pressure primarily through suppression of the renin-angiotensin-aldosterone system. Captopril produces its effect by inhibiting the enzyme responsible for converting angiotensin I to

angiotensin II which is one of the most potent endogenous vasoconstrictor substances.

The dosage of captopril must be individualized according to the clinical response of each patient. In order to avoid a precipitous hypotensive response, patients should be commenced on the lowest possible dosage and then the dosage increased slowly at weekly or biweekly intervals.

Adverse Drug Reactions

Most of the adverse reactions, including rash and loss of taste, are dose related and will often disappear with a dose reduction. Proteinuria can occur and is more common in patients with pre-existing renal disease; proteinuria should be checked for monthly. Neutropenia and agranulocytosis is a serious reversible complication. The white blood-cell count should be monitored fortnightly for the first 12 weeks of therapy in patients with pre-existing renal disease, or with connective tissue diseases.

COMBINED THERAPY

Antihypertensive therapy most often commences with the use of a thiazide diuretic followed by the addition of a beta-adrenergic blocking agent. Drugs from other pharmacological groups may be added and combined for further effect. Combination often reduces the dose required for a single drug and, as a consequence, may reduce the number and severity of adverse effects.

Table 23
Site, Mechanism of Action and Adverse Effects of Antihypertensive Agents

Drug	Site of Action	Mechanism	Adverse Effects
Beta blockers	Mid-brain	Uncertain	CNS: sleep disturbances, blurred vision, drowsiness Respiratory: asthma Cardiovascular: cardiac failure, bradycardia, hypotension, Raynaud's syndrome Metabolic: interference with carbohydrate metabolism Skeletal: cramps, fatigue, gastrointestinal disturbances Haematological: thrombocytopenia, agranulocytosis (rare)
Clonidine	Mid-brain	Reduces sympathetic outflow by stimulation of alpha adrenoceptors	Drowsiness, depression, gastrointestinal disturbances, dry mouth, rebound hypertension on sudden withdrawal
Methyldopa	Mid-brain	Reduces sympathetic outflow by stimulation of alpha adrenoceptors	Postural hypotension, drowsiness, headache, depression, fluid retention, GIT disturbances, nausea, diarrhoea, haemolytic anaemia (positive Coombs' test in more than 20% patients) rashes, nasal stuffiness, sexual dysfunction
Reserpine	Mid-brain	Depletion of transmitter	Depression, nasal stuffiness, lethargy, dreams, increasing weight, diarrhoea
Ganglion blockers (trimetaphan)	Autonomic ganglia	Blockade of sympathetic transmission	Not useful in practice

Adrenergic neurone blockers (e.g. guanethidine, bethanidine)	Adrenergic axons	Inhibition of transmitter release	Postural hypotension, diarrhoea (guanethidine), parotid tenderness, failure of ejaculation
Methyldopa	Adrenergic axons	False transmitter, causes some depletion of transmitter	As above
Prazosin	Alpha adrenoceptors	Postjunctional adrenoceptor blocker	First-dose hypotension, GIT disturbances, nasal congestion, dry mouth, blurring of vision
Labetalol	Alpha adrenoceptors and beta adrenoceptors		
Beta blockers	Beta adrenoceptors	The exact mechanism is uncertain; may include reduction in cardiac output, resetting of baroreceptors	As above
Hydralazine	Vascular smooth muscle	Uncertain, but producing vasodilation	Systemic lupus erythematosus, drug fever, headache, nausea, skin rashes, tachycardia, fluid retention
Minoxidil	Vascular smooth muscle	Uncertain but producing vasodilation	Tachycardia, angina, oedema, hypertrichosis, pericardial effusion pulmonary hypertension
Verapamil	Vascular smooth muscle	Uncertain but producing vasodilation	GIT upsets, cardiac failure, palpitations, aggravation of heart block
Thiazide diuretics	Kidneys	Volume depletion	Hypokalaemia, hyperuricaemia, hyperglycaemia, skin rashes
Captopril	Renin-angiotensin system	Blocks the enzyme responsible for converting angiotensin I to angiotensin II	Rash, loss of taste, proteinuria, neutropenia, agranulocytosis

NURSING IMPLICATIONS

Attention is directed to page 113 for the discussion of nursing implications of diuretic therapy.

Assessment

Establishment of the baseline arterial pressure is essential for monitoring the effects of antihypertensive drugs. The goal arterial pressure must be documented for comparison. A goal of 120/90 to 140/90 mm Hg is common. Because there are so many different types of drugs used to reduce arterial pressure, nurses must check on the adverse reactions reported for each group. Elderly patients are more likely to suffer from adverse effects.

Since non-compliance is a major problem with antihypertensive therapy, the probability of compliance in the long term should be assessed. Other approaches being taken to reduce blood pressure, such as sodium restriction, should be documented and reinforced.

Administration

A regular pattern of administration, which is designed to fit in with the patient's daily routine, will help to increase compliance, especially when multiple drugs are used.

Sodium nitroprusside is administered by continuous intravenous infusion, with flow rates titrated to arterial-pressure response. The use of an infusion-regulating device is vital.

Antihypertensive therapy should not be ceased suddenly.

Evaluation

Evaluation of patients' responses to antihypertensive therapy involves monitoring arterial pressure and the occurrence of adverse reactions.

Arterial pressures must be recorded accurately and under reproducible conditions. The patient should rest for about 10 minutes before the pressure is measured. Recordings taken in the lying, sitting and standing positions will allow for evaluation of orthostatic (postural) hypotension. This problem is manifest by dizziness or faintness on rising and can be avoided by sitting, and then standing, slowly. Several recordings may need to be made at different times of the day. Some institutional policies require that arterial pressure is measured before the administration of each dose. When intravenous routes are used, either continuous arterial-pressure monitoring or recording at short intervals (for example, five minutes) is essential.

Patients should be observed for signs of hypotension, including faintness, dizziness, light-headedness, chest pain and cardiac arrhythmias, which all result from ischaemia. These signs may be evident while the measured pressure is still higher than the goal pressure, or "normal" range, if the pressure has dropped too rapidly for controlling mechanisms to have adapted.

Persistent hypertension should be reported to the prescriber, so that an alternative treatment can be selected. If antihypertensive drugs are withdrawn, or doses changed suddenly, rebound hypertension may sometimes occur.

Nurses must be alert for the adverse reactions reported for each drug, especially bronchospasm in patients taking beta blockers. Reactions may be reduced by dose reduction or a change in the drug regime.

Patient teaching

Several aspects of patient education are important. The medical consequences of uncontrolled hypertension, and the need to take medication regularly and to have regular medical checks are important. Possible causes of non-compliance should be identified, and plans acceptable to the patient made to establish compliance.

Other risk factors, such as high sodium intake and other coronary risk factors should be identified. Risk-factor reduction is an essential part of patient eduction in hypertension.

Patients should be advised of the common adverse reactions they might encounter and told that therapy should not be stopped suddenly. If the adverse effects experienced are unacceptable to the patient, and lead to non-compliance, then a different drug regime should be requested or a non-drug alternative be explored.

A supply of medication should be kept in advance, to avoid missing doses, and doses should not be "doubled up" if they are forgotten or missed.

Family support is usually helpful in establishing a regular dosage regime. Motivation can be increased by telling the patient his or her goal pressure and the actual pressure each time it is recorded. Refusal to reveal the actual pressure can increase a patient's anxiety and frustration with treatment and might even increase blood pressure.

PERIPHERAL VASODILATORS

Another group of drugs acting upon the vascular system are those called *peripheral vasodilators.* As the name suggests, they cause vasodilatation of the blood vessels in the peripheral regions of the body and are therefore used in conditions characterised by poor circulation in such areas, for example, Raynaud's disease and chilblains.

Some drugs, such as ***nicotinic acid, phenoxybenzamine*** (*Dibenyline*) and ***tolazoline,*** cause dilatation by blocking the alpha receptors in vascular walls. The mode of action of others, such as ***rutin derivatives*** *(Paroven),* is not clear. The use of these drugs is not widespread as there is no general consensus as to their effectiveness. However, they all cause a transient warm tingling sensation in the skin and extremities about which the patient should be advised before treatment begins.

Table 24
Drugs Used in the Treatment of Cardiovascular Disease

Drug Group	Drug Name	Use	Action	Adverse Reactions	Nursing Implications
Cardiac glycosides	Digoxin	CCF; arrhythmias	Increases force of contraction, slows heart rate, decreases conduction through the AV node	GIT disturbances, sinus bradycardia, ectopic beats, bigeminy, ventricular fibrillation, fatigue, headache, mental confusion, blurred vision	***Assess:*** apex and pulse rates, ECG rhythm, age, weight, electrolyte status, appetite, respiratory status; other drugs — quinidine. ***Administer:*** review if heart rate less than 60 per minute; give with food, same time each day; check strength and generic name carefully; potassium supplements to prevent toxicity, if hypokalaemic; reduced dose if taking quinidine. ***Evaluate:*** pulmonary and peripheral oedema should decrease; urine output should increase; ECG changes; signs of toxicity — anorexia, vomiting, diarrhoea, arrhythmias, visual disturbances; for hypokalaemia; response to withdrawal of the drug if toxicity occurs. ***Teach:*** signs of toxicity, heart failure; to count pulse rate; generic names.
Anti-arrhythmic drugs	Lignocaine	Ventricular arrhythmias	Stabilises cell membranes and depresses ectopic beats	Paraesthesias, auditory difficulty, drowsiness, agitation, nausea, vomiting, muscle twitching, seizures, hypotension, heart block, psychosis	***Assess:*** vital signs, ECG, previous hypersensitivity, drug interactions possible with digoxin. ***Administer:*** quinidine with food; sustained release tablets to be swallowed whole; with infusion pump if IVI; do not administer brown solutions of quinidine or procainamide; select appropriate lignocaine preparation. ***Evaluate:*** ECG; note

				signs of arterial and pulmonary embolisation; note adverse effects. ***Teach:*** correct dose schedules; direct families to CPR training.
Tocainide	Ventricular arrhythmias	Stabilises cell membranes and depresses ectopic beats	Nausea, vomiting, anorexia, dizziness, tremor, confusion, nervousness, disorientation, CNS toxicity	
Mexiletine	Ventricular arrhythmias	Stabilises cell membranes and depresses ectopic beats	Relatively rare; hypotension, bradycardia, drowsiness, confusion, nausea, vomiting, unpleasant taste	
Quinidine	Atrial and ventricular arrhythmias	Decreases excitability of cardiac muscle; decreases conduction velocity and contractility	High incidence of adverse reactions, nausea, vomiting, diarrhoea, rash, haemolytic anaemia, thrombocytopenia, fever	
Disopyramide	Atrial and ventricular arrhythmias	Action resembles quinidine	Dry mouth and nose, constipation, urinary hesitancy, blurred vision	
Procainamide	Premature ventricular beats, ventricular tachycardia, atrial arrhythmias	Action resembles quinidine	Similar to quinidine	
Phenytoin sodium	Ventricular arrhythmias	Depresses automaticity, improves conduction	Slurred speech, nystagmus, confusion, dizziness, (see Chapter 29)	

continued

Drug Group	Drug Name	Use	Action	Adverse Reactions	Nursing Implications
Anti-anginal Agents					
Nitrates	Glyceryl trinitrate (GTN) Isosorbide dinitrate (ISDN) Isosorbide mononitrate (ISMN)	Angina	Dilates vascular smooth muscle, reduces myocardial oxygen demand	Flushing, headache, hypotension, dizziness, weakness, fainting, drug tolerance may develop	***Assess:*** chest pain — quality, duration, associated activities. ***Administer:*** Sub-lingual — up to three tablets in 15 minutes of GTN 500 mcg or ISDN 5 mg; oral — ISMN, ISDN or GTN slow-release tablets; topical — ¼ to 1 square inch of ointment or one GTN sustained-release patch; avoid contact with own skin; IVI — GTN or ISDN infusions using infusion pump with polyethylene giving set; store away from light, heat, moisture, metal; note expiry dates. ***Evaluate:*** time for relief of chest pain, number of tablets required, adverse effects (particularly hypotension). ***Teach:*** administration method, correct storage, adverse effects, expected to diminish with time, to seek medical attention if pain persists longer than 15 minutes or not relieved by three tablets.
Beta-adrenergic blockers					
Cardioselective	Metoprolol, atenolol	Angina, hypertension, arrhythmias	Decrease heart rate and force of contraction and myocardial irritability, reduce myocardial oxygen demand	Generally well tolerated, bradycardia, hypotension, nausea, vomiting, diarrhoea, lassitude, visual disturbances, nightmares, hallucinations, rashes, paraesthesia, hypoglycaemia	***Assess:*** heart rate, blood pressure, beta adrenergic blockers and calcium antagonists for heart failure, asthma. ***Administer:*** taper off when therapy ceased, check policy for withdrawal before general anaesthetic. ***Evaluate:*** heart rate, arterial pressure, for signs of heart failure, bronchospasm. ***Teach:*** early signs of heart failure,

					hypotension, bradycardia; not to miss doses or to stop treatment suddenly.
Non-selective	Propranolol, oxprenolol, pindolol	Angina, hypertension, arrhythmias	Decrease heart rate, force of contraction and myocardial irritability, reduce myocardial oxygen demand	As above and bronchoconstriction	
Calcium antagonists	Verapamil, nifedipine, lidoflazine, nicardipine, diltiazem	Angina, hypertension	Reduce calcium inflow into cells, thus decreasing ventricular overload and preventing coronary vasospasm	Headache, congestion, nausea, vomiting, hypotension, oedema	***Assess:*** heart rate, blood pressure, beta adrenergic blockers and calcium antagonists for heart failure, asthma. ***Administer:*** taper off when therapy ceased, check policy for withdrawal before general anaesthetic. ***Evaluate:*** heart rate, arterial pressure, for signs of heart failure, bronchospasm. ***Teach:*** early signs of heart failure, hypotension, bradycardia; not to miss doses or to stop treatment suddenly.
Cardiac stimulants	Adrenaline	Cardiac arrest	Stimulates beta-1 receptors, stimulates heart to spontaneous contraction	Flushing, sweating, tremor, headache, tachycardia, palpitations	***Assess:*** note time at diagnosis, ECG, heart rate, arterial pressure, peripheral perfusion when circulation re-established. ***Administer:*** prepare sodium bicarbonate first; do not mix bicarbonate with any drug; check, label and record all doses and times. ***Evaluate:*** ECG rhythm, rate, arterial pressure, respiratory status.
	Isoprenaline	Cardiac arrest	As above	As above	
	Dobutamine	Cardiac arrest	Stimulates beta-1 receptors	Hypertension, vasodilation, nausea, vomiting, headache	

continued

Drug Group	Drug Name	Use	Action	Adverse Reactions	Nursing Implications
	Dopamine	Cardiac arrest	Stimulates alpha, beta and dopaminergic receptors	Ectopic beats, tachycardia, angina, hypotension, nausea, vomiting, headache, dyspnoea	
	Calcium salts	Cardiac arrest	Stimulates myocardium to spontaneous contraction, corrects K and Ca imbalance		
	Sodium bicarbonate	Cardiac arrest	To correct metabolic acidosis	Sodium bicarbonate overload if used to excess.	
Thiazide diuretics	Bendrofluazide Chlorothiazide Chlorthalidone Cyclopenthiazide Hydrochlorothiazide Methyclothiazide	Oedema due to CCF, oedema due to sodium and water retention, hypertension	Inhibition of sodium reabsorption in the diluting segment of the ascending limb of the renal tubule, unrelated antihypertensive action	GIT irritation dehydration, potassium depletion, raised plasma uric-acid and glucose levels	***Assess:*** Peripheral and pulmonary oedema, weight, urinary output, serum electrolytes, cardiovascular status, blood sugar levels in diabetics, hearing function before frusemide or ethacrynic acid. ***Administer:*** early in day, give thiazide with food; potassium supplements — select appropriate dose form; liquids for intragastric instillation. ***Evaluate:*** fluid balance, weight, decreasing oedema; for dehydration if diuresis excessive; potassium, uric acid and glucose levels; hearing with frusemide and ethacrynic acid; for urinary obstruction in prostatic hypertrophy. ***Teach:*** to expect diuresis; to take potassium supplements correctly; signs of adverse reactions.
Loop diuretics	**Frusemide, bumetanide**	More potent and rapidly acting than thiazides	Loop of Henle and proximal sites	Raised serum uric acid, hyperglycaemia, potassium depletion,	

				dehydration, transient deafness	
Potassium-sparing diuretics	Spironolactone	Weak diuretic	Aldosterone antagonist	Drowsiness, lethargy, gynaecomastia, hyperkalaemia	
	Amiloride, triamterene	Weak diuretic	Potassium retention at distal tubule	Hyperkalaemia	
Osmotic diuretics	Mannitol Urea Glycerol	Diuretic mainly in cerebral oedema and raised intraocular pressure	Inhibits water reabsorption along renal tubule	Dehydration, hyponatraemia, hypochloraemia	
Anti-hypertensive agents					
Centrally acting anti-hypertensive drugs	Clonidine	Hypertension	Reduction of sympathetic drive	Dry mouth, sedation, constipation, fluid retention, rebound hypertension on withdrawal, sedation, headache, weakness, orthostatic hypotension, bradycardia, nasal stuffiness, dry mouth, GIT disturbances, impotence	***Assess:*** Baseline arterial pressure, antihypertensive agents, goal arterial pressure, likelihood of compliance, other methods being used to reduce blood pressure; elderly patients more likely to suffer adverse effects. ***Administer:*** establish and reinforce regular pattern; sodium nitroprusside — IVI, titrated to desired arterial pressure; do not cease therapy suddenly. ***Evaluate:*** arterial pressure response; lying, sitting, standing BP for hypotension; continuous monitoring during IVI; signs of hypotension, ischaemia; persistent hypertension; for adverse effects. ***Teach:*** consequences of non-compliance; other coronary risk factors; adverse reactions; not to stop therapy suddenly; not to miss doses or catch-up; goal pressure and progress.
	Methyldopa	Hypertension	Stimulation of central inhibitory alpha-adrenergic receptors		

continued

Drug Group	Drug Name	Use	Action	Adverse Reactions	Nursing Implications
Ganglion blocking anti-hypertensive drugs	Trimetaphan	Hypertension	Prevent action of acetylcholine	Marked anticholinergic effects, orthostatic hypotension	
Adrenergic neurone blocking anti-hypertensives	Guanethidine Bethanidine Debrisoquine	Hypertension	Prevent release of noradrenaline from postganglionic fibres	Orthostatic hypotension, diarrhoea, impotence	
Anti-hypertensive drugs which deplete autonomic transmitter	Reserpine	Hypertension	Depletes noradrenaline in postganglionic neurones	Depression, nasal stuffiness, lethargy, apathy, weight gain, diarrhoea	
Beta-blocking drugs	See anti-anginal agents				
Alpha and beta blocking drugs	Labetalol	Hypertension	Decreases peripheral resistance by alpha blockade	Headache, GIT, disturbances, dizziness, lassitude, bronchospasm	
Postsynaptic alpha blockers	Prazosin	Hypertension	Blocks postsynaptic alpha receptors, thus causing vasodilatation	Postural dizziness, drowsiness, palpitations, urinary frequency, diaphoresis	
Direct-acting vasodilators	Hydralazine	Hypertension	Reduces BP by producing vasodilation and decreasing peripheral resistance	Reflex tachycardia, vomiting, headache, oedema, rash	As above

	Minoxidil	Hypertension	As above	Pericarditis, pericardial effusions, sodium and water retention, arrhythmias, hypotension, rash, dyspnoea, bronchospasm
	Diazoxide	Hypertension	Acts on arteriolar smooth muscle to cause vasodilation; potent drug, useful during crises	GIT upset, hyperglycaemia, sodium and water retention
	Sodium nitroprusside	Hypertension	Dilates arterioles and venules, rapid action, lasts only a few minutes, useful in crises, use continuous infusions	Sweating, muscle twitching, nausea, anxiety, apprehension, thiocyanate toxicity
Angiotensin converting-enzyme inhibitors	Captopril Enalapril	Hypertension	Suppresses renin-angiotensin-aldosterone system	Rash, loss of taste, proteinuria, neutropenia, agranulocytosis

SELF-EVALUATION TEST

1. Define the terms:
   (a) oedema
   (b) diuretic
   (c) antihypertensive agent.
2. Match the following drugs to the disease state in which they are used.

Drug	***Disease or Condition***
Digoxin (*Lanoxin*)	Angina pectoris
Frusemide *(Lasix)*	Hypertension
Methyldopa *(Aldomet)*	Congestive cardiac failure
Isosorbide dinitrate (*Isordil*)	Acidosis
Sodium bicarbonate injection	Cardiac arrhythmias
Quinidine (*Kinidin*)	Oedema

3. Describe in general terms the mechanism of action of:
   (a) diuretics
   (b) anti-arrhythmic drugs
   (c) beta-blocking adrenergic drugs.
4. List the nursing implications inherent in the use of the following drugs.
   (a) digoxin (*Lanoxin*)
   (b) methyldopa (*Aldomet*)
   (c) propranolol (*Inderal*)
   (d) glyceryl trinitrate
5. Beside each of the following drugs list its pharmacological class *or* the disease state for which it is used.

Drug	***Disease State/Class***
Pindolol (*Visken*)	
Bendrofluazide (*Aprinox*)	
Isoprenaline (*Isuprel*)	
Clonidine (*Catapres*)	
Nicotinic acid	
Atenolol (*Tenormin*)	
Procainamide (*Pronestyl*)	

8

DRUGS USED IN THE TREATMENT OF BLOOD DISORDERS

Ross D. MacPherson

OBJECTIVES

At the end of this chapter the reader should be able to:

1. name representative drugs from each pharmacological class discussed;
2. describe the pharmacological action of the drugs acting on the haemopoietic system and list the disease states in which they are employed;
3. give examples of two drugs with a low therapeutic ratio;
4. list the most common adverse effects of the drugs discussed;
5. name the antidotes for heparin and warfarin;
6. list the nursing implications of the use of drugs acting on the haemopoietic system.

PREREQUISITE KNOWLEDGE

Before reading this chapter the students should have a working knowledge of the physiology and pathophysiology of the haemopoietic system, in particular:

1. the clotting response;
2. the mechanism of clot formation and dissolution;
3. lipid productions;
4. disease states associated with deficiency of iron, folic acid and vitamin B_{12}.

ANTICOAGULANTS

Cuts and abrasions that bleed for just a few minutes then heal, are an everyday occurrence. That we are able to sustain such injuries to the body and not haemorrhage profusely is largely due to the life-saving action of the clotting system.

Physiology textbooks explain the "clotting cascade" and indicate the importance of both clotting factors and platelets in the clotting mechanism. It is sometimes necessary, however, to suppress the activity of the clotting system of the body. To accomplish this, agents referred to as ***anticoagulants*** are employed. It would seem obvious that the use of drugs to reduce the body's ability to form clots is not without dangers. The nursing of patients receiving these drugs requires considerable skill, so as to prevent the occurrence of any untoward effects. It must be understood from the outset that anticoagulant medications have a low therapeutic ratio. That is, the difference in the dose required to produce a therapeutic effect and that which could cause a toxic effect is small.

Specific conditions for which anticoagulant drugs may be prescribed include:

1. after implantation of artificial prostheses such as heart valves, where the blood may have a greater tendency to form clots because of the presence of foreign material;
2. in the prophylactic treatment of patients who have developed deep venous thrombosis or pulmonary emboli. It must be emphasised that anticoagulant treatment will not alter the structure of already formed clots, but will prevent the formation of new emboli;
3. following myocardial infarction.

An interesting feature of anticoagulant therapy is that anticoagulant levels are not measured directly to assess their effect. Rather, the clotting function of the blood is measured. A number of tests may be employed for this purpose and each hospital tends to favour one or another of these tests.

To assess the anticoagulant status of patients taking heparin, the following tests may be used: whole-blood clotting time; activated partial thromboplastin time (APTT); and the thrombin clotting time. For patients taking oral anticoagulants, the tests for anticoagulant status include: one-stage prothrombin time; prothrombin and proconvertin test (PTT); and the thrombotest.

There are two main anticoagulant groups in general use: ***heparin,*** an injectable anticoagulant, and a group of ***oral anticoagulants.***

HEPARIN

Heparin is a large mucopolysaccharide molecule which is obtained from sheep, cattle and pigs. Heparin is obtained from animal tissue because the structure of the drug is such that is is far too complicated to make in a laboratory. This is not a unique situation, as insulin is also obtained from animals.

Partly because of this, the dosage of heparin is not measured by weight (for example, milligrams) as you find with most other drugs, but rather is expressed as a number of units. These units are an arbitrary system which allows the anticoagulant activity of the drug to be roughly quantified.

Within the clotting cascade, one of the final steps is the conversion of prothrombin to thrombin. The rate at which this reaction proceeds is controlled by a substance called antithrombin III. This molecule prevents the conversion of prothrombin to thrombin from proceeding, and it is upon antithrombin III that heparin has its direct action. That is, heparin is an antithrombin III agonist. Heparin enhances the activity of this molecule many hundred times and hence prevents the conversion of prothrombin to thrombin.

In concluding this section, it must again be stressed that neither heparin nor the oral anticoagulants have any effect on breaking down clots once they have already formed. The use of anticoagulant drugs is of prophylactic nature only.

Dosage and Routes of Administration

Because heparin is a delicate protein molecule, it is completely ineffective when given orally. Heparin is administered only by the parenteral route. Considerable controversy exists as to the optimum method of administration. An outline of the most common methods is given below.

Intermittent intravenous administration

Heparin is administered intravenously via an IV cannula. It is generally accepted that half of an IV bolus dose of heparin will have been degraded within 90 minutes of administration. Because its length of action is so short, IV bolus injections are given frequently and a dose of 1500 units every 90 minutes is not uncommon, although some practitioners prefer larger amounts given less frequently.

Intravenous infusion

The administration of heparin by intravenous infusion has become increasingly popular over recent years. Usually about 30 000 units or 40 000 units of heparin are added to one litre of infusion solution (most often normal saline) or in approx 50 ml in syringe pump and infused over 24 hours. Some researchers have queried the stability of heparin in solution for such a long period, but it is generally accepted that in saline solutions it will retain its activity for this period. Heparin infusions require the use of specialised equipment to monitor infusion rates accurately.

Subcutaneous injection

The third method by which heparin may be administered is by subcutaneous injection. This method is often used before and after surgery, and the injection need only be administered twice or three times daily.

Adverse Reactions and Precautions

Heparin administration is associated with a low incidence of adverse reactions. Apart from a local irritation, some patients may suffer mild pyrexia, but severe systemic adverse effects are rare. Perhaps the most dangerous complication of heparin use is the danger of haemorrhage. Signs of overzealous heparin administration include haematuria, increased capillary permeability, purpura and more seriously, internal haemorrhage. Because of the short life of heparin in the body, these effects should only be of a transient nature.

However, in severe cases it is possible to antagonise heparin by the use of the specific antidote protamine sulphate. After administration, protamine forms a complex molecule with the heparin, thus inactivating it. To remove the effects of heparin, protamine sulphate is usually administered on the basis of 1 mg for every 100 units of heparin but the use of protamine is not without its own hazards. Not more than 50 mg should be administered over a 10-minute period since its use is associated with depression of the myocardium resulting in hypotension, bradycardia and dyspnoea.

The heparin molecule is too large to cross the placental barrier. It can therefore be used quite safely in pregnant patients (except near to parturition) with no fear of directly harming the foetus.

ORAL ANTICOAGULANTS

This group of anticoagulants includes those which, unlike heparin, may be given orally. The indications and uses of these agents are similar to those of heparin.

Within the clotting cascade there are four factors which depend upon vitamin K for synthesis. These four factors are II, VII, IX and X. The oral anticoagulants ***warfarin*** and ***phenindione*** interfere with the formation of these four factors by inhibiting vitamin K utilisation in their manufacture. ***Dipyridamole*** (*Persantin*) is also available for use as an anticoagulant and acts by depressing platelet aggregation. ***Aspirin*** acts in a similar way to dipyridamole.

General Precautions

Patients on oral anticoagulant therapy must be adequately educated concerning the potency of their medication and the symptoms of toxicity. Educational booklets are published by the major manufacturers of oral anticoagulants and are freely available to patients using these medications.

The general signs of oral anticoagulant overdose are the same as those described for heparin. One of the greatest dangers faced by patients using oral anticoagulants is that of drug interactions. Many drugs can severely interfere with the activity of oral anticoagulants, and patients should be aware at least of those common agents that should be avoided. A brief table of potentially dangerous interactions is given as Table 25.

So far as the dosage of oral anticoagulants is concerned, it is most important to delineate a general dosage schedule. Each patient is treated as an individual, and the dosage is decided by titration against laboratory results of blood coagulability. In most cases it is desirable to have patients' clotting power between 60% and 80% that of normal (using KCCT test) or between 10 and 20% using thrombotest.

Caution is needed in administering oral anticoagulants to patients with pre-existing disease states (for example, peptic ulceration) which may be affected by the therapy. In the emergency situation the effects of the warfarin oral anticoagulants can be rapidly reversed by the administration of the synthetic vitamin K_1, phytomenadione (*Konakion*).

Oral anticoagulants are contraindicated in pregnancy.

Table 25
Some Drug Interactions Involving Oral Anticoagulants

Drug	Interaction
Acetylsalicylic acid *(Aspirin)* in large doses Amiodarone Chloral hydrate *(Noctec)* Clofibrate *(Atromid-S)* Phenylbutazone *(Butzolidin)*	Activity of warfarin increased
Allopurinol *(Zyloric)* Non-steroidal anti-inflammatories (NSAIDs) Nortriptyline *(Allegron, Aventyl)* Thyroxine *(Eltroxin)*	Activity of warfarin possibly potentiated
Phenytoin	Both potentiation and inhibition reported
Barbiturates Griseofulvin *(Fulcin, Grisovin)* Rifampicin	Activity of warfarin decreased
Aspirin Dipyridamole	Anticoagulant effect increased by anti-platelet effects

Source: *British National Formulary*, Appendix 1

HEPARIN/WARFARIN CHANGEOVER

Commonly, patients undergoing anticoagulant therapy will be commenced on heparin owing to its rapid onset of action and ease of dosage adjustment and then be transferred gradually to oral therapy. Many practitioners like to cease heparin and begin oral anticoagulants abruptly, and according to the literature, no ill effects have been elicited by this method of changeover.

NURSING IMPLICATIONS

Assessment

Observation for signs of inappropriate bleeding, or hypersensitivity where animal products are used, form the basis of physical assessment. The possibility of drug interactions should be thoroughly checked when *any* drug is given to a patient on anticoagulants. The conditions for which anticoagulants are used might be life threatening, and the therapy itself could be a source of further anxiety to the patient and his family.

Administration

Careful checking of doses and types of preparations is essential, since a range of concentrations and compounds is available.

Special care should be taken to ensure that subcutaneous heparin is injected into fat and not muscle, and that blood vessel damage is minimised during injection. The site should have a fat fold of at least one inch, when pinched between thumb and finger. A schedule for site rotation will help to minimise tissue damage. The injection site should not be massaged. The patient can be encouraged to participate in maintaining site rotation and reduction of bleeding at the injection site.

With oral anticoagulant therapy, a regular time for the daily dose should be established and adhered to in order to stabilise blood concentration. Action should be taken to prevent the patient from bleeding, by minimising hazards in the environment. Special care should be taken to minimise blood loss from venepuncture sites, since blood tests are common events for these patients. The site may be unsightly and eventually painful. Continuous intravenous therapy with heparin should be regulated by an infusion pump

Evaluation

Evaluation of physiological response to anticoagulants is achieved by frequent clotting tests. Doses might be adjusted on a daily basis, initially. Observation of stools and urine for obvious and occult blood is a useful tool for evaluation of dosage and response. Any spontaneous bleeding must be reported to the medical officer.

Patient teaching

Points to be discussed with patients include:

- reasons for drug therapy;
- frequency of drug interactions with oral anticoagulants, emphasising the possibility of interactions with over-the-counter drugs; the dangers of aspirin and oral-anticoagulant interaction should be stressed and an alternative mild analgesic recommended;
- avoidance of injury, for example, using electric razors rather than safety razors, using soft toothbrushes, and always wearing some footwear;
- the necessity to inform doctors and dentists treating the patient (with other drugs, surgically or in obstetrics) of anticoagulant therapy;

- the advisability of wearing or carrying an identification disc, in case of medical emergencies;
- contraindications to the use of oral contraceptives during pregnancy;
- caution with multiple tablet strengths of oral anticoagulants and the need to check the effects of any newly prescribed drug with the prescriber;
- the importance of complying with blood-test schedules to avoid over-dosage or under-dosage;
- signs of haemorrhage, including back pain which may indicate retro-peritoneal haemorrhage;
- sources of drug information, including the local pharmacist and written information from the drug manufacturers;
- the possibility of frequent dose changes, and the need to make up doses from a range of tablet strengths; the dose schedule might need to be written down;
- the need to adhere strictly to prescribed doses and that missed doses should not be "caught up";
- avoidance of self-medication with non-prescription drugs;

COAGULANTS

Your physiology text shows the clotting cascade, and the clotting mechanisms that cause clot formation. Another system of factors is involved in initiating clot breakdown. Thus, the whole system is in a state of balance; although we want bleeding arrested by clot formation, we don't want the fibrin clot to persist forever. It is the role of substances such as plasminogens which eventually stimulate fibrinolysin activity, which eventually induces clot dissolution.

In general, there are two methods by which drugs can be used to increase coagulability. The first method is to use ***thrombin.*** This preparation is basically the same as the thrombin you have read about in the clotting system. It is applied directly to bleeding surfaces and causes fairly rapid clot formation by enhancing the fibrinogen-to-fibrin reaction. It is often used by dentists to arrest bleeding following tooth extraction. It must never be used systemically.

The second method that can be employed to enhance clotting is to reduce the rate of clot breakdown by inhibiting the substances which are normally involved in the fibrinolytic pathway.

Drugs in this group include ***aminocaproic acid*** *(Epsikapron,* powder and syrup); ***tranexamic acid*** *(Cyklokapron,* tablets, syrup and injection) and ***aprotinin*** *(Trasylol).*

The clotting agents are drugs which are employed to maintain or enhance the clotting ability of blood; that is, their action is the opposite to that of the anticoagulant drugs. These agents, which are not frequently prescribed, are used to arrest internal bleeding from extravascular sites.

In cases of cerebral haemorrhage following trauma or cardiovascular accident, clotting agents can be used to reduce blood loss by decreasing the rate of clot breakdown.

In recent years these agents have been used for a variety of disease states. Tranexamic acid *(Cyklokapron)* may have a place in the treatment of excessive menstrual blood loss in young girls while aminocaproic acid has been extensively used as a prophylactic measure for haemophiliacs prior to minor procedures such as dental extraction. Both agents have been extensively used in the treatment of haematuria following prostatectomy and general urinary-tract surgery.

These drugs are both excreted via renal mechanisms and inhibit the plasminogen-activated urokinase, making them excellent drugs for the treatment of these surgical complications. Finally, clotting agents may be employed as antidotes in the treatment of overdose of the fibrinolytic agents.

The clotting agents inhibit the body's normal mechanisms of clot breakdown, and by doing so, act to decrease further blood loss.

The major uses of clotting agents are: to arrest internal bleeding following trauma or surgical procedures; to prevent excessive menstrual blood loss; as a prophylaxis for haemophiliacs undergoing minor surgical procedures; and an antidote to the fibrinolytic agents.

Adverse Drug Reactions

Adverse reactions to the clotting agents are common. Postural hypotension, pruritus, skin rashes and nausea have been reported following aminocaproic acid use, while gastrointestinal disturbances seem more common with tranexamic acid. An interesting effect, following aminocaproic acid use, is nasal stuffiness and/or conjunctival suffusion. Rapid parenteral administration of aminocaproic acid has been associated with an incidence of cardiac arrhythmias and bradycardia.

Contraindications

1. Dosage should be reduced in patients with renal impairment.
2. Pregnancy is generally considered a contraindication, especially during the first and second trimester.
3. Active intramuscular clotting.

NURSING IMPLICATIONS

Assessment

Patients requiring haemostatic drug therapy are likely to be acutely ill and/or distressed about their conditions. Accurate assessment of blood loss is essential.

Administration

An explanation that most blood losses can eventually be corrected, and that caution with haemostatic drugs is appropriate, will help to relieve the patient's anxiety. Liquid preparations for oral use, especially if mixed with orange juice or other flavouring, could be more acceptable than large numbers of tablets.

Evaluation
Continuous assessment of blood loss and observation for signs of hypercoagulation are appropriate. Signs of renal impairment would indicate that the dose needs to be reduced. Patients should be evaluated for signs of the adverse reactions listed above.

FIBRINOLYTIC AGENTS

Anticoagulants used to prevent clot formation have no activity against thrombi that are already formed. The fibrinolytic agent ***streptokinase*** has activity against formed thrombi.

Streptokinase converts plasminogen to plasmin which then acts to degrade fibrin, fibrinogen and other proteins present in thrombi. Streptokinase can therefore dissolve clots.

The dosage of streptokinase varies, but as a guideline, a loading dose of about 250 000 i.u. is usually given over a 30-minute period. This can be followed by maintenance dose of about 100 000 i.u. per hour and the dose varied according to physiological response. The thrombin clotting time (TCT) is the parameter used to assess the activity of streptokinase preparations.

Streptokinase can be used in a variety of conditions for the dissolution of thrombi, including pulmonary embolism, acute deep venous thrombosis and occluded arteriovenous cannulae. In some hospitals streptokinase is employed in patients following myocardial infarction.

Adverse Drug Reactions

Streptokinase is assocated with a significant number of adverse drug reactions. The most important is the high antigenic potential of the drug. This fact predisposes the patient to two conditions:

1. Repeated administration of the drug is associated with considerable risk of anaphylaxis. It has been reported that 2.5% of patients receiving streptokinase suffered some manifestations of anaphylaxis.
2. Secondly, because of the development of antibodies to streptokinase, excessive doses are often needed to produce a satisfactory response.

Thus, streptokinase resistance is brought about by destruction of streptokinase by antibodies raised to the drug. If more than 1 000 000 i.u. of this drug needed to provide a response, the treatment should be discontinued.

Milder allergic reactions are also common, and urticaria, itching, flushing and nausea have been reported in more than 10% of patients. Patients with a history of allergy appear to suffer more adverse effects.

Contraindications

As a general rule, therapy with thrombolytic agents is contraindicated in patients within 10 days of undergoing most forms of biopsy or other minor surgical procedure. Caution is also advised in using the drug in patients with a history of gastrointestinal bleeding, liver or kidney disease, or endocrine disease of homeostasis. Use of streptokinase is usually reserved for physicians skilled in its administration.

Drug Interactions

Although heparin is often used following streptokinase, the concomitant use of the two should be avoided. Furthermore, any drugs that may interfere with platelet function, such as phenylbutazone, aspirin and indomethacin, should be avoided during streptokinase use.

NURSING IMPLICATIONS

Streptokinase therapy is usually performed under carefully controlled conditions, as in coronary care or intensive care units. Such units will usually have developed a protocol for the administration of streptokinase, and for the observation of the patient during and after the procedure. The principles are outlined below.

Assessment

Patients must be continually observed for signs of mild allergic reactions and for anaphylaxis. An allergy history should be obtained. During therapy, puncture sites (such as peripheral and central intravenous catheter sites), wounds, endotracheal intubation sites and urinary catheters are potential sites for blood loss, so puncture sites must be kept to a minimum. A tissue-perfusion baseline is established in upper and lower extremities. Blood flow may be assessed by a Doppler flowmeter, and colour, temperature, capillary filling and movement are checked.

Patients who have undergone surgical procedures, or who have a history of taking anticoagulants, aspirin, indomethacin or phenylbutazone, might be at increased risk of haemorrhage.

Administration

Unnecessary handling of the patient should be avoided. Intramuscular injections are contraindicated. If invasive procedures must be performed, pressure must be maintained at the injection site for at least 15 minutes and a pressure dressing then applied. This action is especially important if arterial puncture is used to obtain blood samples for gas analysis. Care of the mucous membranes, especially where endotracheal tubes are used, must be scrupulous. Intramuscular and intravenous injections should be avoided for 24 hours after treatment has ceased.

Evaluation

Streptokinase treatment is monitored by frequent clotting tests and by disappearance of the thrombotic lesion. Anaphylaxis and the need for high doses are criteria for discontinuation of treatment. Throughout treatment, the circulation is closely monitored. Bleeding from puncture sites, the gastrointestinal tract and urinary system is constantly monitored until the results of clotting tests return to normal values.

HYPOLIPIDAEMIC AGENTS

Hyperlipidaemia constitutes a group of disorders which are characterised by increased concentrations of various plasma lipoproteins. There are several such lipoproteins in general circulation: these are chylomicrons, very low density, low density and high density lipoproteins. Consequently six different categories of hyperlipidaemias have been classified according to which lipoprotein(s) is/are found in excess. Although a full discussion of hyperlipidaemia cannot be included here, it should be understood that this disease state constitutes a grave risk to health and may predispose the patient to a number of other pathological consequences.

The two hypolipidaemic agents in common use are ***clofibrate*** (*Atromid-S*) and ***cholestyramine*** (*Questran*).

Clofibrate (*Atromid-S*) is probably the most widely used hypolipidaemic agent. Even though it has been in use for over 20 years, its mode of action remains unclear. Certainly it has been shown to inhibit the synthesis of cholesterol, but this is not its only action since it has also been shown to lower plasma triglycerides and increase excretion of sterols. Clofibrate is well absorbed from the gastrointestinal tract and its effect in lowering very-low density lipoproteins (VLDL) becomes apparent within two to five days.

Cholestyramine acts by a completely different mechanism to lower plasma lipoproteins. Firstly, it is a non-absorbed drug which, when taken orally, acts within the gastrointestinal tract. In the intestine, the cholestyramine (*Questran*) binds to bile acids, enabling their removal in faeces. This action causes cholesterol conversion to bile acids to increase. An additional feature of cholestyramine's activity is that bile acids are actually required for the gastrointestinal absorption of cholesterol, so cholesterol uptake by the enterohepatic system will be reduced by this mechanism.

Both drugs are used in the treatment of a variety of hyperlipidaemias. Cholestyramine has the additional advantage of being suitable for the treatment of pruritus induced by elevated levels of bile acids secondary to hepatic dysfunction.

Adverse Drug Reactions

Clofibrate can cause nausea, diarrhoea, muscle cramps and weakness. Cholestyramine causes unpleasant taste, constipation and steatorrhoea.

Drug Interactions

Since cholestyramine is a binding agent, the possibility exists that other substances apart from bile acids may be bound to it and excreted in the faeces.

Clofibrate should be employed cautiously in patients receiving oral anticoagulant therapy since it may enhance the activity of such drugs.

NURSING IMPLICATIONS

Assessment

Treatment with hypolipidaemic agents constitutes one means of reducing risk factors for patients with hyperlipidaemia and is often started before the patient has any symptoms of the life-threatening conditions which can result. Compliance with drug therapy is, therefore, a potential problem. The nurse should assess the patient's knowledge of other risk factors and his appreciation of the need to reduce all of those risk factors that can be reduced. Drugs are not a substitute for the recommended dietary changes or for exercise.

Administration

Cholestyramine has an unpleasant taste and should not be taken as the dry powder. Fruit juice or fruit puree (such as apple sauce) is suitable for mixing to disguise the taste. The powder should be mixed with at least 120 mL of fluid to reach an acceptable consistency and should be allowed to stand for a few minutes for reasonable dispersion to occur. Such actions (taken to increase compliance) are important since doses of up to 30 g a day are not uncommon, and therapy is likely to be long term. It is important in cholestyramine therapy to ensure that regular bowel habits are maintained and that constipation be avoided. The absorption of fat-soluble vitamins can also be impaired, so a vitamin additive to the diet might be required. Patients should know that side effects are usually temporary and decrease with the course of treatment.

To avoid drug interactions through binding, other drugs administered to patients receiving cholestyramine should be given at least one hour before (or no soon than four hours after) the administration of cholestyramine. Dose schedules will have to be adjusted to accommodate this precaution.

Evaluation

Decreased blood-lipid levels and, ultimately, prevention of cardiovascular disease indicate the success of treatment. The patient will be encouraged by measurable differences such as decreased lipid levels and should be informed of the results of blood tests. Compliance wth drug and dietary regimes should be evaluated intermittently.

IRON AND HAEMOPOIETIC AGENTS

When one thinks of drugs affecting erythrocytes, then iron, folic acid and Vitamin B_{12} come to mind. Certainly iron has an important role to play in the synthesis of haemoglobin while the actions of the other two substances are not only concerned with red blood-cell manufacture, but also with many other reactions concerned with DNA and RNA synthesis.

IRON SALTS

Iron can exist in either the ferrous or the ferric state, the former being far more easily absorbed from the gastrointestinal tract. For that reason, almost all commercially available iron preparations are of a ferrous salt.

Ferrous salts have a propensity to degrade, so they are presented in coated tablets or sustained release preparations.

In the treatment of iron deficiency, iron can be given by a number of routes — orally, as already discussed, and by the parenteral route. The use of parenteral iron has fallen out of favour in recent years, as a number of serious adverse reactions such as anaphylaxis have been reported, especially following IV injection. Furthermore, intramuscular iron injections can be particularly painful. Irrespective of how iron salts are administered, haemogloblin will be formed at the rate of approximately 1 g/100 mL/week.

In patients suffering from severe iron-deficiency anaemia, therapy will need to be continued for some time before the haemoglobin and body stores of iron return to normal. Patients should be made aware that they may need to take iron supplements for many months. To enhance iron absorption, the drug is best given in divided doses throughout the day.

Two other points are worth stressing. First, iron preparation can cause stomach upset and should always be taken with food to minimise this. Second, the patient should be made aware that the stools may become quite black and perhaps "tarry" while taking iron supplements as a result of unabsorbed iron being present in the faeces. Commercially available iron preparations are often combined with folic acid.

FOLIC ACID AND VITAMIN B_{12}

Folic acid (folate) and vitamin B_{12} are also important to red blood-cell synthesis, although the incidence of deficiency of these entities is much less than the incidence of iron deficiency in the UK. Where a deficiency is apparent, however, both ***folic acid*** and ***Vitamin B***$_{12}$ are available in tablet form for oral administration. The dose administered and duration of therapy depend upon haematological findings.

In order for Vitamin B_{12} to be absorbed from the small intestine it must first complex with another molecule called "intrinsic factor". Intrinsic factor is secreted from the parietal cells of the stomach wall. Some individuals are deficient not in their intake of Vitamin B_{12} but rather in the quantity or efficiency of the "intrinsic factor" they secrete. When this deficiency is clinically apparent, it is known as pernicious anaemia. To effectively treat pernicious anaemia, Vitamin B_{12} must be administered by a means which by-passes the gastrointestinal tract. Vitamin B_{12} injection (hydroxocobalamin) is available for this purpose.

Adverse Drug Reactions

Iron

Oral iron preparations are associated with gastrointestinal disturbances but taking the medication with meals helps prevent this. Patients should also be advised that stools may become thick and tarry. Iron preparations antagonise tetracycline antibiotics and should not be used with them.

Folic acid

Administration of this agent is practically devoid of any serious adverse effects although there have been some reports that folic acid will antagonise the anti-epileptic effects of phenytoin *(Epanutin)* resulting in an increase in convulsive episodes in those patients.

Vitamin B_{12}

Apart from local injection site discomfort, adverse drug reactions are uncommon.

Note: Overdosage with any of these three agents is potentially dangerous, and long-term therapy should be undertaken only with adequate supervision.

NURSING IMPLICATIONS

Assessments

Where dietary deficiency may have contributed to the disease process, dietary habits need to be assessed. The patient's appreciation of the need for long-term (possibly life-long) treatment and his willingness and ability to comply with treatment should be established. If gastrointestinal bleeding has caused anaemia, signs of further blood loss should be monitored throughout the treatment of anaemia. Vitamin-B_{12} (hydroxocobalamin) doses might require adjustment in the presence of injection.

Administration

Appropriate dietary modifications should be instituted. The patient may require dietary education, and the dietician should be involved.

Giving liquid iron preparations through a straw and diluting them in orange juice will avoid staining of the teeth and lips and promote absorption. Iron salts cause gastric irritation in many people. Dyspepsia and diarrhoea can be avoided by giving iron preparations immediately after food. It should be explained to the patient that black, tarry stools are a harmless side effect of oral iron therapy.

For intramuscular injection of iron, a "Z" track technique is used to prevent staining of the outer tissue layers and to prevent leakage at the injection site. The injection is always given into the gluteal muscle (buttock) and never into the deltoid muscle in the arm. The skin at the injection site is rolled to one side prior to injection and relaxed during withdrawal of the needle.

Folic acid is available in tablet and liquid forms. Care should be taken not to confuse folic acid with folinic acid, which is used for another purpose (see Chapter 27).

Evaluation

Initial evaluation of the effectiveness of therapy can be made by monitoring the blood count and by disappearance of the signs of anaemia. Long-term evaluation involves monitoring of diet, compliance with therapy, and assessment of the potential causes of anaemia, such as recurrent gastrointestinal bleeding.

Patient teaching

Patients requiring iron replacement need to understand that therapy has to be continued for several weeks to allow for the replenishment of iron stores in the body, even after the haemoglobin concentration has returned to normal and the signs of iron-deficiency anaemia have disappeared. If a gastrointestinal disorder exists or is suspected, the patient should be aware of the early signs of anaemia, should the bleeding recur. The appearance of blood in the stools will be masked by the side effects of oral iron therapy.

The patient should be referred to the dietician if dietary education is required. The nurse may be in a position to reinforce the dietician's advice and will be able to help the patient select appropriate foods from the hospital menu.

Pernicious anaemia requies life-long therapy, necessitating periodic intramuscular injections of hydroxocobalamin (Vitamin B_{12}). The patient must understand that the disease is controlled rather than cured and that the symptoms will eventually return if treatment is neglected. If infection occurs, the medical officer should be informed so that the dose can be adjusted if necessary.

Although relatively harmless to adults, iron preparations are potentially fatal if taken in overdose by small children. Such overdoses in children must be treated as medical emergencies. Patients should be aware of the possibility and should store iron preparations well out of children's reach at home. It is because of their potential toxicity to children that iron preparations are packaged in "child-resistant" containers with special closures.

SELF-EVALUATION TEST

1. List two examples of:
   (a) Anticoagulants
   (b) Clotting agents
   (c) Fibrinolytic agents
   (d) Hypolipidaemic agents
   (e) Haemopoietic agents.
2. Name the antidotes for:
   (a) Heparin
   (b) Warfarin.
3. Describe the pharmacological actions of:
   (a) Clofibrate
   (b) Streptokinase.
4. List the disease states in which the following drugs are used:
   (a) Cholestyramine
   (b) Vitamin B_{12}
   (c) Folic acid
   (d) Warfarin.
5. What are the common adverse effects of:
   (a) Iron preparations
   (b) Heparin.
6. List the nursing implications in the use of:
   (a) Warfarin
   (b) Aminocaproic acid
   (c) Iron preparations.

Table 26
Drugs Used in the Treatment of Blood Disorders

Drug Group	Drug Name	Use	Action	Adverse Reactions	Nursing Implications
Anticoagulants	Heparin	DVT, pulmonary emboli, postmyocardial infarct, postprosthesis implantation	Prevents conversion of prothrombin to thrombin	Local irritation, mild pyrexia, bleeding	***Assess:*** for bleeding tendencies, liver disease, recent surgery, gastrointestinal conditions, wounds; probability of compliance; potential for drug interactions; anxiety about condition; laboratory tests. ***Administer:*** check all labels carefully; check for route; do not massage injection site; infusion pump for continuous IV therapy. ***Evaluate:*** blood in urine, stools, other signs of bleeding; for hypersensitivity, drug interactions, for adverse effects. ***Teach:*** importance of compliance with prescription and laboratory tests; common drug and food interactions; to assess for bleeding; to protect from trauma; sources of drug information.
	Warfarin Phenindione	As above	Interfere with production of vitamin-K dependent clotting factors (II, VII, IX, X)	Risk of haemorrhage; *N.B.:* care with concurrent administration of other drugs	
Coagulants	Aminocaproic acid Tranexamic acid	To arrest internal bleeding after trauma or surgery, prevention of	Inhibit normal mechanisms of clot breakdown	Postural hypotension, pruritus, rash, nausea, nasal stuffiness, cardiac	***Assess:*** anxiety, blood loss, pregnancy. ***Administer:*** liquid preparations for oral

		excessive menstrual blood loss, prophylaxis in haemophiliac patients prior to minor surgery, antidote to fibrinolytics		arrhythmias with aminocaproic acid	use, check labels carefully, slow IV infusion. ***Evaluate:*** blood loss, hypercoagulation, for renal impairment, for adverse effects
Fibrinolytics	Streptokinase	Dissolves clots	Converts plasminogen to plasmin	Allergic reactions, anaphylaxis, antibody development, haemorrhage	***Assess:*** allergy history, blood loss, drug history for potential interactions, recent surgery. ***Administer:*** minimal handling of patient, no IM or IV injections, 15 minutes pressure at site of any invasive procedure. ***Evaluate:*** clotting tests, anaphylaxis, for very high doses, drug may have to be ceased.
Hypolipidaemic agents	Clofibrate	Hyperlipidaemia	Inhibits cholesterol synthesis, lowers plasma triglycerides, increases excretion of sterols	Nausea, diarrhoea, muscle cramps, weakness	***Assess:*** risk factors other than hyperlipidaemia; possibility of compliance. ***Administer:*** mix cholestyramine with fruit juice or puree; avoid constipation; add vitamin supplements; give other drugs one hour before or four hours after cholestyramine. ***Evaluate:*** blood lipid levels, other risk factors. ***Teach:*** other risk factors; importance of lowering blood lipid levels; need for compliance; temporary nature of adverse effects.
	Cholestyramine	Hyperlipidaemia	Binds to bile acids in gut, forcing faecal excretion	Unpleasant taste, constipation, steatorrhoea	

continued

Drug Group	Drug Name	Use	Action	Adverse Reactions	Nursing Implications
Iron and haemopoietic agents	Iron salts	Iron-deficiency anaemias	Promotes haemoglobin formation	GIT upset, black, tarry stools	***Assess:*** diet; probability of compliance; gastrointestinal bleeding. ***Administer:*** liquid iron with straw, orange juice; give oral iron with (or just after) food; "Z" track technique for IM injection, into buttock only; do not confuse folic acid and folinic acid. ***Evaluate:*** blood count; for signs of anaemia; recurrent gastrointestinal bleeding; for adverse effects; for infection. ***Teach:*** need for long-term or lifelong therapy; early signs of gastrointestinal bleeding, anaemia; dark stools with oral iron; dietary modification; protect children from iron overdose.
	Folic acid	Folic acid deficiency	Required for synthesis of red blood cells	Rare	
	Vitamin B_{12}	Vitamin B_{12} deficiency, pernicious anaemia	Required for synthesis of red blood cells	Rare; may be some discomfort at injection site	

9

DRUGS IN RENAL FAILURE

Kingsley Ng

OBJECTIVES

At the conclusion of this chapter, the reader should be able to:

1. describe the basic concept of drug management in problems associated with renal failure, with particular reference to renal osteodystrophy, hyperkalaemia, and renal hypertension;
2. name two commonly used immunosuppressive agents and list their main side effects;
3. describe the effect of renal failure and of dialysis on the excretion of drugs.

PREREQUISITE KNOWLEDGE

1. Structure and function of the kidney.
2. The physiological effect of hyperkalaemia, hypokalaemia, hypercalcaemia, and hypocalcaemia.
3. Basic concept of rejection in organ transplantation.

The kidney is responsible for the elimination of a number of products of metabolism such as urea, uric acid and creatinine. It also controls the excretion of electrolytes and water, and thus regulates the internal environment of the body. If the kidney fails, breakdown products of dietary constituents will accumulate in the blood, and water and electrolyte balance can no longer be maintained. Depending on the degree of kidney damage and provided that some renal function remains, the accumulation of metabolic products can be prevented by a careful choice of diet. This usually involves protein, water and salt restriction. However, when a kidney has lost most, if not all, of its function, control by diet is no longer possible. In order to maintain life, the diseased kidney must be replaced with a functional one (that is, transplantation) or have its functions performed by means of artificial or mechanical devices. The technique employed for the latter process is dialysis.

The outlook for patients with end-stage renal disease has been improved substantially over the past two decades by the development of dialysis and renal transplantation. These two techniques enable hundreds of individuals with irreversible renal failure to lead a normal or near-normal life. However, it is not uncommon to encounter problems associated with renal failure in spite of dialysis therapy. Some of these include vitamin deficiency, renal osteodystrophy, hyperkalaemia, hypertension and acidosis.

There are also problems associated with transplantation, such as rejection and the side effects of immunosuppressive therapy. This chapter looks at some of the pharmacological agents which are employed to prevent or manage these problems. A brief discussion on the principles of dialysis is also included.

PRINCIPLES OF DIALYSIS

The principles of dialysis are relatively simple. If a patient's blood is placed on one side of a semipermeable membrane and a solution of known composition on the other, substances to which the membrane is permeable will move from where their concentration is high to where their concentration is low. Thus if the blood levels of substances such as urea and uric acid are high and these substances are absent from the dialysis solution, they will pass from the blood to the solution. Similarly if the blood potassium is low, and the potassium concentration in the dialysis solution is in the normal range, potassium will pass from the solution into the blood. Based on this principle, any abnormal electrolyte levels in patients with renal failure may be corrected by using a dialysis solution which contains the most important electrolytes in concentrations which are normal for healthy individuals. As waste products such as urea, uric acid and creatinine are absent from dialysis solution, they can be removed from the patient's blood by dialysis.

Dialysis can also be used to remove fluid from overhydrated patients. This is done by adding substances such as glucose to the dialysis solution until it is hypertonic with respect to blood. Due to the difference in osmotic pressure, water will move from the patient to the solution.

Not only waste products can be removed by dialysis. Essential body constituents such as the water-soluble vitamins can also be removed by the process. A number of drugs may be removed from the blood by dialysis and this technique has been used to treat certain types of drug poisoning.

Dialysis can be carried out either in the patient's peritoneal cavity (peritoneal dialysis) using the peritoneum as the semipermeable membrane or outside the patient's body (haemodialysis) using an artificial kidney machine with a dialysis membrane.

PROBLEMS ASSOCIATED WITH RENAL FAILURE

VITAMIN DEFICIENCY

It is important to give adequate vitamin supplements to uraemic patients as their vitamin intake can be limited by the dietary restrictions placed on them. It is also necessary to supplement patients on dialysis therapy, since significant amounts of the water-soluble vitamin-B complex, vitamin C and folic acid are lost during dialysis. Supplementation with fat-soluble vitamins such as A and D is unnecessary and risky. On prolonged ingestion, particularly with high doses, they tend to accumulate in the body and cause hypervitaminosis. In the case of vitamin D, some patients may already be taking some form of this vitamin for the management of renal osteodystrophy (see next section); additional amounts of this vitamin in those patients may be undesirable. Similarly, vitamin preparations containing minerals or trace elements, such as magnesium, should be avoided because of the possibility of toxicity from these components. There are a number of preparations containing B complex or B complex with C (ascorbic acid). They vary in composition; hence the number of tablets that must be administered also varies. Commonly used preparations include Vitamin B Compound, Strong tablets and Vitamin capsules BPC.

RENAL OSTEODYSTROPHY

In adults, renal osteodystrophy is largely confined to patients in whom renal failure has been present for a number of years. In these patients, absorption of calcium from the gut is severely impaired as there is resistance to the actions of vitamin D. The failure of the diseased kidney to convert vitamin D into the active form responsible for the absorption of calcium from the gut could be a major contributing factor. Impairment of calcium absorption results in low serum-calcium levels which stimulate the parathyroid glands to secrete parathyroid hormone, which breaks down bone to release calcium into the circulation. Bone demineralisation is, however, only one major aspect of renal osteodystrophy; other factors such as erratic bone formation are also involved. The subject is too complex to be discussed in full here.

The basic principle for the treatment of renal osteodystrophy is to give vitamin D or vitamin-D analogues with the aim of increasing intestinal calcium absorption and hence serum-calcium levels. As high serum-phosphate levels are found in patients with renal failure, a rise in serum-calcium levels tends to produce deposition of calcium phosphate in soft tissues; so if treatment with vitamin D is indicated, the serum-phosphate must be controlled with aluminium hydroxide (see page 156) before starting therapy. Small doses must be used, and any increase in dose should be gradual.

The use of vitamin-D compounds in renal patients must be carefully supervised and frequent biochemical monitoring is essential. Excessive dosage of vitamin D can result in hypercalcaemia and metastatic calcification of soft tissues. The following vitamin-D compounds are commonly used in the treatment or prevention of renal osteodystrophy.

Calciferol
This is available in the form of high-potency tablets (50 000 units). It has a cumulative action, and dosage must be carefully controlled. The effects of changes in dosage may not be apparent for several weeks.

Dihydrotachysterol
This compound is related chemically to calciferol and is equally effective in raising serum-calcium levels. It acts more rapidly and has a shorter duration of action than calciferol, so dosage is more readily controlled.

Calcitriol (*Rocaltrol*)
This is the most biologically active vitamin D derivative which controls the intestinal absorption of calcium. Failure of the kidney to convert precursors to this hormone was thought to be largely responsible for hypocalcaemia observed in patients with chronic renal failure. Calcitriol is available for oral administration, its efficacy having been demonstrated in various clinical evaluations. It is likely that calcitriol will replace other vitamin-D derivatives in the management of hypocalcaemia in patients with renal osteodystrophy.

Aluminium Hydroxide (*Alu-Cap,* Aluminium Hydroxide Mixture)
As mentioned earlier, high serum-phosphate levels are found in patients with renal failure. Increases in serum-calcium levels can produce deposition of calcium phosphate in soft tissues if the serum-phosphate level is not adequately controlled. Aluminium hydroxide is used to reduce serum-phosphate concentration. It is given with meals with the aim of binding dietary phosphate in the bowel and preventing its absorption. There are a number of aluminium hydroxide preparations, both tablets and gels, which contain different amounts of aluminium hydroxide and hence have different phosphate-binding capacities. In general, gel preparations appear to be better binders than tablets. To facilitate stabilisation it is desirable to use the same preparation throughout the treatment.

Compound antacid preparations containing magnesium and other cations (as well as aluminium hydroxide) should not be used as a form of aluminium hydroxide, and their use should be avoided. The most common side effect of aluminium hydroxide is constipation. It can also interfere with the absorption of other drugs and excessive administration can lead to hypophosphataemia.

HYPERKALAEMIA

As urinary potassium excretion is reduced in oliguric renal failure, potassium retention and hyperkalaemia often become a problem. The treatment of hyperkalaemia is a matter of urgency as it can cause cardiac arrhythmias and arrest. Several emergency measures may be followed.

Sodium Bicarbonate
This is administered as an intravenous infusion of 500 mL isotonic sodium bicarbonate. The bicarbonate induces potassium ions to enter the cells, and this reduces plasma potassium. The effect is rapid but temporary, but buys time for other measures such as dialysis to be instituted.

Glucose and Insulin
This is another measure through which serum potassium can be rapidly lowered. Usually 50 mL of 50% glucose together with insulin is given intravenously. When glucose enters the cells under the influence of insulin, it carries potassium with it. The onset of the effect is rapid, and it also wears off quickly.

Polystyrene Resin *(Resonium A, Calcium Resonium)*
Resonium A can be given orally, or rectally as a retention enema. It is a cation-exchange resin which releases sodium ions and hydrogen ions in exchange for potassium ions, the bound potassium ions then being excreted in the faeces. The onset of action is not rapid and the effectiveness depends on the amount of potassium to be removed. Another type of resin which releases calcium instead of sodium, *Calcium Resonium*, is to be preferred when excessive sodium intake is undesirable.

Calcium
Hyperkalaemia can lead to cardiac arrhythmia and subsequent death. The arrhythmia can be reversed or prevented by the administration of calcium, usually in the form of an intravenous infusion of calcium gluconate.

Dialysis is the most effective means for the treatment of hyperkalaemia, but as it often takes time to arrange, the above measures may be used (if severe hyperkalaemia is present) until dialysis can be instituted.

HYPERTENSION

Blood-pressure control is an important aspect in the management of all forms of renal diseases. If hypertension is left untreated, deterioration of renal function is inevitable, and it can also lead to other vascular complications. In some patients hypertension can be relieved by fluid restriction, dialysis and salt restriction. Renal hypertension due to stenosis of the renal artery may be surgically cured in selected patients.

The medical treatment of renal hypertension does not differ in principle from other forms of hypertension. The antihypertensives commonly employed include beta-blocking agents, hydralazine and prazosin. The pharmacology of these agents has been well covered in other chapters of this text. Diuretics, which are frequently used as part of antihypertensive regimens in patients without renal failure, are of limited value in the presence of renal insufficiency. Potassium-sparing diuretics such as spironolactone *(Aldactone)* and amiloride *(Midamor)* may cause fatal hyperkalaemia when given to patients with renal failure and are therefore contraindicated.

ACIDOSIS

The metabolic acidosis of renal failure may be corrected by oral administration of sodium bicarbonate, the dose required varying from patient to patient. Calcium carbonate in adequate doses has been shown to be effective in reducing acidosis, and this may be used when sodium is contraindicated.

PROBLEMS ASSOCIATED WITH TRANSPLANTATION

REJECTION

The main problem of organ transplantation, renal or otherwise, is rejection. The universally accepted method of combating rejection is combined therapy with prednisone and azathioprine. As these suppress the body's immune response, infections (particularly fungal and viral types) are a common problem.

IMMUNOSUPPRESSIVE AGENTS AND THEIR SIDE EFFECTS

Prednisone (or Prednisolone)

As the pharmacology of corticosteroids has been dealt with in other chapters it will not be discussed in detail here.

Prednisone is of value in the treatment of rejection crises as well as maintenance therapy. The dosage schedule and method of administration are subject to variation. One method, for example, is to use high doses at the time of transplantation or when a rejection crisis occurs, that is, 500 mg to 1 g intravenously with gradual (over several months) reduction to maintenance doses of 10 to 20 mg daily, given orally. Whichever method is employed, no patient ever has been completely taken off steroids.

The side effects of steroids are well documented. These include Cushingoid appearance (moon face and buffalo hump), peptic ulceration, sodium and fluid retention, hypertension, psychosis, hyperglycaemia, aseptic necrosis of bone and cataracts.

Azathioprine *(Imuran)*

Azathioprine is the main immunosuppressive drug used to permit long-term acceptance of a graft. However, it lacks the anti-inflammatory and lympholytic actions of prednisone and so is relatively ineffective in treating (as distinct from preventing) acute rejection crises. The side effects of azathioprine include leucopenia, thrombocytopenia and liver damage. When the latter occurs, it is usual practice to substitute azathioprine with other cytotoxic drugs such as cyclophosphamide or chlorambucil. These drugs have similar effects to azathioprine.

Anti-lymphocyte Globulin (ALG)

This is produced by immunising animals (for example, goats and horses) against human lymphocytes. As lymphocytes are of great importance in the rejection process, ALG may be of value in suppressing the phenomenon. The use of ALG as an adjunct to immunosuppressant therapy is somewhat controversial. However, there has been a growing interest of its use in reversing acute rejection episodes. The drug has to be administered intravenously as it is extremely painful to give subcutaneously. Some of the common side effects include fever, thrombocytopenia and anaphylaxis or serum sickness caused by allergy to horse or goat serum.

Anticoagulants and Antiplatelet Agents

Anticoagulants such as ***heparin*** and ***warfarin***, and antiplatelet drugs such as ***dipyridamole*** (*Persantin*), have been used for the prevention and treatment of acute rejection. Anticoagulants inhibit the coagulation of blood by inhibiting the activity (or depressing the synthesis) of various clotting factors. The antiplatelet agents have the properties of inhibiting the adhesion and aggregation of platelets. Neither of these agents has immunosuppressive properties. Their use is based on histological evidence which suggests that the initial damage to a graft in an acute rejection episode may be associated with occlusion of small blood vessels due to aggregation of platelets and fibrin deposition. The efficacy of this type of non-immunosuppressive therapy has yet to be substantiated.

Patients on heparin therapy should be observed for signs of bleeding, particularly if they are being treated with ulcerogenic drugs such as the steroids. With dipyridamole, gastric upset and headache have been associated with its administration in some patients.

Cyclosporin A

This is a new and extremely powerful immunosuppressant. The clinical results so far achieved with this agent indicate that it has an important part to play in future immunosupressant regimens for organ transplantation. In patients who receive cyclosporin A, it is possible to maintain a cadaver graft without the administration of steroids. The side effects include nephrotoxicity, hepatotoxicity, hirsutism, gum hypertrophy and malignant disease. However, most of these side effects are dose dependent and are reversible on stopping administration of the drug.

DRUG ADMINISTRATION IN RENAL FAILURE

Apart from the drugs which are used to treat their basic condition, patients with renal failure also receive a wide variety of pharmacological agents for their intercurrent illnesses. Drugs which are mainly excreted in active form by the kidneys (that is, as unchanged drug or pharmacologically active breakdown products) may accumulate in the presence of renal insufficiency, the result being adverse reactions or toxicity. If toxic effects are to be avoided, modification of dosage regimens and careful monitoring is required. This is particularly important with drugs with a low therapeutic ratio such as digoxin and gentamicin. Dosage modification should take into consideration changes in renal function and dialysis. The latter may result in depletion of therapeutic concentrations of drugs by causing removal from the blood into the dialysate, but in no case will dialytic removal exceed the rate of removal by normally functioning kidneys.

Dosage regimens are usually modified by administering either normal doses at extended intervals or a reduced dose at normal intervals. For drugs whch are highly dialysable, the dose just preceding dialysis and doses scheduled during dialysis are usually omitted, and a supplementary dose is given after dialysis. The factors affecting the removal of drugs during dialysis are molecular size, protein binding in plasma, and distribution between the plasma and other body-fluid compartments. As a generalisation, drugs which are mostly eliminated by the kidneys will undergo significant decreases in concentration during dialysis. For drugs with small molecular weight, losses are less significant with peritoneal dialysis than with haemodialysis because of the lesser efficiency of the peritoneal method.

Drugs which require dose adjustment when administered to patients with renal failure include ***amphotericin B*** *(Fungizone)*; ***co-trimoxazole*** *(Bactrim, Septrin)*, ***digoxin*** *(Lanoxin)*, ***flucytosine*** *(Alcobon)*, ***gentamicin, magnesium-containing antacids, methotrexate, phenobarbitone, potassium salts, procainamide*** *(Pronestyl)* and ***tobramycin*** *(Nebcin)*.

NURSING IMPLICATIONS

Vitamin supplements

Ensure patient awareness of:

(a) the importance of taking the specific vitamin preparation prescribed and of avoiding the use of additional, non-prescribed preparations;
(b) the need for biochemical monitoring during Vitamin-D therapy;
(c) the importance of taking phosphate-binding preparations when prescribed with Vitamin D.

Aluminium hydroxide

Educate the patient of the need to use the specific preparation prescribed. Other drugs taken concurrently should be taken at least two hours before or after aluminium hydroxide, which interferes with the absorption of many drugs.

Watch particularly for constipation. Dietary restrictions may preclude an increase in fibre or fluid content.

Resonium A

Resonium may cause constipation which may be difficult to treat in view of dietary and drug restrictions.

Antihypertensives
See Chapter 7.

Prednisone
See Chapter 11.

Azathioprine
Observe for signs of bone-marrow depression. Protect patient from infection. If stomatitis occurs, use appropriate measures such as mouth washes or a soft, bland diet. Observe for biochemical and/or clinical evidence of liver damage. Educate patient in the reason for immunosuppressive therapy and the necessity to continue therapy as prescribed.

Antilymphocyte Globulin
Store vials of ALG under refrigeration. During and following administration, observe for unwanted effects, including signs of impending anaphylaxis. Have emergency drugs (for example adrenaline, corticosteroids) readily available.

Cyclosporin A
Serum levels of cyclosporin A are monitored during treatment. Observe patient for adverse effects already described; maintain constant vigilance for any other evidence of unwanted drug effects. Cyclosporin A is a relatively new drug, and further aspects of its action may become apparent with time.

General concepts
As patients with renal diseases or on immunosupressive drugs are susceptible to infections, strict aseptic technique should be employed for procedures such as changing of dressings and handling of driplines. Such patients should not be nursed near patients with respiratory, gastrointestinal, wound or skin infections. Dosage intervals for the administration of drugs to patients with renal failure should be strictly adhered to.

SELF-EVALUATION TEST

1. Why is vitamin supplementation necessary for patients with chronic renal failure?
2. Name two drugs which may be used to treat hypocalcaemia in patients with renal osteodystrophy.
3. What are the indications for use of aluminium hydroxide, and what is its main side effect?
4. Name two drugs which may be used to treat hyperkalaemia.
5. Are diuretics of any value in the treatment of hypertension in patients with renal failure?
6. Should potassium-sparing diuretics be administered to patients with renal failure?
7. Name two commonly used immunosuppressive agents, and list their main side effects.
8. Name two drugs which require modification of dosage regimen when administered to patients with renal failure.

10

UROPHARMACOLOGY — THE ROLE OF DRUGS IN BLADDER DYSFUNCTION

Richard J. Millard

OBJECTIVES

At the end of this chapter the reader should be able to:

1. discuss the use of drugs in promoting urinary continence;
2. know the place of drugs in promoting bladder emptying.

PREREQUISITE KNOWLEDGE

Before commencing this chapter, the reader should be familiar with:

1. the anatomy of the bladder and urethra and the nerve supply to each;
2. autonomic physiology and pharmacology.

BLADDER AND URETHRAL FUNCTION

The bladder has two functions. Firstly, it should store urine at low pressure without effort or discomfort. Secondly, when appropriate, it should void to completion under voluntary control. The normal bladder fills to about 500mL capacity and voids at about 20mL/second, emptying in less than 30 seconds. This requires complex control mechanisms coordinated in the brain stem under higher-centre control.

The normal bladder and urethra act together to store urine and maintain urinary continence. Continence is preserved when the bladder neck remains closed and when the pressure within the urethra (the urethral-closure pressure) exceeds the pressure within the bladder (the intravesical pressure). The intravesical pressure is due partly to the intra-abdominal pressure and partly to the detrusor pressure derived from contraction or tonus in the bladder smooth muscle (the detrusor).

The urethral-closure pressure is derived from elastic tissues in the urethral wall and from the urethral sphincter mechanism. This sphincter mechanism is made up of both smooth and striated muscle surrounding the urethra, and from the peri-urethral striated musculature of the pelvic floor and perineal diaphragm. Both smooth and striated components contribute equally to the resting urethral-closure pressure and maintain this during bladder filling.

The bladder neck is usually water-tight and only opens when the bladder contracts. If however the bladder neck is incompetent (for example, after prostatectomy, bladder-neck incision or sometimes after multiple childbirth) or is open as a result of a bladder contraction, continence may be maintained by the distal-sphincter mechanism. If however both are incompetent, stress incontinence can occur with coughing or sneezing.

During filling, the bladder pressure remains low, and the detrusor does not contract until micturition starts. This low pressure occurs because the bladder wall is stretchable and because the bladder is prevented from contracting by inhibitory neural mechanisms. Even under the provocation of bladder fullness, change of posture or exercise, the intravesical pressure remains low due to central inhibition, and micturition can be delayed until it is convenient. The bladder only contracts when voiding is voluntarily initiated at an appropriate time and place. After emptying, the bladder does not contract again until the next time that voiding is started. This cycle of events describes normal and stable bladder function.

Some people cannot inhibit micturition, and unstable bladder contractions may then occur inappropriately during filling or in response to provocations such as exercise, posture change or raised intra-abdominal pressure. These unstable contractions give rise to an urgent desire to void, and urge incontinence occurs if the patient loses control before a toilet can be found.

When micturition is initiated, the distal sphincter mechanism relaxes, and this is followed by a coordinated detrusor contraction. This contraction opens the bladder neck and generates sufficient pressure to overcome the remaining outlet resistance, sustaining that pressure long enough for the bladder to empty. The detrusor then relaxes and the urethral closure pressure is restored. Efficient voiding thus requires both an adequate detrusor contraction and synchronous sphincteric relaxation which is coordinated in the brain stem.

Indeed, the entire bladder cycle is a constant balance between intravesical pressures and forces acting on the urethra. When the bladder pressure exceeds the urethral-closure pressure, urine flows through the urethra, causing micturition (if this occurs intentionally) or incontinence (when the event occurs involuntarily).

THE TYPES AND CAUSES OF INCONTINENCE

STRESS INCONTINENCE is the involuntary loss of urine when the pressure in the bladder excees the urethral-closure pressure in the absence of a detrusor contraction.

Leakage occurs coincident with rises in intra-abdominal pressure such as coughing, sneezing or straining. It implies incompetence of both the bladder neck and the distal sphincter mechanism.

URGE INCONTINENCE is the involuntary loss of urine associated with a strong desire to void.

There are two types: sensory and motor. Sensory urge incontinence is due to discomfort during filling, thus limiting the effective bladder capacity (as occurs with bladder inflammation or infection). Motor urge incontinence is due to involuntary detrusor contractions from an unstable bladder. Unstable detrusor function may occur idiopathically or may result from bladder outlet obstruction, neuropathy or severe intravesical irritation caused by catheters or calculi.

OVERFLOW INCONTINENCE occurs when the intra-vesical pressure exceeds the urethral-closure pressure when the bladder is overfull or distended but is not contracting (that is, in the presence of chronic retention). This may be secondary to obstruction or to detrusor failure.

BEDWETTING is due to an unstable bladder combined with an abnormally deep sleep pattern.

CONTINUOUS INCONTINENCE is the loss of urine usually associated with an abnormal urinary opening. It is associated with fistulae and with ectopia of either the bladder or ureter.

DRUGS USED TO PROMOTE URINARY CONTINENCE

In order to promote urinary continence, it is necessary to achieve either a reduction of intravesical pressure or an increase in urethral closure pressure or both of these. The key to successful management of urinary incontinence is the accurate diagnosis of its cause. A careful history and examination are required to detect incontinence due to fistulae or ectopia requiring definitive surgery. Bladder distension or pelvic-floor weakness may be detected and a neurological examination should be performed.

Urine culture is essential to detect infection, and intravenous urography or cystoscopy may be indicated. Videourodynamic assessment is definitive, accurately detecting unstable contractions, sphincteric weakness and the presence and cause of residual urine or voiding difficulty. Once the cause of the incontinence has been delineated, a rational approach to therapy can be formulated.

THE REDUCTION OF INTRAVESICAL PRESSURE

Indications

Reduction of intra-vesical pressure is indicated when urge incontinence is due to abnormally high detrusor pressures related to the unstable or uninhibited neuropathic bladder (for example, in multiple sclerosis, Parkinson's disease, spina bifida or following a cerebrovascular accident).

Bladder relaxants in such patients reduce the frequency and strength of the unstable contractions by reducing bladder contractility. In so doing, they result in symptomatic improvement by increasing the effective bladder capacity, thus diminishing urinary frequency and nocturia. Urgency is decreased giving the patient more time to get to a toilet or commode. Bladder relaxants do not help when symptoms are the result of intravesical inflammation or infection, and these possibilities should always be excluded and treated appropriately.

Patients with high-pressure bladders (such as the autonomous neuropathic bladder resulting from pelvic nerve, cauda equina or sacral spinal cord lesions), in whom the bladder will not empty, can be managed by intermittent catheterisation combined with bladder relaxants to improve the functional capacity. Patients being managed by intermittent catheterisation due to impaired bladder emptying for any reason may require drug therapy in order to be continent between catheterisations or to reduce the frequency of catheterisation.

Patients who are being managed by an in-dwelling catheter may develop overactive detrusor contractions secondary to mucosal irritation. These contractions give rise to bladder spasms which can be painful and to leakage around the catheter. This sometimes occurs with patients having spinal injury or other neuropathy, in children and adults with catheters after bladder surgery, and in geriatric patients who frequently pull at their catheters. Such patients benefit from bladder relaxants.

Anticholinergic Agents

The detrusor muscle is innervated by postganglionic parasympathetic nerves and is therefore cholinergic with muscarinic receptors. Anticholinergic agents tend to relax the detrusor and lower the intra-vesical pressure. They also impair the ability of the bladder to empty and are thus contraindicated in patients with any degree of obstruction to the bladder outlet.

Atropine is the classic anticholinergic agent, but its use is limited by its cardio-accelerator and mydriatric effects. This agent will not completely paralyse the bladder even at high dosage, suggesting that detrusor muscle contractility is not wholly mediated by muscarinic receptors. Research indicates that beta-adrenergic receptors in the dome of the bladder may have a role in bladder contractility. Stimulation of these receptors causes some detrusor relaxation. Anticholinergic agents however remain the mainstay of drugs used to reduce detrusor tonus or contracility.

Hyoscine and ***hyoscyamine***-containing preparations have been used, and belladonna alkaloids with anticholinergic properties may be tried. ***Propantheline*** *(Pro-Banthine)* is widely used, but some of the more recently introduced synthetic agents appear to be more effective. ***Dicyclomine, penthienate, emepronium*** and ***oxybutynin*** have been found to be as, or more, effective than propantheline in clinical trials.

Penthienate (*Monodral*) is a particularly effective anticholinergic agent for use in treating the unstable bladder. Patients with uninhibited (overactive or hyper-reflexic) neuropathic bladder dysfunction, such as occurs in multiple sclerosis, may be extremely sensitive to this agent and may require only low dosage to get benefit. ***Emepronium bromide*** *(Cetiprin)* is widely available in Europe. It should be taken with plenty of fluid in order to avoid the risk of oesophageal ulceration.

Oxybutynin is a newer agent combining anticholinergic, analgesic and direct smooth-muscle relaxant properties. It is demonstrably superior to the other agents for reducing bladder pressure and enhancing effective bladder capacity and may replace some of the other agents once it becomes available. By contrast, dicyclomine, whilst having some relaxant effect on the bladder and colonic smooth muscle, is disappointing in its effect on urinary symptoms.

Adverse Drug Reactions

The principal side effects of the anticholinergic agents have already been mentioned. Dryness of the mouth is universal, although it is less marked with penthienate than with propantheline. Difficulty in reading small print (due to paralysis of accommodation and dilatation of the pupil) only occurs at high dosage. Constipation and tachycardia may occur.

In the elderly and in patients with neuropathy, the bladder may be very sensitive to these agents and urinary retention may occur. The patient who responds initially and then relapses into incontinence shortly afterwards should be suspected of being in retention with overflow, and the bladder should be checked for residual urine. Dosage reduction or management by intermittent self-catheterisation may then result in continence.

These agents are contraindicated in the presence of bladder outlet obstructions such as prostatic enlargement and stricture. They should not be given to patients with glaucoma or myasthenia gravis.

Tricyclic Antidepressants

The tricyclic antidepressants have weak anticholinergic and ganglion blocking properties which have given them a place in the treatment of urological problems. Traditionally they have been used in the treatment of enuretic children who tend to have two problems, namely an overactive or unstable detrusor combined and an abnormally deep sleep pattern. The tricyclic antidepressants attack both elements of the problem, by promoting a reduction of detrusor pressures and an upward shift of the sleep pattern, making it more likely that the child will wake in the night rather than wetting the bed.

Imipramine in addition to its anticholinergic action also inhibits reuptake of noradrenaline from postganglionic synapses. This leads to an enhancement of adrenergic effects and augments bladder relaxation by an inhibitory action on the dome of the bladder, as well as promoting closure of the male bladder neck and the smooth-muscle component of distal urethral resistance.

Other tricyclic agents have no particular advantage over imipramine in the treatment of urinary disorders. The main place of these agents is in the treatment of persistent nocturnal enuresis. In adults they are useful as adjunctive agents to the anticholinergic agents when these give incomplete urinary control, or as alternative medication when anticholinergics are not tolerated. The sedative action experienced at first quickly becomes less troublesome.

Smooth-muscle Relaxants

Flavoxate has a direct smooth-muscle relaxant effect of unknown mechanism. It has been promoted as having beneficial effects on the overactive bladder. Often the patient must take large numbers of tablets each day to obtain any noticeable benefit.

Beta Sympathomimetics

Beta-adrenergic sympathomimetics such as ***orciprenaline*** *(Alupent)* and ***salbutamol*** *(Ventolin)* have been found to have a detrusor relaxant effect. When used alone, they are seldom clinically effective. Their use is confined therefore to that of adjunctive therapy when one of the anticholinergic agents is incompletely effective in alleviating symptoms.

The results obtained with any of these agents may be disappointing unless high doses are employed. Therapeutic response rates for the various agents range from 30% to 50%. The failure of one anticholinergic agent does not preclude success with another agent, and it is always worth changing drugs and doses or trying combinations to achieve a response. Tachyphylaxis is common with all groups of drugs. Bladder re-education and biofeedback techniques appear to offer a highly successful alternative to pharmaceutical manipulation for the treatment of patients with unstable detrusor function. If this fails, surgery may also be unsuccessful.

NURSING IMPLICATIONS

Assessment

Drugs only help patients to control their bladders by giving them warning of impending micturition. They are not a substitute for motivation or effort. The patient's willingness and ability to cooperate with treatment need realistic assessment. Factors which may decrease motivation should be identified, and ways of increasing motivation considered. The expectation of a positive outcome can act as a motivator.

When there are mobility problems, as with arthritic or bed-ridden patients, the call for assistance needs to be answered promptly. Timed voiding or regular "potting" may still be required.

In the elderly, or in patients with neuropathic bladder dysfunction, these agents can cause retention, especially if there is any degree of urinary obstruction. Therefore, the nurse must know the cause of the patient's incontinence, so that she or he can be alert for this problem.

Leakage around an in-dwelling catheter which is not blocked is usually cured by an anticholinergic agent and by reducing the size of the retaining balloon. The larger the balloon, the more irritating it is to the bladder. A 5-mL balloon is ideal. Securing the catheter so that there is no undue traction on it reduces irritation. The presence of urinary infection as a source of irritation should be assessed. Informed nursing assessment of the causes of catheter leakage and successful management can reduce the need for pharmacological intervention.

Administration
If a patient with a urinary catheter requires anticholinergic agents because of bladder spasms or leakage around the catheter, administration of the drug must be stopped when the catheter is removed, so that normal micturition can be re-established.

Evaluation
The patient's response is expected to be increased continence or decreased leakage around the catheter, but urine retention must be looked for, especially in susceptible patients. Initial response, followed by relapses into incontinence shortly afterwards, may indicate retention with overflow. Residual urine should be checked. Dosage reduction or management by intermittent self-catheterisation may then result in continence. Dry mouth can be distressing to patients, especially the elderly. They should be encouraged to drink and to suck on low-sugar sweets or gum to promote salivation.

Patient teaching
Patients need to know the limitations of drug treatment and that they need to contribute consciously to the treatment program to attain bladder control. Realistic expectations for treatment outcome should be set and conveyed to the patient. Direction to alternative methods of treatment will be appropriate, if drug results are unsatisfactory. They should be instructed to seek medical advice if retention occurs. Patients on imipramine need to be reassured that its sedative effects will diminish with time.

THE ENHANCEMENT OF URETHRAL RESISTANCE

Stress incontinence is the result of incompetence of the usually watertight bladder-neck mechanism which is the chief continence mechanism after detrusor stability. With an incompetent bladder neck, continence is possible if the distal urethral-sphincteric mechanism is passively competent, as found in about 50% of women. When the distal mechanism is incompetent, stress incontinence occurs with coughing, sneezing or any sudden rise in intra-abdominal pressure. The competenece of the distal mechanism relates to the effective urethral-closure pressure which depends upon the elastic and muscular properties of the urethra.

The elastic component of urethral resistance or closure pressure is not amenable to direct pharmacological stimulation. Oestrogens may enhance both the urethral elasticity and muscle tonus in the postmenopausal female.

The distal urethral mechanism is partly adrenergic smooth muscle and partly cholinergic striated muscle. Both types of muscle contribute equally to the maintenance of the urethral-closure pressure. Thus it is possible to enhance the urethral competence by stimulation of either the smooth or striated component of the sphincteric mechanism. Both alpha-adrenergic sympathomimetics and cholinergic agents can achieve this, but since the latter also increase intravesical pressure (nullifying any therapeutic effect on the urethral resistance), they are not used.

Indications

These agents are indicated in the conservative management of minor to moderately severe stress incontinence. They are used as an adjunct to pelvic floor exercises, weight loss and physiotherapy in such cases and when surgery is contraindicated or has been unsuccessful. Post-prostatectomy sphincter-weakness incontinence in males, and in females with a patulous urethra, may respond. Sometimes, urethral stimulation is used in conjunction with anticholinergics in the treatment of patients with both urge and stress incontinence. When drugs fail, treatment is surgical; the most satisfactory operation for stress incontinence is colposuspension.

Alpha-adrenergic Sympathomimetics

Alpha-adrenergic agents increase urethral-closure pressure and resistance. They act on the smooth-muscle component of the urethral sphincter mechanism, causing contraction. In the male, part of the bladder-neck mechanism is alpha-adrenergic smooth muscle, and this is also stimulated.

Ephedrine and ***pseudoephedrine*** preparations can be helpful, particularly in patients with minor degrees of stress incontinence. Unfortunately, many women will not tolerate them due to their unpleasant central effects, such as nervousness, irritability or insomnia, or to the tachycardia and cardiac dysrhythmias which are sometimes induced. ***Phenylpropanolamine*** is tolerated better and causes fewer central and cardiac effects. Several cases of hypertensive reactions have been reported, but these seem to be either idiosyncratic reactions or reactions which have occurred when other adrenergic agents have been taken concurrently. Unfortunately this preparation is not widely available except in combination with antihistamines in various cold remedies *(Sinutabs†,Eskornade†)*. In this form the drowsiness caused by the antihistamine makes long-term therapy unacceptable. In addition, they cannot be prescribed on the NHS.

Midodrine is a long-acting alpha-adrenergic agent which is both well tolerated and therapeutically effective in patients with stress incontinence. Unfortunately it is not available in Britain (at the time of publication).

Adverse Drug Reactions

These agents have the capacity to cause urinary retention in patients with mild degrees of outflow obstruction. This can be of significance when an elderly male requires a decongestant for upper respiratory-tract disease, as nearly all the oral preparations contain sufficient amounts of sympathomimetics to cause an increase in urethral resistance. A topical nasal decongestant in these circumstances is a wiser choice.

Oestrogens

In the postmenopausal or oestrogen-deficient patient, a course of oestrogen therapy over a three-month period may improve urethral competence. This is partly a direct action on the peri-urethral smooth muscle or elastic tissues and partly because oestrogens sensitise the smooth muscle to circulating catecholamines. Any low-dose oral oestrogen preparation may be used. Long-term use is not recommended. The use of topically applied oestrogen creams (such as dienoestrol cream) is helpful in treating concomitant senile (atrophic) vaginitis, but probably does little to improve urethral-closure pressures.

Table 27
Summary of Drugs Used to Promote Continence

Bladder Relaxants	**Urethral Stimulants**
Anticholinergic agents Atropine Hyoscine Propantheline Penthienate Dicyclomine Emepronium Oxybutynin	Alpha-adrenergic agents Ephedrine Pseudoephedrine Phenylpropanolamine
Tricyclic antidepressants Imipramine Amitriptyline	Oestrogens
Beta-adrenergic agents Orciprenaline Salbutamol	
Miscellaneous Flavoxate	

DRUGS USED TO PROMOTE BLADDER EMPTYING

Inadequate bladder emptying may be due to bladder-outlet obstruction or to detrusor failure or to a combination of both disorders. Ultimately, residual urine occurring in any clinical situation results from a failure of detrusor force. That is, the detrusor fails either to sustain sufficient pressure to completely empty, or it fails to generate sufficient pressure to overcome the outlet resistance.

The bladder may be unable to contract, and if this is the case, it is called *acontractile.* In such a bladder, there are no coordinated expulsive contractions of the detrusor and therefore it is unable to empty. Some acontractile bladders can generate some pressure due to abnormal tonus in the bladder wall. The degree of tonus is related to the bladder volume so intravesical pressure rises with bladder filling. If the pressure is high enough, the bladder neck may be opened, and urine may be expelled by abdominal straining.

The atonic bladder which has no tonus and no coordinated contractions is extremely rare. Pharmaceutical attempts to stimulate the truly atonic bladder are futile. This type of detrusor contractile dysfunction is best managed by intermittent self-catheterisation or a permanent indwelling urethral or suprapubic catheter.

Other contractile dysfunctions may respond to pharmacological treatment either by bladder stimulation or by reduction of outlet resistance or both. The causes of contractile dysfunction are shown in Table 28.

Table 28
Causes of Detrusor Contractile Dysfunction

Neurogenic
- Autonomous bladder
  - Sacral/infrasacral cord lesion
  - Cauda equina lesion
  - Autonomic neuropathy
    - Metabolic — diabetes, uraemia, porphyria, hypothyroidism
    - Infectious — Guillain-Barré
    - Toxic — alcoholism, heavy metals
    - Collagen disease — SLE polyarteritis
    - Carcinomatous
  - Pelvic surgery
    - Abdomino-perineal excision of rectum
    - Low anterior resection
    - Cordoma
    - Wertheim hysterectomy
  - Pelvic radiotherapy
- Decompensated neuropathic bladder
- Recovery phase after acute spinal-cord injury

Myogenic
- Overstretch
  - Acute retention
  - Chronic retention
- Radiation
- Outlet obstruction

Psychogenic
- Hysterical retention
- Bashfulness
- Pain
- Postoperative

Pharmacogenic
- Anticholinergic agents
- Ganglion blockers
- Tricyclic antidepressants
- Anaesthetics — general, epidural or spinal

ENHANCEMENT OF DETRUSOR FUNCTION (BLADDER STIMULANTS)

Bladder function can be enhanced by cholinergic agents which stimulate the postganglionic muscarinic nerve endings on the detrusor muscle. Acetylcholine, the classical agent, is too rapidly degraded and too generalised in effect to be useful, and synthetic cholinergic agents are therefore used.

Indications

The main indication for the use of bladder stimulation is non-obstructive urinary retention or impaired voiding efficiency. When this is due to drugs which depress detrusor function, these agents should be discontinued. Outflow obstruction is a contraindication to detrusor stimulation and must be excluded. Postoperative and psychogenic retention may respond to cholinergic agents by injection. Effective voiding function may be restored by bladder stimulation in patients in whom there are ineffective or inadequate detrusor contractions secondary to overstretch of the bladder wall (for example, after prostatectomy for chronic retention), or secondary to neuropathy. Bethanechol is widely used to stimulate the neuropathic bladder either in the recovery phase after spinal injury or when incomplete emptying becomes a problem later in management. Stimulation of the autonomous bladder has been used to facilitate emptying by straining, but management by intermittent self-catheterisation is preferable. In neuropathic bladders in particular, concurrent lowering of outlet resistance by drugs or surgery may be required.

Cholinergic Agents

Carbachol is a choline ester with parasympathomimetic properties. It stimulates neuromuscular junctions of the bladder and bowel. It is a useful and cheap agent which is widely used especially in patients with postoperative retention of urine. Some patients do not tolerate it because of the intestinal colic or diarrhoea which it can induce. This intestinal stimulatory effect makes its use in patients who have had recent bowel anastomosis somewhat hazardous.

Bethanechol *(Myotonine)* is similar in action to carbachol but seems to have more effect on the urinary bladder and less effect on the bowel. It is generally better tolerated and is useful when long-term bladder stimulation is required.

Distigmine (*Ubretid*) is a long-acting anticholinesterase. It is analogous in effect to carbachol and has a pronounced detrusor-stimulating effect especially when given by injection, making it useful for postoperative retention.

Adverse Drug Reactions

The other cholinergic effects of these agents may be troublesome. Stimulation of gastrointestinal muscle and secretion may cause diarrhoea or aggravate peptic ulceration. Sweating, miosis and bradycardia can occur.

They are contraindicated in pregnancy and in patients with asthma or cardiac disease. Retention due to bladder-outlet obstruction is an absolute contraindication to the use of these agents.

NURSING IMPLICATIONS

Assessment

Postoperative urinary retention can often be avoided by good nursing management. Getting male patients to stand to void, ensuring privacy and adequate postoperative analgesia will prevent many problems.

Cholinergic agents should not be used in patients who are pregnant, have bronchospasm, cardiac disease or urinary obstruction. Adrenergic blockers should not be used when congestive heart failure is evident.

Evaluation

During trials of micturition using bladder stimulants, patients should be monitored carefully. Overstretch of the bladder due to prolonged and unsuccessful trials must be avoided.

In spinal-injury patients, cholinergic agents can aggravate dyssynergia (see below), and can result in autonomic dysreflexia, with headache, sweating and profound hypotension. This is a medical emergency, requiring *immediate* catheterisation. Delay in its treatment can be fatal.

The occurrence of intestinal colic or diarrhoea may make cholinergic treatment unacceptable to patients. Cardiovascular and respiratory effects should be evaluated. Arterial pressure response should be monitored when adrenergic blockers are used (cross-reference to Chapter 7 for evaluation of postural hypotension).

REDUCTION OF OUTLET RESISTANCE

Bladder-outlet resistance can be reduced by drugs which act on either the smooth-muscle or striated-muscle components of the distal-sphincter mechanism. Alpha-adrenergic blockers relax the smooth-muscle component, while striated-muscle relaxants act on the voluntary striated component.

Indications

Bladder-outlet obstruction due to urethral strictures, valves or prostatic enlargement requires surgical correction and does not respond to drug therapy. Early or mild degrees of benign prostatic obstruction may be temporarily improved by relaxation of the bladder-neck musculature or the smooth-muscle component of the prostatic capsule by alpha blockers. These agents have also been effective for short periods when patients were unfit for, or unwilling to undergo, surgery. Obstructions such as those which occur at the bladder neck and distal-sphincteric mechanism are amenable to pharmaceutical relief, but this is seldom of a permanent nature.

The normal bladder neck is actively pulled open by detrusor contractions and remains open until the bladder relaxes again. In some men there is a dyssynergia of the bladder neck so that when the detrusor contracts, the neck closes, causing obstruction. These men present between 30 and 50 years of age with symptoms of prostatitis or "prostatism". Definitive treatment for this condition consists of bladder-neck incision, but this carries a risk of retrograde ejaculation and infertility. When fertility is important to the patient, the bladder neck can be reversibly relaxed by alpha-adrenergic blockade and the effect monitored by urinary flowmetry.

The normal distal-sphincter mechanism relaxes synchronously with a voiding detrusor contraction to facilitate emptying. In detrusor-sphincter dyssynergia, there is a failure of this synchronous relaxation; reflex contraction of the distal mechanism occurs during voiding and can produce complete, partial or intermittent outflow obstruction. Detrusor-sphincter dyssynergia occurs in neuropathic bladder dysfunction, particularly in patients with lesions of the spinal cord above the sacral centre for micturition. About 80% of patients with such lesions have this problem, and if untreated, it can cause renal damage. Treatment is surgical endoscopic sphincterotomy. A therapeutic trial of drug treatment may be indicated where surgery is impracticable or hazardous, or when the degree of obstruction is only mild or intermittent. In such cases the therapeutic attack may be directed towards relaxation of either the smooth-muscle or striated-muscle components of the sphincter mechanisms. Logically, in patients with a spastic paraparesis, drugs which relax striated muscle would be expected to be more effective than smooth-muscle relaxants, although both have been employed with clinical success.

In patients with an acontractile bladder such as the autonomous bladder of cauda equina, pelvic nerve or conus medullaris lesions, reduction of outlet resistance can be employed to enable the patient to void by straining. A fine balance is needed between sufficient reduction of outlet resistance to facilitate emptying and its reduction to the point of incontinence. Since the pelvic-floor striated musculature is generally flaccid in such lesions, the use of alpha-adrenergic blockade is the preferred method of lowering the outlet resistance.

Alpha Adrenergic Blockers

Phenoxybenzamine (*Dibenyline*) a long-acting, cumulative alpha blocker, is preferable to phentolamine, which requires parenteral administration and has only a short half-life. Phenoxybenzamine acts at two sites on the bladder outlet, relaxing the adrenergic smooth muscle of the male bladder neck, and the smooth-muscle component of the distal-sphincter mechanism of both sexes. It can take up to 10 days to reach its full effect and has the potential of reducing the resting urethral closure pressure by 50%. ***Prazosin*** *(Hypovase)*, an alpha-1 receptor blocker, has similar effects and is reportedly more effective in lowering bladder-outlet resistance.

Adverse Drug Reactions

Postural hypotension can be a problem at higher doses and requires dosage reduction; hence, stepwise dosage introduction is recommended. Failure of ejaculation is common due to bladder-neck relaxation, allowing retrograde ejaculation to occur, and to the failure of seminal emission which is also under alpha-adrenergic control. Prazosin can induce or aggravate urinary incontinence in the elderly female whose control was already tenuous. Nasal congestion, miosis and reflex tachycardia can occur. These drugs are contraindicated in congestive cardiac failure.

Striated Muscle Relaxants

The striated-muscle component of the distal sphincter mechanism is cholinergic. In trying to reduce outlet resistance, the anticholinergic agents used must not also reduce detrusor contractility. Equally, they should not cause respiratory depression or total paralysis.

Baclofen (*Lioresal*) is an ideal agent to use as it affects both periurethral striated muscle and can alleviate skeletal-muscle spasms of spinal origin. A derivative of gamma-aminobutyric acid (GABA), it produces presynaptic inhibition affecting both polysynaptic and monosynaptic transmission. It also diminishes reflex contractions by reducing gamma efferent activity from the muscle spindles. Generalised hypotonia and drowsiness may be caused and step-wise introduction of the drug is necessary. It can mildly inhibit the detrusor at high dosage. It is the drug of choice for the treatment of sphincteric-outlet obstruction in patients with spinal injuries. It is relatively contraindicated in psychotic or epileptic patients.

Diazepam (*Valium*) is a muscle relaxant, but its central tranquillising effect may make it unacceptable to the patient. It is useful in cases where there is a functional sphincteric-outlet obstruction associated with anxiety, in which case the central effect of the drug may be more therapeutic than its peripheral effect.

Dantrolene sodium (*Dantrium*) reduces skeletal-muscle contractility by an inhibitory effect on excitation-contraction coupling beyond the neuromuscular junction possibly by blocking the release of activator from the sarcoplasmic reticulum. It affects predominantly fast-twitch fibres but also affects slow ones, and its effects are generalised. Profound muscular hypotonia, respiratory depression, hepatocellular damage and drowsiness can occur and limit its usefulness. Dosage titration is necessary, especially when a degree of muscular tonicity is required by the patient for locomotion. Its long-term use cannot be recommended when the only indication for its use is bladder dysfunction.

Methocarbamol reduces skeletal-muscle spasm through a central effect on spinal internuncial neurones. It is claimed not to affect normal muscle tone and to be non-toxic. Its effectiveness in detrusor-sphincter dyssynergia is unknown. ***Orphenadrine*** (*Disipal*) has a parasympatholytic action useful in the treatment of muscular rigidity associated with Parkinson's disease or drug-induced extra-pyramidal muscular dyskinesia. Its use in outlet obstruction is limited by its tendency to reduce detrusor contractility, and therefore it is not recommended.

Table 29
Summary of Drugs Used to Promote Bladder Emptying

Bladder Stimulants	Urethral Relaxants
Cholinergic agents	Alpha-adrenergic blockers
Carbachol	Phenoxybenzamine
Bethanechol	Prazosin
Distigmine	
	Striated-muscle relaxants
	Baclofen
	Diazepam
	Dantrolene

WARNING

None of the agents mentioned in this chapter can be recommended for use in the treatment of functional disorders of the bladder associated with pregnancy. Since these disorders run a self-limiting course, an expectant policy is best adopted after careful exclusion of an infective cause.

SELF-EVALUATION TEST

1. List the types of drugs which can be used to relax the bladder. Give the indications for the use of such agents. What precautions need to be taken?
2. How may the detrusor be stimulated? Under what circumstances are such agents (a) indicated, (b) dangerous, (c) unhelpful?
3. What types of drugs can cause urinary retention?
4. Name the drugs which can be used to lower bladder-outlet resistance. When might they be used, and what side effects do they have?

Table 30
Drugs Used in the Treatment of Bladder Dysfunction

Drug Group	Drug Name	Use	Action	Adverse Reactions	Nursing Implications
Drugs Used to Reduce Intravesical Pressure					
Anticholinergics	Atropine Hyoscine Hyoscyamine Propantheline Dicyclomine Penthienate Oxybutynin	Incontinence	Relax detrusor and lower intravesical pressure	Dry mouth, visual blurring, constipation, tachycardia (see Chapter 5)	***Assess:*** motivation, mobility, urinary obstruction, cause of incontinence, cause of leak around catheter, presence of urinary infection. ***Administer:*** stop anticholinergics when catheter is removed. ***Evaluate:*** for increasing continence, for urine retention, for dry mouth. ***Teach:*** limitations of treatment, need for active participation, alternative methods, to seek medical advice for retention, sedative effects of imipramine will diminish.
Tricyclic antidepressants	Imipramine	Incontinence Enuresis	Weak anticholinergic and ganglion blocking activity; causes relaxation of detrusor	As for anticholinergic sedation (see Chapter 28)	
Smooth-muscle relaxants	Flavoxate	Incontinence	Smooth-muscle relaxation	Drowsiness, blurred vision	
Beta sympathomimetics	Orciprenaline Salbutamol	Adjunctive therapy with anticholinergics	Stimulation of beta adrenoreceptors	See Chapter 5	

continued

Drug Group	Drug Name	Use	Action	Adverse Reactions	Nursing Implications
Cholinergics	Carbachol Bethanechol	Urinary retention	Parasympathomimetic	Diarrhoea, aggravation of peptic ulcer, sweating, miosis, bradycardia	***Assess:*** Cause of postoperative retention, for pregnancy, bronchospasm, cardiac failure, urinary obstruction. ***Evaluate:*** avoid overstretching during long trials; for autonomic dysreflexia in spinal injury, catheterise immediately; for diarrhoea, colic; arterial pressure response to adrenergic blockers; cardiorespiratory effects.
	Distigmine	Urinary retention	Anticholinesterase	As above	
Drugs Used to Treat Urinary Retention					
Alpha-adrenergic blockers	Phenoxybenzamine Prazosin	Urinary retention	Relaxation of bladder neck in male; relaxation of distal sphincter in both sexes	Postural hypotension, failure of ejaculation, nasal congestion, miosis, tachycardia	
Striated-muscle relaxants	Baclofen	Urinary retention	Relaxes periurethral striated muscle	Hypotonia, drowsiness	
	Diazepam	Urinary retention	Muscle relaxant	Sedation (see Chapters 28 and 30)	
	Dantrolene	Urinary retention	Reduces skeletal muscle contractility	Hypotonia, respiratory depression	
	Methocarbamol	Urinary retention	Reduces skeletal muscle contractility	Rare	

SECTION 3

11

DRUGS THAT ACT ON THE ENDOCRINE SYSTEM

Ross D. MacPherson

OBJECTIVES

At the conclusion of this chapter the reader should be able to:

1. list the drugs that may be used to regulate or compensate for altered function of the various endocrine glands;
2. briefly describe the site and mode of action of such drugs;
3. list adverse reactions that may be associated with the use of these drugs;
4. list factors of importance in nursing patients for whom such medication has been prescribed;
5. list factors relating to administration and adverse reactions to such drugs that are important in counselling patients.

PREREQUISITE KNOWLEDGE

Before commencing this chapter you should know:

1. the names and locations of the various hormone-producing glands;
2. the names and actions of the various hormones, together with the effects of under supply and over supply of each on the body;
3. the biological process known as "chemical feedback"

Without effective control and integration of its many internal activities, no organism as complex as the human body could function. This regulation of body processes is provided by the endocrine system.

The endocrine system consists of a number of ductless glands which release their products — hormones — directly into the bloodstream. Hormones may be either proteins or steroids and are large molecules.

They are carried by the bloodstream from their points of manufacture to their sites of action and are the main regulators of metabolism, reproduction and stress responses in the organism. Other functions affected by hormonal activity include those associated with the maintenance of homeostasis — fluid, electrolyte, energy and acid-base balance. Excess or deficiency of any of the various hormones makes the difference between normalcy and abnormality, even, at times, between life and death.

Many students have difficulty in understanding the function of hormonal drugs. This problem need not arise if the student first learns the actions of naturally occurring hormones. Synthetic preparations mimic the effects producted by the naturally occurring substances. This chapter deals with those drugs that may be prescribed to alter, regulate or compensate for abnormalities in function of the various endocrine glands in the following major groups: trophic hormones, adrenocorticosteroids, hypoglycaemic agents, drugs acting on the thyroid gland, sex hormones, and miscellaneous hormonal agents.

TROPHIC HORMONES

Although there is a range of trophic hormones produced by the body and all may be used for specific purposes, only the three most common will be mentioned here.

HUMAN CHORIONIC GONADOTROPHIN OR HCG

HCG is derived from the urine of pregnant women. Its action is similar to that of luteinising hormone. HCG effects gonadal function in both males and females. It induces ovulation in females and the descent of the testes in the male. The actual mode of action is complex. In males the interstitial cells of the testes are stimulated resulting in increased androgen production.

Its main use in females is as a fertility agent to induce ovulation following follicular-development stimulation with FSH (follicle stimulating hormone). To a lesser extent, chorionic gonadotrophin has been employed in the prevention of habitual abortion and in the treatment of secondary amenorrhoea.

In males HCG is used for the treatment of cryptorchidism.

Chorionic gonadotrophin is likely to cause oedema formation and because of this, its use may be hazardous in patients suffering from asthma, epilepsy, cardiac dysfunction or renal dysfunction. Allergic manifestations to HCG are quite common, while its overzealous use in children may result in the development of precocious puberty.

CORTICOTROPHIN AND TETRACOSACTRIN

Natural corticotrophin is responsible for the stimulation and release of the corticosteroids from the adrenal cortex. It is produced in the pituitary in response to the levels of circulating cortisol (hydrocortisone) and is thus an example of a chemical-feedback mechanism. Tetracosactrin is a synthetic substance with similar properties. Because there is a lesser likelihood of allergic reactions with tetracosactrin (*Synacthen*), it is more often used.

Tetracosactrin is used as a diagnostic agent to assess the function of the adrenal cortex, and in the treatment of a variety of disease states for which steroid therapy is routine (for example, collagen disorders, asthma, postherpetic neuralgia). However, tetracosactrin cannot be used in the therapy of adrenocorticoid insufficiency. If a prior deficiency exists in the adrenal cortex, stimulation with tetracosactrin will not produce the release of cortisol.

Commercial preparations of tetracosactrin are available as simple solutions or as depot preparations. Simple solutions are used diagnostically for the evaluation of adrenal function. A small amount, 250 mcg, is administered via IV infusion. The secretion of steroids by the adrenal cortex can then be measured by chemical analysis of plasma corticosteroid levels. Depot preparations are usually employed for therapeutic treatment. Doses of about 1mg for adults are given by IM injection, initially at daily intervals but later less frequently — at three to seven day intervals depending on response.

The adverse effects of tetracosactrin are the same as those for adrenocorticosteroids (see page 183).

THYROTROPHIN OR TSH

Thyrotrophin or thyroid stimulating hormone (TSH) is the substance produced by the anterior pituitary gland that controls the release of thyroid hormone from the thyroid gland. Secretion of TSH is inhibited by high levels of thyroid hormone in the blood and stimulated by a low level, another example of a chemical-feedback mechanism.

TSH is sometimes used as a test to differentiate between myxoedema due to malfunction of the thyroid gland or of the pituitary. TSH is injected by the IV route, and thyroid gland function is measured using a radioiodine uptake test

NURSING IMPLICATIONS

1. Nursing implications of the use of chorionic gonadotrophin relate to its ability to cause oedema and to allergic reactions. Observations of either of these phenomena should be carefully made and reported.
2. As the effects of corticotrophin and tetracosactrin are those of the adrenocorticosteroids, and the effects of thyrotrophin are those of the thyroid hormones, nursing implications will be as for these latter substances (see page 187).

ADRENOCORTICOSTEROIDS

GENERAL

Corticosteroid drugs are a constant source of confusion to the student as they have a multitude of effects, they are used in so many disease states.

An adequate knowledge of physiology in the first instance will make the task of understanding corticosteroid drugs much easier.

In general, steroids excreted from the adrenal cortex have two different major activities: ***glucocorticoid action*** and ***mineralocorticoid action.*** The former implies their ability to influence energy functions by alterations in glucose release and consumption, while the latter activity refers to the actions of steroids in affecting electrolyte balance. Cortisol is the best example of a major glucocorticoid, while aldosterone is the classic potent mineralocorticoid.

Nearly all synthetic-steroid preparations have some degree of mixed effects with respect to glucocorticoid or mineralocorticoid potency. However one of the two types of activity will usually predominate.

In considering the myriad uses of corticosteroids, it must be remembered that in many cases they are used as replacement therapy. That is, they are used in the same manner as insulin, which is given by injection to diabetics who do not produce their own insulin. Likewise, one can give synthetic corticosteroids to people who for one reason or another have a decreased output or malfunction in their own endogenous steroid production.

On the other hand, corticosteroids are also used to treat a multitude of different diseases. Rather than list all these diseases, consider the following list of the different actions which corticosteroids have on physiological processes. This will provide an understanding of how these drugs can be employed in the treatment of disease states as diverse as arthritis and leukaemia.

EFFECTS ON BODY SYSTEMS

The many corticosteroid drugs available include ***cortisone, hydrocortisone, prednisone, prednisolone, methylprednisolone, betamethasone*** and ***dexamethasone.*** The adrenocorticoid steroids have a wide range of actions. The major effects on various body systems are listed as follows.

Carbohydrate and protein metabolism

Glucocorticoids promote gluconeogenesis within the liver. In high doses, adrenocorticoids cause changes in both carbohydrate and protein metabolism which can result in osteoporosis, muscle wasting and increased protein catabolism.

Fat metabolism

Corticosteroids are involved in the movement of fat from peripheral depots and result in a typical pattern of fat deposition in the face and upper back. This is considered to be an adverse reaction rather than a therapeutic effect.

Electrolyte and water balance

Steroid administration is associated, in some instances, with considerable electrolyte retention and subsequent water retention. The extent to which various adrenocorticoids stimulate this fluid retention differs markedly.

Cardiovascular system

In conditions of corticosteroid insufficiency, steroids are employed to maintain cardiovascular status and to prevent reduction in cardiovascular output and capillary permeability. Overuse of adrenocorticosteroids can lead to hypertension and capillary fragility.

Muscle function

Use of steroids for long periods results in muscle weakness and wasting.

Nervous system

Adrenocorticosteroids can exert a powerful effect on the central nervous system. Some patients receiving steroidal drugs undergo psychiatric change, most commonly irritability, depression and apathy. Some may develop true psychotic reactions. Fortunately, these effects subside on cessation of steroid therapy.

Lymphoid tissue

Adrenocorticosteroids induce lymphocytopenia and a decrease in lymphoid tissue mass.

Anti-inflammatory properties

Steroids are often employed for their ability to suppress inflammatory reactions. Although an acceptable explanation for this effect is lacking, the clinical results are often striking. Steroidal agents suppress inflammatory responses in all tissue, resulting in the arrest of the normal occurrence of heat, erythema, swelling and tenderness. In order to achieve this effect, steroids may be given systemically or applied locally as creams or sprays.

Immune response

In general terms, corticosteroids suppress immunological response. This may be due to the retardation of antibody production, although this theory remains controversial. Depending on the use for which the drug is being employed, suppression of the immune response may be considered either an adverse reaction or a therapeutic effect.

USES

Corticosteroids are employed in the treatment of a wide range of conditions.

Replacement therapy

Synthetic steroids are used as replacement therapy in conditions resulting from adrenal insufficiency where, because of either functional or congenital abnormality, insufficient adrenocorticosteroids are produced by the adrenal cortex. Such therapy must be carefully controlled to prevent toxicity. Hydrocortisone or cortisone are usually the drugs of choice.

Anti-inflammatory ability

The ability of steroids to suppress inflammatory reaction makes the drugs ideal for this purpose. As a general rule steroid therapy is withheld until other more conservative measures have failed. Rheumatoid arthritis, asthma and inflammatory diseases of the gastrointestinal tract are all areas in which steroidal agents may be indicated.

Haematological conditions

Because of their antiproliferative effect on white blood cells, adrenocorticoid preparations are often used in the treatment of chronic leukaemias. Steroids may also be useful in helping treat the cachexia and fever associated with the late stages of chronic lymphocytic leukaemias.

Cardiovascular effects

Steroid therapy is of great value in the treatment of cerebral oedema of any aetiology. Large doses — often greater than 100 mg — of prednisone are employed.

Shock

Steroid therapy is a mainstay in the treatment of shock from any cause. Both traumatic and allergic shock will respond to systemic steroid therapy. Again large doses, sometimes up to 1 gram, of hydrocortisone are used.

Diagnostic procedures

Adrenocorticosteroids are employed in a variety of tests to assess function of the adrenal cortex and to assess whether obese patients are in fact Cushingoid.

Adverse Drug Reactions

The list of adverse reactions to adrenocorticosteroid therapy is long. Many of these adverse effects are seen only after prolonged therapy.

Cushing's syndrome

Any overuse or oversecretion of adrenocorticosteroids can lead to the occurrence of the set of symptoms collectively known as Cushing's syndrome. The syndrome can be categorised by the presence of all or some of the signs listed below. In many cases, where long-term steroid therapy is indicated, the eventual appearance of these characteristics is often inevitable.

The physical changes of Cushing's syndrome include moon face; buffalo hump, due to increased fat deposition on the back of the neck; striae, partiularly of the abdomen, due to protein breakdown; hypertrophy of the clitoris; hirsutism and proximal muscle wasting. Biochemical abnormalities include hyperglycaemia, hypokalaemic alkalosis and changes in blood coagulability. Neurological changes include psychoses, mood changes and irritability. Other effects of Cushing's syndrome include hypertension, gastric ulceration, increased susceptibility to infection and osteoporosis.

Dosage

Dosage with steroidal agents should follow a set regime. Steroid therapy is usually commenced with the lowest possible dose, which is increased until improvement in the disease state is achieved. The patient is maintained on this dose for as long as is required. Under normal circumstances such steroid therapy is not continued longer than four to six weeks. The exception is in cases of adrenocorticoid insufficiency.

When therapy is to be discontinued, the dose must be decreased gradually over a period of days or even weeks in some patients. The gradual decrease in dose is required to prevent the onset of acute endogenous adrenal insufficiency, since the body's production of endogenous adrenocorticosteroids will have been suppressed during treatment. Thus, time must be allowed for adrenal-cortex function to return to normal. Large single doses of corticosteroids are unlikely to produce severe systemic adverse effects.

Comparison of strengths

The potency of corticosteroids differs, on a milligram for milligram basis, for each preparation. For example, the following list indicates the relative potencies of some corticosteroid drugs for equivalent anti-inflammatory action:

hydrocortisone	25mg
prednisone	5mg
prednisolone	5mg
methylprednisolone	4mg
dexamethasone	500mcg
betamethasone	500mcg

The difference between prednisone and prednisolone

Prednisone is an inactive drug which is metabolised by the liver to prenisolone, an active substance. Although the drugs are similar in potency and action, they should not be considered interchangeable because such equivalence depends on conversion by the liver. Patients with hepatic dysfunction must be given prednisolone.

NURSING IMPLICATIONS

A discussion of the glucocorticoids necessitates the consideration of the use of these drugs for replacement therapy, immunosuppressive therapy or in the management of a disease process (as anti-inflammatory agents).

Assessment

Assessment includes the establishment of the reason for administering the medication. Concurrent disease, pregnancy and past history of peptic ulceration or tuberculosis should be noted. Baseline vital signs such as BP, pulse rate, temperature, respiration and weight, as well as body-fat distribution, should be recorded. Identify skin colour and texture, nail and hair condition, and presence of bruising. Assess emotional state.

Management

Avoidance of aspirin will minimise the risk of peptic ulceration. Patients on long-term high doses should be treated with care due to the risks of bruising and fractures. This particularly applies during physiotherapy treatment. Care to avoid infection in the patient should be exercised. It should be noted that infection is not always easily identified in patients on glucocorticoid therapy, as body temperature may remain normal in the presence of infection. There may be a need to reduce dietary sodium and increase protein and potassium intake. Therapy should be tapered off slowly and never stopped abruptly.

Evaluation

Consideration of the effectiveness of the drug and dosage is important. Monitor the GIT for signs of gastric bleeding (for example, occult blood in stools). Observe skin for signs of thinning or bruising and wounds for delayed healing. Observe for weakness, muscle pain, backache, weight gain, fluid retention and hypertension. Observe for signs of hypernatraemia, hypokalaemia and protein deficiency. Emotional stress should also be evaluated.

Patient teaching

Patients should be advised not to suddenly cease medication without referral to a physician. They should avoid contact with persons with known active infections and should report to a medical officer any signs of infection, for example, sore throat. The patient should be advised to wear an identification tag and to inform their dentist, any other doctors and pharmacist of the fact they are receiving steroid therapy. Regular medical checks should be advised. Inform patients of adverse effects, especially potassium depletion, oedema and delayed wound healing. Those on long-term high-dose therapy should be warned of the risk of osteoporosis leading to increased susceptibility to fractures.

HYPOGLYCAEMIC AGENTS

INSULIN

It is not in the scope of this chapter to review extensively the physiology of glucose utilisation, but a brief statement is necessary. Glucose is the body's main source of energy, but unfortunately, the molecule is of such a structure that it cannot be stored in the body. That means it will either be used immediately, or it will be inactivated in the body.

In order to counter this problem, the body secretes two hormones from the islets of Langerhans in the pancreas. Insulin is formed in the beta cells, and glucagon is formed in the alpha cells. The main role of insulin is to convert glucose into glycogen, which can be stored as a source of energy in tissue such as liver and skeletal muscle. Glucagon does the opposite. It is responsible for mobilising glycogen and moving it from storage sites to utilisation sites, as glucose. The balance between these two hormones is complex and will depend on the energy need of the body at any particular time.

It is understandable that if an individual is deficient in insulin, he will lack the capacity to lower his blood-glucose level and glucose will be excreted in the urine, producing an osmotic diuresis which is the reason that polyuria and polydipsia are prominent symptoms of insulin deficit. A deficiency of insulin results in the condition known as diabetes mellitus, and the treatment revolves around either replacing the insulin which the individual lacks or stimulating production of small amounts of insulin the body may be able to produce.

Many animals, apart from humans, utilise insulin in exactly the same way, and the structure of animal insulin, although not exactly the same as its human counterpart, is similar and can be substituted in most cases. Thus insulin is obtained from animal sources, mainly from pigs and cows (porcine and bovine insulins), although other species such as fish have occasionally been employed.

A further development in the use of animal insulins has been the refinement of the molecules such that only the portions of the molecule actually necessary for lowering blood sugar are included. These molecules are variously referred to as single peak, purified or monocomponent insulins.

In Chapter 8, under "anticoagulants", the concept of the term "units" was introduced. Insulin is another example of a product obtained from animal sources, so its potency is also measured in arbitrarily defined units rather than by weight. In the U.K., all commercial insulins are 100 units/mL strength.

Most students have been confused at one stage or another by the bewildering range of insulins found in the ward refrigerator, but there is really no cause for alarm.

When naturally occurring animal insulin is injected, it works well in lowering blood sugar, and it starts acting rapidly. The problem is that the action will not last for long. A person with diabetes needs blood-sugar level to be controlled 24 hours a day and does not want to be giving himself or herself injections every hour, which would almost be the case if the only insulin available were the rapidly acting type.

Therefore, drug research has produced a range of insulins. Although they do not lower blood sugar as rapidly as the natural substance, they do so for much longer, even up to 24 hours following a single injection. This is much more convenient for the diabetic patient.

Administration and storage

Insulin is ineffective when given orally because the acid secretion of the stomach rapidly breaks down its protein structure; thus, parenteral administration is necessary. The drug is given by subcutaneous injection although fast-acting insulin (e.g. *Actrapid*) may be given intravenously if indicated.

Table 31
Some Insulin Preparations

Official Name	Other Names
Fast Acting	
Insulin BP	Insulin Soluble, Insulin
Neutral Insulin	Actrapid
Intermediate Acting	
Insulin Zinc Suspension	Semilente
Insulin Zinc Suspension (porcine)	Monotard
Biphasic Insulin	Rapitard
Long Acting	
Insulin Zinc Suspension	Lente
Insulin Zinc Suspension (crystalline)	Ultralente

Insulin should be stored under refrigeration at between 2° to 8°C. It must *never* be frozen. Should ice form in the insulin vial, the insulin molecules will be denatured and become ineffective. In emergency conditions, insulin may be stored at normal room temperatures. Under such conditions the expiry date on the vial becomes meaningless. Thus, diabetics could carry their insulin with them on holiday, for example, for a week with complete safety. However, as soon as practicable, the vial should be discarded and fresh, refrigerated stock used again.

Most insulins are true suspensions. That is, the active ingredients are still in solid form and not dissolved in solution. When such a vial is taken from storage, the white precipitate at the bottom is insulin. Before drawing up the injection, the vial should be rotated gently to resuspend the active substance.

Uses

Patients suffering from diabetes mellitus have either an absolute lack or a relative lack of endogenous insulin, which leads to hyperglycaemia. Insulin injections are used to replace or supplement the natural source in these individuals. Its action is the same as that of endogenous insulin.

Adverse Drug Reactions

1. Insufficient or excess insulin may lead to hyperglycaemia or hypoglycaemia respectively.
2. Localised reaction to insulin injections is often reported. Of these reactions the most common are the lipodystrophies. Repeated injection of insulin into the same site may result in either atrophy or hypertrophy of adipose tissue (lipoatrophy or lipohypertrophy). This is disfiguring and cosmetically embarrassing, and absorption of insulin from these areas may be abnormal. Injection sites should be varied to avoid this occurrence. Local pruritus or swelling at the injection site is also common.
3. Systemic adverse effects are less common. Occasionally a "serum sickness" type of effect is seen. A more serious effect of long-term insulin use is the possible development of antibodies which can lead to insulin resistance. Large doses of insulin must be administered to compensate for this. Monocomponent insulin, being less antigenic, reduces the possibility of antibody formation.

ORAL HYPOGLYCAEMIC AGENTS

During research into the sulphonamide group of antiinfective agents, it was noticed that some of them were capable of producing hypoglycaemia. Further research led to the development of oral hypoglycaemic drugs. Table 32 lists those in use.

Table 32
Some Oral Hypoglycaemic Agents

Generic Name	Trade Name
Sulphonylurea Group	
Acetohexamide	*Dimelor*
Chlorpropamide	*Diabinese*
Glibenclamide	*Daonil, Euglucon*
Gliclazide	*Diamicron*
Tolbutamide	*Rastinon*
Biguanide Group	
Metformin	*Glucophage*

These drugs are not an oral form of insulin and do not directly lower blood sugar. Instead they act in an indirect way, either by causing the pancreas to secrete insulin, or in the case of the biguanide metformin, by promoting the peripheral uptake of glucose.

Uses

The oral hypoglycaemic agents are employed *only* in the treatment of maturity-onset diabetes mellitus. For these agents to exert their effect, there must be some beta cells of the islets of Langerhans functioning. They cannot be used in the treatment of juvenile-onset diabetes mellitus, since such patients have no beta-cell function.

Adverse Drug Reactions

The oral hypoglycaemic agents are a potent group of drugs with a reasonably high incidence of adverse reactions. Because of their potency in lowering blood-sugar levels, the most dangerous adverse effect is hypoglycaemia. This risk is especially high for outpatients whose diet may be inadequate. Oral hypoglycaemic drugs should always be taken with food or at least near a mealtime, which will most often be breakfast. As the drugs are usually taken on a once- or twice-daily basis, patient compliance is not a major problem.

The sulphonylurea group also causes intolerance to alcohol and allergic reactions. The stucture of the sulphonylureas is such that they may cause an inhibition of the enzyme acetaldehyde dehydrogenase within the liver, so that after drinking alcoholic beverages, a build up of acetaldehyde may result, causing nausea, vomiting, flushing and a general feeling of malaise. This is often referred to as the disulfiram (or *Antabuse*) effect, since it has a similar action. Allergic reaction, especially of a dermatological nature, is sometimes seen. Because the structure of the sulphonylureas is similar to that of the sulphonamide anti-infective agents, there may be some cross-sensitivity between the groups.

Metformin, the only biguanide in use, can also cause lactic acidosis in a significant proportion of patients.

Contraindications

The major contraindications to the use of oral hypoglycaemic drugs are juvenile-onset diabetes, renal impairment, hepatic impairment and pregnancy. Metformin is also relatively contraindicated for patients over the age of 65.

Drug Interactions

Many highly protein-bound drugs may displace the sulphonylureas from their body sites resulting in an increased hypoglycaemic effect. Drugs which should be avoided by patients receiving sulphonylureas include aspirin, phenylbutazone and the tetracyclines. The use of beta-adrenergic blocking drugs may also constitute a danger to diabetics, as they tend to mask the symptoms of hypoglycaemia.

NURSING IMPLICATIONS

The hypoglycaemic agents are used to lower the blood-sugar level. Insulin is commonly prescribed for juvenile-onset diabetes in combination with an emphasis on adequate exercise and stable diet. It must be taken into account that change in exercise pattern will necessitate a corresponding insulin and diet adjustment. Insulin may be prescribed for mature-onset diabetes in combination with dietary adjustments, although weight reduction alone may be sufficient. Oral hypoglycaemics may be prescribed to assist in the control of mature-onset diabetes.

Assessment of the patient in terms of pharmacological management will essentially depend on whether the condition has recently presented or whether it has been present for some time. It may be necessary to accurately determine the presence of hypoglycaemic or hyperglycaemic states both by clinical examination and objective blood or urine screening. An assessment should be made of the possible systemic changes that may have occurred as a direct complication of diabetes, for example, leg ulcers or renal failure. Therefore, thorough assessment of the renal, CNS, and cardiovascular systems are essential. Baseline vital signs should be established along with weight and the condition of nails and skin. Previous drug reactions should also be documented. Current medications, alcohol intake and lifestyle parameters must be taken into account. The presence of pregnancy or lactation is an essential feature of assessment.

In terms of management, although insulin may be administered IV, it should be noted that it is unstable when mixed with large volumes of IV fluids, and it should not be given in alkaline fluids. It is best to give it in small volumes via a syringe pump. Diabetic clinics or hospital guidelines should be consulted concerning the protocols for administering insulin either by the IV or SC routes. Insulin should be stored in the refrigerator.

Once the patient has been commenced on hypoglycaemic agents, regular blood and urine screening tests should be evaluated to monitor therapeutic effectiveness. Clinical symptoms and signs of hyperglycaemia must be carefully evaluated. It is important to assess dietary needs and restrictions. Local skin reactions, although rare, should be assessed if they present. Systemic reactions are rare and are mainly associated with sensitivity to the animal tissue from which the insulin has been extracted. In insulin-dependent patients, it is essential to observe for the Somogyi effect. This is characterised by rebound hyperglycaemia that occurs some hours after insulin has been administered.

The education of a diabetic patient should include the education of family and close friends. The patient should be advised that insulin must be taken as prescribed in relation to his/her lifestyle. Any change in lifestyle may necessitate a change in therapy. The patient should also be advised *not* to cease taking the medication without consultation with a diabetic education centre. It is important to ensure that the patient possesses a full understanding of the condition and its possible complications. The patient should be able to identify deviations from the therapeutic effect and differentiate them from complications of the disease process and adverse effects (such as blurred vision, to which tolerance usually develops). Ensure that the patient knows how to treat unexpected effects.

It is essential to inform the patient of those drugs which may induce hypoglycaemia or hyperglycaemia. Teach the patient or family, when appropriate, to identify those conditions in juvenile diabetics which may precipitate hyperglycaemia (such as surgery, menstruation, emotional disturbances, stress or infections) or hypoglycaemia (such as exercise or stress). Part of the education program includes ensuring a full understanding of the medication being used in terms of action, duration and adverse effects. Methods for monitoring blood or urine glucose and ketones should be taught.

Regular medical check-ups are essential, and as minor illnesses may produce instability, patients should be advised to see a medical officer early. Advise the patient to maintain an adequate supply of medication and equipment. Teach the patient and members of the family the technique for administration of the medication. It is important to advise the young female patient that pregnancy will increase the insulin requirements. Ensure a complete understanding of dietary requirements and the need for good general health. A medical identification tag should be worn by people with diabetes.

Note: It is advisable to check with the pharmacist before mixing insulins. As a general rule, the mixing of rapid-acting insulins with long-acting insulins is acceptable. Care must be taken in drawing up such a mixture, so that none of the first insulin drawn into the syringe is allowed to pass into the vial as the second insulin is added. It is recommended that the resultant mixture be injected within five seconds.

Oral hypoglycaemics

Patient education should include relevant points discussed above and the following.

Hypoglycaemia is the major adverse effect in the elderly with poor nutrition, although myocardial infarction has also been implicated. Ensure that the patient can identify deviations from the therapeutic effect and knows what action to take. If unwell, patients should seek advice from the diabetic education centre or medical officer. It is important to stress the dose of hypoglycaemic agent should not be changed or an extra dose taken to catch up if a dose has been missed. Advise that hypoglycaemia can be precipitated when changing from insulin to oral hypoglycaemics or vice versa. Also, insulin may be required in a situation of increased stress, surgery or infection. These medications should not be taken close to retiring for the evening.

THYROID AND ANTITHYROID PREPARATIONS

For individuals not capable of secreting sufficient endogenous thyroid hormone to maintain normal metabolic function, supplementation with thyroid preparations is required. Thus, thyroid preparations are indicated for use in the therapy of hypothyroidism. Conversely, antithyroid drugs are used in the treatment of hyperthyroid conditions to antagonise the production of endogenous thyroid hormone.

DRUGS USED IN THE TREATMENT OF HYPOTHYROIDISM

Drugs used to treat hypothyroidism include ***thyroxine*** *(Eltroxin)* and ***liothyronine,*** also known as tri-iodo-thyronine *(Tertroxin)*.

Thyroxine *(Eltroxin)* is a synthetic thyroid hormone used to supplement simple inadequacy of natural thyronine. ***Liothyronine*** *(Tertroxin)* is synthetic tri-iodo-thyronine (T3), the precursor of thyronine (T4). Both drugs are extremely potent, and doses are normally measured in micrograms. They differ in time of onset and duration of action.

Thyroxine is slow in onset but long acting. Liothyronine is rapidly absorbed from the gastrointestinal tract so its effects are quickly evident, but its action is short and frequent administration is required.

Uses

Both thyroxine and liothyronine are used in the treatment of hypothyroidism. Because of its rapid onset of action, liothyronine is often employed where emergency therapy is indicated. Thyroxine, on the other hand, is usually used for maintenance therapy. Thyroid therapy is also indicated in the treatment of cretinism and juvenile myxoedema.

Adverse Drug Reactions

Common adverse effects include tremor, headache and tachycardia. Less commonly seen adverse effects include gastrointestinal disturbances, weight loss and cardiac arrhythmias. Most of these reactions tend to decrease with time as the patient becomes tolerant to the drug, or subside with a decrease in dosage.

Because thyroid therapy may exacerbate hypertension or cardiac disease, these agents should be used with caution in patients suffering from such conditions.

Drug Interactions

Thyroid replacement agents have been suspected of enhancing the potency of oral anticoagulant preparations.

DRUGS USED IN THE TREATMENT OF HYPERTHYROIDISM

The main drugs used in the treatment of hyperthyroidism are ***carbimazole*** (*Neo-Mercazole*) and ***propylthiouracil.***

Propylthiouracil and ***carbimazole*** exert their antithyroid action by preventing the attachment of iodine to the tyrosine molecule. This prevents the manufacture of di-iodothyronine (T2) in the thyroid gland and so lowers the rate of production of the active T3 and T4 thyroid substances.

Adverse Drug Reactions and Precautions

Adverse reactions to these agents are common, especially during the first two months of therapy. Skin rashes do not necessarily require the cessation of therapy. Other non-specific reactions such as nausea, headache and gastrointestinal upsets have been reported but are usually not serious. The most dangerous adverse reaction associated with the antithyroid drugs is the increased incidence of blood dyscrasias, specifically thrombocytopenia and agranulocytosis. For this reason blood tests are routinely performed.

The nurse should be aware that these drugs also produce a reflex enlargement of the thyroid gland; so they should be used with caution, if at all, for patients suffering any degree of tracheal obstruction, as severe respiratory distress may result.

NURSING IMPLICATIONS

Assessment

Assessment in the pharmacological management of disturbances of thyroid function necessitates the establishment of baseline signs for hypothyroidism or hyperthyroidism. This should include BP, pulse rate, respiration rate, temperature and responses to changes in environmental temperature; weight and weight change, appetite, and bowel activity; mood and general emotional reactions, mood swings, agitation or lethargy; blood and urine glucose, and exophthalmos. Intercurrent cardiac disease and hypertension are important conditions to be noted. Current medications, especially anticoagulants, need to be recorded. Note the presence of pregnancy or lactation. It is important to note the height of children.

Management and Evaluation

Management in hypothyroidism involves consideration of primary pituitary or thyroid disease. In neurosurgical procedures involving the pituitary gland, patients may require postoperative replacement therapy. Correct any adrenal insufficiency before commencing therapy. It may be necessary to readjust steroid medication. Avoid or reduce the use of hypnotics or sedatives. Prevent constipation. Ensure that the patient is warm, and weigh the patient daily. Monitor the pulse rate, and report if in excess of 100 beats/min; follow the appropriate instructions. Evaluate cardiac status and report any angina or dyspnoea. Measure and record height in children.

In terms of administration, it is important to begin with a low dose and slowly increase the dose, administering it before meals. Evaluate the therapeutic effect of the drug, which should appear within 2 to 14 days. Adverse effects of overdose will be observed in the presentation of signs of hyperthyroidism.

The management of patients taking medication for hyperthyroidism will include the following details. Care may need to be taken with the administration of carbimazole and propylthiouracil in pregnancy; as they are excreted in the breast milk, breast feeding is contraindicated. Monitor pulse rate and weight change as indicators of overmedication or undermedication. Regular blood screening may be necessary. Observe and report any sore throat, fever or rash, which may be due to agranulocytosis.

It is important to recognise problems associated with enlargement of the thyroid gland and compression of surrounding structures. The management of thyroid crises with antithyroid drugs and fluids may be necessary along with beta-blocking drugs for cardiac complications. These medications should be administered with meals. It is important to evaluate the therapeutic effectiveness of the drug and to recognise toxic signs which may require a reduction of dose.

Patient teaching

Patient teaching in hypothyroidism will include informing the patient of the signs and symptoms of hypothyroidism and hyperthyroidism so that therapeutic effects can be differentiated from adverse effects. Teach the patient to take his or her pulse and to see a medical officer if there are abnormalities. The patient should be instructed not to discontinue medication as it is usually a long-term replacement form of therapy. They should also be instructed not to alter the prescribed dose without medical supervision.

Patient teaching in hyperthyroidism is similar to hypothyroidism. Teach patients the signs of hypothyroidism and hyperthyroidism and to report any changes to a medical officer. Regular blood screening is necessary, and patients should be told to report any indication of a sore throat to their medical officer as this condition often precedes abnormal haematological findings. Teach the patients to record their own pulse and weight. Ensure an understanding that medications should be taken exactly as prescribed and that doses should never be altered without prior medical advice.

OTHER ANTITHYROID DRUGS

Although the above-mentioned antithyroid agents constitute the main therapy for hyperthyroidism, there are some alternatives. These are discussed briefly.

Iodine

Aqueous iodine solution (Lugol's iodine) was routinely used before the advent of antithyroid drugs. Paradoxically, in patients with hyperthyroidism, administration of large amounts of iodine reduces the production of thyroid hormone by the thyroid gland. This effect is not seen in normothyroid patients. The effect is seen rapidly but may subside within a short period of time. Lugol's iodine is still used prior to thyroid surgery because it reduces friability and vascularity of the gland, making surgery easier. It may be given with a little water or milk.

Radioactive Iodine

Radioactive iodine, I^{131}, emits beta rays and has a half-life of about eight days. When administered to hyperthyroid patients, the radioactive iodine is taken up by the thyroid gland where the beta rays destroy thyroid cells resulting in decreased production of thyroid hormones. I^{131} is usually reserved for the treatment of patients who are not candidates for surgery, for example those with cardiac dysfunction, and elderly or debilitated patients. The use of radioactive iodine is also contraindicated in children, young adults and pregnant women.

Potassium Perchlorate

This substance is rarely used in treatment of hyperthyroidism nowadays. However it will protect the thyroid gland in euthyroid patients when radioactive iodine is to be administered as a diagnostic agent, for example, when radioactive iodine is used for a liver or spleen scan. The potassium perchlorate is given orally prior to administration of the I^{131} and prevents its incorporation into the thyroid gland, thus protecting the patient's thyroid status.

THYROID STORM AND THYROID CRISIS

Thyroid storm or crisis is an acute exacerbation of hyperthyroidism which demands emergency medical treatment. Therapy is instituted with one of the antithyroid drugs in combination with sodium iodide. Supportive therapy is also indicated and may include beta-adrenergic blockade to allay cardiac effects, and steroids. Ice baths may be necessary for hyperpyrexia, if present.

SEX HORMONES

The sex hormones, which are also steroids, fall into the three categories of anabolic steroids, oestrogens and progestogens. See Table 33 for examples.

Table 33
Some Examples of Sex Hormones

Generic Name	Trade Name
Anabolic Steroids	
Nandrolone phenylpropionate	*Durabolin*
Nandrolone decanoate	*Deca Durabolin*
Ethyloestrenol	*Orabolin*
Oestrogens	
Conjugated oestrogens	*Premarin*
Ethinyloestradiol	*Ethinyloestradiol*
Piperazine oestrone sulphate	*Harmogen*
Progestogens	
Hydroxyprogesterone hexanoate	*Proluton Depot*
Norethisterone	*Primolut-N, Utovlan*

Although therapy with any of the above groups is usually given orally, long-acting "depot" preparations are available. These preparations, given by intramuscular injection, have an oil base that gives a slow continual release of drug to the systemic system for up to a month after administration.

ANABOLIC AGENTS

Anabolic steroids imitate the structures and actions of naturally occurring testosterone. They cause an increase in general secondary male characteristics such as growth of hair, penile and testicular development and virilism generally. They possess a second set of effects in their ability to increase protein synthesis and deposition, resulting in a positive nitrogen balance. The overall result is an increase in total skeletal and muscle mass.

They are used to promote growth, to induce weight gain following debilitating illness, in the treatment of eunuchism, hypogonadism and delayed onset of puberty, and in the treatment of some forms of breast cancer, due to their anti-oestrogenic effects.

Adverse Drug Reactions and Contraindications

Apart from the general adverse effects described under the adrenocorticosteroids, masculinisation, although a therapeutic indication, may be an unwanted effect, especially when the drugs are used in females. Masculinisation is characterised by growth of facial hair and deepening of the voice. Anabolic agents are also capable of inducing a cholestatic jaundice.

Considerable expertise is needed in the administration of these drugs, especially for pre-pubescent and adolescent patients. The presence of carcinoma of the prostate or testes is generally considered a contraindication since anabolic agents may promote the growth of such tumours.

OESTROGENS

The oestrogenic steroids have actions related to the naturally occurring oestrogens. They are responsible for maintenance of the menstrual cycle and for the development of secondary female sex characteristics.

Oestrogenic preparations are employed for the treatment of symptoms resulting from failure of ovarian development, and for therapy during menopause when the secretion of endogenous steroid declines, resulting in the characteristic symptoms of menopause. Synthetic oestrogen replacement with ***ethinyloestradiol*** has been shown to be of great use in this condition. Just as anabolic steroids may be used in the treatment of breast cancer, oestrogenic agents are used to treat cancer in the male, for example, carcinoma of the prostate.

In refractory cases of severe acne, oestrogenic agents may be prescribed. This use is generally reserved for female patients.

Adverse Drug Reactions and Contraindications

Long periods of use of oestrogenic preparations as replacement therapy may possibly increase the risk of uterine carcinoma. This warning is found in product data dealing with oestrogenic replacement therapy and in some instances on the product labels. Other adverse effects are as for adrenocorticosteroids (see page 185).

Patients with pre-existing uterine carcinomas should not use oestrogenic steroids as they may stimulate growth of the neoplasm. Patients with a history of thromboembolic disease should use the drugs with caution. Oestrogens are known to depress the activity of clotting factors II, VII, IX and X, and enhance the possibility of embolus formation.

PROGESTOGENS

Progestogenic agents, which also occur naturally, do not possess the wide range of actions of the anabolic or oestrogenic drugs. Physiologically, progesterone is responsible for the maintenance of the second, or secretory, stage of the menstrual cycle.

Both the oestrogens and progestogens may be used as oral contraceptive agents. This use is discussed in Chapter 12. Progestogenic agents are, as a single entity, more commonly used for the treatment of functional uterine bleeding, a condition which may arise at any time during a woman's life. Progesterones have been used in the treatment of dysmenorrhoea and endometriosis.

Some progesterones possess slight androgenic potency and so may be employed in the management of endometrial carcinoma. The usefulness of progesterones in the treatment of threatened abortion has recently been questioned, so is in doubt.

Adverse Drug Reactions

Minor adverse effects due to progesterones may be found in Chapter 12 dealing with oral contraceptives (see page 209). Other adverse effects are similar to those listed for adrenocorticosteroids on page 185 in this chapter.

NURSING IMPLICATIONS

The nursing implications for use of the sex hormones are similar to those for the adrenocorticosteroids (see page 187).

OTHER HORMONE PREPARATIONS

This section briefly examines some miscellaneous hormone preparations which, although not widely used, have a place in the treatment of specific endocrine disorders.

Bromocriptine (*Parlodel*) is an agonist of dopamine. It acts as an inhibitor of prolactin release and can be used in a variety of hormone-induced disease states. One of its uses is in the inhibition of lactation in women who do not wish to breastfeed their child. It has also been used in a number of other areas, including the treatment of Parkinson's disease, acromegaly and gynaecomastia. The drug has also been shown to enhance fertility to some degree.

Physiologically, ***calcitonin*** (*Calcitare*) is responsible for the movement of calcium from the systemic circulation to the bone matrix. This results in increased bone-calcium deposition. Synthetic preparations have a similar activity. They are employed in the treatment of hypercalcaemia and in Paget's disease to increase strength of osteogenic tissue.

Clomiphene citrate (*Clomid*) is used as a "fertility drug". While there may be many other causes of infertility in the female, failure to ovulate and/or failure of implantation are quite common, and clomiphene is used to treat women suffering from ovulatory failure. Its use has been associated with a significant incidence of multiple births. Prescription is restricted to specialists in the gynaecological and obstetric fields.

Glucagon occurs naturally in the alpha cells of the islets of Langerhans in the pancreas. It promotes the conversion of glycogen to glucose, thus raising blood sugar levels. It is available as an injection for either IM or IV use and is used for the reversal of hypoglycaemia.

Table 34
Drugs that Act on the Endocrine System

Drug Group	Drug Name	Use	Action	Adverse Reactions	Nursing Implications
Hypoglycaemic agents					
Insulins	Insulin BP Soluble insulin Actrapid Semilente Monotard Rapitard Lente Ultralente	Hypoglycaemic agent in treatment of diabetes	Lowers blood-glucose levels	Hypoglycaemia or hyperglycaemia, lipoatrophy or lipohypertrophy, serum sickness, insulin resistance	***Assess:*** hyperglycaemic or hypoglycaemic state, baseline vital signs, weight, lifestyle, stress levels, diet and level of exercise, current medication, alcohol intake, pregnancy or lactation. ***Administer:*** SC on an individual basis; medication that has not expired; according to hospital or diabetic-centre protocol. ***Evaluate:*** therapeutic effect and any deviations from this such as hypoglycaemia or hyperglycaemia; adverse effects such as local skin reactions or atrophy of subcutaneous fat at the injection site. ***Teach:*** aspects of the disease process and reasons for the medication; techniques for administering the medication; importance of keeping adequate supplies of medication and equipment; to carry medication and simple carbohydrates for acute hypoglycaemia if travelling; to carry complex carbohydrates if they anticipate problems obtaining suitable meals; to wear a medical identification tag; to adjust insulin requirements according to diet and exercise.

Sulphonylureas	Acetohexamide Chlorpropamide Glibenclamide Gliclazide Tolbutamide	Hypoglycaemic agent in treatment of mature-onset diabetes	Lower blood-glucose levels	Alcohol intolerance, allergy	***Assess:*** Hypoglycaemic or hyperglycaemic state; baseline vital signs, weight; liver, kidney or cardiovascular disease; pregnancy or lactation, current medications and alcohol intake, lifestyle and the degree of emotional or physical stress. ***Administer:*** To prevent nocturnal hypoglycaemia, do not administer just before retiring. ***Evaluate:*** for hypoglycaemia and cardiac disturbances; adverse effects such as GIT irritation, for example, nausea, vomiting and diarrhoea; blood dyscrasias and liver disturbances. ***Teach:*** as for insulin where relevant; avoid the simultaneous use with alcohol; not to take extra medication if a dose is missed; changing from oral hypoglycaemics to insulin, or the reverse, may precipitate hypoglycaemia; to avoid psychosocial and physical stress.
Biguanides	Metformin	Hypoglycaemic agent in treatment of mature-onset diabetes	Lower blood-glucose levels	Lactic acidosis	***Assess:*** as for sulphonylureas, especially alcohol intake. ***Administer:*** as for sulphonylureas. ***Evaluate:*** as for sulphonylureas. ***Teach:*** adverse effects of combining with alcohol, as will induce lactic acidosis.

continued

Drug Group	Drug Name	Use	Action	Adverse Reactions	Nursing Implications
Corticosteroids					
Glucocorticoids	Hydrocortisone Prednisone Prednisolone Methylprednisolone Dexamethasone Betamethasone	Replacement therapy, immunosuppression, anti-inflammatory, haematological conditions, cerebral oedema, shock, diagnostic procedures, skin diseases	Act on: carbohydrate and protein metabolism, fat metabolism, water and electrolyte balance, muscle function, nervous system, lymphoid tissue; are anti-inflammatory, suppress immunological response	Cushing's syndrome, fat redistribution, hirsutism, hyperglycaemia, hypernatraemia, hypokalaemia, psychoses, oedema, hypertension, gastric ulceration, protein depletion, delayed wound healing, osteoporosis, increased susceptibility to infection	***Assess:*** baseline vital signs, BP, weight, sleep patterns, stress, urinalysis (glucose), diet, pregnancy, lactation, cardiac disease, hypertension, peptic ulceration, infection. ***Administer:*** with food; do not cease suddenly. ***Evaluate:*** effectiveness in replacement, immunosuppressive therapy and anti-inflammatory therapy; sleep patterns, alterations in BP, pulse rate and emotional state; urinalysis for glucose, blood sugar; diet for potassium and protein; evaluate for signs of infection (for example, nausea and vomiting, dehydration, lethargy, and for signs of muscle wasting, slow wound healing, bruising and oedema. ***Teach:*** therapeutic effect and how to recognise deviations or adverse effects; not to suddenly cease medication and inherent dangers of doing so; to adhere to advised diet; to prevent infections and inflammation and maintain adequate personal hygiene; care with accidents due to risk of osteoporosis; to wear an identification tag or bracelet.
Thyroid and antithyroid preparations					
Drugs used in hypothyroidism	Liothyronine Thyroxine	Hypothyroidism	Promote thyroid function	Tremor, headache, tachycardia, GIT disturbances, weight loss, hypertension, cardiac arrhythmias	***Assess:*** baseline BP, pulse rate, weight, sleep patterns, presence of pregnancy, lactation, current medications, establish degree of hypothyroidism, past and present history of cardiac disease, hypertension, renal disease. ***Administer:***

					in the morning before meals; ensure accuracy of dose. ***Evaluate:*** therapeutic effects as demonstrated by reversal of hypothyroidism; adverse effects will present as signs of thyrotoxicosis. ***Teach:*** exact dosage; not to confuse micrograms with milligrams; to take own pulse rate and inform medical officer of deviations; not to alter dose without medical supervision; signs of thyrotoxicosis and to inform medical officer if these occur.
Drugs used in hyperthyroidism	Propylthiouracil Carbimazole	Hyperthyroidism	Prevent attachment of iodine to tyrosine molecule and so lowers production of T3 and T4 in gland	Rash, nausea, headache, GIT upset, thrombocytopenia, agranulocytosis, reflex enlargement of thyroid gland	***Assess:*** baseline pulse rate, BP, cardiac status, weight, concurrent medications (especially anticoagulants), presence of pregnancy or lactation, blood screening tests, liver function. ***Administer:*** with meals. ***Evaluate:*** therapeutic effectiveness as demonstrated by decrease in thyrotoxic symptoms; care to ensure that hypothyroidism does not develop; blood screening for thrombocytopenia and agranulocytosis; other adverse effects, for example GIT distress, skin rash, headache, sore throat, thyroid enlargement with respiratory obstruction. ***Teach:*** therapy is often life long, so patients should not alter dose or discontinue therapy without consulting medical officer; teach to take own pulse rate and inform of deviations from the expected therapeutic effect; patients should wear an identification tag or bracelet.

SELF-EVALUATION TEST

1. Name two drugs in each of the following classes:
   (a) antithyroids
   (b) adrenocorticosteroids
   (c) hypoglycaemics.
2. Describe briefly the actions of:
   (a) hydrocortisone
   (b) glibenclamide
   (c) glucagon
   (d) oestrogens.
3. List the adverse reactions to:
   (a) dexamethasone
   (b) thyroxine
   (c) insulin
   (d) carbimazole.
4. What are the nursing implications in the use of:
   (a) oral hypoglycaemics
   (b) insulin
   (c) corticotrophin.

12

CONTRACEPTION AND THE TREATMENT OF INFERTILITY

Claud D. Munro

OBJECTIVES

At the conclusion of this chapter the reader should be able to:

1. list the main female hormones and outline their role in the ovarian cycle;
2. describe the use of synthetic hormones as contraceptives;
3. discuss the side effects of oestrogens and progestogens and apply this information to determine the choice of oral contraceptives for particular patients;
4. name the main causes of infertility and briefly outline their hormonal treatments.

PREREQUISITE KNOWLEDGE

1. Anatomy and physiology of the female reproductive organs.
2. Normal hormonal changes which occur in pregnant and non-pregnant women.

DEFINITIONS

Endometriosis — a disease in which endometrial tissue is located outside the normal lining of the uterine cavity. This condition may give rise to pain, especially during menses, and to infertility.

Menorrhagia — a term used to denote menstrual bleeding which is considered to be in excess of normal, both in terms of number of days (normally five) or amount of blood lost (normally 80 mL).

Amenorrhoea — a term used to denote the absence of menstrual bleeding. In clinical terms, usually important when it lasts for more than six months. In the normal person, the absence of bleeding is expected before menarche, during pregnancy and lactation, and after the menopause.

Galactorrhoea — a term used to denote the inappropriate production of milk. This condition is sometimes associated with the presence of a pituitary tumour, or may be induced by a number of forms of drug therapy. The term is used to distinguish this disorder from the physiological production of milk during lactation.
Progestogen — a synthetic steroid with progesterone-like activity which can be given orally, parenterally or vaginally to promote effects in the endometrium, ovary, breast and hypothalamic/pituitary area. These progestational effects can also be seen during pregnancy.
Nidation — a term used to describe the events surrounding the implantation and early development of the fertilised ovum (zygote and blastocyst). If this occurs in the uterine cavity, it can develop into a normal pregnancy, but if it occurs in a fallopian tube, it can develop into an ectopic pregnancy.
Gonadotrophin — a substance having a stimulating effect on the gonads. In the female, the pituitary hormones FSH and LH are said to have a gonadotrophic effect on the ovaries.

FEMALE HORMONES

The female gonads (ovaries) maintain ova, maintain nutrition and the mature size of female reproductive organs, and sensitise the mucous membrane of the uterus so that it responds to the contact of the developing ovum and assists in implantation.

Two pituitary hormones directly affect the ovary: ***follicle stimulating hormone (FSH)*** which controls the production of oestrogen, and ***luteinising hormone (LH)*** which, together with FSH, controls ovulation.

Prolactin, also found in the pituitary, is responsible for the secretion of milk. Lactation occurs when the fully developed breast is released from the inhibitory influence which oestrogen and progesterone exert during pregnancy upon the action of prolactin. With the rapid decline of oestrogen and progesterone levels that follow delivery, prolactin from the pituitary gland is able to exert its full effect upon the mammary tissue, and milk production commences.

The two principal female sex hormones are ***oestrogen*** and ***progesterone.*** Oestrogen is produced throughout the entire menstrual cycle and is responsible for the regrowth of the lining of the uterus after each menstruation (the proliferative phase). Oestrogen is necessary to stimulate the endometrium just prior to its conversion to a secretory state. Progesterone is produced from the ruptured egg follicle (the corpus luteum) after ovulation, and is therefore present only in the latter half of the menstrual cycle. It is responsible for maintaining pregnancy and is mainly involved in the secretory phase of the menstrual cycle.

Fertility drugs fall into two categories: those which by various means stimulate ovarian activity and those which suppress it. Whereas most drugs are foreign to the body, hormones (used to a large extent in the first category and used entirely in the second) are natural secretions of the endocrine glands which exert effects on specific tissues. However, a number of compounds which have pronounced hormonal activity have been synthesised. Stilboestrol and ethinyloestradiol are synthetic oestrogens, and norethisterone and levonorgestrel are synthetic progestogens.

CONTRACEPTION (OVARIAN SUPPRESSION)

The main use for these drugs is antifertility or contraception, although the suppression of ovulation is often indicated in the treatment of gynaecological disorders such as endometriosis and menorrhagia.

Progesterone by injection as a means of suppressing ovulation was in use in the 1930s, but the era of oral contraception did not begin till 1951 in the USA when Pincus had developed work on progestogens. Oral contraceptives, unlike most other drugs, are prescribed for healthy women and are taken for long periods so that the chance of toxic manifestations is increased. Either oestrogen or progestogen taken orally can be used to inhibit ovulation. Chemical and mechanical methods do not stop ovulation but prevent fertilisation of the ripened eggs. The natural oestrogen, oestradiol, is not sufficiently active orally, so synthetic ethinyloestradiol is used.

The menstrual bleeding pattern produced by oestrogen alone, however, is irregular, often prolonged, and unpredictable. For this reason, progestogen is administered with oestrogen for part of the second half of the cycle. This usually produces a predictable and satisfactory menstrual pattern. Thus, the most commonly prescribed type of oral contraception is a "combined pill", taken from the fifth day for 21 to 22 days of the cycle.

THE "COMBINED PILL"

Early types of the combined pill used a combination of various forms of oestrogens and progestogens. For example, one of the early pills, *Anovlar* (1961), was a combination of ethinyloestradiol 50 mcg and norethisterone acetate 4 mg. Later developments led to improved oral progestogens, such as levonorgestrel, which permitted lower dosage of both hormones, such as *Microgynon 30* released in 1975, containing ethinyloestradiol 30 mcg and levonorgestrel 150 mcg. More recent changes sought to imitate the changing hormonal levels of a normal cycle, leading to the biphasic concept *(BiNovum)* and the current triphasic or three-step concept *(Trinordiol, TriNovum, Logynon)* which would appear to be the final development of the combined type of pill. This triphasic concept was designed "by a woman, for women" and closely imitates the changing levels of oestrogen and progestogen during the monthly cycle.

THE PROGESTOGEN-ONLY PILL OR "MINI-PILL"

Small doses of progesterone, such as levonorgestrel 30 mcg or 350 mcg of norethisterone, find special application in the immediate postpartum period for lactating mothers and have been used also to minimise the adverse side effects of oestrogen, such as thrombosis.

How oral contraceptives work

Oral contraceptives that combine the hormones oestrogen and progestogen are thought to prevent conception on different but interrelated levels: they prevent FSH and LH release from the pituitary; the ovarian follicles are not stimulated to maturity by FSH and ovulation is not triggered by LH; the cervical mucus thickens and prevents sperm penetration; and they prevent the thickening of the endometrium, making nidation difficult.

Adverse Drug Reactions

Most of the side effects due to oral contraceptives are reversible.

Adverse effects of Oestrogens

1. Nausea – maximal on commencing oestrogen and improving as tolerance develops.
2. Reduction of lactation – only progesterone should be used for fertility control during lactation.
3. Water and salt retention – oestrogen increases the osmotic pressure of the tissues, and patients may have difficulty in wearing contact lenses due to tissues holding more fluid. Diuretics, however, are rarely needed.
4. Leg cramps – especially at night.
5. Leucorrhoea – oestrogen stimulates the cervical glands to increased activity.
6. Migraine – attributable to the withdrawal of oestrogen at the completion of a course of tablets.
7. Hypertension – frequently due to family history of hypertension; also found in patients who develop pre-eclampsia during pregnancy.
8. Thrombosis – the most important irreversible side effect of oral contraceptives is thrombosis, with possible death due to pulmonary embolism. Studies done suggest the risk of thrombosis is increased about eight times with women taking oral contraceptives.
9. Slight breast development and deposition of fat on thighs are stimulated by oestrogen.

Adverse effects of Progestogens

1. Weight gain — all types of progestogens facilitate fat deposition but nor-testosterones, in addition, stimulate appetite. This is of particular importance in women who develop diminished glucose tolerance. Progestogen also decreases physical activity.
2. Breakthrough bleeding — this often occurs, and the menstrual flow is reduced. Oral contraceptives predispose to monilial infections, and

nystatin gives little relief unless progesterone is reduced at the same time. Progestogen in high doses can cause breast discomfort, headaches, migraine and tension premenstrually.

3. Acne — young patients with a tendency to acne should be given an oestrogen type of preparation.
4. Depression, chronic fatigue, irritability and a diminished glucose tolerance can be the result of progesterone therapy. Patients may also develop side effects of alopecia, gingivitis, loss of libido, hirsutism, jaundice and chloasma.

Clinical assessment for choice of oral contraception

From this discussion, it is clear there is not one "pill". From the range of formulations available, a suitable choice should be possible after consideration has been given to age, length of menses, length of cycle, breast size, fat and hair distribution, history of acne, lactation, and any history of thrombosis. For lactating mothers, the progestogen-only pill is recommended, especially the levonorgestrel type *(Microval* and *Neogest)* to minimise any possible effects from oestrogen metabolites during the infant's first year of life.

OTHER HORMONAL METHODS OF CONTRACEPTION

Progesterone injection (*Depo-Provera*)
Medroxyprogesterone acetate, a potent inhibitor of the gonadotrophins, can be given intramuscularly. Slowly absorbed, it results in prolonged activity (150 mg given at three-month intervals produces a reliable method of contraception).

Progesterone implants
Dimethyl polysiloxane (DPS) can be used subcutaneously but cannot be immediately withdrawn if side effects are encountered.

Special precautions and contraindications

It seems likely that women on oral contraceptives have impaired vitamin B_6, vitamin C and vitamin A metabolism. Concurrent administration of various drugs may impair the contraceptive efficiency of hormonal preparations. The commonest mechanism appears to be that of enzyme induction causing accelerated steroid breakdown. Among drugs which are known to increase steroid breakdown are rifampicin, barbiturates, cyclophosphamide, phenytoin and sulphonamides. Other drugs reported to have a similar effect are chloramphenicol, ampicillin and nitrofurantoin. Serum folate is significantly reduced in women on oral contraceptives.

TREATMENT OF INFERTILITY (OVARIAN ACTIVATION)

The discovery of the gonadotrophic hormones of the pituitary as separate identities (FSH and LH) was not made until 1933, although as early as 1900 it was known that the pituitary was a gland which regulated and controlled growth. Today we know that these hormones control the ovary, but also that by feedback mechanisms the ovary exerts an effect on the pituitary. Infertility can be treated with drugs only when hormone abnormality is the cause. Causes of sterility also include hypothyroidism, tubal blockage and severe mental strain, but we will deal only with drug treatments involving sex hormones. Low hormone levels are frequently the cause of infertility, and therefore oestrogen and/or progesterone replacement therapy is all that is required.

The natural oestrogen, oestradiol, is not sufficiently active by oral administration so a synthetic form, ethinyloestradiol, is used for sterility caused by low oestrogen levels, for example, genital underdevelopment. It is slowly metabolised and then excreted in the urine.

Adverse Drug Reactions

Side effects are gastrointestinal disturbances, nausea, vomiting, headache, dizziness, breast tenderness and sodium and water retention. Its use is contraindicated in pregnancy, jaundice and patients with a previous history of blood clotting or impaired liver function.

Impaired fertility due to failure of nidation may be treated with progesterone replacement therapy in the form of allyloestranol (*Gestanin*). It may be given safely long term since this drug is without androgenic activity. Oestrogen given by mouth can produce contraception by stopping ovulation. But if oestrogen levels are too high and we give an antioestrogen, it follows that ovulation may take place. In other words, it is the "pill" in reverse.

CLOMIPHENE (CLOMID) has been described as an anti-oestrogen or a weak or impeded oestrogen. Clomiphene competes for hypothalamus and pituitary receptor sites and replaces endogenous oestrogen with weak or impeded oestrogen. This interferes with the feedback mechanism causing an outpouring of gonadotrophic hormones FSH and LH with resultant increased prospects of ovulation. It enlarges the ovary (reversible side effect) and ovulation can be obtained in a high proportion of patients with amenorrhoea. It is slowly excreted through the liver into the bile.

In normal rats, clomiphene stops the oestrous cycle and reduces the size of the ovaries, and in the male it reduces spermatogenesis, thus producing a contraceptive effect in both sexes.

Just as lower levels of oestrogen at the menopause cause hot flushes, depression, insomnia and weight gain, so menopausal side effects are often produced by this drug since the oestrogen levels are lowered. High doses produce ovarian cysts and visual blurring. The incidence of multiple pregnancy is increased. This drug is contraindicated for patients with liver disease, ovarian cysts and endometrial carcinoma.

TAMOXIFEN (NOLVADEX) is also an anti-oestrogen with an action similar to clomiphene. It is used to stimulate ovulation in women who are menstruating regularly, but have anovular cycles. It is also used as a palliative treatment for breast cancer. It competes with oestrogen for uptake at specific receptor sites and has a strong affinity for tissue dependent on oestrogen activity, such as breast tissue.

Adverse Drug Reactions

Side effects include oedema, gastrointestinal upsets, vaginal bleeding and dizziness. It is metabolised by the liver and excreted in the faeces.

BROMOCRIPTINE (PARLODEL) is a peptide ergot alkaloid which does not have the vasoconstricting effect of other ergot compounds. It is described as a dopaminergic receptor stimulant, as it mimics the action of dopamine which suppresses secretion of prolactin by the anterior pituitary. Bromocriptine also acts at the hypothalamic level by stimulating dopaminergic receptor sites in the hypothalamus, as well as either enhancing the release of gonadotropic hormones (LH and FSH) or restoring the sensitivity of the ovary to gonadotropic stimulation. As elevated prolactin levels cause amenorrhoea and galactorrhoea, treatment with bromocriptine returns pituitary production of prolactin to normal, the gonadal sensitivity to gonadotrophins promptly returns and normal ovulation occurs. It can also hasten the return to ovulation following childbirth, so patients who have bromocriptine prescribed for the suppression of lactation should be advised of the need for appropriate contraceptive measures.

GONADOTROPHINS (PREGNYL), given parenterally, are also used for sterility. After the menopause, the ovaries become insensitive to gonadotrophin activity, while before puberty such activity causes undesirable stimulation of the ovaries. When endometriosis is a cause of sterility in the female, oral therapy preventing the maturation of the follicles and ovulation is obtained by combined doses of oestrogen and progesterone. These two hormones maintain amenorrhoea, reduce pain and cause regression of ectopic endometrial growths.

DANAZOL (DANOL), a new synthetic derivative of ethisterone, is the latest treatment for endometriosis. Oral administration of danazol results in reduced plasma levels of the pituitary gonadotrophins LH and FSH with suppression of ovulation and menses. It is devoid of progestational and oestrogenic effects, but possesses weak, impeded androgenic activity and associated anabolic properties. Danazol is indicated for the treatment of visually proven (for example, laparoscopy) endometriosis if surgery has been unsuccessful or contraindicated and the required end-point of treatment is pregnancy. Also used to treat various endocrine and gynaecological disorders where the control of pituitary gonadotrophins would be expected to have a beneficial effect.

Its use is not recommended for longer than six months and should not be given during pregnancy or lactation. Treatment should start during menstruation, and a diuretic is sometimes needed for fluid retention. Androgenic effects such as hirsutism, acne and decrease in breast size may occur.

NURSING IMPLICATIONS

Ovarian activation

Assessment will include consideration of the physical health of both partners and psychosocial aspects. The response of the couple to success or failure of fertility treatment should be assessed. When ovarian activating drugs are to be prescribed for whatever reason, the patient must be assessed for the presence of pregnancy and/or lactation and past familial history of gynaecological malignancy, also past history of drug reaction and hypersensitivity.

Administration of HCG should be by intramuscular injection. Clomiphene should not be given to patients with liver disease, ovarian cysts or endometrial carcinoma. Tamoxifen should not be given to women with functioning ovaries. Danazol should not be given during pregnancy or lactation. Treatment should commence during menstruation, and diuretics may need to be given concomitantly.

Evaluation is essential, and the following should be taken into account: observe for adverse effects, especially sodium and water retention with ethinyloestradiol, signs of ovarian enlargement or cysts and visual blurring with clomiphene. With tamoxifen, oedema and vaginal bleeding may occur; with danazol, the patient should be assessed for signs of oedema, acne and hirsutism.

Patient education is important, and patients should be informed of possible adverse effects of ovarian activators. Important aspects of education include timing of coitus in relation to courses of treatment and informing the patient of the increased incidence of multiple births following treatment with drugs such as clomiphene. Instruction should be given as to basal-temperature monitoring and collection of urine for determination of oestrogen levlels.

Ovarian suppression

Assessment will include blood pressure, pulse rate, weight and medical history (especially of cerebrovascular disease, hepatic disease, oestrogen-dependent tumours, fluid retention and hypertension) present health, smoking habits and possibility of pregnancy or existence of lactation.

Administration is cyclical and normally self-administered.

Evaluation is important and should include consideration of adverse effects, for example, nausea, chloasma (which responds to reduction in sun exposure) and headache, which may be assisted by simple analgesics. Note the incidence of migraine, which may necessitate a change in the type of oral contraceptive. Weight gain may be helped by reduction in salt and calorie intake. Oedema and hypertension should be constantly watched for, and their presence may necessitate a change in the method of contraception recommended. Patients who wear contact lenses may experience difficulty and may need to wear glasses. Evaluate for break-through bleeding, mood changes, moniliai infection and acne. Current medication should be evaluated because rifampicin, phenytoin, a variety of antibiotics (including ampicillin) and barbiturates have been implicated in reducing the effectiveness of oral contraceptives. Haematological tests and endocrine tests may be affected by oral contraceptive therapy.

Teaching should include the need for regular medical checks (at least annually) for patients on long-term therapy. Patients should be made aware of the major adverse effects of these drugs and the correct steps to take should any of these occur. Patients should be instructed in correct administration of oral contraceptives and how to manage when doses are missed.

SELF-EVALUATION TEST

1. List the main female hormones.
2. Describe the role of these hormones in the normal ovarian cycle.
3. What types of contraceptive "pill" are available, and what factors would determine the type of "pill" to be chosen for a particular patient?
4. Which of the following are adverse effects of oestrogen?
   (a) acne, depression, weight gain.
   (b) leucorrhoea, hypertension, water retention.
   (c) migraine, acne, leg cramps.
   (d) hypertension, thrombosis, breakthrough bleeding.
5. List the main causes of infertility and briefly outline the treatments available for hormonal abnormalities.

PREGNANCY TESTING

Human chorionic gonadotrophin (HCG) is produced by the trophoblast as soon as implantation occurs. HCG takes over from the pituitary the job of stimulating the corpus luteum of pregnancy to produce both progesterone and oestrogen. These prevent further ovulation and menstruation and maintain implantation until about the end of the first trimester.

HCG forms the basis for the diagnosis of pregnancy in the early stages. It is excreted in the urine probably as early as the first missed period. The test is usually done immunologically (see Figure 3).

FIGURE 3: DIAGRAMMATIC REPRESENTATION OF PREGNANCY TESTING – INTERPRETATION OF RESULT

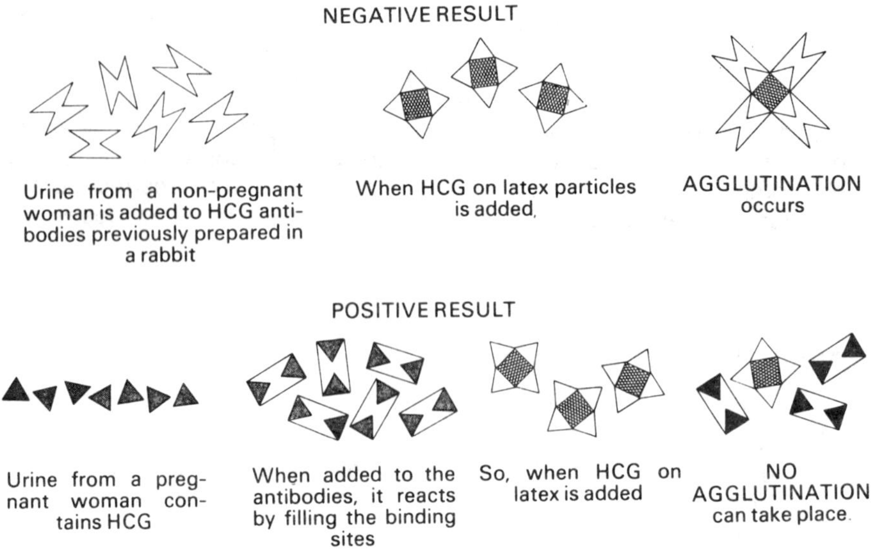

13

MATERNAL AND INFANT CARE

Claud D. Munro

OBJECTIVES

At the conclusion of this chapter, the reader should be able to:

1. discuss the risks and benefits of drug usage during pregnancy;
2. list the drugs commonly used to treat problems associated with labour and at the time of delivery;
3. describe the principles involved in drug transfer to the neonate through breast milk and how potential problems can be minimised;
4. discuss the use of drugs in the treatment of common neonatal conditions in intensive care nurseries.

PREREQUISITE KNOWLEDGE

1. Anatomy and physiology associated with pregnancy and the puerperium.
2. Basic neonatal care and treatment of common medical conditions in the newborn.

DEFINITIONS

Puerperium — the period of time following the birth of a child; traditionally the six-week period from confinement to the postnatal examination and discharge from medical care.

Teratogen — a substance that causes major malformations in the developing foetus, literally, "monster originating or producing", usually reserved for gross abnormalities such as anencephaly, phocomelia (caused by thalidomide) and serious structural malformations.

Dysmorphogen — a substance causing minor or less obvious congenital abnormalities; commonly used in recent literature to describe agents or medications that produce functional abnormalities or minor structural changes such as cleft palate, hare lip, skin folds and so on. Literally, it means "form or shape altering"

Sympathomimetic — a term used to describe a group of drugs that mimic the effects produced by adrenaline, hence also referred to as adrenergics. Beta-2 sympathomimetics are drugs such as salbutamol and ritodrine which have a powerful relaxant effect on smooth muscle such as the bronchioles and uterus, but minimal effect on the heart.

Myometrial relaxant — a substance that causes relaxation of the uterus or a ceasing of contractions, for example, beta-2 sympathomimetic agents and ethyl alcohol, as well as general anaesthetic agents (especially halothane) and rapidly acting vasodilators used in hypertensive crises, such as hydralazine and diazoxide.

Oxytocic — a term used to refer to the group of drugs that mimic the effects of oxytocin, with respect to increasing uterine contraction. Common examples are the synthetic oxytocin syntocinon and the ergot alkaloid, ergometrine.

DRUG USAGE IN PREGNANCY

Just over 20 years ago, one word — thalidomide — brought anxiety and a new realisation of the harmful potential of drugs to the public and health care professionals. Prior to that, drug usage in pregnancy was considered almost exclusively in terms of the mother, the foetus being viewed merely as an integral part of the maternal organism requiring little separate consideration with regard to medication therapy. Since then, there has been an increasing awareness in the medical profession and among lay people of the potentially harmful effects of drugs taken during pregnancy. At the same time, a balanced outlook is most important, as many untreated medical conditions would pose a greater threat to the continued welfare of the foetus than would the use of the drugs indicated to treat such conditions. Typical examples include infections, hypertension, diabetes, epilepsy and the toxaemias of pregnancy.

DRUG TRANSFER TO THE FOETUS

What actually happens when a drug is consumed by a pregnant woman? In almost every case, two persons are affected, the mother and the foetus. Drug transfer occurs normally across the placenta from the maternal arterial blood supply by way of intervillous space into the umbilical vein. (Figure 4).

For any substance to pass from the maternal blood stream to the foetal blood supply, it must traverse what used to be called the "placental barrier". In fact, it must be transferred through the syncytiotrophoblast, which is a single layer of multinuclear syncytium with no distinct cell boundaries, and the cytotrophoblast, a single layer of cuboidal cells with distinct cell boundaries (also called the layer of Langhans). There may be some scattered mesoderm beneath this layer of cells (Figure 5).

FIGURE 4 THE PLACENTAL WALL – SITE OF DRUG TRANSFER

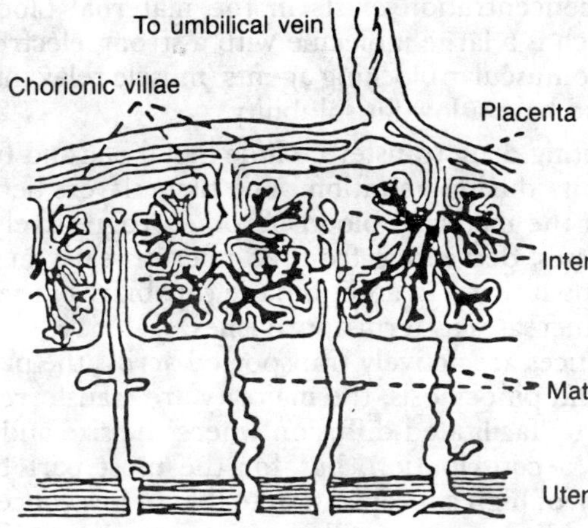

FIGURE 5 PLACENTAL-FOETAL MEMBRANES – CROSS SECTION OF PLACENTAL TISSUES

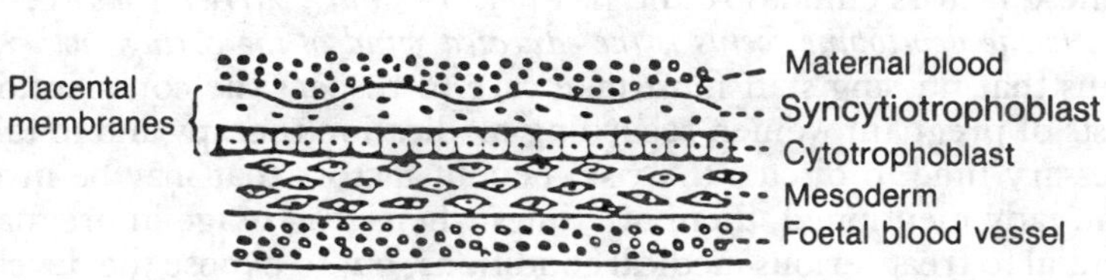

In common with other semipermeable cell membranes, these two primary layers are composed in large part of phospholipid or lipoprotein and carry a surface charge. There is also a pH difference between maternal blood and foetal blood. Foetal blood is slightly more acid, about 0.15 pH units lower than maternal blood. For these reasons, substances that are fat (lipid) soluble and in their non-ionised form will be transferred most readily. The transfer of drugs that are weak bases will be promoted, as these will ionise more readily in the more-acid foetal blood and will thus produce a higher concentration in the foetal bloodstream at equilibrium than in the maternal bloodstream. This knowledge finds important application in the timing of administration of narcotics for pain relief, such as pethidine, as these are commonly used drugs that are weak bases. Other drugs that are also quickly transferred to the foetus include alcohol, barbiturates, anaesthetic agents and phenothiazines. On the other hand, drugs that will be unlikely to pass to the foetus (unless an extremely high concentration exists in the maternal bloodstream) include heparin, which is a large molecule with a strong electronegative charge, and the neuromuscular blocking agents (muscle relaxants), which are highly ionised and have a low fat solubility.

Other factors affecting drug transfer include metabolic and functional changes of the placenta during gestation. The tissue layers between the foetal capillaries and the maternal blood become progressively thinner as pregnancy progresses, decreasing from 25 microns early in gestation to around two microns at term. In addition, the capability of the placenta to metabolise drugs increases as term approaches.

While some substances are actively transported across the placenta by enzymatic reaction and pinocytosis, the majority are transferred by passive transport, some by facilitated diffusion where the size and shape of the molecule makes a contribution, but for the most part by simple diffusion from an area of high concentration to that of low concentration. This means that virtually any drug will pass from mother to foetus if a sufficiently high concentration gradient is produced, unless it is destroyed or altered during passage. For these reasons, the meaning of the term "placental barrier" is largely believed to be untrue, and discontinuance of this expression is recommended. The placental "sieve" appears in recent literature and is more in accord with current understanding of placental function.

These factors emphasize the fact *that the final "barrier" to any potential harm to the developing foetus is the educated mind of the caring mother.* This means that nursing staff must take care to respect the conscientious requests of pregnant women regarding medication therapy and to take the necessary time to discuss the risk/benefit factors that may be involved. As already mentioned, there are times when drug usage in pregnancy is essential to treat serious medical conditions, but to expose the developing foetus to risk for trivial reasons, such as those associated with the casual usage of sedatives and tranquillisers, is sheer folly in view of the known risks and the potential of harmful effects that may yet be recognized in the future.

It is already well recognized that some of the earlier benzodiazepines have pharmacologically active metabolites with extremely long half-lives that accumulate in the foetus. Thus, long-term use of diazepam (*Valium*) in pregnancy will often give rise to hypotonia and hypothermia in the foetus, with the condition persisting long after birth. This can result in the "flat baby" syndrome, characterised by lethargy and poor sucking reflexes.

Which drugs should be avoided during pregnancy?

This is not a question that can be answered simply. Many matters are involved, such as the time during pregnancy when the drug is given, the dose of the drug, the medical condition of the mother and any known allergic and genetic factors from both parents. As a general rule, every effort should be made to totally avoid medications of any kind during the organogenesis period (the first eight weeks of pregnancy) except where serious medical conditions require urgent treatment, with risk/benefit factors being carefully evaluated by prescriber and patient. The same special care should be exercised in the period just before delivery when physiological systems of mother and baby can be modified by drug therapy such as aspirin, long-acting sulphonamides and the non-steroidal anti-inflammatory medications.

There is still considerable discussion in the world literature about the list of drugs that have been proven to be teratogenic or dysmorphogenic. For this reason, the following table lists *examples* of such medications. For specific information about a particular drug, the reader is referred to publications that are continually updated with current information, such as the *British National Formulary.*

Table 35
Examples of Drugs to Avoid During Pregnancy

Name of drug	**Effect produced in foetus**
Androgens	Masculinisation of female foetus
Cytotoxic agents	Severe malformations, abortion
Ethyl alcohol (chronic)	Foetal alcohol syndrome (includes craniofacial malformations)
Etretinate *(Tigason)** and Isotretinoin *(Roaccutane)*	Structural deformations, limb-reduction deformities, cranio-facial anomalies, spontaneous abortion
Iodides and antithyroid drugs	Foetal goitre
Stilboestrol	Carcinoma of vagina after 15 to 20 years in female offspring; reproductive disorders in males
Tetracyclines	Enamel hypoplasia and staining of teeth; skeletal growth retardation (reversible)
Thalidomide	Phocomelia; cardiovascular defects

*It is essential for every woman of child-bearing age to avoid pregnancy during treatment with etretinate and for at least one year after its discontinuation.

Retrospective problems

A further important aspect for consideration by everyone involved in patient welfare is the possibility of dangers learnt in retrospect. How many drugs in use may prove to have been harmful to the foetus, with the adverse effect becoming apparent only after the passing of several years?

Such has been the experience with administration of ***stilboestrol*** during pregnancy. Fifteen to 20 years after their mothers had received stilboestrol, female offspring have incurred an increased incidence of adenocarcinoma of the vagina, as well as abnormalities of the reproductive system, including irregular menstrual cycles and vaginal adenosis. Recent reports indicate that male offspring were also affected, with about one-quarter of males who had been exposed in utero to stilboestrol suffering reproductive system abnormalities, including epididymal cysts, hypotropic testes, capsular induration and pathologic semen.

So how many medications being used today may prove to be a future problem? In this regard, the information supplied by the manufacturers of nitrofurantoin shows the importance of patient counselling and subsequent referral of any potential problem back to the prescriber for further evaluation.

Nitrofurantoin has been commonly prescribed in pregnancy for urinary-tract infections, but recent information calling attention to possible future problems has by no means been widely publicised. In man, nitrofurantoin can decrease sperm counts and produce abnormal testicular histology suggestive of arrested spermatogenesis. Nitrofurantoin is mutagenic in certain bacterial systems and although it is not known how far this relates to the clinical situation the possibility of a permanent mutagenic effect on spermatozoa-producing cells requires that careful consideration be given to its use in young males. The potential for mutagenic effect should normally contraindicate the use of nitrofurantoin during pregnancy at any stage.

A parallel example is the current usage of the ***progesterone-only "pill"*** as a contraceptive for feeding mothers. Recent papers have called into question the nor-ethisterone type because of the production of oestrogen metabolites which may have the potential of affecting the sex-differentiation role in the brain in the first months of life. Even if subsequent investigation shows this is not the case, surely if any element of doubt exists at the present time, it would be wise to avoid any possible damage to future generations.

Another situation where good patient care is involved is well illustrated by the ***tetracycline group*** of drugs.

The potential dangers to the foetus from the tetracyclines are well documented and among the best known in the general community because of the obvious effect of teeth staining. Tetracyclines are concentrated in chelated form in the enamel and dentine of developing teeth, resulting in irreversible discolouration and enamel hypoplasia. They also cause a reversible inhibition of skeletal growth in premature infants. It is rare for a pregnant woman to be given tetracyclines to treat an infection. It is fairly common practice for women in their late teens to be prescribed tetracycline for acne, often over a long period. Should they continue taking such medication well into their pregnancy, unnecessary exposure of the foetus may take place during a critical period. As is common practice in radiography, nursing staff should have no reservations about routinely asking patients receiving such medication: "Are you pregnant, or is there a possibility that you could become so during the course of this treatment?"

This question should actually become a part of the standard counselling procedure used by all health-care workers for all women of child-bearing potential. Most drug manufacturers have a standard warning for their products against usage during "the first trimester", but how often is this warning actually passed on to the consumer? We must never forget that the greatest dangers to the foetus are posed during the early weeks of organogenesis, during the period that pregnancy may not even be suspected, and even when it is, the woman may not be aware that her former daily routine of drug taking could present a threat to her developing child. There are few other areas where appropriate counselling could have such a profound effect upon future life prospects and the quality of life for an individual.

Self-administered drugs

In addition to prescribed medications, many pregnant women regularly consume a variety of self-administered drugs. It is important for nursing staff, especially midwives, to be aware of the patient's total medication profile so adverse reactions and interactions of drugs can be recognised. Examples of self-administered medications are alcohol, aspirin, iodides and nicotine (tobacco smoking).

Alcohol

A number of recent papers have called attention to the problems resulting from the injudicious use of alcohol during pregnancy. The "foetal alcohol syndrome" describes symptoms such as growth failure, facial abnormalities, cardiac defects, joint and limb deformities as well as delayed development and microencephaly.

Major investigations in Europe indicate that the syndrome may be caused by the chronic ingestion of alcohol, causing an accumulation of the metabolite of ethyl alcohol, acetaldehyde, in the maternal bloodstream, with subsequent transfer to the foetus. It has been claimed that two glasses of spirits per day during pregnancy will decrease foetal weight by 90 g. So while an occasional social drink appears to cause no problems, mothers can well be advised to avoid a level of consumption of alcohol during pregnancy that could cause long-term hardships for their children.

Aspirin

The effect of aspirin on blood coagulation mechanisms is well documented. When mothers consume more than 300 mg of aspirin in the week prior to delivery, diminished factor XII and impaired platelet aggregation have been observed in umbilical cord blood. In addition, by inhibiting prostaglandin synthesis in the mother, unnecessarily prolonged labour may result, while the inhibition of prostaglandin synthetase in the foetus may cause premature closure of the ductus arteriosus and consequent cardiac failure. To avoid these problems and potential dangers of maternal and neonatal haemorrhage, it would appear wise to recommend that mothers avoid ingestion of aspirin for at least the week before delivery.

Nicotine

The effects produced by nicotine as a result of smoking during pregnancy are well recognised and documented. The degree of effect has been shown to be directly proportional to the number of cigarettes smoked, with resulting symptoms including low birth-weight infants, miscarriage, premature delivery, stillbirth and neonatal death, as well as increased incidence of bleeding during pregnancy, abruptio placentae, placenta praevia and premature and prolonged rupture of the membranes.

In addition to these immediate problems, recent follow-up studies have reported postnatal growth deficiency and impaired mental development. Such children score lower on tests for reading ability, vocabulary, perceptual motor skills, IQ, cognitive ability and mathematics. Sound medical evidence therefore continues to accumulate that the threat to foetal well-being is so great that women should be encouraged to "break the habit" as soon as pregnancy is recognized, or better, when the possibility of pregnancy may exist.

Iodides

Excessive intake of iodides during pregnancy may result in foetal goitre, leading to airway obstruction and interference with brain function because of inadequate thyroid hormone production.

It can often be overlooked that many common cough mixtures contain iodides, as do a number of "health preparations" such as kelp tablets. Such information may be of benefit to the mother and her unborn child.

THE USE OF DRUGS IN LABOUR

PRETERM LABOUR (THREATENED PREMATURE DELIVERY)

The incidence of premature deliveries is about 8% of all births, yet prematurity accounts for approximately 75% of the perinatal mortality rate. In other words, less than one-twelfth of all births accounts for three-quarters of the deaths associated with childbirth. Consequently, the discovery of medications that can suppress premature labour has been welcomed by everyone involved with the practice of obstetrics. While some controversy exists about the indications for use of such drugs (for example, the management of pregnant women with ruptured membranes and preterm labour), the following are examples of medications that have been used to inhibit labour, referred to as myometrial relaxants.

Ethanol (Ethyl alcohol)

The site of action of ethanol in suppressing premature labour has not been positively demonstrated. It has been postulated that the primary effect is the inhibition of oxytocin release from the pituitary, while other groups have suggested a direct suppression of uterine muscle contractions, a release of endogenous labour-inhibiting catecholamines such as adrenaline or a prevention of prostaglandin synthesis or release. While future research may clarify its specific site of action, ethanol is seldom used because of the undesirable side effects typical of over-use of alcohol.

Magnesium Sulphate

Commonly known as *Epsom's salts* and as a laxative, magnesium sulphate has been recognized as an inhibitor of uterine contractions for over half a century. It has also been widely used in the treatment of pre-eclamptic toxaemia (PET) and recently has again become the drug of choice for this indication in some obstetric centres. While the magnesium ion causes paralysis of skeletal muscle, it appears to have a relaxant effect on smooth muscle by a direct effect on the muscle cell. While it is a relatively safe drug with a vast obstetric experience in its use, its role in the suppression of labour has been overshadowed by the more common use of the beta-2 sympathomimetic agents such as salbutamol and ritodrine.

Beta-2 sympathomimetic agents (beta-adrenergic receptor stimulants)

The study of adrenergic receptors goes back to the work of Langley and Dale around 1905 to 1906. Since that time, the well-known "fight or flight" syndrome of effects produced by adrenaline has been taught to generations of students in health care professions. Further investigations by Ahlquist in 1948 provided the current concept of alpha and beta adrenergic receptors, with activation or stimulation of alpha receptors causing vasoconstriction, while stimulation of beta receptors promotes vasodilatation, cardiac stimulation and relaxation of smooth muscle.

In 1967 the concept was elaborated on by Lands and associates, who described a sub-division of beta receptors into two types, called beta-1 and beta-2. Stimulation of beta-1 receptors resulted in increased heart rate and output as well as lipolysis (breakdown of fat) while beta-2 activation produced vasodilatation, bronchodilatation and muscle glycogenolysis (breakdown of glycogen), with resulting relaxation of smooth muscle. While further clarification is still needed, it was shown that beta-1 receptors were dominant in the heart, small intestine and fatty tissue, while beta-2 receptors dominated in the smooth muscle of the uterus, blood vessels, diaphragm and bronchioles. Reasoning on these basic principles will explain the use of salbutamol and terbutaline as a bronchodilator in the treatment of asthma and a uterine relaxant in obstetrics, as well as the reverse role of beta-blockers for the treatment of hypertension.

Isoxsuprine (*Duvadilan*) is one of the early examples of the beta-sympathomimetic group of drugs. It is not so specific in beta-2 activity as ritodrine and salbutamol and consequently is no longer in common use for obstetric indications.

Ritodrine (*Yutopar*), because of its beta-2 sympathomimetic activity, is a potent inhibitor of uterine contractions. It is used as an intravenous infusion and orally. Dosage by infusion is 50 to 350 mcg/min depending on cardiovascular response. One recommended regime is an initial infusion rate of 50 mcg/min, increasing by 50 mcg every 10 minutes until adequate uterine relaxation occurs, with a maximum infusion rate of 350 mcg/min. If disturbing palpitations or maternal heart rate in excess of 120/min are observed, the infusion rate is reduced by similar steps until an acceptable heart rate is obtained. When appropriate, the patient can be transferred to oral therapy with a dosage regime of 10 mg, four times a day, or more if necessary.

Salbutamol (*Ventolin*) is one of the beta-2 sympathomimetic agents in common use in hospitals. *Ventolin solution for intravenous infusion* is a special presentation of salbutamol for obstetric use, as ampoules containing 5 mg in 5 mL as distinct from *Ventolin* ampoules for use in the treatment of asthma, containing 0.5 mg of salbutamol in 1 mL. To produce uterine relaxation, a suitable solution for infusion may be prepared by diluting the contents of *Ventolin solution for intravenous infusion* in 500 mL of normal saline, dextrose injection, or dextrose saline injections. (The contents of the ampoule should never be injected undiluted by any route.) A dosage regime of 2.5 to 50 mcg/min then can be administered, with careful monitoring of maternal cardiovascular effects. When maternal heart rate in excess of 140/min occurs, the dose rate should be reduced or administration of the drug discontinued. When appropriate control has been established, the patient can be maintained on oral salbutamol therapy, with a recommended initial dose of 8 mg every six hours and suitable adjustments as necessary. It has also been suggested by some workers that oral therapy can be used to initiate treatment rather than the intravenous route.

Terbutaline (*Bricanyl*) and ***fenoterol*** (*Berotec*) are recent additions to this group of medications, with similar nursing considerations for appropriate dosage regimes.

Adverse Drug Reactions

Adverse drug reactions can include hand tremor, tachycardia, hypotension, headaches and flushing, dizziness, nausea and vomiting. A more severe complication that has been reported in recent articles is pulmonary oedema.

Contraindications:

Beta-2 sympathomimetics are contraindicated in hyperthyroidism, diabetes, foetal acidosis (pH 7.1 to 7.2), active uterine bleeding, maternal cardiac disease and hypersensitivity to this group of drugs. Great care should be exercised when administering these drugs to patients with hypertension and cardiac abnormalities.

NURSING IMPLICATIONS

1. Close monitoring of infusion strength and rate of administration is necessary.
2. Careful monitoring of maternal pulse rate and blood pressure is essential.
3. Careful observation of foetal heart rate and the status of the infant is recommended.

Miscellaneous

Other items that have been suggested for tocolytic purposes include ***diazoxide*** (*Eudemine*) and ***hydralazine*** (*Apresoline*). Both are well known for their roles in the treatment of hypertension, and when used in this capacity in late pregnancy, it was observed that women in labour experienced a dramatic inhibition of uterine contractions. Various mechanisms of action have been suggested, but neither drug is commonly recommended for this purpose. Similar observations have been made when general anaesthetic agents are administered to women in labour, particularly the gaseous inhalation type such as ***halothane*** (*Fluothane*). A practical application of this has been the use of halothane to assist the manual removal of retained placentas in the third stage of labour.

An adjunct to the use of tocolytic agents has been the discovery that administration of corticosteroids to the mother with threatened premature delivery may result in early maturation of the foetal lungs and avoidance of the respiratory distress syndrome (hyaline membrane disease). In the normal pregnancy, the surfactant that promotes respiration (gaseous exchange in the alveoli of the lungs) is present from about 36 weeks of gestation and is indicated by a lecithin-sphingomyelin ratio (L/S ratio) of two to one or greater. It is understood that adminstration of corticosteroids activates choline phosphotransferase which catalyses the conversion of choline to lecithin. While dexamethasone has been recommended in some centres, the preferred regime has been the administration of ***betamethasone*** in two injections of 12 mg, twelve hours apart. This should produce pulmonary maturity within 24 hours and subsequently safe delivery within 48 hours. Considerable discussion exists in the world literature about the application of such use of corticosteroids, but generally it is believed that the technique is of value up to 34 weeks of gestation. Such treatment should not be employed when infection is present, in severe hypertensive conditions, when the mother has diabetes or in the presence of ruptured membranes, except in the latter case when delivery is planned within 48 hours. Also avoid treatment when the L/S ratio is found to be good. In the case of diabetic mothers, an Israeli study recommends the use of intra-amniotic thyroxine to ensure foetal-lung maturity, but the technique has not been generally accepted. Other workers have claimed that foetal stress may also contribute toward early pulmonary maturity, as well as medications used to treat maternal hypertension such as the alpha-beta blocker labetalol (*Trandate*).

NORMAL LABOUR

A normal human pregnancy lasts approximately 40 weeks, when delivery of the infant and the placenta (the afterbirth) are brought about by strong rhythmical contractions of the uterus. This process ordinarily takes place automatically under the influence of endogenous oxytocin and prostaglandins.

Oxytocin and Ergometrine

For controlled induction of labour, ***synthetic oxytocin*** may be administered. At the completion of labour, oxytocic drugs are used routinely. It is at this time and in the puerperium that the oxytocics are especially useful.

The drugs available include ***synthetic oxytocin*** (*Syntocinon*, 1 unit/mL, 5 units/mL and 10 units/mL), ***ergometrine maleate*** (oral tablets 250 mcg and 500 mcg and injection of 500 mcg) and a combination of both for intramuscular use (*Syntometrine*, containing synthetic oxytocin 5 IU and ergometrine maleate 0.5 mg in 1 mL).

Oxytocin stimulates the rhythmical contractions of the uterus. In lactation it also stimulates milk let-down. The postpartum use of oxytocics causes the uterus to become firm and active. This reduces the incidence and extent of postpartum haemorrhage.

Oxytocin is used for induction of labour, stimulation of inadequate uterine effort, management of the third stage of labour, and for disorders of lactation.

Ergometrine maleate is used for the production of rhythmic contractions which increase in both frequency and force and for the treatment of postpartum haemorrhage.

When oxytocin is used for induction or stimulation of labour, it is given by a well-controlled intravenous infusion in dextrose 5% in water. For the management of the third stage of labour, an intramuscular injection is given at the birth of the anterior shoulder. A nasal spray is used for disorders of lactation (*Syntocinon Nasal Spray*, oxytocin 40 IU/mL, 5 mL).

Uterine contractions occur almost immediately and subside within one hour following IV administration of oxytocin. IM injection produces uterine response within three to five minutes, which persists for two to three hours.

Ergometrine initiates uterine contractions within five to 15 mintues when given orally, within two to five minutes by IM injection and virtually immediately by IV administration. Contractions persist for three hours or more for the oral and IM routes and for 45 minutes after IV use. Because of the severity of contractions produced by ergometrine when given by the IV route, it is seldom given in this manner, except when needed to control severe postpartum haemorrhage. The combination of oxytocin and ergometrine, *Syntometrine*, is given routinely with the birth of the anterior shoulder, except in cases of elevated blood pressure when the diastolic reading is more than 90 mmHg.

Various regimes are used for oxytocin infusion for induction or augmentation of labour, so nursing staff should take care to become thoroughly familiar with the procedure used in each particular hospital. Close patient observation is essential, with attention being paid to duration of contractions, interval between contractions, foetal heart rate and the possibility of water intoxication, in addition to routine obstetric observations. When a patient receives more than 3.5 litres of infused fluid, the risks of water intoxication increase.

Prostaglandins

The most recent additions to the list of drugs that promote uterine contractions are the prostaglandins. The term refers to a group of 20-carbon compounds that are produced by the action of the enzyme, prostaglandin synthetase, on the precursor substance, arachidonic acid. While many prostaglandins are known, only two types have become commonly used in international practice, the E_2 (PGE_2) and the F_2 alpha (PGF_2). They can be prepared for extra-amniotic and intra-amniotic use respectively and find special application in the case of intrauterine foetal death to initiate uterine contractions to expel the contents of the uterus. The specific site of action of prostaglandins has yet to be defined, although inhibition of the formation of cyclic AMP or an effect on calcium release have been suggested as possible mechanisms. Prostaglandin E_2 is available as vaginal tablets which are used to "ripen" the cervix.

Adverse Drug Reactions

Oxytocin has been known to cause some serious reactions when given in large or excessive doses, including violent uterine contractions with rupture of the uterus, soft tissue damage, foetal bradycardia and arrhythmias; severe hypertension and subarachnoid haemorrhage; water retention and intoxications with convulsions, coma and death; allergic reaction, nausea and vomiting.

Ergometrine maleate may cause nausea and vomiting, an occasional increase in blood pressure, and peripheral vascular constriction and gangrene.

Oxytocics should be used with caution in patients with toxaemia.

Prostaglandins have been reported to cause cardiac arrhythmias, including sudden cardiovascular collapse.

Contraindications

Oxytocin is contraindicated in severe toxaemia, hypertonic uterine inertia, abnormal foetal posture, placenta praevia, foetal distress or mechanical obstruction of delivery.

NURSING IMPLICATIONS

1. During administration of oxytocics, the foetal heart rate, duration and amplitude of contractions should be kept under constant supervision.
2. Closely monitor the drip rate.
3. Ergometrine, like most ergot alkaloids, has some tendency towards causing peripheral vascular constriction from which gangrene may result. Be alert to symptoms, which would indicate this effect — the patient's feet may become cold, numb or even purple.
4. Be sure not to confuse the oxytocic injections with any injection intended for the infant, for example, vitamin K.

Other drugs in common use at the time of delivery

Phenothiazines, such as chlorpromazine (*Largactil*), promazine (*Sparine*) and prochlorperazine (*Stemetil*) are used as adjuncts to pain relief in labour as well as for sedation and treatment of nausea. Promethazine (*Phenergan*) can be employed similarly, with the added benefit of its antihistamic effect for itch and rash therapy, which is a fairly frequent adverse effect of narcotic epidural anaesthesia.

Metoclopramide (*Maxolon, Primperan*) is used as an antiemetic, and recently, to assist in the promotion of lactation, because of its effect of elevating serum prolactin levels.

Lignocaine (*Xylocaine*) is used for local anaesthesia prior to episiotomy, and also in combination with bupivacaine (*Marcain*) for epidural anaesthesia.

Narcotics, especially pethidine and papaveretum (*Omnopon*) are used for pain relief during labour and following caesarean section. Less severe pain, particularly following delivery, is commonly treated with paracetamol (*Panadol*), paracetamol and codeine (co-codamol and dispersible tablets) and dextropropoxyphene with paracetamol (co-proxamol).

Laxatives are administered for postpartum constipation. Agents such as lactulose† (*Duphalac*) and dioctylsodium sulphosuccinate with danthron (co-danthrusate capsules) may be used, the former to soften faeces and the latter to soften faeces and promote peristalsis. Senna fruit derivatives† (*Senokot*) may also be used.

Antibiotics are given for postpartum and postcaesarean infection and for the treatment of mastitis. Amoxycillin (*Amoxil*) is for general gram-positive and gram-negative cover, and metronidazole (*Flagyl*) is used to treat anaerobic infection such as bacteroides.

DRUGS AND BREAST FEEDING

As in the case of drug consumption during pregnancy, the past 20 years has witnessed a growing awareness of the need for caution when recommending medication for mothers while they are breast feeding. While only a small list of items are totally contraindicated, many others will produce undesirable side effects in the nursing infant. As an example, many sedative and tranquillising drugs will be transferred to the baby, causing drowsiness and poor feeding habits. This may result in increased anxiety on the part of the mother thus negating the original intent of the maternal therapy. So during breast feeding, it is important to restrict drug therapy to essential medical indications and to avoid the casual use of medications when realistic alternatives such as patient education, re-assurance and attention to physical comfort are all that are needed.

The same basic principles exist for transfer of drugs in breast milk as in transplacental passage of drugs. Milk can be viewed as an oil-in-water emulsion containing droplets of fat in an aqueous medium in which lactose, inorganic salts and protein are in solution. Within the breast, this emulsion is separated from the mother's blood by a semipermeable membrane that is lipid in composition and allows a similar exchange to the membranes involved in placental transfer. It is understood that water, electrolytes and small water-soluble molecules are able to pass through small pores in the membrane, while larger molecules, including most drugs, traverse the lipid membrane by simple passive diffusion, from an area of high concentration to one of low concentration.

Additionally, breast milk has a lower (more acid) pH than maternal serum, so many drugs, such as those that are weak bases, will be more ionised on the milk side of the membrane, thus encouraging a higher concentration of total drug in milk compared with serum. Drug binding to plasma proteins is a further factor, as most drugs are significantly more bound to plasma proteins than to milk proteins. In summary, this means that fat-soluble drugs in their non-ionised form will transfer readily into breast milk, especially when the dosage given produces a high maternal-serum level of the drug. Also, the nature of the drug will affect the degree of transfer, as will the amount of protein binding of the drug in the mother's bloodstream. It has been demonstrated that "back-diffusion" of drugs can take place from milk to maternal plasma as the concentration falls in the mother's bloodstream due to metabolism and excretion of the drug; so timing of infant feeding in relation to the time when the mother consumes the medication is another important factor for consideration.

This brief summary of the principles involved in drug transfer into breast milk illustrates that it is often difficult to give a simple "yes" or "no" answer to an enquiry about whether breast feeding should be stopped when the mother has a course of drug therapy prescribed for her. As in the case of drugs used in pregnancy, it is wise to check with a local Drug Information Centre about the most recent findings about any particular drug and relate this information to the individual patient's medical condition to evaluate the risks and benefits that could be expected in each case. Prescribers who include the mother in the decision-making process gain the benefit of optimal patient compliance and minimal parental anxiety when adjustments need to be made to the normal routine.

Publications vary when listing drugs that should be totally avoided while breastfeeding, but the following table lists *examples* of drugs that are generally contraindicated during lactation.

Table 36
Some Drugs Contraindicated during Lactation

Drug	Comment
Anticoagulants (except warfarin and heparin)	Can cause bleeding tendencies in the breast-fed infant
Antithyroid drugs and iodides	Supression of thyroid function and goitre in the infant
Benzodiazepines (early types, such as diazepam)	"Flat baby" syndrome; lethargy, poor feeding habits, possible jaundice
Chloramphenicol	Possible infant blood dyscrasias
Ergot preparations	May cause symptoms of ergotism (vomiting, diarrhoea)
Lithium compounds	Hypotonia, difficulty in feeding, failure to thrive
Oestrogens	Hormonal effects on infant
Radioactive preparations	May resume feeding when milk is no longer radioactive
Reserpine	Nasal stuffiness, respiratory difficulty, poor feeding habits
Sulphonamides	Can cause neonatal jaundice and kernicterus

Ways to minimise infant drug intake from breast milk

1. For a drug that can be given as a single daily dose, this should be administered just before the longest sleep period for the child. Feeding can thus be avoided during peak milk levels of the drug.
2. To minimise the amount of drug received even further, the first feeding after the drug has been taken can be of milk that has been expressed earlier in the day and saved. Engorgement can be avoided by expressing milk at the usual feeding time and discarding it.
3. If a drug must be given several times a day, the mother should consume the drug immediately after nursing. The pharmacokinetics of most drugs ingested by breast-feeding women are such that administration of the drug at this time will allow back-diffusion to take place and will result in the lowest amount of drug in the milk at the subsequent feeding.

NURSING IMPLICATIONS

A survey carried out in 1980 by Martin and Monk suggested that 65% of mothers in the UK attempt to breastfeed their babies, and 52% are still breastfeeding two weeks after giving birth. Encouragement and reassurance are therefore most appropriate, as well as expert advice when adjustments have to be made because of the mother's medical condition. Specific information about a particular drug can be obtained from the pharmacy department within each hospital.

Avoid uninformed personal opinion that may cause subsequent confusion or concern.

Careful observation of all breast-fed infants whose mothers are receiving drug therapy should be routine. Make sure both Paediatricians and Obstetricians are made aware of any adverse effects or any change from normal neonatal functions.

DRUG USAGE IN THE NEONATE

Neonatology has been one of the most dramatic and exciting "growth areas" in medical science in recent decades. Infants delivered prematurely, often after as little as 26 weeks of gestation and weighing less than one kilogram, now have reasonable prospects of survival in modern special-care nurseries, and those of longer gestation are regularly aided to proper development and discharge from hospital by the time birth would have occurred normally.

While improved technology and intensive care techniques have played a large role in such improvements, drug therapy has also been involved and has made a major contribution toward treatment of specific functional defects and problems associated with hepatic immaturity and enzyme deficiency. An example is the previously mentioned use of corticosteroids to enhance foetal lung maturity and the application of the prostaglandin synthetase inhibitor indomethacin, to assist closure of patent ductus arteriosus.

The following are examples of drugs for special application which are regularly used in Intensive Care Nurseries in Obstetric Hospitals.

Dosages will of course vary considerably depending on the gestational development and condition of each neonate, but the figures given will indicate the approximate range of dosage in common use in Intensive Care Nurseries.

Aminophylline is used in the treatment of neonatal apnoea. An initial loading dose of 5 to 7.5 mg/kg is common, followed by 2 mg/kg twice daily, by slow IV infusion.

Ampicillin (*Penbritin*) has been widely used for routine gram-positive and gram-negative infections. Recommended dosage is 100 mg/kg/day, in two divided doses. Recently amoxycillin (*Amoxil*) which is hydroxy-ampicillin, has become the drug of choice in many centres. It is effective in smaller dosages and can be given orally, independent of time of food intake.

Calcium gluconate is a means of supplying calcium to correct hypocalcaemia which is common in preterm infants. Calcium glubionate injection (*Calcium Sandoz 10%*) contains 1.375 g calcium glubionate in 10 mL which is equivalent to 10% w/v calcium gluconate. Dosage aims to supply 27 mg of elemental calcium per kilogram per day (3 mL of 10% solution).

Digoxin (*Lanoxin*) is used in thc treatment of cardiac failure to increase the force of myocardial contraction. Dosage is 30 micrograms/kg to digitalize, then 5 micrograms/kg twice daily.

Dopamine is a precursor of noradrenaline and is used to correct haemodynamic imbalance resulting from acute hypotension associated with renal failure and low cardiac output. Dopamine (*Intropin*) stimulates beta-1 adrenergic receptors in normal doses and alpha-adrenergic receptors in higher doses. Dosage is 5 micrograms/kg/min and upwards, depending on desired response.

Gentamicin (*Garamycin, Cidomycin*) is commonly used for suspected gram-negative infections. Dosage is 2.5 mg/kg twice daily, IM or by slow IV injection, also used in association with ampicillin or amoxycillin for broad spectrum cover.

Indomethacin (*Indocid*) has become the treatment of choice to facilitate the closure of patent ductus arteriosus. Recommended dosage is 0.2 to 0.3 mg/kg every eight to 12 hours for two or three doses.

Isoprenaline (*Isuprel*) is a synthetic sympathomimetic agent that acts almost exclusively on beta receptors (beta-one and beta-two). Known as isoproterenol in the US, it is part of the group of drugs referred to as catecholamines because of the amine structure in the molecule. Hence, adrenaline, noradrenaline, dopamine and isoprenaline are sometimes referred to as sympathomimetic amines. Isoprenaline is used to correct peripheral circulatory failure, particularly in conjunction with bradycardia. Dosage recommendations vary, but 0.1 to 0.4 micrograms/kg/min administered in 5% dextrose injection is common. Dopamine is often given in association with isoprenaline to maintain cardiac output.

Metronidazole (*Flagyl*) is used for suspected anaerobic infections: 7.5 mg/kg three times a day, by slow IV infusion.

Latamoxef sodium (*Moxalactam*), described as a "third generation cephalosporin", is a semisynthetic broad-spectrum beta-lactam antibiotic. It finds special application in the treatment of neonatal meningitis due to gram-negative bacteria. Dosage is 25 to 50 mg/kg, every 12 hours for the first week of life, reverting to a dose every eight hours for weeks 1 to 4. Cefotaxime (*Claforan*) is another recent "third generation cephalosporin" with similar applications.

Naloxone (*Narcan*) is a narcotic antagonist described as "essentially pure". That is, it does not possess the "agonist" or morphine-like properties of earlier narcotic antagonists. Indicated for the complete or partial reversal of narcotic depression, including respiratory depression in the neonate following medical or illicit administration of narcotics to the mother. Usual initial dose is 0.01 mg/kg by IM, IV or SC injection, repeated as necessary to produce the required degree of counteraction and improvement in respiratory function.

Phenobarbitone is used in the first-line treatment of seizures: 10 to 20 mg/kg initially, then 3 to 6 mg/kg every 12 hours, IV or IM.

Phytomenadione provides routine prophylaxis for haemorrhagic disorders of the newborn: 1mg following delivery for all birth weights.

Known as Vitamin K_1, phytomenadione (*Konakion*) injection is 1 mg in 0.5 mL.

Prostaglandin E_1 (alprostadil; *Prostin VR*) is indicated for palliative therapy to temporarily maintain the patency of the ductus arteriosus until corrective or palliative surgery can be performed in neonates who have congenital heart defects and who depend upon a patent ductus for survival.

Presentation is 500 mcg in 1 mL and administration is by continuous IV infusion, beginning with 0.1 mcg/kg/minute; when the intended effect is achieved, reduce to the lowest possible dose while maintaining desired effects.

Sodium bicarbonate, for correction of metabolic acidosis, is used in neonatal therapy to increase the buffering capacity of the blood, which is diminished following episodes of hypoxaemia, anaemia and ischaemia. Initial dosage is 2 mmol/kg to an upper limit of 6 to 8 mmol/kg over 24 hours. The 8.4% sodium bicarbonate injection BP contains 1 mmol sodium and 1 mmol bicarbonate in 1 mL.

Theophylline is used as an oral alternative to aminophylline in neonatal aponea; 5 mg/kg is given initially, then 1 to 2 mg/kg every eight or 12 hours.

Tolazoline is well known as an oral peripheral vasodilator. It now finds a new application in neonates in the treatment of pulmonary hypertension, which contributes to persistent foetal circulation after delivery, instead of normal progression to "mature" circulation; 1 to 2 mg/kg initially, then 1 to 2 mg/kg/hr, by infusion.

Vitamin E is used to reduce the severity of toxic effects associated with long-term use of oxygen in preterm infants. Neonates with respiratory distress syndrome (RDS, also known as hyaline membrane disease) require increased concentrations of oxygen, which may result in bronchopulmonary dysplasia and retrolental fibroplasia (retinopathy of prematurity). Evidence suggests that vitamin E, also known as alpha tocopherol, may diminish the toxic effects of oxygen, one of the causal factors of bronchopulmonary dysplasia. Recommended dosage is up to 25 mg (25 i.u.) daily IM or up to 20 mg/kg daily by oral administration.

NURSING IMPLICATIONS

Extreme care must be exercised constantly to avoid error in dosage. Many products have both neonatal and adult strength presentations and may be located near to each other in obstetric and neonatal units. (Examples are digoxin, phytomenadione and naloxone). Pay close attention to the strength of the solution (mg/ml) and the prescribed dosage requirement (mg/kg). If any doubt exists, double check with the prescriber or other experienced nursing staff. Be sure other important factors are clearly understood such as intended route (I.M., I.V. or oral) and the duration of therapy (single dose, until a defined response is achieved or for a fixed period).

Be alert to recognize and report any suspected adverse reactions or side effects. Cultivate good observation techniques.

Avoid confusion of milligrams (mg) and micrograms (mcg).

SELF-EVALUATION TEST

1. Describe the mechanisms involved in drug transfer to the foetus. Which drugs will be more likely to accumulate in the foetal bloodstream?
2. List some of the drugs that should be avoided during pregnancy and those where caution should be exercised.
3. Discuss the use of drugs for a mother with premature labour at 30 weeks gestation. What changes would be considered if the patient was also a diabetic or was diagnosed as pre-eclamptic?
4. Which drugs can be used to induce uterine contractions?
   (a) In normal labour.
   (b) In the case of intra-uterine foetal death.
5. What other drugs are commonly used at the time of delivery, and for what indications? What additional considerations exist if the mother is breast-feeding?
6. Name some of the new drugs or new uses for older drugs in the treatment of neonatal conditions.
7. Outline some aspects of special nursing care that must be exercised when administering drug therapy to neonates.

SECTION 4

14

PAEDIATRIC THERAPEUTICS

Elizabeth Creber

OBJECTIVES

At the end of this chapter, the student should be able to:

1. discuss factors which should be considered in paediatric drug therapy;
2. discuss reasons why a neonate handles drugs differently from children and adults;
3. name some of the benefits achieved monitoring drug concentrations in serum.

PREREQUISITE KNOWLEDGE

1. An understanding of drug action (Chapter 1).
2. A knowledge of drug administration.

INTRODUCTION

Drug therapy in paediatrics can be complex because children are not just little adults who respond to therapy proportional to their age, height or weight with respect to adults. Children have changing organ function, body size and composition in relation to adults. At birth, a baby may weigh about 3 to 3.5 kg. This weight will be doubled by about five months, doubled again by about 9.5 years, and again by about 16 years. A baby's height (length) may not be doubled till about four years, and in most cases, a person will not double his or her four-year-old height even by maturity.

A number of different rules based on weight, age, or body surface area as a basis of calculating paediatric doses (as a fraction of the adult dose) have been used, but none have proved truly satisfactory for all drugs.

Most drugs used in day-to-day paediatric practice are relatively non-toxic (that is, there is a wide margin between the therapeutic and toxic dose), and the "mg/kg" method for each drug is the most suitable method of dose calculation, although mg/m² (body surface area) may also be used. The more toxic drugs with a narrow margin between therapeutic and toxic dose (for example, ***digoxin*** and ***aminoglycoside antibiotics***) require a more sophisticated knowledge of drug handling by the body. Recent developments in analytical methods for measuring concentrations of drugs in different tissues and in plasma have contributed to knowledge on specific drugs and their interactions with other drugs, and has provided a detailed knowledge of patient and organ variables in drug handling. Doses of the more toxic drugs are usually based on a mg/kg rule, and serum levels of the drugs are then monitored to test that rule's accuracy for that particular adult or child.

FACTORS INFLUENCING PAEDIATRIC DRUG THERAPY

The important factors to be considered in paediatric drug therapy are:

administration
absorption
distribution
metabolism
excretion
adverse effects and toxicity

DRUG ADMINISTRATION

Oral

Oral administration of drugs to the newborn child may result in aspiration, especially with strong-tasting medicine, and older children may fight vigorously to avoid taking medicine. Mixtures can be flavoured, but if the drug is unpleasant to taste, even the flavoured mixture may be unpleasant. On the other hand, if the mixture is too pleasant, this may encourage the toddler to overdose. Sugar content of many mixtures is high to increase patient acceptability, but this may increase the development of dental caries. Addition of any medicines to milk should be discouraged for three reasons: first, if the infant does not like the taste, he may reject it and subsequent milk feeds; second, feeds are not always finished, so dosage may be suboptimal; third, some drugs may have their activity decreased when mixed with milk.

Many drugs are not available in mixture form because of decreased stability in solution, lack of stability information or because they are rarely used in paediatrics. Most tablets can be crushed, or capsules pulled apart and mixed with jam, honey, apple sauce or peanut butter immediately before administration. Capsules containing enteric-coated granules (for example, pancrease) may be pulled apart and the contents administered by sprinkling them on soft food. The reason for administration with soft food is so that the granules will be swallowed whole and not crushed. If crushed, the enteric coating would be destroyed, and the drug would be released in the stomach which would then lead to possible destruction of the drug's activity.

Compliance in paediatrics depends not only on the convenience of dosage schedule but on patient acceptability.

Inhalation

Many drugs, especially those used in treating patients with respiratory disease, are effective by inhalation. A metered aerosol is appropriate for children over seven or eight years of age, but below this age the drug could be administered as a dry powder by inhalation from a Rotacap, for example, ***salbutamol***. In children under four years of age, aerosols are administered using a compressed air pump and nebuliser to deliver a fine mist which is inhaled by breathing naturally.

Intramuscular

Intramuscular administration should be avoided where possible in infants, since sciatic neuropathy and subsequent stunting of leg growth has been reported after IM injection.

Intravenous

Intravenous therapy carries most of the same problems for children as for adults (drug instability, phlebitis). Accurate administration of small volumes (for example, 1mL per hour) may be a problem in neonates, and trying to restrain an active toddler or young child often causes problems.

Unintentional

Before birth, some drugs given to the mother will have crossed the placenta, leaving the neonate to detoxify and/or excrete the drug. Some of these drugs may have adverse effects, for example, ***salicylates*** may cause bleeding problems, and ***diazepam*** may cause newborn apnoea, hypotonia, hypothermia and poor feeding.

Many drugs ingested by a nursing mother may be excreted in her milk. The amount excreted, however, is usually so small (about 1% of ingested maternal drug) that it is detected only with difficulty. Some conditions requiring drug treatment (for example, malignancy) and treatment with some drugs known to have caused problems in breast-fed infants (for example, ***isoniazid***) will preclude the mother from breast feeding and unintentionally administering the drug to her infant.

DRUG ABSORPTION

Oral

The neonatal gastrointestinal tract undergoes significant changes from birth. At birth, the pH of the stomach is approximately 6 to 8. Within

24 hours, it falls to values of 1 to 3 but acid secretion is depressed to low levels for about 10 days until the gastric mucosa matures. The pH gradually decreases to adult levels by about two years. The relatively achlorhydric situation of the infant stomach may partially explain the higher bioavailability of some penicillins and the decreased absorption of acidic drugs, phenobarbitone and phenytoin in the newborn. Gastrointestinal enzyme action may also contribute to differences in drug action, for example, ***chloramphenicol palmitate*** must be hydrolysed in order for free active ***chloramphenicol*** to be liberated, which explains why peak serum levels may take about 12 hours to occur in newborns compared to two hours in infants. At birth the stomach holds about 10 to 20 mL, after two weeks about 80 mL, and at the end of the first month about 100 mL. The relatively smaller size of the stomach may explain the frequent regurgitation and vomiting characteristic of neonates.

Intramuscular

The marked changes in relative blood flow to various muscles (due to developmental adaptation, the relative insufficiency of muscle contractions, the reduced skeletal-muscle mass and subcutaneous fat of the infant, relative to children) lead to altered, unpredictable absorption from this route in neonates and infants.

Topical

Absorption of drugs through the skin is significantly enhanced in the very young due to the relative thinness of the stratum corneum and the degree of skin hydration. Toxic effects have been noted in neonates from application of ***boric acid*** in powder (which can cause severe diarrhoea), ***hexachlorophane emulsions*** (which have been reported to cause neurotoxicity), and repeated applications of ***corticosteroids,*** which may produce significant adrenal suppression.

DRUG DISTRIBUTION

When a drug is administered to a patient, it is distributed to various compartments of the body. The following factors affect this distribution.

Body water and fat

Body water and fat composition alter disproportionately in relation to age and weight. Total body water as a percentage of body weight is approximately 80% at birth, 65% at 12 months and 60% for a young adult male. Total body fat as a percentage of body weight is approximately 1% to 3% in the premature infant, 12% to 15% at normal birth, 30% at 12 months and 18% for a young adult male. Some drugs are distributed more readily into fat stores and others more readily into body water. For water-soluble drugs, for example, ***benzylpenicillin,*** the dose required to achieve the same plasma concentration decreases during childhood.

Protein binding

Drug protein binding is diminished in neonates due to a lower concentration of plasma proteins (particularly albumin) and a lower drug-binding capacity of foetal albumin. This may lead to an increase in the fraction of unbound pharmacologically active drug in the plasma. Examples showing the lower percentage of drug bound to plasma proteins in newborns compared to adults are ***ampicillin*** (9% to 11% compared to 15% to 29%) and ***phenobarbitone*** (28% to 36% compared to 46% to 48%). These differences in protein binding lead to differences in the apparent volume of distribution of a drug, making the interpretation of plasma drug levels more complex. In newborn infants the hepatic conjugation of bilirubin is limited and increased plasma levels of bilirubin often occur. Acidic drugs, for example, ***salicylates*** and most ***sulphonamides*** which are highly bound to plasma albumin, compete with — and can displace — bilirubin from albumin binding sites. If hepatic metabolism is already compromised, the increased unbound, unconjugated lipid-soluble bilirubin may cross the blood-brain barrier and lead to kernicterus.

Blood-brain barrier

Immaturity of the blood-brain barrier at birth, leading to an increased permeability by lipid-soluble drugs, may be one of the factors causing increased uptake of ***barbiturates*** and ***morphine*** in young infants.

Drug receptor sensitivity

The newborn child has an increased sensitivity to non-depolarising neuromuscular blocking agents, for example, ***tubocurarine***, but response to neuromuscular blocking agents alters during the neonatal period.

DRUG METABOLISM

The various metabolic reactions occurring in the mature liver are not fully developed at birth. Oxidation and glucuronide conjugation are decreased at birth, but the same patient may have a relatively good ability to demethylate compounds and good capacity for sulphate conjugation. ***Lignocaine***, ***phenobarbitone***, ***phenytoin*** and ***diazepam***, which are metabolised by oxidation, and ***chloramphenicol***, which is glucuronidated, show decreased metabolism in the neonate, resulting in increased drug half-life. The plasma half-life of phenytoin is 30 to 70 hours for a full term baby, six to 15 hours for a neonate aged five to 10 days, two to seven hours for infants, five to 30 hours for a child, and 24 hours for adults. Chloramphenicol given in "usual doses" based on body weight for a term baby may cause serious toxicity (circulatory collapse or "grey baby" syndrome) in a premature baby due to defective glucuronidation. The plasma half-life for chloramphenicol is 15 to 28 hours for a premature baby, 6 to 10 hours for a term baby, and 1.5 to 4 hours for a baby aged 10 to 15 days. Cardiac insufficiency and respiratory distress also contribute to decreased metabolic activity. During the first 15 days of life in premature and full-term babies, a decrease in metabolism is evident, but this is followed by a dramatic increase in metabolism.

In older children, 1 to 10 years, evidence has shown hepatic microsomal oxidation is more rapid than in adults, thus helping to explain the fact that ***phenobarbitone, phenytoin*** and ***theophylline*** have shorter plasma half-lives in children than in adults.

DRUG EXCRETION

At birth, renal function is significantly less developed in premature and full-term newborns than it is in children and adults. Glomerular filtration, tubular reabsorption and tubular secretion mature at different rates, but functional values comparable with adults are usually reached between six and 12 months providing these are corrected for body surface area. The relative lack of renal function in the newborn affects those drugs which are excreted by the kidney, especially ***aminoglycosides, digoxin*** and ***penicillins***, all of which have prolonged half-lives during the first week of life. The half-life of ***gentamicin*** for premature babies less than seven days of age is five to six hours, and for full-term babies less than seven days of age, the half-life is four to five and one-half hours. But by 7 to 14 days of age, the half-life has decreased to three and one-half hours, with the adult value being about two to three hours.

ADVERSE DRUG REACTIONS AND TOXICITY

Many newer drugs have been tested in adults but not in children. Therefore, side effects specifically related to children have not been reported. This emphasises the importance of reporting adverse drug reactions to a central bureau for data collection.

Some adverse effects of drugs are related to growth and development.

1. Identical drug doses may be toxic in one age group (***chloramphenicol*** in newborn) and yet may be insufficient to give the desired therapeutic results two to three weeks later.
2. Neonates with breathing disorders may require therapy with a high concentration of oxygen, which can lead to retrolental fibroplasia and possible blindness if not carefully monitored.
3. ***Tetracyclines*** are distributed and deposited in teeth and bone, which means that when ingested during the period of tooth development, they will produce permanent yellow-brown discolouration of teeth. All teeth formed during administration of tetracycline are stained; therefore, use of this drug should be avoided in all children under eight years.

Other adverse effects are related to altered metabolism and usually appear during childhood when drugs are first encountered.

1. Glucose-6-phosphate dehydrogenase deficiency is responsible for the haemolysis of red blood cells that occurs after exposure to certain drugs, for example, sulphonamides. Clothes stored with naphthalene (to deter moths) have caused haemolysis when worn by patients with this disorder.

2. Many tablets and capsules use lactose as a filler, and many mixtures contain sucrose or lactose. In certain diseases, for example, disaccharide intolerance, patients cannot metabolise these sugars and often suffer severe adverse effects.

A child's or infant's disease state may affect the body's response to a drug. The state of hydration is important in drug distribution, and dehydration is common in sick infants, as is acidosis. These factors may lead to toxicity even when a standard dose is given, for example, of salicylates.

Paradoxical reactions may occur in children, for example with ***phenobarbitone.*** Some children, especially those with lesions of the central nervous system, react with increased irritability and excessive activity following a standard sedative dose.

Some children may be less able to tolerate well-known side effects of drugs. For example, gum hyperplasia and increased hair production associated with ***phenytoin*** therapy can cause serious embarrassment in adolescent girls.

Most adverse reactions, toxicity and drug interactions occurring in infancy and childhood are similar to those occurring in adults. However, because fewer children receive complex or multiple drug therapy, interactions appear to occur less often.

COMMON PAEDIATRIC DISORDERS

In the UK the majority of children are healthy and have occasional acute disorders (infection, pain, fever) requiring therapy. Three common problems are briefly discussed here.

FEVER

It is not known whether fever may sometimes be beneficial and therefore whether treatment is necessary. Fever is of diagnostic value; therefore, treatment should only be commenced after consideration has been given to a diagnosis. Fever due to dehydration should be treated with fluids rather than an antipyretic like ***paracetamol***.

One reason for treating fever is to help prevent febrile convulsions. Seizures associated with fever occur primarily in children between six months and six years of age, with a maximum incidence during the second year of life. The higher the fever, the greater the risk of convulsions, so children who have suffered a previous febrile convulsion need aggressive therapy to decrease fever, for example, ***paracetamol***. Therapy with an anticonvulsant may also be instituted depending on the patient's history.

Aspirin is metabolised differently by children compared with adults. Dehydration and acidosis are common in febrile infants and children, and this will decrease salicylate excretion by the kidneys which may lead to accumulation. Gastrointestinal irritation and bleeding, haemorrhage, change in blood clotting processes, and metabolic side effects have been reported in children who have taken normal doses of aspirin.

In June 1986, the CSM advised that aspirin should not be used for children under 12 except under medical supervision. This was because of an association between the use of aspirin and the incidence of Reye's syndrome.

Paracetamol (10 mg/kg) is a safe drug, and toxicity only occurs in doses greatly in excess of the therapeutic range.

Aspirin and paracetamol have an onset of action of about one-half hour and a duration of action of about four hours. Paracetamol is available in a mixture form, with a long shelf life.

INFECTION

Some infections require little or no therapy, while others require immediate therapy. Initial therapy will depend on the physician's knowledge of the infecting organism, and subsequent therapy will depend on results of bacterial cultures.

Penicillin may be used to treat most common bacterial infections of the upper and lower respiratory tract. Penicillin V needs to be taken four times a day on an empty stomach. In the case of follicular tonsillitis caused by beta-haemolytic streptococci, treatment should be continued for 10 days to prevent the occurrence of rheumatic fever or glomerulonephritis. Benzyl penicillin (administered intravenously) may be used in meningitis, septicaemia, and other serious infections. The semi-synthetic penicillin, ***amoxycillin***, has a broader spectrum and only needs to be administered every eight hours, but significant diarrhoea has been reported in up to 48% of children under two years of age. Effective blood levels of ***benzathine penicillin*** injection are maintained for at least seven days in children, but injections are painful and the risk of fatal anaphylactic reactions is slightly greater than with oral therapy.

Co-trimoxazole has a broad spectrum of activity, and the advantage of being effective when given twice a day. It contains a sulphonamide, and skin rashes (including the Stevens-Johnson syndrome) have been reported.

Erythromycin has a similar spectrum of antibiotic activity to penicillin and may be used in patients with penicillin sensitivity.

Chloramphenicol is used in severe infections, especially epiglottitis and meningitis. Serum levels should be monitored.

Aminoglycoside antibiotics are effective against a wide range of gram-negative bacteria and some gram-positive organisms. They are often used in septicaemia or meningitis in newborn infants. Serum levels should be monitored.

ASTHMA

Determining whether a child has asthma and consequently needs bronchodilator therapy may not always be easy. Bronchodilator drugs used in asthma include the sympathomimetic agents and theophylline.

Beta-2 sympathomimetic drugs (for example, ***salbutamol, terbutaline***): few patients aged less than six months respond well to these agents; however, most patients aged over 18 months will respond. There is no way to predict which patients between 6 and 18 months will respond. The most effective method of administration is by inhalation (by metered aerosol, Rotacap or compressed-air pump and nebuliser), although oral and parenteral preparations are available. Failure to respond requires urgent medical assessment for additional therapy.

Theophylline and its analogues can be used in conjunction with beta-2 sympathomimetic agents. Monitoring of theophylline serum levels has led to a greater understanding of the body's handling of this drug. Dosage is 5 mg/kg for patients up to 45 kg. Higher doses may be used if serum levels are monitored. Slow-release preparations have recently been developed and have proved effective when given in dosages of approximately 10 mg/kg every 12 hours. Adverse effects include nausea and vomiting, and in higher doses, arrhythmias and convulsions.

Sodium cromoglycate, administered as a dry-powder inhalation, may be added when the response to bronchodilator drugs is inadequate.

Corticosteroids should be added if bronchodilator therapy is ineffective. These may be administered as ***beclomethasone*** by metered aerosol or Rotacap. This method of administration minimises the risk of systemic side effects. If inhalation therapy is ineffective, corticosteroids may be administered orally or parenterally.

SUMMARY

The choice of drug and dosage form for paediatric patients depends on:

(a) knowledge of the drug, its dosage, and its therapeutic index; if the therapeutic index is narrow, serum level monitoring should be performed;
(b) a knowledge of the drug and how it is handled by the body;
(c) drug-handling capacity of the patient, age, organ function and disease state;
(d) patient acceptability, route and form of dose.

NURSING IMPLICATIONS

Assessment

The child should be approached in a manner appropriate to his or her age and experience, with thought for the extent to which the patient can understand and participate in the treatment. A young child may respond to make-believe and the use of favourite toys, while the older child, with chronic disease, may already be participating in the management of his therapy.

The child's weight, accurately recorded, is essential to calculate the drug dose.

Administration

Consideration should be given to the child's ability to cope with the drug, the dose, the dose form, and the route of administration. Some drugs for example, chloramphenicol, digoxin (see previous discussion), are particularly hazardous in newborn infants. Institutional policies may require double checking and may restrict administration of such drugs to authorised staff members.

A dose form suitable to the child's age will aid compliance. If a tablet is unacceptable, a paediatric mixture may be available. Some tablets may be crushed and given in jam, but care must be taken not to crush slow-release formulations.

In children under two years, the gluteal muscles are insufficiently developed to be used for intramuscular injection. Alternative sites are deltoid or vastus lateralis muscles. Paediatric institutions may have specific policies regarding intramuscular injections.

Keeping of medications under lock and key is particularly important in a paediatric context. Equipment, particularly syringes, must also be inaccessible to children.

Evaluation

Even very young children may convey subjective response to drug therapy, for example, whether analgesia has been effective or whether the drug makes them nauseated. Careful, continuous observation is necessary to evaluate the effectiveness of therapy and possible adverse effects. Unwanted effects, especially of new drugs, may be less predictable in the child than in the adult.

Monitoring of serum drug levels is used in the neonate when the therapeutic ratio is narrow and may be used in some instances of continuing therapy, notably with phenytoin. If these serum levels are to be useful, standard protocol must be observed for collection times and their relationship to time of drug administration.

Patient teaching

The older child will be able to understand a specific drug regimen, for example, whether the drug is to be taken with food or not. Parent education will, of course, be extremely important in ensuring drug compliance.

Information will be given to the younger child at a level appropriate to his or her age, possibly through play, stories and the use of toys. Failure to explain may create and reinforce attitudes of fear towards health care and the people who give it.

The child (for example, the diabetic or epileptic child) must be offered a well-organised program for education and continuing support: As he grows older, he will gradually assume increasing responsibility for management of his own treatment. Other family members, preferably the whole family, should be offered the same learning opportunities.

SELF-EVALUATION TEST

1. Name three factors affecting drug absorption in the neonate.
2. Why is caution needed when chloramphenicol is administered to a premature baby?
3. Why does excretion of gentamicin vary with age in young babies?
4. What drugs are used to treat a fever?
5. What factors must be considered when choosing which drug to use in the treatment of fever in babies and children?

15
GERIATRIC THERAPEUTICS

Ian Kilminster

"Do not cast me off in the time of old age." Psalms 71:9

OBJECTIVES

At the end of this chapter, the reader should:

1. be able to describe the changes taking place in people as they age and how these changes are affected by drug action.
2. know what practical steps to take, as a nurse, to help the older person use his or her medication correctly, the aim being to maximise the aged person's independence and to avoid unnecessary hospital admissions;
3. be able to name the signs and symptoms of important adverse drug reactions which occur frequently in the elderly.

PREREQUISITE KNOWLEDGE

1. Pharmacology and use of drug groups and commonly used drugs listed in previous chapters.
2. General concept of diseases and conditions of old age.

DEFINITIONS

Ageing — senescence (ageing) in the individual is a progressive loss of physiological adaptability to the environment, culminating in death (Rowland and Pranks). Though age means little, 70 years or more is often mentioned as the time of onset of old age. Some, like Artur Rubenstein, are outstanding at 94. It is an individual matter. From a drug therapy viewpoint, Birkett and Wing suggest 75 years onward as a guide.
Confusion — reduced alertness, inability to think with usual speed and clarity.
Delirium — a condition of mental excitement, confusion and clouded

sensorium, usually accompanied by hallucinations and delusions. Delirium is acute in onset and reversible.
Dementia — gradual decline in mental powers, including reasoning power, memory, and the will. It is characterised by confusion, disorientation, apathy and stupor in varying degrees.
Therapeutic index — ratio of therapeutic or desired dose to toxic dose; the larger the therapeutic index, the better. It gives an idea of a drug's safety margin.

INTRODUCTION

There is an increasing proportion of ageing people in the populations of Western countries. In the UK there were 6.8% over 60 years of age in 1911 and 16.8% in 1981. By contrast, India has about 2% over 65 years. There are twice as many aged women as men in UK, and an even higher proportion in the US. Elderly people use proportionately more drugs then the rest of the population and hence are more prone to adverse drug reactions. The risk of adverse drug reactions is higher in women than in men. A person with a history of allergy is more likely to have an adverse drug reaction than a person with no such history.

Most research recommends that the elderly should not be prescribed more than 3 medications per day, but in a recent study, 25% of patients admitted to geriatric units were on 4-6 a day on admission, and approx. 15% in another study were on 10 or more medications.

Drug induced conditions account for a significant number of admissions to hospital among the elderly. One medical team found that 10% of their admission beds were occupied by people suffering from drug-induced Parkinsonism. Other common offenders are diuretics, antihypertensive agents, sedatives and digoxin.

It must be remembered that people, as they get older, suffer increasingly from chronic degenerative and terminal diseases.

Common findings in those older than 75 include: anxiety, mental depression, deafness, stroke, heart failure, diabetes, rheumatic diseases, chronic bronchitis, hip diseases and cancer. It is no wonder that elderly people take more drugs than younger people.

Many suffer loss of independence, loss of driver's licence, difficulty managing the steps on the bus or at home, incontinence, poor eyesight and poor memory. The cult of youth may make an older person feel unwanted and useless, especially when this is reinforced by family members.

Isolation, be it in nursing homes or living alone at home with the TV as companion, reduces the ability to converse, shop and relax with others. These factors can reduce the ability to take one's medications intelligently. A forgetful or confused person can easily take another warfarin or digoxin tablet, possibly resulting in a fatal bleed or fatal arrhythmia. Overdosing with insulin could be disastrous, and poor eyesight can make the graduations on a syringe difficult to see. Conversely, some people are inclined to self-prescribe and to "try out" their friends' medications. Imagine the outcome should an asthmatic take propranolol.

SOME PHYSIOLOGICAL CHANGES WHICH OCCUR WITH AGE

IMPAIRMENT OF HOMEOSTASIS

Deterioration in function occurs in several organs causing the body's homeostatic mechanisms to be less effective. Examples include: maintenance of normal blood pressure, electrolyte and fluid balance, insulin response, body water, and body temperature control. Healing, haemostasis and resistance to infection are likely to be impaired. There is a higher incidence of auto-antibodies in the aged. In short, environmental insults become harder to handle.

DIFFERENT DISEASE PRESENTATION

Diseases may present differently. Myocardial infarction may make the person feel off colour or confused. There may be little pain. The organs tend to "suffer in silence". Some authorities say that geriatric medicine is dominated by the four 'I's: intellectual failure, instability, immobility and incontinence. From a drug therapy point of view, the main physiological changes are: reduced renal function, lower body weight and changes in the tissues' responsiveness to drugs. Reduced liver function and increased body fat are important factors when taking some drugs.

BODY WEIGHT

The ageing person tends to lose protein, and the proportion of body fat increases. The volume of body water is usually lowered. Therefore, drugs which are poorly water soluble but very fat soluble (for example, diazepam) will tend to accumulate in body fat.

In a hypothetical 75-year-old patient, one might expect a 12% decrease in total body weight, a significant decrease in total body protein due to muscle wasting, up to 100% increase in body fat, and total body water decreased by about 15%.

CARDIAC FUNCTION

Cardiac output tends to decline with age, perhaps at 1% per year from 40 to 80 years. Lower cardiac output means less blood flowing through the kidneys and liver. Some drugs like propranolol, lignocaine and chlormethiazole are so rapidly metabolised by the liver that age-related reduction in liver blood flow results in larger amounts of the drugs in the circulation. To avoid toxicity, smaller doses of these drugs may be required, at least when treatment is initiated.

LIVER FUNCTION

Drug metabolism (transformation) occurs mainly in the liver.

From the few studies done, it appears that drugs which are metabolised in the microsomal fraction of the liver cell are metabolised more slowly in old age, for example, amylobarbitone and phenylbutazone. Drugs inactivated by enzymes in the cytoplasm of the liver cells appear to be unaffected by increasing age, for example, ethanol. More studies are required, however.

Other factors may be more important than age alone. Smoking and disease are factors in reduced metabolism of propranolol, for example. Diet may affect drug metabolism. A high-carbohydrate, low-protein diet has been shown to reduce theophylline's inactivation, with the possibility of accumulation and toxicity of the drug.

KIDNEY FUNCTION

With increasing age, the kidneys shrink in size, nephrons are lost, renal blood flow is reduced, and glucose reabsorption capacity is reduced. Glomerular filtration rate at age 70 is about two-thirds that of age 20 years, in the absence of renal disease. Many drugs are excreted by the kidneys, and in the ageing kidney, they will be removed at a slower rate. This is important for drugs with a low therapeutic index, that is, little difference between therapeutic and toxic dose. Examples of these are digoxin, gentamicin and other aminoglycosides, lithium, quinidine and chlorpropamide. Smaller doses of these drugs tend to be needed. Dehydration, congestive heart failure and renal disease will further reduce renal function and increase the risk of drug toxicity.

Measurement of renal function

Do not assume that a "normal" serum creatinine level means adequate renal function. The serum creatinine level does not rise until creatinine clearance (and renal function) is significantly reduced. Production of creatinine from muscle is reduced with ageing.

TISSUE RESPONSIVENESS AND AGE

The effect of a drug at its site of action may be altered in the elderly person. For example, the incidence of agitation instead of sedation from barbiturates and nitrazepam is higher with older people. Some body systems become more sensitive to the effects of drugs. For example, effects of warfarin on the haemostatic system are increased with age.

ABSORPTION OF DRUGS IN THE ELDERLY

Absorption appears to be little affected by age as most drugs are absorbed by passive diffusion from the duodenum.

SOME DRUGS COMMONLY USED IN ELDERLY PATIENTS

CARDIOVASCULAR DRUGS

Congestive heart failure is common in the elderly. Older people are particularly susceptible to unwanted effects of cardiac drugs, so the question should be asked, "Is drug treatment still needed?"

Digoxin has a low therapeutic index. Since the drug is excreted by the kidney and lean body weight is less in the elderly, smaller doses are usually needed. Hypothyroidism, hypokalaemia and advanced lung disease or heart disease necessitate small doses. Therefore, 62.5 micrograms per day is often sufficient, although a higher dose may be necessary for atrial fibrillation.

Toxic effects of digoxin

Cardiac effects include arrhythmias (look for sudden changes in pulse rates), heart block to some degree, and slowly *worsening* heart failure. Sometimes the only way to decide if toxicity is present is to withdraw the drug while the patient is hospitalised. CNS effects include confusion, depression, facial pain, blurred vision, light flashes and coloured haloes around lights. Delirium and even psychosis have been reported. Nausea, abdominal discomfort or vomiting need not be present with digoxin toxicity. Several studies have shown that many people taking digoxin who are in sinus rhythm may be taken off the drug under medical supervision. Thus, digoxin may not be necessarily a lifetime "sentence".

Selected patients can be taught to take their own pulse rate and to notify their doctor directly or via their District Nurse if the pulse rate is too slow (for example, less than 60/min). A change from a rapid and irregular rate to one which is slow and steady may indicate an *increasing* degree of heart block.

Diuretics

These drugs are commonly prescribed for the elderly to treat oedema and hypertension. They may cause unwanted effects from excessive diuresis. Urinary incontinence may occur when diuretic therapy is instituted. Thiazides are gentler than frusemide and are usually taken early in the morning to fit in with the daily routine of the patient, so there will be no diuresis to cope with during the night. Dose reduction may overcome incontinence, for example, half of a chlorothiazide (500 mg) tablet. Long-acting thiazides (for example, chlorthalidone) can cause nocturnal incontinence. Patients who are heavily sedated often do not wake in time or are too sleepy to take appropriate action. Excessive diuresis causes dehydration, haemoconcentration, hypotension and weakness from hyponatraemia and hypokalaemia and other electrolyte losses. Frusemide's intense action and short duration can overstretch the bladder causing retention and the patient may require catheterisation. Frusemide may be required regularly and the lowest possible dose used. Frusemide is available in 20 mg tablets, which are suitable for use in elderly patients.

Diabetes and gout may first appear while the patient is on diuretics.

Hypokalaemia may be diuretic induced. Body potassium may be depleted before hypokalaemia is noted with symptoms of tiredness and muscle weakness. Hypokalaemia must be prevented when digoxin is prescribed, in order to reduce the risk of digoxin toxicity.

Potassium

If the patient finds large sustained-release potassium chloride tablets *(Slow K)* difficult to swallow, effervescent tablets *(Sando-K)* or well-diluted elixir *(Kay-Cee-L)* can be taken at mealtimes. Potassium-rich diets may be sufficient in the long term.

Alternatively, potassium-conserving diuretics can be used instead of the potassium supplements, for example amiloride or triamterene.

They are often prescribed with hydrochlorothiazide as *Moduretic* and *Dytac*. Serum-potassium levels should be regularly checked as there is a risk of hyperkalaemia, particularly if potassium supplements are given at the same time.

Drug induced oedema

The following drugs have been implicated in oedema: ***Anti-inflammatory*** drugs such as phenylbutazone and prednisolone, ***antihypertensive*** drugs such as methyldopa, prazosin, clonidine and hydralazine, and, ***steroid*** drugs such as fludrocortisone (used to correct hypotension) and oestrogens.

Antihypertensive drugs

Uncontrolled hypertension can cause heart failure and stroke in elderly patients. It is hoped that widespread screening programs will detect people with hypertension before irreversible changes occur. Drug treatment should be accompanied by regular medical examinations. If doses of antihypertensive drugs become excessive, the patient may experience unpleasant side effects. Some of these side effects are listed as follows.

(a) Side effects of beta-blocker drugs: fatigue, unmasking of latent airways obstruction, nightmares, and cold extremities.
(b) Side effects of methyldopa: drowsiness, lethargy and sedation.
(c) Side effects of clonidine: gum "ulcers" from ill-fitting false teeth and dry mouth, urinary retention in males with prostatic enlargement; rebound hypertension is likely in the forgetful or unsupervised patient, due to missed doses.

Drugs which have been shown to be effective and well tolerated in the elderly include: thiazide diuretics in low dosages; prazosin; calcium antagonists, verapamil and nifedipine; labetalol; some beta-adrenergic blockers, and combinations of these. Oral doses of beta blockers and verapamil may cause severe bradycardia in the older patient.

Postural hypotension with attendant fainting and fractures is a risk of excessive antihypertensive treatment.

Drugs which may cause postural hypotension include:

(a) ***antihypertensives*** in excessive doses; prazosin on first dose; excessive dosage of diuretics;
(b) ***antidepressants*** such as amitriptyline;
(c) ***vasodilators*** such as glyceryl trinitrate and isosorbide dinitrate *(Isordil);*
(d) ***levodopa*** and ***neuroleptics*** such as chlorpromazine, haloperidol and prochlorperazine

In the absence of a treatable cause of hypotension drugs are sometimes used to raise blood pressure, for example, fludrocortisone (*Florinef*) 0.1 mg, once or twice daily.

Anti-arrhythmic drugs

All anti-arrhythmic drugs are capable of causing cardiac arrhythmias when given in high doses. Quinidine tends to be more slowly metabolised and excreted in the elderly. Signs of accumulation are termed "cinchonism" and include ringing in the ears, nausea, headache and blurred vision. Disopyramide causes strong anticholinergic effects of dry mouth, blurred vision, constipation and urinary hesitancy, particularly in the presence of prostatic enlargement. With quinidine and disopyramide, a slow pulse rate may indicate a degree of heart block. Lignocaine, as mentioned before, requires smaller doses in the older age groups.

Anticoagulants

Deep vein thrombosis and pulmonary emboli are common and often silent. Treatment is with heparin administered IV, which is replaced by warfarin, as in younger patients. The haemostatic system is more sensitive to warfarin's effects in the aged patient, so that smaller starting doses are used, for example, 2 mg. It takes up to two weeks for the system to stabilise after the dose has been altered. The prothrombin ratio, or index, shows what has been happening two days previously.

Bleeding from excess warfarin intake may not be obvious. Haematoma in the bowel can cause colic and obstruction; and cerebral bleeding has been reported. Heart failure, liver disease and drug therapy increase the risk of bleeding (see Chapter 8).

RESPIRATORY DRUGS

Bronchodilator drugs are used for acute and chronic bronchitis, emphysema, asthma and any condition where breathing is difficult. Elderly patients often experience difficulty coordinating the use of aerosols. The resulting poor response to aerosol therapy may force the clinician to switch unnecessarily to oral corticosteroid therapy. Watch how the aerosol is used — many elderly patients fail to use it properly. This can be partly overcome with use of a plastic tube on the end of the mouthpiece, as with *Bricanyl*. Even a disposable cup with a suitable hole in the bottom for the aerosol mouthpiece has been effective. For other patients, inhalation of dry powder from capsules in the *Ventolin Rotohaler* system can be effective. The same *Rotohaler* system applies for *Becotide*, which of course must be used regularly. Some people require bronchodilator administration via a mask in a respirator solution. Home respirators are available.

Theophylline has an additive effect when used with the aerosols. Though its clearance rate has been shown to be reduced in the older patient, the dose varies widely with other factors such as severe lung or liver disease, which slows elimination from the body. The sustained-release forms of the drug are usually well tolerated. Lower starting doses are advised.

Respiratory failure can be caused by overuse of CNS depressants such as barbiturates, benzodiazepines, opiates, neuroleptics, hypnotics, anxiolytics, antidepressants and alcohol. Patients suffering from chronic bronchitis, emphysema, asthma or other obstructive airways disease are susceptible to respiratory depression.

DRUG THERAPY IN RHEUMATIC DISEASES

The incidence of most rheumatic disease rises with age, often beginning in middle age. Osteoporosis (reduction of bony substance), osteomalacia (reduction in mineral content, bone 'softening') and fractures of the forearm and femur are more common in older people.

The most common diseases are osteoarthritis, rheumatoid arthritis, polymyalgia rheumatica and gout.

Non-steroidal anti-inflammatory drugs (NSAIDs)

Aspirin is commonly used in rheumatoid arthritis. Like all NSAIDs, it can cause sodium-retention oedema and even heart failure. Effervescent forms of aspirin contain sodium bicarbonate and may add to this risk. Symptomless ulcers and iron-deficiency anaemia from gastrointestinal blood loss are also seen in patients taking these drugs. The older person with underlying hearing loss does not get tinnitus from excessive doses of aspirin, so that this warning sign of toxicity is not heard. Small doses of aspirin may cause an acute attack of gout, by interfering with uric-acid excretion. As studies have shown a reduction in renal function with salicylates, caution is wise in prescribing salicylates for those with renal disease, heart failure or dehydration. Anaphylactic reactions can occur rarely on restarting treatment with NSAIDs.

Low starting doses of ***indomethacin*** can sometimes prevent the headaches, dizziness and hallucinations reported in elderly people. Psychosis has also been reported in the elderly. The suppository form is useful to relieve morning joint stiffness, as are naproxen suppositories. Indomethacin tends to reduce the effect of antihypertensive drugs.

Other NSAIDs may be indicated. Simple twice-daily regimes of naproxen, sulindac and diflunisal are easier to remember than some more complex drug regimes.

Slow-acting antirheumatic drugs

Penicillamine is as effective in the older patient as in the younger patient but produces a higher incidence of skin disease and taste abnormality in the older age group according to one study. Gold and chloroquine therapy is as effective in the elderly as it is in younger patients.

Corticosteroids

Because of toxic effects (see Chapter 11) and because of difficulty in withdrawing treatment, corticosteroids (for example, prednisolone) are used reluctantly. There are exceptions, such as in polymyalgia rheumatica, temporal arteritis and other vasculites. Some practitioners believe corticosteroids are no more effective than aspirin in the long-term management of rheumatoid arthritis.

The risk of developing cataracts is high, at or above a dose of 20 mg prednisolone daily for four years or more. Regular X-ray examination of the spine may detect and prevent the development of vertebral-compressing fractures from osteoporosis, particularly in postmenopausal women.

DRUGS ACTING ON THE CENTRAL NERVOUS SYSTEM

Common analgesics

For the relief of mild to moderate pain, ***paracetamol*** 500 mg to 1000 mg repeated every four hours (taking up to eight doses per day) is effective, though rare liver toxicity has been reported after several months of regular use. Generally, it does not cause GI upsets and is safe to use with warfarin. ***Effervescent aspirin*** is effective for short-term analgesia, if tolerated. ***Dextropropoxyphene*** *(Doloxene)* is probably no better than aspirin or paracetamol, and being a weak narcotic, it carries the risk of dependence. It may constipate bed-fast patients. The non-steroidal anti-inflammatory drugs should not be given to people recovering from a gastric ulcer. The pain threshold appears to be higher, and pain perception is less in elderly patients compared to younger people. However, this does not mean that the older person should be denied pain relief.

Opioids

For postoperative pain relief, small doses (for example 10 to 20 mg ***pethidine***) given IV just prior to the end of anaesthesia and at first sign of discomfort is effective, and the risk of respiratory depression and hypotension is minimal. Normal adult doses of pethidine may result in exceptionally high blood levels of drug in the over-70 age group (up to four times the blood level anticipated in younger patients). For this reason, doses as low as 25 to 50 mg IM may be effective postoperatively. Chronic administration of methadone can give rise to respiratory depression and coma due to accumulation.

Alcohol, sedatives, hypnotics and other respiratory depressants add to this effect. Naloxone effectively and specifically reverses respiratory depression from opioids, in doses up to a maximum total dose of 5-10 mg SC, IM or IV. The dose may have to be repeated because the duration of action of naloxone is short.

Pain relief in terminal illness

This should be part of a regular regime tailored to the patient's needs. This can vary from ***aspirin*** or ***paracetamol*** for mild pain, to ***morphine mixture*** in varying doses every four hours. Regular use of a bulk or stimulant laxative should prevent constipation. Nausea and vomiting respond to metoclopramide or drugs of the prochlorperazine type. Suppositories of oxycodone or prochlorperazine can be considered if oral or IM administration is impractical.

Hypnotics

Many older people need as much sleep as they had 50 years ago, despite reduced physical activity and frequent afternoon naps. Other causes of sleeplessness should be remedied before prescribing sleeping tablets, for example, anxiety, depression, breathlessness, full bladder or bowel, drinks containing caffeine at bedtime, or hypoglycaemia in diabetic patients.

A warm comfortable bed and a hot milk drink may suffice. Brandy in the milk or a glass of sherry could be useful, but not in combination with hypnotics. The routine use of hypnotics (for example, in some nursing homes) is liable to cause daytime sedation and confusion. Confusion from CNS depressants (sedatives, anti-anxiety agents and so on) add to this risk. Hypnotics should, ideally, be given for a limited period and then reviewed. The withdrawal effects from diazepam after chronic treatment in conventional doses is well documented (see Chapter 28).

The unsteadiness experienced in old age is increased by the use of many hypnotic drugs, making falls more likely, especially if the person is confused already.

Barbiturates should be avoided in the elderly as they cause more paradoxical reactions (restlessness and excitement) than in younger people. Other unwanted effects of barbiturates are falls from muscle weakness, hangover and psychosis. Sudden withdrawal of high doses, for example, 50 mg of pentobarbitone taken at night, has resulted in epileptic fits.

Benzodiazepines should be used in low doses, for example, 2.5 to 5 mg for ***nitrazepam***, 7.5 to 15 mg for ***oxazepam***, 10 mg for ***temazepam*** and 1 mg for ***lorazepam***. Administration of higher doses increases the risk of nightmares and hallucinations. Diazepam can make people weak and prone to falls due to its muscle-relaxant properties.

Chloral hydrate (*Noctec Caps* 500 mg, and mixture, usually 1g/10 mL) should be taken with milk, food or fluids to reduce gastric irritation. This drug is probably best avoided in patients with gastric or duodenal ulcers. Most hypnotic drugs lose their effectiveness after several weeks of continuous therapy.

Neuroleptic drugs, for example, ***thioridazine*** (*Melleril*) 10 to 50 mg at night, or ***haloperidol*** (*Serenace*) 0.5 to 5 mg at night, are frequently prescribed for confused elderly patients.

Chronic treatment with neuroleptic drugs has caused tardive dyskinesias (abnormal tongue, facial and chewing movements). Appearance of these effects may call for cessation of the drug. Anticholinergic effects, hyperthermia, hypothermia and hypotension may also be troublesome.

Anti-depressant drugs

Depressive illness is common but often well disguised. For severe depression, the tricyclic antidepressants are of proven benefit. The sedative ***amitriptyline*** is useful when agitation is prominent. Doses required are lower and need to be introduced more slowly than in younger people. They are best given just before the evening meal and/or at bedtime, in the hope of minimising the unwanted effects. For debilitated people, a starting dose of 10 mg daily of amitriptyline may suffice.

Common unwanted effects include dizziness and postural hypotension, anticholinergic effects (constipation, dry mouth, blurred vision, urinary retention), oedema, fine muscle tremor in 10% of patients, delirium, weakness and fatigue. Amitriptyline and imipramine have strong anticholinergic effects, while trazodone and mianserin (newer antidepressants) have less anticholinergic activity and therefore are more frequently prescribed for geriatric patients.

Drugs for Parkinson's Disease

Levodopa has benefited many sufferers, slowing though not reversing the devastating symptoms of Parkinson's disease. Patients who have been totally dependent may, with this form of drug therapy, improve sufficiently to feed and dress themselves.

Levodopa, combined with decarboxylase inhibitors and marketed as *Sinemet* in various strengths, lessens the nausea and hypotension that occur when levodopa is given alone (see Chapter 29).

Abnormal facial movements and arrhythmias are troublesome side effects. Dose reduction may alleviate these. Administration of too much levopoda can cause agitation, delirium, visual hallucinations and paranoia. These effects are reversible and are more common in patients with a history of mental disorder or dementia.

The anticholinergic drugs, though helpful in reducing tremor, are liable to cause confusion in high doses. Side effects of anticholinergic drugs have been discussed previously.

Antimania drugs

The elderly are more sensitive to ***lithium*** toxicity, often requiring lower plasma levels (0.6 to 0.8 mmol/L) for maintenance. A toxic confusion state of muscle twitching, coarse tremor, slurred speech and ataxia may arise particularly if diuretics have been started or if excessive sweating or diarrhoea occurs.

Lithium can cause hypothyroidism mimicking depression. The drug is more slowly excreted in the older person.

Neuroleptic drugs

These are used to relieve the distressing symptoms of dementia and psychoses. For dementia, small doses are administered initially, for example, chlorpromazine and thioridazine 10 to 25 mg three times a day, haloperidol 0.5 to 5 mg three times a day. These drugs and others in their class are effective for daytime restlessness or irritability. For severe delirium, haloperidol 5 to 10 mg IM is effective. Neuroleptic drugs cause dose-related sedation (less with haloperidol) and postural hypotension, and interfere with temperature regulation causing heat exhaustion in summer, hypothermia in winter. They can also cause Parkinsonian tremor and tardive dyskinesias (less with thioridazine). Excessive doses can result in an immobile, withdrawn and drooling person in the "chemical strait-jacket". Others suffer from akathisia (anxiety, jitters).

Where anticholinergic effects are troublesome, thioridazine may be an alternative. When it is necessary to stop the drug in chronic users, this should be done gradually or withdrawal symptoms may occur.

Toxic confusion or delirium

Excessive doses of sedatives (for example, barbiturates and benzodiazepines), anticholinergics (for example, benzhexol in Parkinson's disease), and levodopa may give rise to toxic confusional states and delirium. Alcohol withdrawal (for example, prior to elective surgery), corticosteroids, digoxin and antidepressants also may be responsible for these effects. Alcohol withdrawal symptoms are exacerbated by poor diet.

DRUGS AND THE EYE

Many elderly patients have difficulty in reading and doing fine motor movements, hence the need for large-print labels. Cataracts and glaucoma become more common with increasing age. Anticholinergic drugs (for example, atropine) have an increased effect on the senile eye and may cause acute glaucoma in those people with shallow anterior chambers.

Drugs can have adverse effects on the eye. Long-term administration of corticosteroids can cause cataracts and glaucoma, which is genetically mediated, in one-third of the population.

Antipsychotic drugs taken chronically in high dose (for example, thioridazine 1000 mg/day), deposit on the retina. Night blindness is an early sign of retinal deposits. Anyone having a photosensitive reaction (such as unduly severe sunburn) from drugs of this type should be examined for retinal deposits and lens opacities. Fortunately, blindness from this cause is rare.

DRUGS AND THE EAR

Hearing, especially at high frequencies, declines with age. Conversation should be enunciated clearly (not shouted) and slowly for people so affected. Drug-induced deafness and dizziness (labyrinthine damage) are more common with elderly people due to slow renal excretion of antibiotics such as gentamicin and streptomycin. Neomycin-induced deafness has been reported due to wound and colonic irrigation and from oral use in people with ulcerative colitis or gastroenteritis, when prolonged high doses were administered.

Salicylates, quinidine and quinine cause reversible dizziness and hearing loss. Patients should be observed for dizziness, nausea and hearing loss even after administration of these drugs has been ceased.

GASTROINTESTINAL TRACT

Treatment and prevention of constipation

Constipation is a frequent complaint of old age. Bowel transit times are delayed in the elderly, but it is unknown whether this is an effect of age, of low-residue diet or other causes. Reduced physical activity is probably another factor. Each person's bowel patterns are individual. Chronic laxative abuse and the abuse of slimming tablets containing the laxative phenolphthalein are difficult to treat. Many elderly people are obsessed with the need to open bowels daily but forget that when less food is eaten, less waste is excreted. Excessive laxative use causes dehydration, weakness and hypokalaemia. Regular bowel habit, not necessarily daily, without discomfort is the aim. Any change in bowel habit should be investigated by the doctor.

If there is insufficient fibre and fluid in the diet, then the bulk-forming laxatives (for example, bran or the proprietary lines such as *Fybogel* or *Normacol)* may be suitable alternatives to the irritant laxatives. For some people, a glycerin suppository may be sufficient.

Faecal impaction can delay postoperative recovery, and manual evacuation may lead to a damaged anal sphincter with resulting incontinence. Soap enemas and olive-oil enemas are still commonly used, but there is now a wide range of oral drugs, such as *Dioctyl* and *Lactulose,* that can be used very effectively to prevent and relieve constipation.

Disposable phosphate enemas may be difficult to retain, and care must be exercised when introducing the rectal catheter so that perforation of the bowel wall does not occur. Regular use of phosphate enemas has caused sodium-retention oedema.

Drugs causing constipation include anticholinergics, antidepressants, antihistamines, antispasmodics, opiates and derivatives (such as codeine, dextropropoxyphene and morphine) and some antacids.

Faecal incontinence can be secondary to impaction or damage to anal sphincter from frequent manual evacuations due to poor bowel habit. Prolonged use of paraffin emulsion has caused anal leakage and vitamin malabsorption.

Laxative abuse is a frequent cause of diarrhoea and incontinence, with possible dehydration and electrolyte losses. Offending drugs include cascara and magnesium sulphate (Epsom salts). Other causes are broad-spectrum antibiotics such as tetracyclines, ampicillin and co-trimoxazole.

Upper gastrointestinal tract

The incidence of ulcer rises with age, as does the use of anti-inflammatory drugs which aggravate gastric ulcers. Oesophageal reflux and hiatus hernia are more common in the elderly. Anticholinergic drugs slow peristalsis, delay stomach emptying and often worsen these complaints. For reflux, antacids, bethanechol or metoclopramide are frequently used.

DRUGS USED IN DIABETES MELLITUS

The incidence of diabetes mellitus rises with age. The insulin response to a specific concentration of sugar in the blood is reduced with ageing. Many factors are involved. Thiazide diuretics and frusemide may unmask undiagnosed diabetes, as can corticosteroids. When possible, dietary restriction is preferable to hypoglycaemic drugs. Hypoglycaemic drugs should always be taken at mealtime as there is a risk of hypoglycaemia and unconsciousness if food is not ingested. Glibenclamide and tolbutamide have shorter duration and are preferable to chlorpropamide which can cause prolonged hypoglycaemia. Propranolol and other non-selective beta-blocking drugs may mask the symptoms of an approaching hypoglycaemic episode (palpitations and sweating) in insulin-dependent, unstable diabetics. They may also aggravate or induce latent diabetes. The cardioselective beta blockers (such as metoprolol) do not have this effect and are preferred therapy.

DRUGS ACTING ON THE SKIN

Epidermal changes, such as loss of water and collagen and thinning, in the aged skin are usually obvious. Excessive dryness is responsible for most of the itchings of the aged. Bath oils and simple creams give symptomatic relief. Healing of ulcers and tissue repair are slowed and are practically at a standstill when vascular disease is present or when corticosteroids are taken. Ulcer remedies are great in number. The aim is to promote a clean granulating surface with debriding agents and to use non-adherent non-allergic dressing when needed. Naturally, underlying vascular disease should be treated where possible.

NURSING IMPLICATIONS

As ageing and disease are not synonymous, the combination of several drugs may mean that the final outcomes are unpredictable. Several diseases may be present. Therefore in many cases, several different types of drugs may be taken by the patient. There is often an increased incidence of adverse drug reactions or interactions, including an increased potentiation of some drug effects. In the elderly, oesophageal clearance time may be delayed, due to weakness of smooth-muscle contraction. Also, the lower oesophageal sphincter may fail to relax after swallowing. As cardiac output is often decreased, the result is an increased circulation time. This in turn means a delayed onset of drug action. Altered circulation to the liver will result in altered drug metabolism and may lead to an increase in drug toxicity. A decrease in renal function may impair drug excretion.

Assess

The following should be recorded and assessed: age, height, weight, fat distribution, food and drug allergies, diet and nutrition, liver function, renal function, blood screening, present medications (especially the need for drug therapy, the dose, preparation and label).

The adverse effects of medications must be noted, including the expected outcome, the possibility of self-medication, and perhaps the discontinuation of some medications. Record baseline behavioural parameters and baseline vital signs such as BP, pulse rate, and ECG.

Assess the patient's understanding of his or her disease process and medications, vision, hearing, memory, mobility and level of dependence.

Administration

Often the elderly have difficulty in swallowing large tablets or capsules. Administer these with a full glass of water if possible. Sit the patient upright.

Ensure that an appropriate dose form is available — this may require a new prescription for a liquid. Do not crush or dissolve any solid medication without prior referral to a pharmacist. Medication should begin at low doses and be slowly increased to a therapeutic level to prevent toxicity. As few drugs as possible should be administered.

Evaluate

The therapeutic effect of the drug, the adverse effects of the drug, and evidence of any interaction must be evaluated, as well as renal function and liver function. Hypoproteinaemia will result in an increase in the free, unbound fraction of the circulating drug.

Changes in body weight and composition (for example, amputation) may change drug distribution and effect. The situation varies, but peak levels can increase, and drug half-lives may be prolonged, resulting in increased drug effect.

Patient teaching

Teach the patient to recognise the therapeutic effects of the drugs and to recognise adverse effects and interaction effects. The patient must know the action to take if doses are missed and the reason for taking each drug.

Warn the patient against self-regulation of medication or sudden discontinuation. Inform relatives (or persons who may be assisting) about administration of medication.

Ensure that the drug bottles are clearly labelled and that the patient can understand the instructions.

SELF-EVALUATION TEST

Consider the following case study. A 75-year-old retired bank manager, Mr B, and his wife have lived a quiet suburban life since their family left home. Mr B recovered from a myocardial infarction 10 years ago and was placed on quinidine tablets, 750 mg twice a day, to suppress ventricular ectopic beats.

Two months ago, Mr B's doctor noticed some ankle oedema and prescribed chlorothiazide 500 mg each morning and potassium chloride 600 mg, two tablets twice a day (which Mr B took when he remembered). He found them too big to swallow. Besides, his friend at the club has "heart trouble", and he did not take those big yellow tablets.

Some months ago whilst gardening, Mr B tore his right ankle, and the injury developed into an ulcer. He is having the dressing done by the district nurse. Mr B was recently commenced on digoxin 0.25 mg daily for atrial tachycardia and heart failure. In the past few days, the district nurse has noticed his deteriorating condition; he has ankle oedema again and complains of breathlessness at night and is more confused. His wife complains that he is "not with it" and that he must need glasses again since he is not reading the paper and does not even like to watch TV lately. At times he is confused, restless and complains of blurred vision and ringing ears.

Yesterday his pulse was 50/min and regular. It is usually more rapid and irregular. The district nurse discusses the problem with the doctor, who subsequently admits him to hospital. After a physical examination is performed and blood samples are taken, all of Mr B's drugs are stopped. Serum electrolytes were normal except for a serum potassium of 2.5 mmol/L, serum sodium 120 mmol/L, and serum albumin 30 g/L. Enzymes, thyroid function and the results of other routine studes were within normal limits.

Questions

1. Mr B's condition is most likely the result of:
   (a) poor diet
   (b) heart failure due to ageing
   (c) his drug regime
   (d) excessive physical activity while gardening
2. Mr B was taking:
   (a) quinidine
   (b) chlorothiazide tablets
   (c) potassium chloride
   (d) digoxin
   (e) alcohol — 1 to 2 drinks per day
   (f) aspirin for headaches, usually 6 per week

   Which of the above list has been shown to cause:

1. hypokalaemia
2. the non-specific symptoms of listlessness, anorexia and malaise
3. worsening heart failure
4. tinnitus
5. blurred vision?

For further reading

1. Drug Treatment of the Elderly Patient. Judge TG, Caird FI. Pitman Medical, 1978.
2. Essentials of Geriatric Medicine. 2nd ed. Chapter 4. Adams GE. Oxford Medical Publications, 1981.

SECTION 5

16

ANALGESICS

Rhondda Figgis Close

OBJECTIVES

At the conclusion of this chapter the reader should be able to:

1. define the term "analgesic";
2. describe the different types of analgesics with examples from each group;
3. list the signs of overdosage in each group.

DEFINITIONS

Analgesic — a drug which alleviates pain.
Antipyretic — a drug which allays or prevents fever.

INTRODUCTION

Pain is defined in *New Gould Medical Dictionary* as "a disturbed sensation causing suffering or distress". The degree of pain experienced by any one person is dependent not only on the stimulus and its perception but also on its interpretation by the sufferer, and this may be entirely different for any two people.

In the first century AD, Marcus Aurelius wrote: "If thou art pained by any external thing, it is not this thing that disturbs thee, but thy own judgment about it." Each patient should be assessed individually. A stereotyped approach to the degree of painfulness of each condition, and bias to the usefulness or uselessness of the analgesics, should be avoided.

It is extremely difficult to measure pain, and any assessment of it must necessarily be subjective.

Analgesics are usually divided into two main groups.

"Simple" or "weak" or "mild" analgesics

This group tends to exert its action peripherally by influencing the production of the pain-producing substance at the site of injury.

"Strong" or narcotic analgesics

These exert their effect through the central nervous system in two ways: by reducing the ability of the patient to perceive the sensation, and by altering the emotional reaction to it so that it is no longer perceived as an unpleasant sensation probably by acting on the cerebral cortex.

The use of analgesics has been known at least since the time of Hippocrates who recommended the leaves of the willow in childbirth. The use of salicylate-bearing barks, leaves and fruits for therapeutic purposes has been referred to throughout the early Christian era, the Middle Ages and the Renaissance. In 1763, the then President of the Royal Society, the Reverend Edward Stone, reported using salicylate as an antipyretic agent, though its use in home remedies had no doubt predated this.

Aspirin (acetylsalicylic acid) was first prepared by Van Gerhardt in 1853. Salicylic acid became available in 1874 but it was not until alternatives for long-term use were researched that the advantages of aspirin were noticed. In 1899 Wohlgemut a Dreser used aspirin in the treatment of rheumatic disease when the powerful analgesic effect was soon noted. It was then more than half a century after aspirin was first prepared that its clinical use was introduced. It is still, weight for weight. the most potent of the non-narcotic analgesics.

THE SALICYLATES

ASPIRIN

The salicylates are more widely used for pain relief than any other class of drugs. ***Aspirin*** is the most important drug in this group. It is analgesic, antipyretic and anti-inflammatory in action. Estimates have been made that between 10 to 20 thousand tons of aspirin are consumed annually in the US. It is non-addictive and chronic use does not lead to tolerance. Its toxicity is lower than that of other analgesics. However, over 10 000 cases of serious intoxication occur in the US every year so that it is indeed not the harmless household remedy as often thought. Because of its ready availability, it tends to be underestimated as an analgesic. In double-blind cross-over studies, 650 mg of aspirin was more effective than eight other oral analgesics in managing pain for cancer.

Analgesic action

The analgesic action of aspirin is thought to be both a central action (possibly hypothalamic) and peripheral action. It is thought to exert its effect by influencing some pain-producing substance released at a site of injury or disease. The inhibition of prostaglandin synthesis by aspirin and related drugs has been postulated as an explanation of many of the actions and side effects of these analgesic drugs. These actions include the antipyretic effect, anti-inflammatory action, analgesic effect, gastric irritation and ulceration, sodium retention, effect on reproductive function and perhaps the observed prevention of cholera-induced diarrhoea by aspirin.

Antipyretic action

Moderate doses of aspirin reduce elevated body temperature by means of a predominantly central effect — that is, by influencing the body's "thermostat" in the brain in the hypothalamus region. It is unusual for normal body temperature to be affected, however — the antipyretic effect appears to be due not to a direct effect on the hypothalamic neurons, but rather, like the analgesic effect, to involve inhibition of the synthesis of prostaglandins. Toxic doses of aspirin, however, produce a rise in body temperature, or pyretic effect, due to increased oxygen consumption and metabolic rate. This results in sweating, and enhances the dehydration that occurs in salicylate intoxication.

Anti-inflammatory action

Aspirin and the salicylates have long been known by rheumatologists to reduce inflammation, but the precise mechanism remains obscure. The effect of these drugs on prostaglandin metabolism is probably significant. Other actions of salicylates include the increase of urinary excretion of urates when given in large doses, while small doses may cause a decrease in the excretion of urates. Thus, gout may be precipitated in susceptible patients. The salicylates cause a reduction of the plasma level of prothrombin due to a reduction of factor VII when the metabolic rate is increased by fever.

Use

The use of the salicylates is related to their effects. They are used for their analgesic effect in the treatment of pain, their antipyretic effect in reducing body temperature in fever and their anti-inflammatory as well as analgesic effect in rheumatoid arthritis.

Adverse Drug Reactions and Allergy

Ingestion of aspirin produces a measurable blood loss from the alimentary tract, probably due to an alteration of platelet stickiness. This blood loss is mostly of no significance, but would be contraindicated in patients with a history of abnormal bleeding (for example after tooth extraction), gastric ulceration or alcoholic gastritis. An alternative analgesic could be used in these cases.

Studies in the US show that aspirin intolerance occurs in about 0.9% of normal subjects and in about 4.3% of asthmatic patients. Allergy appears more likely over the age of 50 and in women more than men. Other adverse effects include nausea, vomiting, diarrhoea and angioneurotic oedema.

Drug Interactions

Sulphonylureas (for example, tolbutamide) may be displaced from serum-protein binding sites, thus releasing more free tolbutamide and causing a hypoglycaemic reaction. Salicylates may cause reduction in blood sugar so possibly an additive effect is involved as well. Salicylates may compete with probenecid in the renal tubule and so antagonise the uricosuric effect of probenecid.

Kernicterus, which carries with it a risk of mental retardation, may be produced in neonates. The raised level of free serum bilirubin is produced by displacement of the bilirubin from serum albumin by salicylates.

A table of the more common drug interactions of aspirin may be seen in Chapter 17 (Table 42).

NURSING IMPLICATIONS

As most of the aspirin for analgesic and antipyretic use is purchased over the counter on a non-prescription basis as treatment for self-diagnosed illness, the primary nursing implications are involved with patient teaching.

Nurses should make certain that their patients are familiar with the contraindications and adverse effects of aspirin. Persons who experience mild dyspepsia should be advised to take aspirin with milk or food. If this fails to give relief, they should be advised to use paracetamol. People who have a history of bleeding or ulcerative gastrointestinal conditions, blood dyscrasias or are taking anticoagulants should be advised that aspirin is contraindicated in these situations. If they need analgesia, they should seek the advice of their physician or pharmacist. Paracetamol is usually considered a safe alternative in these situations.

Patients should be informed of the signs of salicylate toxicity (for example, tinnitus, dimness of vision, dizziness and confusion) and that if these occur, they should reduce or cease their dose, as deafness may result.

Nurses need to be familar with any other drugs their patients are taking so they can correctly advise them concerning any potential drug interactions which may occur with aspirin (see Table 42, Chapter 17).

As with all medications, aspirin should be kept out of the reach of children due to the high incidence of accidental overdose which has occurred with this product.

MISCELLANEOUS ANALGESICS

PARACETAMOL

This analgesic is an alternative when aspirin is contraindicated. However, it does not have the marked anti-inflammatory or antirheumatic effects of aspirin. It is rapidly absorbed from the gastrointestinal tract in the majority of patients, conjugated in the liver and rapidly excreted in the urine, 3% as unaltered drug and the rest as the conjugated form. It is known as acetaminophen in the U.S.

Paracetamol is available as both plain and soluble tablets, capsules, and for paediatric use as drops and elixir. It also exists in combination with other analgesics in such compound products as *Panadeine* (paracetamol and codeine).

Paracetamol should be given with care to patients with impaired kidney or liver function. Paracetamol is normally well tolerated though gastric irritation and haemorrhage are possible. Side effects are commonly experienced.

Overdosage is dangerous and can cause irreversible damage to the liver unless treated within the first 12 hours. The observed hepatotoxicity is due to the formation of a toxic metabolite which is thought to cause damage and necrosis of the liver cells. Overdosage is treated with ***Acetylcysteine*** (*Parvolex*) which protects the liver possibly by restoring depleted hepatic glutathione or by acting as an alternative substrate for the toxic paracetamol metabolite.

NURSING IMPLICATIONS

As this drug is such a widely used over-the-counter analgesic, nursing implications relate mainly to patient and community teaching. This drug is becoming an increasing vehicle of attempted suicides which may in fact be successful if not treated promptly. Some patients choose paracetamol because of its ready availability and the fact that the general public see it as a mild analgesic and are not aware of its dangerous effect on the liver. It should be noted that the paracetamol victim may present without any symptoms and, because of this, is often sent home without treatment. Such action can have disastrous consequences.

Because the effects of overdose can often be irreversible and fatal, there must be even greater emphasis on preventing the accidental access of children to this drug. Tablets and especially the attractively coloured elixirs should have child-proof tops and should be stored in a safe place.

Assess: History for previous allergy; establish baseline descriptions of pain and fever.
Administer: Orally.
Evaluate: Relief of pain and fever.
Teach: Dangers of overdose; keep out of reach of children.

PHENACETIN (no longer available)

This analgesic has antipyretic properties which are said to be similar to those of aspirin. However, the drug does not have the anti-inflammatory or antirheumatic effect of aspirin. Because of the implication of its role in the production of acute renal nephropathy with analgesic abusers, its use which was commonly in combination with aspirin and caffeine in the old APC tablets has been discontinued. Phenacetin is metabolised in the liver to paracetamol and acetaldehyde.

Adverse Drug Reactions include acute and chronic renal failure from prolonged use of analgesic compounds (for example, powders) containing phenacetin. The incidence of renal papillary necrosis was found to be higher in analgesic abusers – phenacetin was suspected to be the culprit.

ANALGESIC–SEDATIVE COMBINATIONS

Sedatives have no analgesic activity and compound sedative/analgesic preparations have a high abuse potential, especially those of the barbiturate class. In 1971 the Misuse of Drugs Act was passed. The penalties applicable to offences concerning "Controlled Drugs" were graded broadly according to the harmfulness attributable to a drug when it is misused. Barbiturates are in Schedule 3, so the prescribing of barbiturates is now regarded as being undesirable. Dependency develops easily.

During the past few years, many workers in geriatric medicine have indicated that short-acting barbiturates are not the most suitable hypnotics or sedatives for geriatric patients. Frequently, old people treated with these preparations become restless and disorientated which may lead in some instances to an apparent increased need for sedation, thus instituting a vicious circle.

In most instances, analgesic tablets alone would be adequate to dispel aches and pains, thereby allowing relaxation and the development of a normal sleep pattern without the necessity for a hypnotic.

Algologists (specialists in the relief of pain, from the Greek *algos* meaning pain) uniformly agree that there is no place for barbiturates in the management of pain. In an article on the management of intractable pain, Professor Les Brophy mentions the antianalgesic effect of the barbiturates. Indeed in small doses, the barbiturates are hyperalgesic and increase the reaction to painful stimuli. In view of the poor clinical record of barbiturates, barbiturate/analgesic compounds and the abuse of these drugs in the community, it is advisable not to give the ***paracetamol/codeine/pentobarbitone*** combinations for simple pain relief. Sedation will not override pain. If sufficient analgesia is given so that the pain is relieved, most people do not require sedating. Those that do require sedating can be prescribed a safer sedative than a barbiturate, such as one of the benzodiazepines, for example, temazepam or nitrazepam.

MEFENAMIC ACID

Mefenamic acid, which is produced as capsules (*Ponstan*), has antipyretic properties as well as analgesic properties. It is used in arthritis, soft-tissue pain and dental pain and has been particularly useful in primary dysmenorrhoea and menstrual pain due to its inhibitory effect on prostaglandin release.

Adverse Drug Reactions include drowsiness, dizziness, headache, nausea and skin rashes. Less commonly, ulcerations of the stomach and intestinal tract have been reported, as well as severe diarrhoea, bleeding and haematemesis. Mefenamic acid is therefore contraindicated in patients with ulceration or inflammation of the gastrointestinal tract.

Care should be taken in giving the drug to asthmatics, in pregnancy (as the effect on the foetus is unknown), and with the oral anticoagulants, the effect of which may be enhanced with mefenamic acid. The drug should be ceased if diarrhoea or skin rash occurs.

Table 37
Some Proprietary Preparations Containing Aspirin

Trade Name	Form	Contents in Milligrams			
		Aspirin	Paracetamol	Codeine Phosphate	Other
1. Actron	BST	267	133		Caffeine 40
2. Alka-Seltzer	BST	324			
3. Anadin	T	325			Quinine Sulph. 1; caffeine 15
4. Anadin Soluble	ST	325			Caffeine 30
5. Anadin Extra	T	300	200		Caffeine 45
6. Anadin Max. St.	T	500			Caffeine 32
7. Antoin	ST	400		5	Caffeine citrate 15
8. Askit	T	230			Aloxiprin 110; caffeine citrate 20
9. Askit	Pd	530			Aloxiprin 140; caffeine citrate 110
10. Aspergum	T	227			
11. Aspav	BST	500			Papaveretum 10
12. Aspro	T	320			
13. Aspro Clear	ST	300			
14. Bayer's	T	300			
15. Beecham	Pd	600			Caffeine 50
16. Beecham	T	300			Caffeine 25
17. Breoprin	EC	648			
18. Caprin	EC	324			
19. Claradin	ST	300			
20. Codis	ST	500		8	
21. Cojene	T	300		8	Caffeine 95
22. Disprin	ST	300			
23. Dolasan	T	325			Dextropropoxyphene 100
24. Doloxene Co.	C	375			Dextropropoxyphene 65; caffeine citrate 30
25. Duralin	BT	500			
26. Duralin	BC	500			
27. Equagesic	T	250			Ethoheptazine 75; meprobomate 150
28. Fynnon Calcium	ST	500			
29. Hypon	T	325		5	Caffeine 0.01
30. Laboprin	T	300			Lysine 245
31. Levius	SRT	500			
32. Mrs. Cullen's	Pd	600			Caffeine 62
33. Myolgin	ST	200	200	5	Caffeine citrate 15
34. Napsalgesic	T	500			Dextropropoxyphene 50
35. Nurse Syke's	Pd	165.4	120		Caffeine 60
36. Nu-Seals	EC	300			
37. Nu-Seals	EC	600			
38. Paynocil	ST	600			Glycine 300
39. Phensic	T	325			Caffeine 50
40. Phensic	ST	325			
41. Powerin	CT	300	200		Caffeine 45
42. Robaxisal Forte	T	325			Methocarbamol 400
43. Safapryn	EC	300	250		
44. Safapryn Co.	EC	300	250	8	
45. Solmin	ST	300			Glycine 133
46. Solprin	ST	300			
47. Trancoprin	T	300			Chlormezanone 100
48. Veganin	T	250	250	6.8	

T — Tablet; ST — Soluble or Dispersible Tablet; Pd — Powder; C — Capsule; SR — Slow or Sustained Release; EC — Enteric Coated; B — Buffered.

Table 38
Some Proprietary Preparations Containing Paracetamol (No Aspirin)

Trade Name	Form	Contents in Milligrams		
		Paracetamol	Codeine Phosphate	Other
1. Cafadol	T	500		Caffeine 30
2. Chilvax	T	400		Caffeine 10
3. Codanin	T	500	10	
4. Codural	T	250		Homatropine 0.75; caffeine 50
5. Cox Pain Relief	T	450	8.1	Caffeine 15
6. Delimon	T	400		Morazone 150
7. De Witts Pills	T	330		Caffeine 30
8. Distalgesic	T	325		Dextropropoxyphene 32.5
9. Distalgesic Sol.	ST	325		Dextropropoxyphene 32.5
10. E.P.	T	300	8	Caffeine 50
11. Femerital	T	250		Ambucetamide 100
12. Feminax	T	500	8	Hyoscine 0.1; caffeine hydrate 50
13. Fennings Adult	Pd	180		Caffeine 30
14. Fennings Child	Pd	50		
15. Fortagesic	T	500		Pentazocine 15
16. Hedex	C	500		
17. Hedex Soluble	Pd	1000		
18. Hedex Plus	C	500	8	Caffeine 30
19. Hedex Seltzer	Pd	1000		Caffeine 60
20. Disprol Junior	ST	120		
21. Lobak	T	450		Chlormezanone 100
22. Medised	T	500		Promethazine 10
23. Medocodene	T	500	8	
24. Migraleve Pink	T	500	8	Buclizine 6.25; docusate 10
25. Migraleve Yellow	T	500	8	Docusate 20
26. Norgesic	T	450		Orphenadrine 35
27. Panadeine	T	500	8	
28. Panadeine Forte	T	500	15	
29. Panadeine Sol.	ST	500	8	
30. Panadol	T	500		
31. Panadol	C	500		
32. Panadol Soluble	ST	500		
33. Panasorb	T	500		
34. Paracodol	ST	500	8	
35. Parahypon	T	500	5	Caffeine 10
36. Parake	T	500	8	
37. Paralgin	T	450	6	Caffeine 20
38. Paramol	T	500		Dihydrocodeine 10
39. Pardale	T	400	9	Caffeine hydrate 10
40. Paxalgesic	T	325		Dextropropoxyphene 32.5
41. Persomnia	T	500	8	
42. Pharmidone	T	400	10	Diphenhydramine 5; caffeine 50
43. Propain	T	400	10	Diphenhydramine 5; caffeine 50
44. Q-Panol	T	500		
45. Resolve	Pd	500		
46. Salzone	T	500		
47. Solpadeine	ST	500	8	Caffeine 30
48. Solpadeine Forte	ST	500	15	Caffeine 30
49. Syndol	T	450	10	Doxylamine 5; caffeine 30
50. Tramil	C	500		Caffeine 32
51. Unigesic	C	500		Caffeine 30
52. Zefringe	Pd	800		Caffeine 60

T — Tablet; ST — Soluble or Dispersible Tablet; Pd — Powder; C — Capsule; SR — Slow or Sustained Release; EC — Enteric Coated; B — Buffered.

DIFLUNISAL

Diflunisal is produced as tablets of 250 mg (*Dolobid*). It is an analgesic for acute pain of musculoskeletal origin. Dosage is two tablets initially followed by one or two tablets twice a day when necessary. It can also be used for short-term treatment of osteoarthritis (two tablets for the first dose followed by one tablet twice daily — maximum daily dose being no more than 750 mg).

Adverse Drug Reactions include possible hypersensitivity in patients who have had asthmatic attacks precipitated by salicylates or non-steroidal anti-inflammatory agents and gastrointestinal bleeding. The drug should not be used during pregnancy or lactation.

OTHER NON-NARCOTIC DRUGS

Other non-salicylate non-steroidal anti-inflammatory drugs such as ***oxyphenbutazone, phenylbutazone, indomethacin, sulindac, naproxen*** and others are not recommended primarily for the relief of non-inflammatory pain and so are not included here. They will be discussed in Chapter 17.

NARCOTIC ANALGESICS

Analgesia with the narcotic analgesics is produced through an interaction between the narcotic analgesics and the so-called narcotic receptors in the CNS. The analgesia probably occurs through an elevation in pain threshold and an alteration in the patient's physical reaction to the stimuli.

Narcotics are the most important agents in the management of post-operative pain and may be given continually by small injections intravenously or by the use of a continuous intravenous solution. Visceral pain is treated especially effectively by narcotic analgesics which appear to be more effective against dull continuous pain than sharp intermittent pain.

The main disadvantages are depression of respiration (mostly dose-related), dependence with repeated use and constipation. Apart from preoperative and postoperative use, the use of narcotics for a period longer than a few days may produce psychic and physical dependence. Its hallucinogenic and euphoric effects are the factors which lead to the abuse potential.

Opium, which contains a group of alkaloids, has been known in medical practice for many centuries. Thomas Sydenham in 1680 wrote: "Among the remedies which it has pleased almighty God to give to man to relieve his suffering, none is so universal and so efficacious as opium." Opium is obtained by cutting the seed heads of the opium poppy and collecting the dried exudate after 24 hours. The opium poppy grows best in warm sunny climates and has long been cultivated in the Middle and Far East.

The drug was used as crude extract until 1803 when Friedrich Serturna distilled it and tried out the various fractions on animals. He tried the ***morphine*** fraction (named after Morpheus, god of sleep) on himself and some others. Opium has been used until recent times in a tablet (*Ipecacuanha and Opium Tablet BPC*) to promote sweating and sleep in fevers, and may still be occasionally called for in its tincture form to produce *Chalk and Opium Mixture* (BPC) to control diarrhoea.

Dr Thomas Dover, who set up in medical practice after retiring from his career as a licensed pirate and rescuing Robinson Crusoe (Alexander Selkirk) in 1709, invented *Dover's Powders* which were available until recently. These consisted of a mixture of opium and ipecacuanha, that is, a built-in safety device so that overdosage would be accompanied by vomiting.

The alkaloids derived from opium include ***morphine*** and ***codeine,*** and the lesser-used ***papaverine*** and ***noscapine. Papaveretum*** is a purified mixture of the alkaloids.

These analgesics share some of the properties of naturally occurring peptides, namely enkephalins and endorphins.

CODEINE

Codeine is one of the opium alkaloids. It is active orally and is approximately two-thirds as effective by this route as when given by injection. It has all the pharmacological properties of morphine or similar drugs although it is far less potent weight for weight, and so has become regarded as one of the mild analgesics; 30mg is said to be approximately equivalent in analgesic potency to 600 mg aspirin.

Codeine is particularly good for pain of visceral origin. For somatic pain it is commonly given in combination with aspirin and the combined effect is said to be more than additive. It is also used as a cough suppressant as *Linctus Codeine.*

Adverse Drug Reactions are the same as with other opium derivatives: nausea, anorexia, confusion, sweating, and constipation. This latter effect has been often exploited therapeutically by using the drug for severe diarrhoea although this practice is not recommended.

Table 39
Commonly Used Analgesics Containing Codeine

Trade Name	Aspirin	Paracetamol	Codeine
Codis	500	0	8
Panadeine	0	500	8
Panadeine Forte	0	500	15
Veganin	250	250	6.8

DIHYDROCODEINE TARTRATE (or BITARTRATE)

This drug, which is related to codeine, is an analgesic and antitussive which may produce dependence of the morphine type in susceptible individuals. The usual dose is 30 to 60 mg as an analgesic (60 mg being claimed to be equivalent to 10 mg morphine). As an analgesic the drug is available as tablets (*DF 118*† 30 mg) and in combination as *Co-dydramol* with 500 mg paracetamol.

Adverse Drug Reactions are the same as for morphine, for example, nausea, anorexia, confusion and sweating.

MORPHINE

Morphine is the most potent derivative of opium and acts to relieve pain. It acts on the CNS both as a depressant (leading to analgesia, respiratory depression, depression of cough reflex and sleep) and as a stimulant (leading to vomiting, miosis, convulsions and some hyperactive spinal-cord reflexes). It can stimulate smooth muscle leading to spasm of gastro-intestinal muscle (causing constipation by delaying passage of contents), biliary tract, and possibly renal tract. It may be given by SC, IM or IV injection, 10 mg usually being adequate for an adult dose.

Morphine is used after surgery for the relief of pain, in terminal diseases such as cancer and was formerly used in cough mixtures as a cough suppressant (***Linctus Morphine***). The use of ***Brompton Mixture*** or ***Brompton Cocktail*** containing morphine, cocaine, alcohol and chloroform-water has largely fallen into disrepute. Studies have shown that a simple flavoured morphine mixture is as effective in pain control as a standard Brompton mixture without the side effects of cocaine (schizophrenic-like paranoid psychoses) and alcohol (CNS effects such as impairment of judgement and coordination).

Adverse Drug Reactions are as stated below in the general description of narcotics, the most important being depression of respiration, nausea and vomiting. Hypotension and bradycardia may occur in patients taking antihypertensive drugs by stimulation of the vagal centre and impairment of the sympathetic vascular reflexes.

Morphine is potentiated by neostigmine and chlorpromazine and, it is thought by some authors, by MAOIs and tricyclic antidepressants. Overdosage may lead to death by respiratory depression.

PAPAVERETUM (Omnopon)

Papaveretum acts on the CNS. It is a purified mixture of the opium alkaloids (anhydrous morphine, codeine, noscapine and papaverine). It has the analgesic and narcotic properties of morphine.

Papaveretum is a convenient means of administering the total alkaloids of opium by injection and may be used in all cases in which morphine is indicated. It is commonly used with hyoscine for preoperative medication.

Adverse Drug Reactions are as with morphine, but it is claimed to produce fewer side effects.

DIAMORPHINE (Heroin)

Diamorphine is still available to doctors in Great Britain but not available for therapeutic use in many countries. It is a semisynthetic drug first made from morphine (to which it is metabolised in the body) in 1874 in London. It was first introduced 24 years later (1898) as a remedy for cough and for morphine addiction. It was some time before it was realised that its efficiency in treatment of the latter was by substitution of one dependence-producing drug for another. It is commonly said that heroin is the most potent of all dependence-producing drugs.

Adverse Drug Reactions are similar to morphine, although it causes less vomiting, restlessness and fidgeting.

PETHIDINE

Pethidine (***meperidine,*** *Demerol* in the US) is a synthetic strong analgesic which was introduced in 1939. It has some morphine-like properties, but it does not cause constipation, suppress cough or constrict the pupils.

This drug can be used for pain which requires a stronger analgesic than codeine, but not great enough to require morphine. Pethidine is relatively ineffective if given orally and this combined with its short duration of action (two to three hours) make it unsuitable for chronic pain.

Adverse Drug Reactions are the same as for morphine. It may cause vomiting, dry mouth and blurred vision but the psychic effects are not as marked as with morphine. Death from overdose is by respiratory depression.

METHADONE (Physeptone)

Methadone is a synthetic morphine-like compound with properties similar to those of morphine including its abuse potential. It is, however, much more active orally than morphine. Its high potency and long duration of action (the plasma half-life being 22 to 72 hours) means that the danger of accumulation in the elderly or ill patient is great. It should not, therefore, be given more often than once every six hours.

It has been used as a cough suppressant, and as a strong oral analgesic. Methadone has had a place in the past few years in the treatment of heroin and morphine addicts.

Adverse Drug Reactions include vomiting, sedation and dependence, which is less severe than with morphine and heroin. Because of its dependence-producing properties, methadone treatment of long-term chronic complaints should be avoided if possible.

PENTAZOCINE (Fortral)

This is a synthetic analgesic of about one-third the potency of morphine. It is an opiate antagonist and can therefore induce withdrawal symptoms in addicts. It can cause dependence as it also has a partial opiate agonist activity, but the potential for producing dependence is less than with other morphine-like drugs. It may need to be given more frequently than morphine (for example, every three hours) and is available by injection and orally.

Adverse Drug Reactions include nausea, vomiting, hypertension, sweating, dizziness, palpitations, tachycardia and CNS disturbances (euphoria, restlessness, hallucinations, delusions, distorted body image, depersonalisation, nightmares and depression).

DEXTROMORAMIDE

Dextromoramide (*Palfium*) is a narcotic analgesic which is claimed to be equally effective by the oral route as by injection. It is used as a potent analgesic in, for example, inoperable tumours.

It is claimed to be twice as potent as morphine but produces short-lasting analgesia of about two hours and therefore requires close monitoring for chronic use. It is used as a potent analgesic in exacerbations of acute and chronic pain in terminal illnesses.

BUPRENORPHINE (Temgesic)

This is a narcotic with agonist-antagonist activity. It is well absorbed sublingually, about 0.4 mg being equianalgesic with 10 mg of morphine. It is thought to have less abuse potential than that of morphine. It also appears to have a lower incidence of side-effects and psychotomimetic effects than pentazocine, and about double the duration of action of morphine.

NURSING IMPLICATIONS

Narcotic Analgesics

Assessment

The nursing care of the patient in pain involves more than just giving the ordered analgesic. An holistic approach to the patient as an individual should always be used. Full assessment of the patient should include documenting the type and frequency of pain, the underlying cause and the patient's psychological reaction to the pain and the type of drug to be used for its relief.

The patient may not verbalise his or her pain, and the nurse needs to be able to recognise the various signs that the individual patient may manifest when experiencing pain, such as increased pulse rate and respiratory rate, facial expression, posture, guarding muscular action, restlessness, sweating or pallor.

The nurse should also realise that some patients may not desire to have their awareness reduced by drugs, and this right should be respected. Alternative measures such as the application of heat or cold or massage should not be overlooked. Sometimes such simple nursing measures as changing the position, loosening a tight dressing, a back rub, or talking with the patient may do a great deal to promote comfort and alleviate anxieties and fears.

Pain is what the person experiencing it says it is, and nurses should avoid having fixed ideas about what they think the patient is experiencing. People, especially those with a terminal illness, should be given adequate analgesia as required. It is not appropriate to withhold pain relief in this class of patient because of fear of addiction.

The nursing implications are essentially the same for all narcotic analgesics. Initially, prior to administration, the patient's drug profile should be assessed for the concurrent use of drugs such as alcohol, phenothiazines or antidepressants, as the combined use of any of these with a narcotic will cause a cumulative CNS depressant effect.

Patients, whose histories reveal chronic respiratory disease, liver disease, convulsive disorders, Addison's disease or myxoedema, are at increased risk of adverse effects and should therefore be subject to rigorous evaluation following administration.

Where it is vitally important to monitor the patient's neurological state, (for example, raised intracranial pressure, head injuries, diabetic ketoacidosis), the administration of potent narcotics will usually be contraindicated as they will mask the true neurological state of the patient.

Administration

Narcotics are most effective if they are administered to the patient before the pain reaches its greatest level of intensity. Administration should be scheduled so that the peak effect is reached when painful procedures are being done. Aspirate the syringe carefully before injecting intramuscular or subcutaneous doses to avoid accidental intravenous administration. Do not mix narcotics with other drugs due to the potential physical and chemical drug incompatibilities which can occur.

Note: Nurses must strictly observe the rules relating to the administration of Controlled Drugs. All controlled drugs must be ordered by a medical officer (who must specify and limit the amount of the drug which can be given on any particular order). Any loss must be reported to the appropriate person as defined by your particular district — usually to the principal pharmacist in a hospital.

Evaluation

Following administration, the nurse must assess the efficacy of the drug used for degree and duration of relief. Monitor the patient carefully for signs of adverse effects and toxicity. Respirations should be checked regularly and narcotics should not be given if the respiration rate falls below 10/min. Watch for abdominal and bladder distension and prevent constipation and impaction, especially in terminal-care patients. Be alert for signs of dependence and tolerance such as coryza and itching nose, which usually will appear 24 to 48 hours after the last dose. Assist patients to sitting positions slowly due to the postural hypotension which can occur with narcotics.

Patient teaching

Patients should be reassured that the side rails are for their protection against falling, due to narcotic-induced altered sensory preceptions. They must be encouraged to deep-breathe and cough and change position regularly as the antitussive and respiratory depressant properties of most narcotics can produce other respiratory complications.

DEXTROPROPOXYPHENE

This is a synthetic analgesic structurally related to the narcotic analgesic methadone. However, it is less analgesic, antitussive and dependence producing than methadone. Used alone, it is only marginally more effective than placebo and requires 120 mg to achieve analgesia equivalent to 600 mg of aspirin. It is available as dextropropoxyphene capsules (*Doloxene*); dextropropoxyphene plus aspirin (*Doloxene-Co*, the Co standing for "compound" not "codeine"); and dextropropoxyphene plus paracetamol (*Cosalgesic, Distalgesic†, Paxalgesic†).*

Dextropropoxyphene is a centrally acting analgesic and is believed to act in the same way as morphine, although the mechanism is not clear. It has an onset of action and duration similar to that of codeine but with a less potent analgesic effect. Dextropropoxyphene can be useful in viscerally engendered pain or in somatic pain when in combinations with other drugs (for example, *Doloxene-Co, Distalgesic†*).

A variety of side effects may occur, including headache, drowsiness, dizziness, insomnia, habituation and abdominal pain. It has become a much-abused drug and despite the early claims that dependence would not occur, this has happened in some patients, the incidence being about the same as with codeine. An increased number of deaths in which the drug has been implicated has been reported. In the US, the Food and Drug Administration estimates that 1000 to 2000 deaths each year are associated with dextropropoxyphene, and it ranks second only to the barbiturates associated with drug fatalities.

NURSING IMPLICATIONS

As compound analgesics containing dextropropoxyphene are widely used, the nurse needs to be fully aware of the individual properties of each drug contained in the formulation, so that appropriate assessment, evaluation and patient teaching can be carried out.

Due to the narcotic-like component, dextropropoxyphene, there is the potential for abuse.

Patients should be warned not to take alcohol with compounds containing dextropropoxyphene as the central nervous sytem depressant effects of both drugs will be greatly potentiated.

Nurses should know that *Doloxene-Co* contains aspirin (not codeine) and that all nursing implications for aspirin will also apply. Constipation can be a problem with dextropropoxyphene-containing compounds.

Table 40
Equivalent Doses of Analgesics

Weak Analgesics		
Aspirin	600mg	All are approximately equivalent to 1.5mg morphine IM, or 1.5mg oral dextromoramide, 3mg oral methadone, 4.5mg oral oxycodone or 3mg to 9mg oral morphine.
Paracetamol	1 gram	
Codeine	30mg	
Pethidine	45mg	
Pentazocine	30mg	
Dextropropoxyphene	60mg	
Strong Analgesics		
Morphine	10mg IM	20mg to 60mg oral
Methadone	10mg IM	20mg oral
Pethidine	75mg IM	Unsatisfactory by mouth
Dextromoramide	5mg IM	10mg oral

These data have been combined, and in some cases extrapolated, from information published by Coates, Houde, Brophy, Twycross and others. They are useful only as a starting point when changing analgesics. There is much variation between individual patients, as well as between published studies. Half-lives also vary from one agent to another.

NARCOTIC ANTAGONISTS

NALORPHINE

Nalorphine is used to reverse overdosage of the opiates with which it competes at the site of action. It was often used in an attempt to avoid respiratory depression caused by the narcotic analgesics in both mother and child at childbirth. The introduction of the antagonist to the narcotic is complex, and great care is needed in combining the two so that the respiratory depression is not made worse. It is closely related to morphine with some of the same actions (for example, analgesia), but it has tended to become obsolete as it produces unpleasant abnormalities of mood and hallucinations. It is of no use in reducing the respiratory depression of other drugs such as the barbiturates.

It is no longer available in the UK.

NALOXONE

Naloxone (*Narcan*) has to a great extent replaced nalorphine. It reverses the action of relatively large doses of any narcotic and is the only specific antagonist to pentazocine.

NURSING IMPLICATIONS

Narcotic Antagonists

Nursing assessment includes documenting the extent of the narcotic induced respiratory depression and the determination of any existing addiction by the patient.

Evaluation following administration focuses on monitoring the patient's respiration and level of consciousness. When naloxone is administered to narcotic addicts to reverse the effects of overdose, they may be expected to manifest signs of withdrawal.

SELF-EVALUATION TEST

1. Define the terms "analgesic" and "antipyretic".
2. List some of the salicylates.
3. Describe the ways in which aspirin acts.
4. What is the contraindication to giving paracetamol?
5. List the uses of codeine.
6. What would you advise a patient who has been prescribed dextropropoxyphene?
7. List the naturally occurring opium derivations commonly used and the synthetic narcotics.
8. State the nursing implications of giving narcotic drugs.

Table 41
Summary of Analgesics

Drug Group	Drug Name	Use	Action	Adverse Reactions	Nursing Implications
Salicylates	Aspirin Sodium salicylate	–Minor pain –Fever –Inflammatory conditions –Prevention of platelet aggregation	Analgesic Anti-inflammatory Antipyretic Antiplatelet	GIT bleeding, allergy especially in asthmatics, nausea, vomiting diarrhoea, angioneurotic oedema	***Assess:*** history of previous allergy, intestinal lesions, dyspepsia, peptic ulceration, anticoagulant therapy, use of oral hypoglycaemic drugs and uricosurics, for kidney or liver disease,pregnancy, lactation, coagulation disorders or bleeding tendencies: establish and document baseline observations of location and degree of pain and or fever. ***Administer:*** as required or as ordered, preferably with food or milk to reduce the risk of GIT irritation. ***Evaluate:*** for relief of pain, reduction in pyrexia, for signs of allergy, toxicity, GIT distress and bleeding tendencies in long-term use. ***Teach:*** self-evaluation for side effects and toxicity, potential drug interations, to take with food or milk, not to break or dissolve enteric-coated or slow-release formulations, to keep out of the reach of children.

continued

Drug Group	Drug Name	Use	Action	Adverse Reactions	Nursing Implications
Narcotic analgesics	Morphine Pethidine Papaveretum Methadone Pentazocine Dextromoramide Buprenorphine Codeine phosphate Dextropro-poxyphene	Severe pain, such as in terminal disease or after surgery	CNS depressant	Respiratory depression, nausea, vomiting, hypotension, bradycardia, constipation, suppression of cough reflex.	***Assess:*** for concurrent use of alcohol and other CNS depressant drugs, history of chronic respiratory disease, liver disease, convulsive disorders, Addison's disease, myxoedema, head injury, raised intracranial pressure, severe debilitation, pregnancy, lactation; establish base-line observations of vital signs, especially respiratory rate; document extent and severity of pain. ***Administer:*** prior to development of severe pain; observe legal and/or hospital policy requirements during administration procedure; intravenous administration by slow, dilute infusion; intramuscular or subcutaneous administration — aspirate syringe to avoid accidental IV administration. ***Evaluate:*** for relief of pain and duration of analgesic effect, for hypersensitive reactions, toxicity and side effects, for developing dependence; monitor vital signs especially respiratory rate; institute nursing measures to prevent and/or treat constipation. ***Teach:*** to ambulate with assistance; that if side rails are used, they are for patient's safety; not to smoke while under the influence of drugs; to cough, deep breathe and change position regularly.

17

DRUG TREATMENT OF MUSCULOSKELETAL DISORDERS

Jennifer Liege Benzie and Craig Serjeant

OBJECTIVES

At the conclusion of this chapter the reader should be able to:

1. identify drugs used in the treatment of musculoskeletal disorders;
2. state either the mode of action or the disease state for which drugs in this class are used;
3. list the common adverse reactions to drugs used in treating musculoskeletal disorders;
4. write brief notes describing the nursing implications of the drugs mentioned.

PREREQUISITE KNOWLEDGE

1. Anatomy and physiology of the musculoskeletal system.
2. Disease states of the musculoskeletal system.

DEFINITIONS

Counter-irritation — superficial irritation intended to relieve some other irritation.
Rubefaction — reddening of the skin.
Rubefacient — an agent that reddens the skin.

NON-STEROIDAL ANTI-INFLAMMATORY DRUGS

The non-steroid anti-inflammatory drugs (NSAIDs) are used for the symptomatic relief of pain and inflammation in a wide range of musculoskeletal conditions such as arthritis, rheumatoid arthritis, ankylosing spondylitis and osteoarthritis. The number of NSAIDs on the market has increased rapidly in the past decade. All these drugs have anti-inflammatory, analgesic and antipyretic properties.

ACETYLSALICYLIC ACID (Aspirin) and SODIUM SALICYLATE

The anti-inflammatory effect of ***aspirin*** is obtained in the plasma salicylate-concentration range of 150 to 300 mg/L, and this is usually achieved with doses of 2.6 to 6 g of aspirin per day.

Action

Pain relief is effected by both a central and peripheral action. The types of pain eased are usually those of low intensity from bone and joint. A large variety of pains are eased, ranging from headache and toothache to acute rheumatic fever. Aspirin and the salicylates inhibit the synthesis of prostaglandins in inflamed tissues and so prevent sensitisation of pain receptors to substances that appear to mediate the pain response.

Absorption is rapid, partly from the stomach and mostly from the upper small intestine and appreciable plasma concentrations are attained within 30 minutes. After absorption, aspirin is rapidly distributed throughout the body tissues, and it readily crosses the placenta.

Adverse Drug Reactions

Headaches, dizziness and tinnitus are common, particularly at continued high dosage, with difficulty in hearing, dimness of vision, mental confusion, hyperventilation, sweating, thirst, worsening of gout and a number of other adverse reactions. Overdosage with salicylates initially causes overbreathing with increased respiration rate, and respiratory alkalosis occurs. In infants and children this may easily be missed.

Hypersensitivity reactions

These are not common, but may occasionally be severe and even fatal, as in acute asthma and anaphylactic reactions. Aspirin hypersensitivity may occur after taking only small amounts of the drug.

Drug Interactions

The scope for interactions of aspirin with other drugs is potentially great, but fortunately interactions are seldom clinically important. Nevertheless, in the use of a drug which can be taken freely by the patient without prescription, it is important to know of the potential interaction problems. See Table 42.

Clinical Use

Aspirin was traditionally the drug of first choice in rheumatoid arthritis, but it is of relatively little help in the treatment of acute gout and severe ankylosing spondylitis. Aspirin may be used in individual doses of 0.6 to 1 g as required, purely as an analgesic. However, to exert an anti-inflammatory effect, regular dosage every three to four hours is necessary, total dosage being around 4 to 6 g daily. The aim is to use the lowest effective level, which is often the highest tolerated. Only about half the patients who tolerate a lower dosage will continue at a higher dosage of 4 to 6 g for any period of time, and many of these experience troublesome adverse reactions.

Table 42
Some Common Potential Drug Interactions with Aspirin

Drug	Possible interaction
Alcohol	Increased gastrointestinal irritation with risk of gastric haemorrhage.
Ammonium chloride Ascorbic acid	Increased salicylate levels due to decreased urinary clearance.
Antacids	Decreased plasma salicylate levels due to increased urinary clearance. Therapeutic plasma levels may not be maintained.
Anticoagulants	Increased risk of gastric haemorrhage with both oral anticoagulants and heparin.
Antidiabetic drugs (oral)	Increased hypoglycaemic effect with sulphonylureas and large doses of aspirin.
Corticosteroids	Accumulation of salicylate with toxicity when long-term steroid therapy is withdrawn and dose of aspirin not reduced.
Uricosuric agents	Low doses of aspirin inhibit uricosuric action of probenicid, sulphinpyrazone and phenylbutazone.

PHENYLBUTAZONE (Butazolidin) and OXYPHENBUTAZONE (Tanderil)

Action

Phenylbutazone has anti-inflammatory, analgesic and antipyretic properties, but it also causes considerable sodium chloride and water retention and so may precipitate heart failure and acute pulmonary oedema. ***Oxyphenbutazone*** is an analogue of phenylbutazone and one of its major metabolites. It has the same general properties and the same action, therapeutic uses, interactions and toxic effects as the parent drug.

Adverse Drug Reactions

Some undesirable effects are seen in 20% to 30% of patients, and the treatment will have to be withdrawn in about half of these. Nausea, vomiting and epigastric discomfort may occur. Skin reactions are not common. Blood dyscrasias such as agranulocytosis and aplastic anaemia are dangerous but rare.

Drug Interactions

Drug interactions are very important. Phenylbutazone has the potential to inhibit the hepatic metabolism and renal excretion of certain drugs which, combined with its ability to displace some highly bound drugs (for example warfarin, tolbutamide, chlorpropamide) from plasma-albumin binding sites, greatly increases the risk of important drug interactions. Phenylbutazone markedly enhances the activity of oral coumarin anticoagulants and oral sulphonylurea hypoglycaemic drugs such as tolbutamide *(Rastinon)* and chlorpropamide *(Diabinese)*. The salt and water retaining effect of phenylbutazone may lead to inhibition of the action of diuretics and antihypertensive drugs.

Clinical Use

Phenylbutazone and oxyphenbutazone are effective in almost all the rheumatic disorderss. Nevertheless, it is wise, because of the risk of adverse reactions and drug interactions, to use them only where a less potentially dangerous agent fails to control symptoms. They should not be used to treat mild conditions such as trivial sports or other injuries where less-toxic agents would suffice. Phenylbutazone should always be given with or after food.

INDOMETHACIN (Indocid)

Actions

Indomethacin has anti-inflammatory and antipyretic properties. Its therapeutic action begins about two hours or less after an oral dose and lasts some six hours or more. Indomethacin is perhaps, with phenylbutazone, the most potent non-steroidal anti-inflammatory agent available today and will, if tolerated, reduce inflammatory swelling and lessen pain in the inflammatory arthropathies.

Adverse Drug Reactions

Headaches, vertigo, mental "muzziness", confusion and a number of other cerebral sensations are dose-related and diminish or disappear with reduction of dosage. Gastrointestinal symptoms, abdominal pain, vague discomfort, anorexia or peptic ulceration may occur at any time on any dose. Blood changes have been reported but are rare. Severe depression, hallucinations and even psychoses have been reported. The use of suppositories may diminish, but does not entirely prevent, gastrointestinal irritation.

Clinical Use

Indomethacin is useful throughout almost the entire field of rheumatoid disorders, but it is most helpful in ankylosing spondylitis, gout, rheumatoid arthritis and osteoarthritis, particularly of the hip.

SULINDAC (Clinoril)

Sulindac is a derivative of indomethacin, which appears to have similar effects without some of the characteristic adverse reactions. It is given on a twice-daily basis.

Adverse Drug Reactions

Sulindac causes less adverse reactions than aspirin. Those which occur tend to be mild and seldom lead to withdrawal of treatment. It does not cause headaches (as indomethacin does). Constipation, epigastric pain and nausea are nevertheless the most common problems, occurring in 25% of patients.

Clinical Use

Sulindac is as effective as aspirin in rheumatoid arthritis. It is more effective than ibuprofen and comparable with naproxen and is a useful alternative to indomethacin.

A dose of 200 mg twice daily is usually required in severe rheumatoid arthritis. The dose can often be reduced to 200 mg daily in milder conditions and should be given in the lowest effective maintenance dose.

PROPIONIC ACID DERIVATIVES

Drugs in this group include ***ibuprofen*** *(Brufen)*, ***naproxen*** *(Naprosyn)*, ***fenoprofen*** *(Fenopron)* and ***ketoprofen*** *(Orudis)*. One of the major mechanisms of actions of these drugs is to reduce the production of prostaglandins and their metabolites and thus lower concentrations of potent joint "inflammogens".

Adverse Drug Reactions

Side effects include gastrointestinal upsets (nausea, indigestion), and gastrointestinal bleeding is being reported more commonly. Rashes, headaches and lightheadedness have been reported. Toxic amblyopia has been reported with ibuprofen, but this responds rapidly to drug withdrawal. A rare hypersensitivity reaction has been reported with fenoprofen.

Clinical Use

Propionic acid derivatives are useful in a wide range of rheumatic disorders. They should be used to suppress pain when there is evidence of inflammation – heat, redness and swelling. The spectrum of effects and side effects of propionic acid derivatives is similar, though patients respond individually to them, both in terms of pain relief and adverse reactions.

FENEMATES

Mefenamic acid *(Ponstan)* has analgesic, antipyretic and mild anti-inflammatory actions.

Adverse Drug Reactions

Gastrointestinal irritation is not uncommon. Dyspepsia, abdominal discomfort and diarrhoea are the most frequently reported side effects. Rashes occur rarely. Mefenamic acid has been reported to cause haemolytic anaemia, and in aspirin sensitive patients, it may cause bronchoconstriction.

Drug Interactions

Mefenamic acid binds strongly to plasma protein and may potentiate the activity of coumarin anticoagulants. It should therefore be used with caution in patients receiving warfarin.

Clinical Use

Mefenamic acid is used mainly as an analgesic agent to relieve pain arising in any rheumatic condition.

DIFLUNISAL (Dolobid)

Diflunisal is a salicylate with higher potency, longer duration of action and better tolerance than aspirin.

Adverse Drug Reactions

Side effects are relatively uncommon with diflunisal, with gastrointestinal upsets being the most frequent. Skin rashes and pruritus are uncommon. Gastrointestinal bleeding has been reported. Diflunisal should be avoided in patients with salicylate hypersensitivity.

Drug Interactions

Diflunisal may cause some prolongation of prothrombin times when given with oral anticoagulants. Patients receiving such a combination should be closely monitored.

Clinical Use

It is a useful analgesic for short-term relief of postoperative, dental and post-traumatic pain, and it is also useful in long-term treatment of osteoarthritis and rheumatoid arthritis.

NURSING IMPLICATIONS

Assessment

Prior to the administration of NSAIDs to individuals with rheumatoid arthritis, the nurse should assess the patient's history for any indication of allergy, peptic ulceration or other intestinal lesions or previous GIT bleeding. Concurrent use of drugs which may interact with the NSAID (especially anticoagulants and sulphonylurea hypoglycaemic drugs) should also be determined. In all of these cases, the drug must be withheld and the physician informed. If the potent anti-inflammatory drugs (for example, indomethacin or phenylbutazone) are to be used, the patient's history should also exclude evidence of renal or hepatic impairment and blood dyscrasias. If the patient is prescribed phenylbutazone, the base line weight should be recorded, as this drug can cause fluid retention. Document baseline observations concerning the degree of joint pain, swelling and movement.

Administration
To reduce irritation to the intestinal mucosa, all of these drugs are best given with food. Note that antacids can reduce plasma salicylate levels. Do not dissolve or crush slow-release or enteric-coated formulations.

Evaluation
When aspirin is being used in rheumatic disorders, it must be remembered that high doses are needed to obtain the anti-inflammatory effect required. Therefore, there is often a fine line between the therapeutic and toxic levels of the drug. Thus, these patients need to be watched closely for signs of salicylate toxicity, such as hyperventilation, tinnitus, dimness of vision, confusion, headache, sweating, thirst, nausea, vomiting and diarrhoea.

Observe all patients for signs of drug effectiveness, that is, relief of pain, reduction of swelling and improved joint mobility.

All patients on non-steroid anti-inflammatory drugs are at risk of incurring GIT upsets and GIT bleeding; therefore the nurse needs to be alert for signs of these. Patients on more potent drugs, such as phenylbutazone or indomethacin should also be watched for signs of bone-marrow suppression, such as reports of sore throat, bleeding mucosa, bruising and signs of infection. Watch for CNS effects with indomethacin and signs of oedema with phenylbutazone.

Evaluation of patients who have been on aspirin for a long time should also include observations for tarry stools, haematemesis, petechiae and bruising, which could occur due to the fact that aspirin reduces prothrombin levels and platelet adhesiveness.

Patient teaching
This will include teaching the importance of taking the correct dose regularly to maintain blood levels necessary for therapeutic effect, to evaluate for adverse effects and toxicity, and to report these if they occur. To reduce the risk of gastrointestinal upsets, patients should be advised to take their medication with food or milk.

It should be stressed to patients on the potent anti-inflammatory drugs to report a sore throat or any other symptoms of blood dyscrasias to their physician immediately. These patients should be made aware of the importance of keeping appointments to monitor their blood count at regular intervals if on long-term therapy. Patients taking phenylbutazone should be advised to reduce the amount of salt in their diet so as to decrease the risk of oedema, and those on indomethacin should be warned of the potential dangers of driving or operating power machinery due to the mental confusion this drug may cause. It may be necessary to explain to patients taking aspirin why such large doses are needed. The importance of keeping these drugs out of the reach of children should be stressed.

PENICILLAMINE (Distamine, Pendramine)

Penicillamine is another substance used in the treatment of rheumatoid arthritis. Although its mechanism of action is unknown, it appears to suppress disease activity. Its use is reserved for those patients with active rheumatoid arthritis who have failed to respond to an adequate trial of conventional therapy. Response is slow, usually taking about three months for the first signs of remission to occur, and maintenance therapy may be indefinite.

Adverse Drug Reactions

Reported adverse reactions are many and often serious, including haematological changes, gastrointestinal upsets, allergic response and renal problems.

GOLD

Gold in the form of ***sodium aurothiomalate*** *(Myocrisin)* is used as a specific treatment for rheumatoid arthritis. The mechanism of action is not clear. Treatment usually begins with doses of 1, 5 and 10 mg at intervals of one week (to test tolerance), and then 20-50 mg weekly until remission occurs or a total of 1 g has been given. The interval between injections can be varied between 2 and 4 weeks depending on response.

Adverse Drug Reactions

Minor reactions such as rashes are frequent, but must not be taken lightly as they may be early signs of toxicity. The most serious and frequent complication is renal failure. Blood disorders may also occur.

Clinical Use

The use of gold is limited to patients with active, progressive rheumatoid arthritis which cannot be satisfactorily controlled with NSAIDs alone.

NURSING IMPLICATIONS

Assessment

Prior to the administration of gold or penicillamine, the nurse will be required to test the urine for protein and ensure that current laboratory tests of blood counts and renal function are at hand, as these drugs can be extremely toxic to bone marrow and renal function.

Evaluation

Patients on these drugs will usually have regular appointments at their rheumatology clinic for checks on their dosage regime, administration of gold injections, evaluation of improvement in their condition or adverse effects. The nurse will be required to test the urine for protein and report the result. Blood will possibly be taken for laboratory tests, including ESR and full blood count. Nursing evaluation will also include observation of the patient for any other signs of adverse drug effects, including signs of skin reactions, evidence of blood dyscrasias (such as bruising, haematuria or evidence of infection) and reports of tiredness and lethargy.

Patient teaching

The patient needs to be reassured that these drugs are slower acting than other anti-inflammatory drugs he may have taken in the past and that it may take some time for benefit to be apparent. The patient should be asked to report skin rashes, mouth ulcers, or evidence of bleeding or infection to his physician. The importance of keeping regular appointments for urine tests, blood tests and assessment of dosages and progress should be stressed.

GOUT

AETIOLOGY

Gout is a clinical syndrome characterised by recurrent attacks of acute monoarticular arthritis which is associated with an elevation of serum urate (hyperuricaemia) and abnormal accumulation of urate within the body. The upper limit of normal for the serum urate concentration is usually defined as 0.44 mmol/L in males and 0.37 mmol/L in females.

The hyperuricaemia which invariably precedes gouty arthritis is due to either metabolic over-production of urate or a reduced ability of the kidney to excrete urate. Precipitation of urate crystals into joint, renal tubules and tissues may result in acute arthritis, renal calculi and tophi.

TREATMENT

Non-steroidal anti-inflammatory agents are used for the treatment of acute attacks of gout, while long-term treatment is based on the use of ***uricosuric agents*** and ***agents preventing uric acid formation.***

Treatment of the acute attack

Indomethacin is most frequently prescribed for the treatment of acute gouty arthritis. The recommended dose is 50 mg three or four times daily until all symptoms and signs subside. The dose should be reduced as the attack comes under control. ***Naproxen*** has also been used successfully for the treatment of acute gouty attacks. It is usual to give 750 mg for the first dose, followed by 250 mg every eight hours. Treatment with naproxen results in a marked reduction in pain, tenderness and swelling. Other non-steroidal anti-inflammatory agents such as ***sulindac*** have also been used with good results.

Anti-inflammatory drugs such as indomethacin and naproxen should be administered with or after food to reduce the incidence of gastrointestinal distress or peptic ulceration.

Colchicine is sometimes used to relieve the pain and inflammation of gout, relief usually occurring within a few hours. In acute gout a dose of 1 mg is given initially followed by 500 mcg up to every 2-3 hours until either relief or toxic effects (nausea and diarrhoea) occur. A total of 4 to 8 mg is usually needed, and it is unwise to exceed 10 mg for the acute attack.

Long-term treatment

Long-term treatment is aimed at reducing the uric acid in the body either by increasing renal excretion with uricosuric drugs or by decreasing its synthesis in the tissue by the use of ***allopurinol*** *(Zyloric)*. This may take many months. Success is shown by a reduction in acute attacks, a lowering of serum uric acid, and absorption of tophi. Long-term treatment may be given concurrently with treatment for an acute attack. Treatment can be continued indefinitely.

There is a tendency for acute gout to be precipitated by treatment with uricosuric agents or allopurinol at the initiation of therapy, but this can be treated with anti-inflammatory agents as outlined above, and the condition usually subsides.

Allopurinol *(Zyloric)* reduces the formation of uric acid from purines by inhibiting the enzyme xanthine oxidase. Since there is less uric acid to be excreted, the drug has a special place for use in patients with impaired renal function. The average dose is in the range of 200 to 600 mg daily, and troublesome side effects are unusual. The action of allopurinol is not antagonised by salicylates.

Probenecid *(Benemid)* is a uricosuric agent that increases the elimination of uric acid via the kidney. Therapy should be initiated at 250 mg twice daily for one week and increased by weekly increments of 250 mg until a daily dose of 2 g is achieved. The common adverse reactions of probenecid are gastrointestinal distress and skin rashes. The serious adverse reactions, such as nephrotic syndrome, bone-marrow depression and hepatic necrosis are rare. Probenecid cannot be used in patients with renal insufficiency.

Sulphinpyrazone *(Anturan)* also has a uricosuric action. It should be initiated at a dose of 100-200 mg twice daily and gradually increased at weekly intervals, according to plasma uric acid concentration, up to 600-800 mg in daily divided doses. Adverse reactions to sulphinpyrazone are similar to those of probenecid, with gastrointestinal distress and skin rashes being the most common.

Salicylates (aspirin and sodium salicylate) in large doses of 5 to 6 g daily decrease serum urate levels by inhibiting renal tubular reabsorption of uric acid. (*Note:* Salicylates in low doses of 1 to 2 g daily have the reverse effect, and decrease urate secretion by inhibiting tubular secretion.) However, the adverse effects of salicylates in high doses are frequent and limit their use in the treatment of gout. The uricosuric action of probenecid and sulphinpyrazone is antagonised by the salicylates, and they should not be used in combination. See Table 43 for other drug interactions.

Colchicine may also be administered prophylactically (500 mcg twice daily) when initiating therapy with hypouricaemic agents.

Table 43
Drug Interactions in the Treatment of Gout

Drug	May Interact With	Potential Result
Allopurinol	Ampicillin	Increased incidence of skin rash
	Thiazide diuretics	Therapeutic efficacy of allopurinol inhibited
	Azothiaprine Mercaptopurine	Activity of antineoplastic agent increased (reduce dose to 25% usual)
	Anticoagulants (coumarin) e.g. warfarin	Activity of coumarins increased
Probenecid	Salicylates Thiazide diuretics	Therapeutic efficacy of probenecid inhibited
Sulphinpyrazone	Salicylates Thiazide diuretics	Therapeutic efficacy of sulphinpyrazone inhibited
	Anticoagulants (coumarin)	Activity of coumarin increased

NURSING IMPLICATIONS

Uricosuric drugs, colchicine and allopurinol

Assessment

Initially the nurse should establish baseline observations of joint pain, swelling and frequency of attacks. Depending on which type of drug is used, the patient's history should be checked for presence of liver or renal impairment, ulcerative gastrointestinal disorders, pregnancy, history of renal calculi and known hypersensitivity to the drug being used.

Administration

As gastric irritation and upset is often a problem with these drugs, they should always be given with food.

Evaluation

This is primarily concerned with observing for therapeutic effect of the drug such as relief of pain, reduction of swelling and return of serum urate levels to normal. The nurse should also observe for adverse reactions such as allergic reactions, GIT upsets, including nausea, vomiting, diarrhoea and abdominal pain. Severe GIT disturbance is a sign of toxicity with colchicine and will necessitate discontinuing the drug. Reports of retroperitoneal pain may indicate the presence of kidney stones which are especially likely to occur with uricosuric drugs, as the increased clearance of uric acid by these drugs tends to promote stone formation. As the effects of the oral hypoglycaemic drugs are enhanced by the uricosuric agents, diabetic patients taking these drugs should be watched for signs of hypoglycaemia.

Patient teaching

If the patient is to take colchicine for acute attacks, he should be advised to initiate therapy at the earliest indication of the attack and to continue therapy until relief is obtained. However, if signs of toxicity such as nausea, vomiting or diarrhoea occur, he must discontinue taking the drug and seek advice from his physician.

It should be stressed to patients taking any of these drugs that a high fluid intake (at least three litres daily), is vitally important to prevent formation of kidney stones and the formation of new deposits of uric acid.

Patients taking uricosuric drugs or allopurinol should be advised that they may initially experience transient attacks as the uric acid is being mobilized from the joints, but that this will pass once serum urate levels approach normal.

Patients taking a uricosuric drug should also be advised to avoid aspirin or over-the-counter preparations which contain it, as this will reduce the effect of the drug.

MUSCLE RELAXANTS

Muscle relaxant drugs can be divided into four main groups: neuromuscular blocking agents; centrally acting muscle relaxants; directly acting skeletal-muscle relaxants; and indirectly acting muscle relaxants. The first of these groups, neuromuscular blocking agents, is discussed in Chapter 30 on anaesthetic agents, so is not covered here.

CENTRALLY ACTING MUSCLE RELAXANTS

Centrally acting muscle relaxants act on the central nervous system. They are used mainly for relieving painful muscle spasms or spasticity occurring in musculoskeletal and neuromuscular disorders.

Methocarbamol *(Robaxin)* and ***orphenadrine*** *(Norflex)* are agents with centrally acting muscle-relaxant properties. Centrally acting muscle relaxants commonly produce drowsiness, dizziness, headache, blurred vision, weakness, lethargy, ataxia and nystagmus.

Benzodiazepines such as ***diazepam*** *(Valium, Atensine)* and ***lorazepam*** *(Ativan)* also have central muscle-relaxant properties. They are used in the treatment of skeletal-muscle spasm and pain associated with rheumatoid arthritis, spastic cerebral palsy and bone fractures.

Adverse Drug Reactions to benzodiazepines include drowsiness, impairment of psychomotor performance, sometimes frank confusion, paradoxical excitement, ataxia and dysarthria. Benzodiazepines should be used with caution in elderly patients. Their use is not recommended in early pregnancy as they have been suspected of causing a slightly increased risk of cleft palate.

DIRECTLY ACTING SKELETAL MUSCLE RELAXANTS

Dantrolene *(Dantrium)* is a directly acting skeletal-muscle relaxant. It produces relaxation and reduces contraction of skeletal muscle by decreasing the amount of calcium released from the sarcoplasmic reticulum. It does not alter neuromuscular transmission.

Dantrolene is used for the symptomatic treatment of skeletal muscle spasm due to multiple sclerosis, spinal-cord injury, cerebral palsy and stroke. Dantrolene is not indicated for muscle spasm associated with rheumatoid disorders.

Adverse Drug Reactions may be seen in the gastrointestinal system (nausea, diarrhoea); nervous system (drowsiness, dizziness, lightheadedness, speech and visual disturbances, mental depression and confusion); urogenital system (urinary frequency, incontinence, nocturia and urinary retention); and in the cardiovascular system (tachycardia, erratic blood pressure and phlebitis).

Dantrolene should be used with caution in patients with impaired pulmonary and hepatic function or severe myocardial disease. The central effects of dantrolene may be enhanced by sedative drugs or anti-anxiety drugs.

INDIRECTLY ACTING MUSCLE RELAXANTS

Baclofen *(Lioresal)* is an indirect muscle relaxant and antispasticity agent which acts at the spinal level. Although the mode of action is not fully known, its major effect is presynaptic inhibition. Baclofen is indicated for suppression of voluntary muscle spasm in conditions such as multiple sclerosis and lesions of the spinal cord. Patients must be hospitalised during the initiation of treatment in order to monitor usage and adverse reactions.

Adverse Drug Reactions are likely to be encountered early in therapy if the initial dose is too high. The incidence appears to be higher in the elderly and in cerebral forms of spasticity. The more common adverse reactions are: gastrointestinal system (nausea, vomiting, diarrhoea and dyspepsia); musculoskeletal system (asthenia, muscle weakness, hypotonia, muscle incoordination, tremors); nervous system (daytime sedation, lethargy, vertigo, headache and dizziness).

Baclofen is contraindicated in patients with a history of epilepsy or convulsive disorders. Baclofen is excreted largely in the urine; thus, a reduction in dosage may be necessary for patients with impaired renal function. It should be used with caution in patients with a history of gastric and duodenal ulcer, severe psychiatric disorders and in patients receiving antihypertensive therapy.

NURSING IMPLICATIONS

Assessment

The nurse should be familiar with the types of muscle-relaxant drug being used, so that assessment relates to the mode of action, precautions and contraindications specific to that drug. It is important to establish baseline observations of the degree of physical incapacity and any other signs and symptoms which are present, before administration of the drug, so that any adverse reactions which may occur will not be confused with the pre-existing disease state.

Evaluation

Monitor the patient carefully for signs of drug effectiveness and adverse effects.

Patient teaching

Patients should be warned that due to the motor incoordination, drowsiness and other CNS effects which may occur, they should take extra care when negotiating stairs and performing daily activities in order to avoid falls and subsequent injury.

COUNTER-IRRITANTS AND RUBEFACIENTS

There is probably little difference between the counter-irritant effects produced by physical and chemical methods. Pain, whether superficial or deep seated, is relieved by any method which produces irritation of the skin. Counter-irritation is comforting in painful lesions of the muscles, tendons and joints and of non-articular rheumatism. A large number of substances have been and still are used as counter-irritants. Essentially they act through the same mechanism.

The essential oils, when applied to the intact skin, have irritant and rubefacient actions, causing first a sensation of warmth and smarting, followed by a mild local anaesthesia. For this reason they are used as counter-irritants and cutaneous stimulants in the treatment of chronic inflammatory conditions, and to relieve neuralgia and rheumatic pains. Clove oil, eucalyptus oil, thyme oil and turpentine oil are commonly used in counter-irritant formulations.

Other pharmaceuticals used in formulations include camphor, methyl salicylate and capsicum. Camphor is applied externally and acts as a rubefacient and mild analgesic and is employed in liniments as a counter-irritant in fibrositis and neuralgia. Methyl salicylate is employed only for cutaneous counter-irritation in the form of ointments and liniments, and capsicum is used as a counter-irritant in lumbago, neuralgia and rheumatism.

A wide range of proprietary preparations of this nature is available. Although the formulations vary, their action is similar. They include *Finalgon, Deep Heat* and many others.

TOPICAL ANAESTHETICS

Topical anaesthetics are compounds which produce insensitivity by preventing transmission of impulses along nerve fibres and at nerve endings. The effects are reversible. In general, loss of pain (analgesia) occurs before loss of sensory and autonomic function (anaesthesia) and loss of motor function (paralysis).

Surface or topical anaesthesia blocks the sensory nerve endings in the skin or mucous membranes, but to reach these structures, the drug must have good powers of penetration. There are a number of special uses for topical anaesthesia, including anaesthetising the cornea during ophthalmological procedures and the throat and larynx before intubation and bronchoscopy. However, the application to the skin is likely to give rise to allergic reactions; such reactions may be avoided by changing to a local anaesthetic of the alternative chemical type.

There are two chemical types of topical anaesthetics: the ***ester type*** includes amethocaine, benzocaine, cocaine and procaine, and the ***amide type*** includes bupivacaine, cinchocaine, lignocaine, mepivacaine and prilocaine.

ESTERS

Amethocaine

A potent local anaesthetic whose action is greater than that of lignocaine. It is mainly used as a surface anaesthetic in ophthalmology and otorhinolaryngology. A 1% ointment is used in painful conditions of the anus or rectum.

Benzocaine

This is used in concentrations of 1%-2% in ointments as a local anaesthetic applied to ulcerated surfaces, burns, or wounds, or for the relief of intractable pruritus. Proprietary preparations include *Medilave gel* and *Nestosyl.*

Cocaine

A surface anaesthetic used almost entirely in ophthalmology and otolaryngology.

Procaine

Procaine is useless for surface application because of its poor penetration of intact mucous membranes and so is used chiefly by injection.

AMIDES

Bupivacaine

This is a long-acting local anaesthetic used mainly by injection for different types of nerve block.

Cinchocaine

This is a local anaesthetic with a longer duration of action than lignocaine and can therefore be used in lower concentrations. A 1% cream or ointment has been used for the relief of painful skin conditions. Proprietary preparations include *Nupercaine*.

Lignocaine
Lignocaine is a widely used local anaesthetic. Anal or genital pruritus and painful haemorrhoids may be relieved with suppositories or a 5% ointment or cream. A 2% gel may also be applied prior to cystoscopy or catheterisation, and a 2-4% solution may be used before bronchoscopy. Proprietary preparations include *Xylocaine*, *Xylotox* and *Bismodyne*.

Mepivacaine
This is a local anaesthetic used for different types of nerve blocks; not used in cream or ointment preparations.

Prilocaine
This local anaesthetic is used for surface anaesthesia as well as for nerve blocks. A 4% topical solution is used for surface anaesthesia of mucous membranes in bronchoscopy and minor surgery of the mouth, nose and throat. The proprietary preparation is known as *Citanest*.

ENZYME PREPARATIONS

Enzyme preparations are often used in treating trauma of the soft tissues, such as sprains and bruises. Some are available in oral form while others are applied topically. While the mode of action of proteolytic enzymes has not been fully established, it seems most probable that breakdown of fibrin and permeability modifications of venules and lymphatics underlie the action. Some doubt has been expressed however as to their degree of usefulness.

Enzyme preparations are used in the treatment of traumatic injuries (contusions, sprains, ecchymoses, haematosis); infections and other inflammatory disorders (abscesses and other local infections, phlebitis and thrombophlebitis, thrombotic and postpartum haemorrhoids, varicose ulcers and bursitis); allergic reactions (allergic rhinitis, urticaria and angioneurotic oedema); respiratory disorders (to facilitate the liquefaction of mucoid sputum); and for induced trauma (resulting from dental, obstetrical and general surgical procedures, including instrumentation).

ORAL PREPARATIONS

Trypsin
This is a proteolytic enzyme (protease) obtained from mammalian pancreas. It is used for the removal of coagulated blood, exudates and necrotic tissue and as an adjunct in the treatment of necrotic wounds and

ulcers, abscesses, empyemas, haematomas, sinuses and fistulae. It has negligible effect on viable tissue because of the presence of inhibitors.

Allergic reactions with symptoms of fever, skin rash and occasionally angioneurotic oedema may occur. Reactions may be diminished by prior administration of an antihistamine. Application of the dry powder to surface lesions may cause a severe burning sensation.

Proprietary preparations include *Chymoral* – tablets of trypsin and chymotrypsin, activity in a ratio of 6 : 1.

Chymotrypsin

This is a proteolytic enzyme obtained from bovine pancreas. It is used mainly in ophthalmology, but is also used to reduce soft-tissue inflammation and oedema from abscesses and ulcers, or associated with traumatic injuries. It has been used to promote liquefaction of secretions of the upper respiratory tract in asthmatic and bronchitic patients.

When administered by mouth, it is usual to give 20 000 to 40 000 units (USP) four times daily. Chymotrypsin may cause nausea, vomiting, diarrhoea and skin rash. Local irritation has occurred occasionally after buccal administration. Chymotrypsin is antigenic and severe allergic reactions have followed its use. It should be used with caution in patients with abnormal blood-clotting mechanisms, in patients taking anticoagulants, or with severe hepatic disease. Proprietary preparations include *Chymar* and *Deanase DC*.

Streptokinase with streptodornase *(Varidase)*

This enzymatically transforms plasminogen into the physiological plasmin. Plasmin, by digesting the fibrinogen or fibrin (or both) which can be found in areas of inflammation and in blood clots, has the physiological function of clot lysis and reduction of oedema and inflammation.

Varidase is an anti-inflammatory agent and may aid in the relief of such symptoms of inflammation as pain, swelling, and tenderness and may assist in the resolution of extravasated blood. It is useful in the management of oedema associated with infection or trauma in such conditions as abscesses, thrombophlebitis, haematomas, contusions, sprains and fractures.

Varidase oral tablets contain streptokinase 10 000 units and streptodornase 2500 units. The average oral dose is one tablet four times daily for four to six days. Streptokinase with streptodornase has been used topically in solutions containing 5000 to 10 000 units streptokinase and 1250 to 2500 units streptodornase per mL applied as a wet dressing.

Varidase is contraindicated in patients with reduced plasminogen or fibrinogen. Allergic manifestations are rare, but proper precautions should be taken. There have been some reports of nausea, vomiting, diarrhoea, skin rash and urticaria associated with the use of *Varidase*, which rarely require cessation of treatment.

Heparinoid compounds

Heparinoid compounds may be applied topically for their anticoagulant and anti-inflammatory effects. They should be gently massaged into the affected areas several times daily, avoiding any areas of broken skin. Slight reddening of the skin is a favourable response and indicates an improvement in local blood flow. Examples of this type of product include *Hirudoid* and *Lasonil.*

NURSING IMPLICATIONS

Topical enzyme preparations

Assess type of lesion to which substance is to be applied, and plan appropriate equipment needed. Before applying fresh ointment, clean area thoroughly and debride as necessary. Apply fresh ointment, avoiding healthy skin areas. Enzyme preparations should be applied at least once daily.

Evaluate for effectiveness of treatment, note allergic reactions and document progress and results.

Heparinoid compounds

Assess area to be treated, and note any areas where skin is broken. Apply by gently massaging into skin, avoiding any broken areas. Evaluate for effectiveness of treatment.

SELF-EVALUATION TEST

1. Which of the following drugs are used in musculoskeletal diseases?
   (a) phenylbutazone
   (b) pheniramine
   (c) aspirin
   (d) ibuprofen
   (e) chlorthalidone
   (f) indomethacin
   (g) penicillamine
   (h) phenmetrazine
2. List one disease state for which each of the following drugs is used.
   (a) fenoprofen
   (b) sodium aurothiomalate
   (c) chymotrypsin
   (d) lignocaine
   (e) methyl salicylate
   (f) baclofen
   (g) probenecid
   (h) naproxen
3. List two adverse effects often seen with the following drugs.
   (a) indomethacin
   (b) baclofen
   (c) colchicine
   (d) sulindac
4. Write brief notes on the nursing implications of the use of:
   (a) non-steroidal anti-inflammatory drugs
   (b) drugs used for the treatment of gout
   (c) counter-irritants and rubefacients.
5. List four drugs whose action may be altered by concomitant administration of aspirin.

Table 44
Drug Treatment of Musculoskeletal Disorders

Drug Group	Drug Name	Use	Action	Adverse Reactions	Nursing Implications
Non-steroidal anti-inflammatory drugs	Aspirin Sodium salicylate	Anti-inflammatory analgesic, in inflammatory diseases and conditions	Central and peripheral analgesic action, inhibition of prostaglandin synthesis in inflamed tissue	Headache, dizziness, tinnitus, GI bleeding, worsening of gout	***Assess:*** history for previous allergy, intestinal lesions, dyspepsia, peptic ulceration, anticoagulant therapy, use of oral hypoglycaemic drugs and uricosurics, for kidney or liver disease, pregnancy, lactation, coagulation disorders or bleeding tendencies; establish baseline description of joint pain, inflammation and degree of mobility. ***Administer:*** with meals at times ordered regularly. ***Evaluate:*** for relief of pain, inflammation and improved mobility, signs of allergy, GI distress, increased bleeding tendencies, signs of salicylate toxicity. ***Teach:*** self-evaluation for side effects and toxicity, the need for compliance in maintaining adequate blood levels to achieve therapeutic benefit, to take with food or milk and not to break or dissolve enteral-coated or slow-release formulations.

Indomethacin	Anti-inflammatory, uricosuric	Prostaglandin inhibition, promotes excretion or uric acid	Headache, vertigo, confusion, GIT discomfort, GIT bleeding, peptic ulceration, blood dyscrasias, depression	***Assess:*** history for previous allergy or sensitivity, dyspepsia, peptic ulceration, renal, hepatic dysfunction, asthma, bleeding tendencies, concurrent use of anticoagulants and uricosurics; establish baseline documentation of joint pain, inflammation and immobility. ***Administer:*** oral – with food, suppositories per rectum, usually at night. ***Evaluate:*** for relief of pain, inflammation and improved mobility, for adverse effects such as rash, GI disturbances, GI bleeding, dizziness, increased bleeding tendencies, blood dyscrasias and CNS side effects. ***Teach:*** self-evaluation for adverse effects, potential danger of driving or working with power tools and industrial machinery (due to CNS effects), to take with food and to keep out of the reach of children.
Sulindac	Anti-inflammatory, uricosuric	Prostaglandin inhibition, promotes excretion of uric acid	Constipation, epigastric pain, nausea	As for indomethacin.

continued

Drug Group	Drug Name	Use	Action	Adverse Reactions	Nursing Implications
	Ibuprofen Naproxen Fenoprofen Ketoprofen	Anti-inflammatory uricosuric	Prostaglandin inhibition, promote excretion of uric acid	GIT disturbances, GIT bleeding, rash, headache, light headedness	***Assess:*** as for aspirin. ***Administer:*** as for aspirin. ***Evaluate:*** for relief of pain, inflammation and improved mobility, for signs of allergy, GI distress, increased bleeding tendencies. ***Teach:*** self-evaluation for side effects, the need for compliance in maintaining adequate blood levels to achieve therapeutic benefit, to take with food or milk.
	Mefenamic acid	Analgesic, anti-inflammatory	Prostaglandin inhibition	GIT irritation, rash, haemolytic anaemia, bronchoconstriction	***Assess:*** history of previous allergy to fenamates or aspirin, pregnancy, lactation, dyspepsia, peptic ulceration, concurrent use of coumarin-type anticoagulants, e.g. warfarin; establish baseline description of pain and degree of mobility. ***Administer:*** with food. ***Evaluate:*** for drug effectiveness, e.g. relief of pain and improved mobility; for adverse effects including allergy, (rash, asthma, bronchoconstriction), GIT upsets and bleeding. ***Teach:*** self-evaluation for side effects, the need for compliance to achieve therapeutic benefit; to take with food or milk.
	Diflunisal	Analgesic, anti-inflammatory	Prostaglandin inhibition	Relatively uncommon, may include GIT upset, rash, GIT bleeding	As for salicylates.

	Sodium aurothiomalate	Rheumatoid arthritis	Mechanism of action is unclear, but can control active, progressive disease	Renal failure, blood disorders, rash	***Assess:*** for pregnancy, lactation; for history of liver or renal insufficiency; test urine for protein; for previous hypersensitivity; establish baseline observations of degree of joint function, mobility and pain; baseline blood count may be required. ***Administer:*** by intramuscular injection – dose as ordered at proper intervals. ***Evaluate:*** for improvement in clinical condition; monitor laboratory reports including ESR and blood counts; observe for adverse effects such as pruritus, exfoliative dermatitis, mouth ulcers, bone-marrow suppression, renal impairment; test urine for protein; watch for postinjection vasomotor reactions such as flushing, anxiety or palpitations. ***Teach:*** self-evaluation for improvement and adverse effects; stress importance of keeping appointments for regular checks on urine and blood count and to report adverse effects to physician.
	Penicillamine	Rheumatoid arthritis	Appears to suppress disease activity	Haematological changes, GIT upsets, allergic reactions, renal failure	***Assess:*** as for gold. ***Administer:*** orally – initially low dose increasing to daily maintenance dose as ordered. ***Evaluate:*** as for gold. ***Teach:*** as for gold.

continued

Drug Group	Drug Name	Use	Action	Adverse Reactions	Nursing Implications
Antigout preparations	Colchicine	High dose, in acute gout attack; low doses for long-term prophylaxis	Uricosuric – promotes renal excretion of uric acid	Nausea, diarrhoea	***Assess:*** for history of kidney, liver, heart disease, ulcerative gastrointestinal disorders; document baseline observations of joint swelling and pain and frequency of attacks. ***Administer:*** with food at prescribed intervals until relief is obtained. ***Evaluate:*** for relief of joint pain and swelling; for signs of toxicity – nausea and diarrhoea and abdominal pain; fluid intake and output. ***Teach:*** to initiate therapy at earliest indication of acute attack; to maintain high fluid intake; to self-evaluate for adverse effects and to discontinue therapy when pain is relieved or at signs of toxicity.
	Allopurinol	Long-term gout prophylaxis	Suppress synthesis of uric acid by inhibition of xanthine oxidase	Rash, fever, nausea, diarrhoea, abdominal pain, bone-marrow depression in patients with renal disease	***Assess:*** for pregnancy, hepatic or renal dysfunction. ***Administer:*** with food. ***Evaluate:*** for skin rash, drowsiness, GIT upsets. ***Teach:*** that transient initial increase of attacks may occur and that drug effectiveness may require several weeks; to self-evaluate for adverse effects; to maintain high fluid intake; warn that drowsiness may occur initially and to avoid driving or using power equipment during this time.

	Probenecid Sulphinpyrazone	Long-term gout prophylaxis	Increases renal excretion of uric acid	Probenecid: headache, GIT upset, urinary frequency, anaphylaxis, flushing, dizziness, haemolytic anaemia Sulphinpyrazone: GIT bleeds, rash, anaemia, blood dyscrasias (rare)	***Assess:*** for history of renal calculi, renal disease, hypersensitivity, use of hypoglycaemic drugs or aspirin; establish baseline observations of joint pain, swelling, frequency and severity of attacks. ***Administer:*** with meals. ***Evaluate:*** for adverse effects, especially signs of renal calculi – observe urine for calculi, report complaints of retroperitoneal pain; monitor effects of drug including improvement in condition and/or further attacks. ***Teach:*** to drink at least three litres of fluid per day; may experience fleeting attacks of gout initially as drug starts to take effect; to continue taking drug as prescribed at regular intervals unless otherwise instructed by physician; not to take aspirin or other over-the-counter medication without consulting physician.
Centrally acting muscle relaxants	Methocarbamol Orphenadrine Benzodiazepines, e.g. diazepam	Painful muscle spasm, spasticity	Act on CNS	Drowsiness, confusion (benzodiazepines)	Methocarbamol *(Robaxin)* – ***Assess:*** degree of physical incapacity and current disease state, pregnancy, history for liver, renal, neurological dysfunction. ***Evaluate:*** for drug effectiveness, for adverse effects such as drowsiness, dizziness, blurred vision, weakness, lethargy, ataxia and nystagmus. ***Teach:*** self-evaluation for adverse effects and that motor coordination may be impaired and to take appropriate precautions.

continued

Drug Group	Drug Name	Use	Action	Adverse Reactions	Nursing Implications
					Orphenadrine *(Norflex)* – ***Assess:*** degree of physical incapacity and current disease state; establish baseline observations relating to degree of muscle spasm; general assessment as for anticholinergic drugs. ***Evaluate:*** for drug effectiveness, i.e. improvement in spasm; for anticholinergic side effects. ***Teach:*** as for anticholinergics.
Direct acting muscle relaxants	Dantrolene	Painful muscle spasm, spasticity	Reduces amount of calcium released in muscle	Nausea, diarrhoea, drowsiness, dizziness, speech and visual disturbances, depression, confusion, urinary problems, tachycardia, erratic blood pressure	***Assess:*** history for cardiopulmonary insufficiency, concurrent use of anxiolytic or sedative drugs, pregnancy, renal or hepatic disease, degree of muscle spasm. ***Evaluate:*** for relief of spasm and adverse effects, e.g. GIT upset; check blood pressure and pulse regularly, urine output for signs of retention or frequency; observe for CNS side effects. ***Teach:*** as for methocarbamol.
Indirect acting muscle relaxants	Baclofen	Muscle relaxant, spasticity	Presynaptic inhibition of impulses	Nausea, vomiting, diarrhoea, dyspepsia, asthenia, muscle weakness, hypotonia, tremor, sedation, lethargy, vertigo, headache	***Assess:*** history for convulsive disorders, psychiatric disorders, renal dysfunction, gastric or duodenal ulceration; establish age, pregnancy, lactation, concurrent use of antihypertensive drugs; establish baseline observations for blood pressure, degree of muscle spasm and disability. ***Evaluate:*** for drug

					effectiveness and monitor for adverse effects related to GIT muscle weakness, ataxia, and CNS effects. ***Teach:*** as for methocarbamol.
Enzyme preparations	Trypsin	Removal of coagulated blood and exudates	Proteolytic enzyme	Allergic reactions, angioneurotic oedema	***Assess:*** for known hypersensitivity. ***Administer:*** local as powder or orally, as ordered. ***Evaluate:*** for drug effectiveness and for signs of allergic reaction.
	Chymotrypsin	Ophthalmology, reduction of soft tissue inflammation and oedema	Proteolytic enzyme	Nausea, vomiting, diarrhoea, rash, local irritation	***Assess:*** for known hypersensitivity, hepatic disease, disorders of blood-clotting mechanisms, concurrent use of anticoagulants, pregnancy; establish baseline observations of inflammatory condition. ***Evaluate:*** for drug effectiveness, GIT side effects; monitor carefully for signs of allergy as severe allergic reactions may occur.
	Streptokinase with streptodornase	Lysis of blood clots, resolution of extravasated blood	Converts plasminogen to plasmin	Allergic reactions, nausea, vomiting, diarrhoea, rash, urticaria	***Assess:*** for known hypersensitivity, disorders of blood clotting; establish baseline observations of inflammatory condition. ***Evaluate:*** for drug effectiveness, signs of allergy and adverse effects, usually GIT upsets.

SECTION 6

18
DRUGS USED IN OPHTHALMOLOGY

Margaret P. Shaw

OBJECTIVES

The student should be able to comprehend the following points after reading this chapter:

1. the pharmacological action, use and side effects of drugs used in ophthalmology;
2. the correct storage, dosage, and method of instillation of eye medications.

PREREQUISITE KNOWLEDGE

1. An understanding of the anatomy and physiology of the eye.
2. Common disease states of the eye.
3. The mode of action of antibacterials, corticosteroids and antihistamines.

INTRODUCTION

The following types of preparations may be used in treating problems affecting the eye.

1. ***Eye drops*** for quick local penetration (suitable for daytime use).
2. ***Minims*** — single dose eye drops without preservative.
3. ***Eye ointments*** (suitable for night use); the medication is more slowly released and therefore longer acting.
4. ***Subconjunctival injection*** which gives optimum local effect (antibiotics and steroids).
5. ***Retrobulbar injection*** (for local anaesthetics and alcohol).
6. ***Oral medications,*** for example, antibiotics, steroids.
7. ***Parenteral medications,*** for example, antibiotics and antifungals in sight-threatening infections
8. ***Sustained-release devices*** — the drug is released gradually over a period of time *(Ocusert).*

STANDARDS NECESSARY FOR ALL TOPICAL EYE PREPARATIONS

STERILITY

This is necessary to stop the growth of bacteria. The following methods are used to sterilise eye preparations:

(a) autoclaving if the drug is heat stable;
(b) using a micropore filter;
(c) using aseptic technique if the drug is insoluble, for example, hydrocortisone. The addition of a preservative such as benzalkonium or chlorhexidine helps maintain sterility once the bottle has been opened. Drops with preservative may be used for a week or even up to one month after opening. Drops without preservative should be refrigerated and discarded three days after opening.

STABILITY

This ensures that the drug keeps its full strength and is comfortable on instillation into the eye. It is brought about by adjusting the pH with a buffer, usually borate or phosphate. Drugs unstable to heat should be refrigerated, for example, penicillin.

HOW TO INSTIL EYE DROPS

When an eye drop is instilled, four things may happen.

1. It may run out of the eye and be lost.
2. It may be diluted by tears and lose its effect.
3. It may run down the tear duct and throat into the stomach to give systemic side effects.
4. It may be absorbed into the eye to give the desired effect.

Therefore, the correct method of usage is important. The patient's head should be tilted slightly backwards. Hold the bottle so that it does not touch the lids, and instil one drop into the outer quadrant. Tell the patient to close his eyes. For an ointment, insert it 6 mm inside the lower lid. Replace the cap immediately. Pressure over the puncta will prevent systemic side effects of the more potent drops, for example, mydriatics and timolol.

NURSING IMPLICATIONS

Assessment

Initially the ophthalmic patient should be assessed for any existing visual disability to establish a baseline for observations, plus appropriate nursing actions to assist him or her where necessary. Before the administration of any ophthalmic preparations, a check should be made for any previous allergic reactions to the drug to be used. Of vital importance is the correct and careful identification of the patient. The nurse should be fully conversant with the patient's ophthalmic diagnosis and history, the presence of (or previous history of) other diseases, and the action of the drug to be administered. For example, if a pupil is wrongly dilated this could precipitate a glaucoma attack in some patients. Not only is correct identification of the patient important, but the nurse must make doubly sure which eye is to be treated.

Administration

Because of the delicate nature of the eye, great care must be taken to avoid infection. Precautions to observe during administration relate to keeping the medication from becoming contaminated and avoiding cross-infection between patients. Do not allow the medication container to come into contact with the patient's eye or eyelid. Promptly replace lids on containers. Use individual medication for each patient. Observe proper storage conditions according to manufacturer's directions. Check expiry dates and discard drops one month after opening, or according to the hospital's policy. Ensure the patient receives the correct drug and the correct dose. Ophthalmic drugs are often available in a variety of strengths, so check names and strengths of preparations carefully.

The correct administration procedure is important, as it is concerned with not only preventing infection but also ensuring maximum effect of the medication. (Refer to previous description on how to instil eye drops and ointments.) Systemic side effects of the more potent drugs can be prevented by putting pressure over the puncta. Medications in suspension should be shaken before use. In order to ensure that the drug is given at the correct time, check dosage schedules carefully, and if the patient is to receive more than one medication in the same eye, these may have to be spaced two or more minutes apart to ensure the correct effect of each.

Evaluation

This should include observation of the patient for the required effect of the drug, local signs of allergy, optic or systemic side effects. If it is expected that the drug will have some effect on the patient's vision (for example, photophobia, accommodation difficulties or decreased visual field), ensure the patient understands this, and take appropriate nursing measures to assist him where applicable.

Patient teaching

Ensure the patient (or a member of his family) understands the correct way to instil his eye drops or ointment. Make sure he understands his dosage regime and, if on multiple drops, which one to instil first and the correct time to wait between each installation of drops. Instruct him to report to his doctor any untoward local or systemic effects which could be due to the drug.

THE AUTONOMIC CONTROL OF OCULAR FUNCTION

In order to understand the action of drugs on the eye, here is a brief summary of the autonomic nervous system.

SYMPATHETIC NERVOUS SYSTEM

Noradrenaline and adrenaline released at nerve endings contract the dilator pupillae to produce mydriasis (dilatation of the pupil). Drugs which have the same action are termed sympathomimetic, for example, adrenaline and phenylephrine.

Drugs can be used to block the action of adrenaline at its alpha and beta receptors. The most common one used in the eye is the beta blocker, timolol.

PARASYMPATHETIC NERVOUS SYSTEM

Acetylcholine released at nerve endings contracts the sphincter pupillae to produce miosis (contraction of the pupil). Drugs which have the same action are termed parasympathomimetic or cholinergic, for example, pilocarpine and carbachol.

The action of acetylcholine is terminated by cholinesterase. If a drug is used to combine with or destroy cholinesterase, this allows an accumulation of naturally occurring acetylcholine, thus producing prolonged miosis. Such drugs are called anticholinesterases, for example, physostigmine and ecothiopate.

Drugs that block acetylcholine at its receptors are called anticholinergic, and they dilate the pupil, for example, atropine, homatropine, hyoscine, cyclopentolate and tropicamide. This last group is also cycloplegic (they paralyse the muscles of accommodation).

THE MYDRIATIC DRUGS

ANTICHOLINERGICS

Drugs in this group block the action of acetylcholine and produce mydriasis and cycloplegia. They are used to dilate the pupil preoperatively and postoperatively, after trauma, in the treatment of inflammatory eye conditions (such as iritis and uveitis), to relax the ciliary muscle and to aid healing.

The naturally occurring drug is atropine. It is extracted from *Atropa belladonna* (Deadly Nightshade). Its action may last up to 14 days and is too strong to be reversed by a miotic. Strengths used are 0.5% and 1% drops and 1% ointment. Dosage varies from once or twice a day to four times daily for severe inflammation. Diagnostically it is used for three days before ocular refraction is measured in children. For children up to two years, use 1% ointment twice a day: for two to five years, use 1% ointment or 0.5% drops three times a day: for five to ten years, use 1% drops three times a day.

Related but shorter-acting drugs include ***homatropine*** 1% and 2% drops (lasts 12 to 24 hours) and ***hyoscine*** 0.25% and 0.5% drops (lasts 48 to 72 hours). These may be used when a patient is sensitive to the toxic effects of atropine.

Other mydriatics include ***cyclopentolate*** *(Mydrilate* 0.5% and 1%), and tropicamide *(Mydriacyl* 0.5% and 1%). (*Note:* 0.5% *Mydriacyl* is not a cycloplegic.) Because of their quick onset and shorter duration of action (up to 24 hours and nine hours respectively), they are used when adult refraction is measured. The dosage is one drop repeated in 5-10 minutes if required. Side effects are much less common than with atropine. Cyclopentolate is also used therapeutically when a patient is allergic to atropine or a shorter-acting mydriatic is required.

Adverse Drug Reactions

Possible side effects of the mydriatics

1. Locally: redness, swelling, photophobia and increased intraocular pressure.
2. Systemically: dry mouth, nausea, tachycardia, restlessness and confusion.

NURSING IMPLICATIONS

This is a potent group of drugs, therefore correct and careful identification of the patient is vitally important. For example, the administration of an anticholinergic drop to a patient who has glaucoma could have disastrous consequences.

Be aware of the duration of action of the drug used. If the effect is not to be reversed, ensure that the patient understands that the drug is affecting his vision and accommodation. Take appropriate nursing measures to help him cope with this when necessary. When the pupil is dilated, photophobia can be distressing to the patient, and the use of sunglasses can help alleviate this discomfort.

Systemic side effects of the longer-acting mydriatics can be minimised by putting pressure on the puncta during administration. Use only one drop.

SYMPATHOMIMETICS

This group of drugs are weak mydriatics. They do not produce cycloplegia (for example, ***adrenaline*** (*Eppy* 1%, *Simplene* 0.5% and 1%). They lower intraocular pressure by decreasing the production of aqueous humour and in lower strengths act as a vasoconstrictor.

Adrenaline *(Eppy* 1%, *Simplene* 0.5% and 1%) is used in the treatment of open-angle glaucoma. The usual dosage is one drop twice daily. It is contraindicated in narrow-angle glaucoma as the mydriatic effect could precipitate angle closure. It should be used with caution in hypertensive patients. Protect solutions from air and light, and discard if coloured brown. Prolonged use may cause a brown discolouration of conjunctiva and lens.

Dipivefrin *(Propine* 0.1%) is a new pro-drug. It is not active until converted into adrenaline in the aqueous humour. Local and systemic side effects are less with this drug.

Phenylephrine 10% decreases intraocular pressure in the normal and glaucomatous eye. It is especially good for breaking synechiae (adhesions) in the eye and is used in combination with other mydriatics for intensive dilatation. A 0.125% solution produces a blanching effect only on a red eye. This drug will sting the eye on instillation.

Adverse Drug Reactions

Systemic side effects of the sympathomimetics include nausea, dizziness, headache, tachycardia and increased blood pressure.

Contraindications

Adrenaline is contraindicated in narrow angle glaucoma.

NURSING IMPLICATIONS

Prevent systemic side effects by correct instillation of one drop only. Do not use adrenaline drops if they have turned brown.

THE MIOTICS AND OTHER DRUGS USED IN GLAUCOMA

PARASYMPATHOMIMETICS (CHOLINERGICS)

Drugs in this group simulate the action of acetylcholine. They constrict the pupil to produce miosis, and contract the ciliary muscles to increase the outflow of aqueous humour. Accommodation is also increased. Their main use is in open-angle glaucoma and to reverse the action of mydriatics more rapidly (with the exception of atropine).

Glaucoma is a condition in which there is increased intraocular pressure due to excessive retention of aqueous humour. This is accompanied by a decrease of visual field and changes in the optic disc. The causes of glaucoma are as follows.

1. Obstruction of the flow of aqueous humour in the trabecular network.
2. Narrowing or closure of the filtration (irido-corneal) angle.
3. Congenital.
4. Secondary to injury or drugs (mydriatics or steroids).

If glaucoma is not treated, blindness will result. The aim of treatment is to increase the outflow of aqueous humour or to decrease its production.

Pilocarpine 0.5% to 4% drops are used for chronic open-angle glaucoma. A two-week trial will indicate which strength is suitable. The dose is one drop every 6 hours. In acute glaucoma crises, pilocarpine is used every 15 minutes for 1 to 2 hours, every hour for the next 5 to 6 hours, then every 4 hours for 12 hours to help lower pressure prior to surgery.

Carbachol 3% is slightly more potent than pilocarpine and may be used where a patient does not respond or has become sensitive to pilocarpine.

Adverse Drug Reactions

The parasympathomimetics may cause brow ache, headache, accommodative spasm and decreased visual field. Systemic effects include nausea, diarrhoea, weakness, salivation, sweating and asthma.

Contraindications

Acute iritis and (according to some authorities) narrow angle glaucoma.

NURSING IMPLICATIONS

Identify the patient carefully as, for example, it would be dangerous to administer a miotic to a patient with acute iritis.

Make sure that the patient understands the effects the drug may have on his vision, and take appropriate nursing action to help him cope should these effects occur.

If a cholinergic is combined with adrenaline instil the adrenaline last, five minutes apart. This slight mydriatic effect of adrenaline decreases the miotic effect of the cholinergic to give better vision.

ANTICHOLINESTERASES

These drugs allow the accumulation of naturally occurring acetylcholine by preventing its destruction by cholinesterase. Like the cholinergics, they produce miosis and increase the outflow of aqueous humour but are long acting. They are used for more resistant cases of open-angle glaucoma and in the treatment of accommodative strabismus.

Physostigmine (0.25%, 0.5%) is used every six hours. It should be protected from light. If the solution turns pink, it will be irritant and should be discarded.

Ecothiopate (*Phospholine Iodide* 0.03%, 0.06%, 0.125% and 0.25%) is much longer acting. The dosage is one drop twice a day, and the effect lasts up to four weeks.

Adverse Drug Reactions

These are the same for anticholinergics as for the cholinergics. In addition, ecothiopate can cause pupillary cysts from prolonged constriction, also cataracts. Physostigmine may cause depigmentation of eye lid skin in black patients.

Precautions

Avoid exposure to organo-phosphate compounds (for example, those used during crop dusting). Discontinue therapy for six weeks before a general anaesthetic, as the effect could be fatal if succinylcholine is used in conjunction with an anticholinesterase.

Contraindications
Anticholinesterase drops are contraindicated in narrow-angle glaucoma.

BETA BLOCKERS

The beta blocker commonly used in open angle glaucoma is ***timolol*** (*Timoptol* 0.25% and 0.5%) which acts mainly by decreasing aqueous humour production. The dosage is one drop once or twice a day. It differs from previous glaucoma therapy in that there is no change in pupil size. It may be used alone or in conjunction with a miotic or acetazolamide. If instilled before adrenaline it prevents the mydriatic effect of this drug.

Adverse Drug Reactions
Ocular effects are rare, and systemic effects include asthma and bradycardia.

Contraindications
Timolol is contraindicated in cardiac and asthma patients.

CARBONIC ANHYDRASE INHIBITORS

Carbonic anhydrase is an enzyme which regulates bicarbonate absorption. In the eye, bicarbonate is necessary for the production of aqueous humour. Acetazolamide and dichlorphenamide are drugs which inhibit carbonic anhydrase, thereby modifying bicarbonate absorption. They therefore decrease production of aqueous humour and so lower intraocular pressure. Acetazolamide *(Diamox)* is available as 250 mg tablets or 500 mg sustained release capsules. Maximum daily dosage is 1g in divided doses. It is used for all types of glaucoma, usually in combination with a miotic or adrenaline. For glaucoma patients, before and after surgery, a 500 mg injection is available for IV or IM use. The dose of dichlorphenamide *(Daranide* 50 mg) in a glaucoma crisis is four tablets immediately, then two tablets every 12 hours until controlled. The maintenance dose is one-half to one tablet up to three times a day.

These drugs are also used to lower intraocular pressure after injury or after administration of certain drugs, for example, mydriatics and steroids.

Adverse Drug Reactions
These include nausea, vomiting, diarrhoea and tingling of the extremities. Gastric irritation may be prevented by giving the drug after food, and tingling of the extremities may be remedied by administration of a potassium supplement. Potassium loss may be greater with dichlorphenamide than with acetazolamide.

Contraindications
Acetazolamide is contraindicated in renal failure and acidosis.

NURSING IMPLICATIONS

Because these drugs are derivatives of the sulphonamides, it is important to check for previous history of allergy to any drugs in this group.

The nurse should also be aware of the effect of carbonic anhydrase inhibition on the electrolyte and acid-base balance of the individual. If the drug is to be used for more than one or two doses, there may be increased potassium excretion leading to hypokalaemia and increased bicarbonate excretion (due to retention of hydrogen ions). This can cause a systemic acidosis plus an alkaline urine, which may predispose the patient to stone formation.

The mechanism which causes drowsiness and depression with these drugs is not fully understood.

OSMOTIC DIURETICS

Osmosis occurs when water is drawn through a semipermeable membrane from a region of lower concentration to a region of higher concentration. When an osmotic agent enters the blood stream, it draws water from the aqueous and vitreous humours to reduce intraocular pressure. Osmotic agents are used in glaucoma crises and to restore a flat anterior chamber after operation.

Glycerol is given orally as a 50% flavoured mixture, the dosage being up to 1.5 g/kg. It should be stored under refrigeration and administered cold as it is unpleasant to taste.

For rapid diuresis, a 20% solution of ***mannitol*** is given IVI, the dosage being 1.5 to 2 g/kg. If the solution crystallises, redissolve it by warming before use. The action lasts from 40 minutes up to five or six hours. Another drug is ***urea***, the dosage being 1 g/kg IVI.

Adverse Drug Reactions

Adverse drug reactions of osmotic diuretics include dizziness, headache, nausea and hypokalaemia. Glycerol may raise blood sugar in diabetics.

DRUGS USED IN INFECTIONS OF THE EYE

Eye infections may be bacterial, viral or fungal in origin. A mild infection should be treated topically only, while severe infections and trauma require the addition of systemic medication.

ANTIBACTERIAL DRUGS

The first group of antibacterial drugs act by inhibiting protein synthesis within the bacterial cell. ***Chloramphenicol*** (*Chloromycetin*) drops and ointment have intraocular penetration and a broad spectrum of activity. They are used for conjunctivitis, before and after surgery and after foreign-body removal. Drops must be stored under 8°C. ***Gentamicin*** is particularly effective against pseudomonal endophthalmitis. The drops are used every one to two hours by day and the ointment is used at night. ***Neomycin*** is broad spectrum, and combined with gramicidin and bacitracin, it is known as *Neosporin* and is effective against most gram-positive and gram-negative infections as well as being used before and after surgery.

Polymyxin B acts by restricting bacterial cell-membrane function and is used for pseudomonal corneal ulcers. It is combined with bacitracin as *Polyfax* ointment for broader spectrum. Drops should be stored in the refrigerator.

Penicillin and ***bacitracin*** act on the bacterial cell-wall structure. Penicillin drops are rarely used as they often cause allergies, especially in patients who have had oral penicillin. Their use is restricted to venereal disease affecting the eye, where initial treatment is intensive (every half hour until some improvement, then decreasing to every four hours). Drops should be freshly prepared and refrigerated.

Systemically, penicillin is given in large doses for streptococci and pneumococci, and flucloxacillin is used for resistant "staph" infections. Endophthalmitis may be treated with a combination methicillin and gentamicin or one of the cephalosporin group, for example, cephalothin *(Keflin)* and gentamicin.

Adverse Drug Reactions

Side effects of topical eye treatment are mainly of the allergic type, but precautions should be taken with those drugs that could have systemic side effects. Chloramphenicol can cause aplastic anaemia, and gentamicin may cause hearing damage or kidney damage if too much of the drug is absorbed.

SULPHONAMIDES

The sulphonamides are bacteriostatic and act by interfering with the synthesis of folic acid. ***Sulphacetamide*** *(Albucid)* is used for conjunctivitis. It is likely to cause stinging. Other uses are before and after surgery and after foreign-body removal.

Adverse Drug Reactions

The main side effects are redness, swelling, tear production and stinging.

ANTIVIRALS

The virus *herpes simplex* affects the cornea producing superficial punctate keratitis, and later dendritic ulcers. The lesions may become chronic and result in scarring which impairs the vision. To prevent the initial or epithelial stage of herpes simplex infection from spreading, ***idoxuridine*** *(Kerecid)* drops are used every one to two hours by day and the ointment at night for a maximum of 21 days. It should be used with caution during pregnancy. Intraocular penetration is poor, and for stromal or deeper lesions, ***vidarabine*** *(Vira-A)* should be used. The ointment is instilled five times a day. It penetrates the vitreous humour as the metabolite Ara-Hx and terminates the viral chain.

Acyclovir *(Zovirax)* is a new antiviral ointment. Used five times a day, it differs from the above drugs in that it does not penetrate all the eye tissues, only the viral cells. ***Trifluorothymidine*** is thought to be effective on any Herpes simplex virus infection which is resistant to idoxuridine.

ANTIFUNGALS

Fungi can penetrate the eye via the cornea or posterior chamber. The most common causes of fungal infections are garden matter, cosmetics, and contaminated needles used by drug addicts. Antifungals act by binding to a sterol in the membrane of the fungal cell.

Clotrimazole 1% is effective against *Candida* and *Aspergillus* infections. ***Natamycin*** *(Pimafucin)* has a broader spectrum, but is less effective. ***Amphotericin*** is a strong irritant, and is best avoided because of toxicity to the epithelium.

Antifungal agents are not generally available as eye drops in the UK. Information can be obtained from the District Pharmaceutical Officer or Moorfields Eye Hospital, City Road, London EC1V 2PD (01-253 3411).

Adverse Drug Reactions

When administered parenterally, amphotericin has a number of undesirable effects including fever, headache, nausea, bone marrow depression and renal damage, so it should only be used parenterally as a last resort.

Precautions

Amphotericin I.V. should be protected from light and refrigerated. Intravenous ***miconazole*** *(Daktarin)* may be used parenterally, the dosage being up to 3600 mg daily in three divided doses.

Fungal infections of the eye are difficult to treat, as topical and systemic penetration into the eye is poor, and the fungus may continue to spread even after the corneal wound has healed.

MISCELLANEOUS EYE PREPARATIONS

CORTICOSTEROIDS

Anti-inflammatory steroids used topically inhibit redness, swelling and capillary dilatation in the eye. They also inhibit deposits of collagen (a protein substance that can cause corneal scarring) after chemical burns or trauma. Minor inflammation such as contact dermatitis or allergy is treated with ***hydrocortisone*** 0.5% or 1% drops and ointment. Iritis, uveitis and chemical burns may require a stronger agent such as ***fluorometholone*** *(FML)*, ***prednisolone*** 0.5% *(Predsol)* or ***dexamethasone***

(Maxidex). With the exception of *Predsol*, all are suspensions and should be shaken before use.

Systemically, corticosteroids are given in large doses for optic neuritis, temporal arteritis and as immunosuppressants in sympathetic ophthalmia and thyroid exophthalmos.

Adverse Drug Reactions

The higher the dose, the more likely are adverse effects, so dosage should be kept to a minimum. Adverse effects include corneal thinning, raised intraocular pressure and cataracts after long term usage.

Precautions

Corticosteroids can mask infection and delay wound healing. Antibiotic cover should be added if there is any risk of infection. Corticosteroids should never be used in Herpes simplex infection, but may be used with caution in Herpes zoster, once ulceration is controlled. Corticosteroids must be used with great care in glaucoma patients.

LOCAL ANAESTHETICS

Local anaesthetics act by blocking the conduction of superficial nerves. They also increase the permeability of the cornea. This aids the absorption of other drugs, for example, homatropine and fluorescein. They are used to anaesthetise the cornea before applanation tonometry (a test for intraocular pressure), before the removal of foreign bodies, and for some operations.

Cocaine 1% to 4% acts in 10 minutes, and superficial anaesthesia lasts about two hours. It is also a mydriatic, and blanches the sclera. Combined with homatropine (both in a 2% solution), it is used before surgery to examine the fundus.

Amethocaine is not quite so long acting. It is used before surgery and foreign-body removal. ***Oxybuprocaine*** *(Benoxinate)* acts within 1 minute and corneal sensitivity is normal again after about 1 hour. It is less damaging than amethocaine to the cornea. Three drops at 90 second intervals produce sufficient anaesthesia after 5 minutes to allow minor operations to be carried out.

The short-acting ***proxymetacaine*** *(Ophthaine)* acts in about 20 seconds and lasts for about 15 minutes. It causes less initial stinging, so is useful for children.

Lignocaine (*Xylocaine* 4%) can be used for welding burns, up to six times in 24 hours. The patient should be hospitalised for observation, as anaesthetic drops easily damage the cornea. They also cause loss of blink reflex, so that a foreign body may easily enter the eye. If the eye is rubbed, this will cause further damage. Always tell the patient not to rub his anaesthetised eye. Lignocaine is also used as a retrobulbar injection for local anaesthetic before surgery. The addition of adrenaline prolongs the anaesthetic effect. Lignocaine 4% combined with fluorescein sodium 0.25% is used to aid foreign-body detection.

Adverse Drug Reactions

These include excitement, confusion, headache, nausea, convulsions and respiratory arrest.

STAINING AGENTS

Fluorescein is a phthalein dye that has intense fluorescence in dilute solution. It stains tissues not protected by living epithelium and is available as 1% and 2% minims or sterile impregnated strips. The strips are inserted into the conjunctival cul-de-sac to release the drug. It is used to diagnose abrasions and foreign bodies in the cornea, to check the fit of contact lenses and to check the lachrymal system. After examination, the eye is irrigated with normal saline eye lotion.

Fluorescein injection is used intravenously to examine retinal blood flow and to diagnose retinal detachments.

Adverse Drug Reactions

These include transient nausea, and occasionally urticaria and collapse.

Bengal Rose has more affinity for staining destabilised conjunctival cells. It is available in minims and is used to detect keratoconjunctivitis sicca.

CONJUNCTIVIAL DECONGESTANTS

Decongestants are used to constrict superficial blood vessels of the eye after minor irritation or allergy. A red eye rapidly regains its white look. ***Phenylephrine*** 0.125% may be instilled three or four times a day but should be used with caution, as even this strength may cause mydriasis.

Zinc sulphate 0.25% is an astringent and antiseptic drop used to soothe non-specific irritation. Sometimes it is combined with adrenaline as a vasoconstrictor. ***Adrenaline*** 1:20 000 and 1:1000 solution can be used as a decongestant prior to surgery.

ANTIALLERGY PREPARATIONS

Sodium cromoglycate *(Opticrom)* is prescribed prophylactically to prevent allergies. It acts by stopping the mast cells from rupturing and releasing histamine and is effective for vernal (spring) keratoconjunctivitis. Both antazoline and sodium cromoglycate may be used four times a day.

LUBRICANTS

Lubricants are used to soothe dry eyes, which can result from lack of tears, prolonged periods of unconsciousness, or the inability of the eye lids to close properly after facial palsy or thyrotoxicosis. Lack of treatment may lead to formation of corneal ulcers. Drops used include ***hypromellose*** *(Isopto Alkaline* and *Isopto Plain)* and ***polyvinyl alcohol*** *(Liquifilm)*. They may be used as often as required. For longer contact or night-time use, the ointment *Lacri-Lube* is instilled.

ENZYME PREPARATIONS

Alpha-chymotrypsin is an enzyme used in cataract surgery to dissolve the zonules or ligaments holding the lens in place. This aids easy extraction of the lens in patients over 20 years. The solution is diluted and instilled into the posterior chamber, and afterwards irrigated out of the eye with normal saline eye lotion. Trade names of the preparation include *Chymar-Zon* and *Zonulysin. Chymar-Zon* and *Zonulysin* should be stored in the refrigerator. A possible side effect is increased intraocular pressure.

Urokinase is used to dissolve clots in retinal arteries or veins. It should be refrigerated and protected from light.

CHELATING AGENTS

These drugs remove heavy-metal ions by forming a complex with them. This is necessary if the metal is imbedded in the cornea and cannot easily be extracted or washed away. Calcium deposits after lime burns may be treated with ***disodium edetate*** (EDTA). ***Desferrioxamine*** *(Desferal)* chelates iron deposits in the eye.

MUCOLYTICS

A mucolytic is used to decrease viscid secretions. In the eye it is used to treat chronic ulcerative keratitis. ***N-acetylcysteine*** 10% *(Ilube)* is mixed with ***hypromellose*** eye drops *(Isopto Plain)*, and the drop used four times a day. Once prepared, the product is stable for one month under refrigeration.

COLLAGENASE INHIBITORS

Collagenase is an enzyme which in the epithelium of the eye can break down collagen and cause ulceration. It is released after trauma such as chemical burns, especially lime burns. The newly forming epithelium becomes changed in nature, and the fibrous tissue formed causes scarring. To prevent the action of collagenase, treatment is started with ***L-cysteine*** approximately 48 hours after injury. One ampoule of L-cysteine is mixed with one ampoule of borate buffer and used as an irrigation every two hours. It must be freshly prepared to prevent precipitation. L-cysteine must be stored in the refrigerator.

SYSTEMIC DRUGS WHICH CAUSE OCULAR SIDE EFFECTS

Some drugs taken in large doses over a prolonged period have the potential to cause ocular side effects. In most cases this will be reversible if the dosage is reduced or the drug withdrawn.

The phenothiazines can cause corneal and lens pigmentation and impair vision, especially ***thioridazine*** (*Melleril*) and ***chlorpromazine*** (*Largactil*). ***Trifluoperazine*** (*Stelazine*) can cause oculogyria (the eyes roll back in the head and fixate upwards).

The benzodiazepines, because of their anticholinergic effect, can increase intraocular pressure, for example, ***diazepam*** *(Valium)*. Tricyclic antidepressants have the same effect, for example, ***amitriptyline*** *(Tryptizol)* and ***nortriptyline*** *(Aventyl)*. These two groups should be used with caution in glaucoma patients.

Monoamine oxidase inhibitors (*Parnate* and *Parstelin*) cause blurred vision. ***Chloral hydrate*** (*Noctec*) can cause diplopia (double vision) and miosis.

Barbiturates used long term can paralyse extraocular muscles. In early barbiturate poisoning, the pupils are constricted but react to light. In later stages, the pupils are oblated.

Amiodarone therapy can result in corneal microdeposits.

SELF-EVALUATION TEST

1. List the main use for the following drugs: homatropine, timolol, cyclopentolate, ecothiopate, adrenaline, phenylephrine.
2. Give side effects for: atropine, pilocarpine, adrenaline, phenylephrine, acetazolamide, mannitol.
3. What are the contraindications for: timolol, atropine, adrenaline?
4. In what order would you instil the following:
   (a) adrenaline and pilocarpine;
   (b) chloramphenicol and hydrocortisone. Why?
5. What should you do before instilling a suspension eye drop?
6. How long should you keep eye drops once opened:
   (a) with preservative;
   (b) without preservative.

Table 45
Drugs Used in Opthalmology

Drug Group	Drug Name	Use	Action	Adverse Reactions	Nursing Implications
Anticholinergics	Atropine Homatropine Hyoscine Cyclopentolate Tropicamide	Pupil dilatation	Block acetylcholine, produce mydriasis, and cycloplegia N.B. Tropicamide is not a cycloplegic	Ocular: redness, swelling, photophobia, increased intraocular pressure Systemic: dry mouth, nausea, tachycardia, restlessness, confusion (see Chapter 5)	***Assess:*** correct patient, eye, dose, strength; history of glaucoma, retention of urine; concurrent use of other anticholinergic drugs. ***Administer:*** dose as ordered; use correct administration technique; compress puncta to avoid systemic side effects. ***Evaluate:*** for drug effectiveness in relation to purpose for which it was given; watch for systemic side effects such as dry mouth, tachycardia, restlessness or confusion (cross-reference anticholinergic drugs, Chapter 5). ***Teach:*** make sure the patient understands the effects of the drug and to report any systemic side effects if they occur; instruct on correct administration technique if he is to administer medication himself.
Sympathomimetics	Adrenaline Dipivefrin Phenylephrine	Mydriasis, lower intraocular pressure in glaucoma	Weakly mydriatic, not cycloplegic	Nausea, dizziness, headache, tachycardia, hypertenstion	***Assess:*** correct patient, eye, dose, strength; pulse rate and blood pressure. ***Administer:*** dose as ordered; use correct administration technique. ***Evaluate:*** for drug effectiveness and systemic side effects, including nausea, dizziness, headache, tachycardia or raised blood pressure. ***Teach:*** as for anticholinergics.

continued

Drug Group	Drug Name		Action	Adverse Reactions	Nursing Implications
Parasympatho-mimetics (cholinergics)	Pilocarpine Carbachol	Pupil constriction, miosis, open-angle glaucoma, reversal of mydriatics	Stimulation of acetylcholine, contraction of ciliary muscle, increased aqueous humour outflow	Brow and headache accommodative spasm, nausea, diarrhoea, weakness, salivation, sweating, asthma	***Assess:*** correct patient, eye, dose, strength. ***Administer:*** as ordered; check dosage regime and timing of doses carefully; use correct instillation technique. ***Evaluate:*** for drug effectiveness, for ocular side effects such as brow ache, headache, accommodative spasm, decreased visual field; evaluate for systemic side effects such as nausea, diarrhoea, weakness, salivation, sweating and asthma. ***Teach:*** correct dosage regime and administration technique if patient is to administer medication to himself; ensure he understands the effect of the drug on his accommodation and visual field and reports any untoward local or systemic effects of the medication.
Anticholinesterases	Physostigmine Ecothiopate	Resistant open-angle glaucoma, accommodative strabismus	Prevent enzymatic destruction of acetylcholine, causing miosis and increased aqueous outflow	As for sympathomimetics, Ecothiopate can cause pupillary cysts and cataracts	***Assess:*** as for cholinergics. ***Administer:*** as for cholinergics; do not administer physostigmine if it has turned pink as it will irritate. ***Evaluate:*** as for cholinergics; be aware of the duration of action of these drugs. ***Teach:*** as for cholinergics.

Beta-adrenergic blockers	Timolol	Open-angle glaucoma	Decreases aqueous production	Ocular ADRs are rare, systemic ADRs, see Chapter 5	***Assess:*** correct patient, eye. dose; previous history of asthma or heart failure, establish baseline pulse rate. ***Administer:*** dose as ordered; use correct administration technique. ***Evaluate:*** for drug effectiveness; note there is no change in pupil size with timolol; watch for signs of asthma and bradycardia. ***Teach:*** correct administration technique and to report systemic side effects if they occur.
Carbonic anhydrase inhibitors	Acetazolamide Dichlorphenamide	Lower intraocular pressure in glaucoma	Inhibition of carbonic anhydrase so modifying bicarbonate absorption	Nausea, vomiting, diarrhoea, gastric irritation, tingling of extremities	***Assess:*** hypersensitivity to sulphonamides, pregnancy, weight, intraocular pressure, hepatic or renal disease, fluid and electrolyte balance, cardiac disease. ***Administer:*** dose as ordered, give oral doses after food to prevent gastric irritation. ***Evaluate:*** for drug effectiveness; check pH of urine, ensure adequate fluid intake to prevent stone formation (long-term use); watch for signs of hypokalaemia including paraesthesia, muscle weakness, cardiac irregularities; signs of acidosis include fatigue, confusion, hyperventilation. Drowsiness and gastric irritation may occur. ***Teach:*** that drowsiness may occur and to avoid activities where full alertness is required; teach to replace potassium in diet.

continued

Drug Group	Drug Name		Action	Adverse Reactions	Nursing Implications
Osmotic diuretics	Glycerol Mannitol Urea	Glaucoma crisis	Draws water by osmosis from aqueous and vitreous humours	Glycerol may raise blood sugar levels. Dehydration and electrolyte imbalances if therapy too vigorous	Glycerol — ***Assess:*** fluid and electrolyte balance; intraocular pressure, weight, urine for sugar, history of diabetes. ***Administer:*** orally as 50% flavoured mixture — up to 1.5 g/kg; store in refrigerator and give cold. ***Evaluate:*** reduction in intraocular pressure, tolerance to unpleasant taste, urine output, signs of dehydration, hypokalaemia, dizziness, headache, nausea. ***Teach:*** ensure patient understands reason for this type of therapy and that his urine output will increase. Mannitol — ***Assess:*** fluid and electrolyte balance, intraocular pressure, weight. ***Administer:*** IV — as ordered. ***Evaluate:*** as for glycerol. ***Teach:*** as for glycerol.
Antibacterials	Chloram-phenicol Gentamicin Neomycin Polymyxin Penicillin Bacitracin	Bacterial eye infections	See Chapter 22 for mode of action of various antibacterials	Mainly allergic reactions; caution with drugs which may be absorbed systemically, e.g. chloramphenicol which may cause aplastic anaemia and gentamicin which may lead to renal damage and damage to 8th cranial nerve	***Assess:*** history of hypersensitivity to drug; correct eye, dose, dose regime. ***Administer:*** use correct instillation technique; observe correct dosage regime and correct storage precautions. ***Evaluate:*** effectiveness of drug (reduction in the signs of infection); signs of allergy, signs of systemic side effects with the more toxic drugs, e.g. chloramphenicol, gentamicin. ***Teach:*** correct administration procedure, dosage regime and storage precautions.

Sulphonamides	Sulphacetamide	Bacterial eye infections	Bacteriostatic, interferes with bacterial folic-acid synthesis	Redness, watering, swelling, stinging	***Assess:*** as for antibacterials. ***Administer:*** as for antibacterials. ***Evaluate:*** effectiveness of drug, signs of allergy or irritation. ***Teach:*** as for antibacterials; drops may sting on application.
Antivirals	Idoxuridine Vidarabine Acyclovir Trifluoro-thymidine	Viral eye infections	Antiviral (see Chapter 24)	Local stinging	***Assess:*** as for antibacterials; caution in pregnancy. ***Administer:*** as for antibacterials. ***Evaluate:*** drug effectiveness. ***Teach:*** as for antibacterials.
Antifungals	Natamycin Amphotericin Miconazole Clotrimazole	Fungal eye infections	Antifungal, see Chapter 24; penetration of the eye by antifungals is poor, topically and after IV administration	See Chapter 24	***Assess:*** as for antibacterials. ***Administer:*** as for antibacterials; shake suspensions before use. ***Evaluate:*** as for antibacterials. ***Teach:*** as for antibacterials; shake suspensions.
Corticosteroids	Hydrocortisone Fluoro-metholone Prednisolone Dexamethasone	Redness, swelling, capillary dilatation, after burns and trauma to prevent corneal scarring, minor inflammation, allergy	Anti-inflammatory (see Chapter 11)	Corneal thinning after long-term use; raised intraocular pressure masking of infection, delayed wound healing, may be systemically absorbed	***Assess:*** presence of infection, intraocular pressure, presence of glaucoma, herpes simplex; identify correct patient, eye, dose. ***Administer:*** as ordered; use correct technique, shake suspensions; instil suspension drops last if other drops being used. ***Evaluate:*** for reduction in inflammation (lessening of redness, swelling and capillary dilatation); observe for signs of infection, raised intraocular pressure, visual impairment. ***Teach:*** to use these drugs only as ordered by the doctor, and to report any unusual visual effects, e.g. pain, visual impairment.

continued

Drug Group	Drug Name		Action	Adverse Reactions	Nursing Implications
Local anaesthetics	Cocaine Amethocaine Oxybuprocaine Lignocaine Proxymetacaine	Anaesthesia of eye	Block conduction along superficial nerves, increased corneal permeability	Corneal damage, loss of blink reflex, excitement, confusion, headache, nausea, convulsions, respiratory arrest	***Assess:*** correct patient, eye, dose and reason for use. ***Administer:*** use correct technique; administer at ordered intervals where applicable; be aware of type of local anaesthetic drops being administered and duration of action of the drug; advisable to protect eye with a pad. ***Evaluate:*** for required effect; ensure the cornea is protected as the blinking reflex will be lost, and the cornea could easily be damaged; observe for systemic side effects such as excitement and confusion. ***Teach:*** instruct the patient not to rub anaesthetised eye as the cornea could be damaged.
Staining agents	Fluorescein	Diagnosis of abrasions and foreign bodies in cornea, checking lachrymal system, IV to examine retinal blood flow	Stains tissues not protected by living epithelium	Local ADR: rare; IV: transient nausea, urticaria, collapse	***Assess:*** for local application — correct patient, eye, dose; for IV fluorescein — establish baseline vital signs and skin colour. ***Administer:*** local — as ordered, after examination irrigate eye with normal saline; IV fluorescein — as ordered, use freshly prepared solutions. ***Evaluate:*** after IV fluorescein — vital signs, watch for nausea, signs of allergic reactions, observe for yellowing of

					skin. ***Teach:*** ensure that patient understands that his skin may be coloured yellow after IV fluorescein, but that this fades after 24 hours.
	Bengal rose	Detection of kerato-conjunctivitis sicca	Stains destabilised conjunctival cells	Rare	
Conjunctival decongestants	Phenylephrine	To reduce redness after minor irritation or allergy	Constriction of superficial blood vessels (sympathomimetic)	Slight stinging on instillation, Systemic: as for sympathomimetics	***Assess:*** correct patient, eye dose, strength; establish baseline pulse rate and BP. ***Administer:*** correct dose and interval as ordered; use correct technique. ***Evaluate:*** for desired effect of drug, mydriasis, signs of increased intraocular pressure, systemic side effects such as tachycardia, raised blood pressure. ***Teach:*** correct instillation technique and that these drugs should only be used as ordered and for a limited period.

19

DRUG TREATMENT OF COMMON DISEASES OF THE EAR, NOSE, THROAT AND MOUTH

Julie Hilditch

OBJECTIVES

At the conclusion of this chapter the reader should be able to:

1. outline briefly the use of drugs in the treatment of:
   (a) rhinitis (allergic, vasomotor and infectious)
   (b) sinusitis
   (c) otitis externa (acute and chronic)
   (d) otitis media (acute, chronic and secretory)
   (e) acute pharyngitis, tonsillitis and laryngitis
   (f) mouth ulcers
   (g) fungal infections of the mouth
   (h) *herpes simplex* infections of lips and oral cavity;
2. explain why nasal decongestant sprays or drops should not be used for prolonged periods or more frequently than directed;
3. give the reason why sodium cromoglycate and beclomethasone should be used regularly and not whenever necessary;
4. detail the instructions which should be given to patients or their parents to minimise the risk of recurrence of chronic otitis externa;
5. state two reasons why nasal decongestants are useful in otitis media;
6. list three reasons to avoid prolonged use of topical antibiotics such as framycetin, gentamicin, and neomycin in chronic ear disease;
7. list three preparations which can be used in the ear to soften wax.

PREREQUISITE KNOWLEDGE

1. Structure and functions of the ear, nose, throat and mouth.
2. Common disease states of the ear, nose, throat and mouth.

COMMON DISEASES OF THE NOSE

In this section we will look at the drug therapy of the following common diseases of the nose.

Allergic rhinitis

This can be either seasonal — the symptoms of rhinitis are due to allergy to inhaled pollens of grasses and flowers (popularly known as "hay fever") — or perennial, resulting from allergy to house dust, dust mites, moulds and foods.

Vasomotor rhinitis (sometimes called non-allergic rhinitis)

This is a poorly understood entity which seems to be due to an imbalance between the parasympathetic and the sympathetic nerve supply to the nose.

Infectious rhinitis (viral and bacterial)

Acute viral rhinitis is exceedingly common and usually presents as a manifestation of the common cold and upper respiratory tract influenzal infections. Bacterial infections are less common and are generally secondary to viral infections.

Sinusitis

This is usually a viral infection which often originates as an acute viral rhinitis and spreads to the sinuses.

ALLERGIC RHINITIS — TREATMENT

Avoidance

Elimination or avoidance of known allergens is the ideal method of treatment of allergic rhinitis. However, it is rare that patients are allergic to one allergen only, and the identification and elimination from the patient's environment and/or diet of all offending allergens may be very difficult.

Desensitisation (Hyposensitisation)

If, after the allergens are identified, it is impractical to eliminate or avoid them, desensitisation treatment can be considered. Specific desensitisation is carried out by administering a carefully estimated dose of the allergen to a patient by subcutaneous injection or by a sublingual drop method. The dose is gradually increased at weekly intervals. Good results have been seen with careful and adequate desensitisation in seasonal allergic rhinitis. It is less likely to help in the perennial allergic rhinitis. All forms of desensitisation carry the risk of an anaphylactic reaction. Therefore, adrenaline, hydrocortisone and an antihistamine injection should always be readily available.

If avoidance or desensitisation is not practical one or more of the following medications can be tried.

Nasal Decongestants

The drugs which are classified as nasal decongestants may be either topical or oral. Topical presentations (nose drops and spray) include ***phenylephrine*** *(Neophryn)*, ***oxymetazoline*** *(Afrazine, Vicks Sinex)*, and ***xylometazoline*** *(Otrivine)*. Oral preparations of ***ephedrine*** and ***pseudoephedrine*** *(Sudafed)* are available.

Action

Normal nasal patency depends on a constant sympathetic nervous stimulation to nasal blood vessels. This sympathetic stimulation causes vasoconstriction and enlarges the nasal airway. All of the decongestants are sympathomimetic, that is they mimic the action of the sympathetic nervous system. Therefore, the decongestants cause vasoconstriction of the blood vessels and promote shrinkage of swollen nasal mucosa, thus increasing the airway and improving ventilation. The decongestants are sometimes called vasoconstrictors.

Uses

The decongestants provide relief of congestion of the nasopharyngeal mucous membranes in allergic, infective and vasomotor rhinitis. Remember that only symptomatic relief is provided and chronic use is to be avoided. (These agents also reduce congestion and facilitate drainage from the eustachian tube. Thus they are used as adjunctive therapy in otitis media).

The topical decongestants act selectively on the nasal mucosa and have the advantage of a faster onset of action than the oral forms. However, they are also associated with some problems peculiar to their topical applications

Adverse Drug Reactions

The most significant adverse reaction associated with the locally applied decongestants is a rebound oedema of the nasal mucosa. This can lead to further use of the decongestant and a pattern of repeated use established. Eventually, repeated use can lead to irreversible changes in the vasomotor structure and mucous membrane. This is sometimes called rhinitis medicamentosa.

The topical decongestants interfere with ciliary activity and decrease mucosal blood flow. Therefore, it has also been suggested that their excessive use could interfere with normal body mechanisms for eliminating toxins and prolong or add to disability. Topical decongestants are thus only indicated for short-term use, that is, five to seven days. They should not be used more frequently than directed.

The systemic decongestants can cause typical sympathomimetic effects, that is, an increase in blood pressure, tachycardia, palpitations, nervousness, insomnia, urinary retention, sweating or flushing, and tremor. Systemic absorption is usually not significant with the topically applied drugs. However, in sensitive patients or in overdosage, adverse sympathomimetic reactions as described may be noted.

Contraindications and Precautions

These drugs should be administered cautiously to infants and children, the elderly and hypertensive and cardiac patients. In patients with prostatic enlargement, there may be increased urinary retention. Patients who are taking monoamine oxidase inhibitors for treatment of depression should be warned to avoid these nasal decongestants as there is a danger of an exaggerated sympathomimetic reaction.

Antihistamines

The antihistamines are dealt with in detail elsewhere (see page 356). They may be used to relieve the sneezing and rhinorrhoea of allergic rhinitis. They are of most use in mild bouts of seasonal allergic rhinitis but are less effective in perennial allergic rhinitis. Drowsiness is the major adverse reaction. Numerous antihistamine-decongestant drug combinations are available. Common combinations are listed in Table 46.

Table 46
Common Antihistamine-Decongestant Combinations

Trade Name	Antihistamine	Decongestant
Actifed	Triprolidine	Pseudoephedrine
Congesteze	Azatadine	Pseudoephedrine
Dimotane	Brompheniramine	Phenylephrine Phenylpropanolamine

Sodium Cromoglycate (*Rynacrom*)

Sodium cromoglycate is used primarily in the treatment of asthma. It has been formulated as a capsule for nasal insufflation and as a nasal spray for use in allergic rhinitis. Eye drops are also available for the eye symptoms of allergic rhinitis.

Actions

Sodium cromoglycate acts to inhibit the release of chemical mediators, such as histamine, from mast cells. It is these chemical mediators which, when released in response to exposure to an allergen, cause the familiar local "allergic" reactions.

Use

Sodium cromoglycate is used as a prophylactic agent to prevent the development of allergic rhinitis, both seasonal and perennial. The sodium cromoglycate must be available to the mast cell at, or before, exposure to the allergen so it should be used regularly and not on development of the symptoms of rhinitis.

Adverse Drug Reactions

The only adverse reaction reported in the use of intranasal sodium cromoglycate is irritation of the nasal mucosa.

Intranasal Corticosteroids

Intranasal corticosteroids include the drug ***betamethasone*** *(Betnesol)*, ***beclomethasone*** *(Beconase)*, and ***flunisolide*** *(Syntaris)*.

Action

Administration of a corticosteroid directly into the nose provides high concentrations of steroid in nasal tissues but low systemic levels, therefore minimising the risk of adverse systemic effects. Intranasal corticosteroids act to decrease inflammation and oedema of the nasal mucosa. Their exact mode of action is unknown.

Uses

The intranasal corticosteroids are generally used only in severe rhinitis where symptoms cannot be controlled by alternative methods. The onset of action is delayed, taking three to seven days to decongest a swollen nose. Dosage should be regular and not "when required" for symptomatic relief.

Adverse Drug Reactions

The only common reaction noted is a burning or stinging sensation and sneezing on administration. Haemorrhagic secretions and an increased incidence of nasal and sinus infections have also been noted, but less commonly. Long-term high-dose topical steroid use has the potential to produce increased capillary fragility and mucosal atrophy. However, nasal mucosal atrophy has not been reported with use of intranasal corticosteroids at recommended dosages.

There appears to be little systemic absorption from the intranasal corticosteroids at regular doses. However, excessive doses may lead to suppression of the hypothalamic-pituitary-adrenal axis. A total daily dose of beclomethasone of 1 mg (20 puffs) should not be exceeded. (Administration of beclomethasone inhalant into the lungs should also not exceed 1 mg per day.) For flunisolide, a total daily dose of 0.4 mg (eight sprays in each nostril) in adults, and 0.2 mg in children under 15 years, should not be exceeded.

Gross overdosage has not been reported, but it could give rise to signs and symptoms of Cushing's Disease. Because there is not adequate data on long-term safety of the intranasal corticosteroids it is recommended that their use be of a limited duration.

VASOMOTOR RHINITIS

Drug treatment of vasomotor rhinitis is difficult. Patients with this disorder are often abusers of topical decongestant sprays or drops and rhinitis medicamentosa is typical. ***Oral decongestants*** can be used, but in high doses tachycardia may be a problem. ***Antihistamines*** are of little use although some antihistamines with anticholinergic and vasoconstrictor activity may help relieve rhinorrhoea or nasal congestion. Perhaps more effective is the use of intranasal beclomethasone.

Ipratropium bromide *(Atrovent),* a topically active anticholinergic drug, decreases the excessive watery secretions found in vasomotor rhinitis. It acts within a few minutes and thus can be used when symptoms occur. It is available in the UK as an aerosol for treatment of asthma, but it is not yet approved for use in rhinitis.

INFECTIOUS RHINITIS

There is no known specific treatment for acute viral rhinitis, but symptomatic treatment can mitigate the severity of the attack. Local symptoms of rhinitis can be treated with ***topical decongestants***, although excessive use should be avoided. ***A steam inhalation*** can help liquefy secretions, decreasing their viscosity and thus promoting drainage and easing the nasal congestion. ***Menthol*** or ***benzoin tincture, compound*** are sometimes added to a steam inhalation but their therapeutic value is questionable.

Antihistamines will not reduce or abolish the symptoms but may have a place in treatment of the allergic patient who is often particularly susceptible to such infections.

Bed rest, if possible, and analgesics and antipyretics such as ***aspirin*** or ***paracetamol*** may help the general malaise, aching and feverishness of the cold. Copious fluids should be ingested.

Antibiotics are not indicated in a viral infection and should only be used if secondary bacterial infection supervenes. Congestion persisting for seven to 10 days or purulent discharge suggests bacterial involvement. Appropriate oral antibiotics, as determined by culture and sensitivity tests should be commenced immediately.

The most common bacteria responsible for rhinitis are pneumococci and streptococci, so ***benzylpenicillin*** or ***phenoxymethylpenicillin*** are drugs of choice. If *E. coli* or *H. influenzae* is suspected, ***ampicillin*** or ***amoxycillin*** is more effective. ***Cloxacillin*** or ***flucloxacillin*** may be necessary if the penicillinase-positive *Staphylococcus aureus* is cultured.

SINUSITIS

Acute sinusitis is usually associated with a viral rhinitis. Unless a secondary bacterial infection supervenes treatment is symptomatic and similar to that indicated in acute viral rhinitis.

If secondary bacterial infection does supervene, an appropriate antibiotic should be commenced. The most likely pathogens are pneumococci, streptococci, *Staphylococcus aureus,* or *Haemophilus influenzae.* Antibiotics of choice are ***ampicillin, amoxycillin*** or ***co-trimoxazole.*** A tetracycline such as ***doxycycline*** can be used but it is not appropriate for children in view of its adverse effects on tooth development. ***Erythromycin*** can be used in penicillin-allergic patients.

NURSING IMPLICATIONS

Assessment

The nurse should be aware of the diagnosis and predisposing causes of the patient's condition, allergy, or infection. Assessment should also include a check on the concurrent use by the patient of other drugs (including alcohol), in order to exclude the risk of drug interactions occuring, especially if the medication is to be administered systemically or there is the risk of systemic absorption. Where the latter is concerned, the existence of pre-existing disease states, which could be exacerbated by the drug, should be excluded.

Administration

As with all medication administration, correct identification of the patient, drug, dosage and time is essential. Use correct technique for instilling drops, drugs by insufflation and metered aerosols. Ensure that sympathomimetic decongestants are administered only as ordered and for no longer than five to seven days, due to the risk of rebound rhinitis.

Evaluation

Observe the patient for relief of symptoms and any adverse effects of the medication such as insomnia or palpitations with sympathomimetic decongestants, or drowsiness with antihistamines. If the patient is administering the medication himself (for example, an insufflation) make sure he is doing it correctly.

Patient teaching

Make sure the patient understands his condition and its treatment. This goes a long way towards gaining his cooperation and ensuring compliance. If allergic rhinitis is the problem and the allergen(s) have been identified, discuss with him how these can best be avoided in his environment and/or diet.

If he has a nasal or sinus infection, he should be warned against blowing his nose too forcefully as this could spread the infection. If topical decongestants are being used, make sure the patient understands that they should not be used for longer than five to seven days and to use no more frequently than at the times ordered.

Teach the patient the correct administration techniques for topical applications, and where topical corticosteroids are prescribed, make sure the patient understands that these do not produce an immediate effect.

Where antihistamines are prescribed, warn the patient that drowsiness may occur and to avoid driving or operating machinery. He should also be warned that alcohol and other CNS depressant drugs such as tranquillisers potentiate the sedative effects of antihistamines.

If there is a risk of systemic side effects occurring where the patient is prescribed a sympathomimetic decongestant, he should be advised to report any of these effects if they occur.

COMMON DISEASES OF THE EAR

In this section, drug treatment of the following common ear conditions will be discussed: **otitis externa** (acute and chronic), **otitis media** (acute, chronic and secretory), **mastoiditis** and **impacted wax.**

OTITIS EXTERNA

Two main classifications of otitis externa are recognised: acute (localised) otitis externa (furunculosis), an acute infection around the hair follicles of the ear canal with subsequent boil formation; and chronic or diffuse otitis externa, which may be due to a primary infection (bacterial, viral or fungal) or may be a secondary infection of a generalised dermatitis. Recurrences are often precipitated by scratching and/or wetting of the ear canal. "Swimmer's ear" is a recurrent oedematous otitis externa.

Drug treatment of acute localised otitis externa

Treatment of otitis externa initially involves scrupulous cleansing of the ear by curettage, suction or syringing, followed by careful drying and wiping with a solution of 70% to 95% alcohol. As most of these infections are due to either *Staphylococcus* or *Streptococcus,* oral ***cloxacillin*** or ***flucloxacillin*** should be commenced. In severe cases parenteral cloxacillin may be necessary. Treatment should be continued for seven to 10 days. Systemic analgesics such as ***aspirin*** or ***paracetamol and codeine*** will often be necessary. In severe cases narcotic analgesics may be required for the first 24 hours. Local heat such as a covered hot water bottle, electric heating pad or heat lamp can help to relieve pain.

Drug treatment of chronic or diffuse otitis externa

Again scrupulous cleansing and drying of the ear canal is necessary. No topical therapy is effective unless the outer ear is free of debris. Many products have been used topically to treat the infection, inflammation and swelling of diffuse otitis externa. Drugs commonly used include ***ichthammol, aluminium acetate solution, alcoholic solutions, antibiotics, antifungal agents*** and ***corticosteroids.***

Ichthammol is a weak antiseptic agent with emollient properties. Ear drops of ichthammol 10% in glycerine are used to treat local inflammation and swelling of the external ear. Aluminium acetate solution is an astringent which, when applied to the external ear canal, dries it and forms a protective layer on the mucosa. The aluminium acetate solution is also acidic and helps to restore the normal acidity of the ear canal. (The skin of the ear canal should have an acidic surface which inhibits bacterial growth. Changes in this acidity can allow infections to develop). Alcoholic ear drops (70% to 90% ethanol) exert a local bactericidal action as well as drying the external ear canal.

Antibiotic ear drops are often prescribed to treat the infectious component in diffuse otitis externa. As the infection is commonly due to a gram-negative organism the antibiotic employed is usually an aminoglycoside such as ***gentamicin***, ***framycetin*** or ***neomycin*** sometimes combined with ***polymyxin***, ***gramicidin*** or ***bacitracin***. A corticosteroid is often included in the formulation. Examples of such ear drops include *Betnesol-N*, *Otosporin* and *Sofradex*.

The use of topical antibiotics is associated with certain problems. The main problems are local skin sensitisation especially to neomycin; emergence of resistant strains of bacteria and overgrowth of yeast and fungi with prolonged use.

A combination antiseptic/corticosteroid ear drop containing the antiseptic ***clioquinol*** *(Locorten-Vioform)* can be used as an alternative to the antibiotic/corticosteroid ear drops.

Topically applied antibiotics will not penetrate into abscesses and thus are not usually indicated in acute localised otitis externa.

In cases of otomycosis, antifungal ear drops containing clotrimazole are required. Corticosteroid ear drops act to decrease inflammation and swelling.

The majority of cases of diffuse otitis externa can be controlled by aluminium-acetate solution or acetic acid in 70% alcohol. In severe cases the exudate should be cultured for antibiotic sensitivity to ensure an appropriate agent is being used.

Occasionally systemic antibiotics (determined by swabs for culture and sensitivities) are necessary, but generally local drugs will suffice. In cases where there is severe swelling, oral or parenteral corticosteroids may be required in order to reduce the oedema enough to allow penetration of topical medications.

Symptomatic treatment will usually be required as well. Simple oral analgesics should be given as required. For itchy ears, crotamiton cream or lotion (*Eurax*) may be rubbed in gently. Corticosteroid creams have a similar action but because long-term application can cause atrophy of the skin, their unnecessary use is best avoided. An oral antihistamine may also be required for the itching. In severe cases a sedative may sometimes be required for a couple of nights.

Recurrent crusting or itching of the meatus after the course of ear drops is completed may necessitate prophylactic use of steroid drops.

If the otitis externa is associated with other conditions, for example, dermatitis, this must also be treated.

Prevention of relapse

The patient should be advised to avoid scratching or rubbing in and around ears. This includes over-enthusiastic cleansing of the canal.

The ear canal must be kept dry. Cotton wool or gauze plugs smeared with soft paraffin should be used in the ears whenever there is a danger of water entering the canal, for example, when washing hair or showering. Using such ear plugs and a bathing cap, limited swimming is also possible. If accidental wetting occurs, the ears should be dried immediately and drops such as ***acetic acid 5%***, or ***aluminium acetate 8% (in ethanol 70%)*** instilled. (As previously mentioned, these drops dry the skin, are bactericidal and fungicidal, and maintain the normal pH of the skin). The prophylactic use of these drops, especially in patients liable to have repeatedly wet ears (for example, swimmers) can be useful in the prevention of recurrence.

OTITIS MEDIA

Otitis media, one of the most common illnesses encountered by the general practitioner, is essentially a disease of childhood. It may be classified as acute, chronic, or secretory; or as mastoiditis. The basic aims of treatment are to control infection in the middle ear, restore normal eustachian-tube function and ventilation to the middle ear, and to provide symptomatic relief of pain.

Drug treatment of acute otitis media

Treatment of acute otitis media is by systemic antibiotics, nasal decongestants and analgesics.

The common infecting organisms of otitis media are pneumococci, *Haemophilus influenzae,* beta-haemolytic *Streptococcus* and less commonly *Staphylococcus aureus.* In children under six years old, *Haemophilus influenzae* is the most common pathogen.

The antibiotic of choice in acute otitis media is ***ampicillin*** or ***amoxycillin.*** In patients who are allergic to penicillins, ***erythromycin,*** a ***sulphonamide*** or ***co-trimoxazole*** is used. Recently there have been increasing reports of an ampicillin-amoxycillin resistant *H. influenzae,* necessitating a change of antibiotic treatment. In this instance erythromycin, a sulphonamide or co-trimoxazole is recommended. A 10-day course is advisable to prevent the development of secretory otitis media, although there is some evidence that a shorter course may be equally effective.

Nasal decongestants are used to clear the nose and the eustachian tubes. The middle ear and eustachian tubes are extensions of the upper lateral part of the back of the nose. The opening of the eustachian tube allows ventilation and drainage of the middle ear, therefore it is important to establish a clear nasal passage and eustachian patency. Note also that the eustachian tube only opens with swallowing. A patient who breathes through his or her mouth swallows infrequently. Thus mouth breathing will exacerbate a problem of poor middle-ear ventilation and drainage and prevent or delay resolution of middle-ear function.

Nasal decongestants, either nose drops such as ***phenylephrine, oxymetazoline*** or ***xylometazoline*** or oral agents such as ***ephedrine*** or ***pseudoephedrine*** will clear the nose and the eustachian tubes, thus facilitating nose breathing and promoting natural drainage and re-aeration of the middle ear. (For more details about nasal decongestants see page 338).

Rest and sedation are required. Local application of heat will help ease pain. ***Glycerin*** or ***olive oil*** warmed to body temperature is an effective heat-retaining ear drop which will also help relieve ear ache. If the tympanic membrane is ruptured, however, oily ear drops are contraindicated. Topical solutions containing local anaesthetics such as ***benzocaine*** or ***lignocaine*** can also be used, warmed to body temperature, to fill the ear canal. Such drops should be used with caution as they tend to obscure the tympanic membrane and may be mistaken for discharge.

Systemic analgesics such as ***aspirin*** and ***paracetamol*** are often required. ***Codeine phosphate*** can be added if pain becomes severe.

Treatment of a ruptured membrane

The pressure within the middle ear can increase to the point where the tympanic membrane ruptures, resulting in a mucopurulent discharge. If the discharge persists after thorough cleaning and drying, an anti-infective ear drop or powder should be used. The purpose of this is to disinfect the macerated skin which would otherwise provide an ideal bacterial incubator encouraging a secondary bacterial external otitis infection. Topical agents such as described for the treatment of chronic or diffuse otitis externa are usually used (see page 343). With adequate treatment, the ruptured tympanic membrane should heal spontaneously, but in some instances the perforation may remain open and chronic otitis media may develop.

Drug treatment of chronic otitis media

Chronic otitis media is the chronic or recurrent discharge of pus or mucopus through a pre-existing eardrum perforation. It is usually the result of repeated unresolved bouts of acute otitis media. Reinfection occurs via upper respiratory-tract infections by way of the eustachian tubes or by water entering the middle ear via the patent perforation.

A course of systemic antibiotic may be necessary to clear any residual infection. The choice of antibiotics should be determined by culture and sensitivity tests. Treatment is then directed at ensuring a healthy nose and paranasal sinuses. Causes of nasal and eustachian obstruction must be corrected — for example, nasal allergy should be treated, adenoidectomy and nasal-septal operations performed if required. Once the nasal airway has been cleared, children should be educated to breathe through it rather than the mouth. At the same time careful local aural toilet should be maintained. Topical application of antibacterial drops or powder once daily for several weeks may be necessary. Swabs for culture and sensitivities should be performed to isolate the causative bacteria. The organism is commonly a *Pseudomonas* or *Proteus*. Topical antibacterials commonly used include ***alcohol 70%***, ***acetic acid 1% to 5%***, or an antibiotic ear drop such as ***gentamicin*** or ***chloramphenicol***. Occasionally a yeast infection will be found in which case clotrimazole should be used. If the exudate does not clear up after six weeks of intensive therapy, tympanomastoid surgery may be required.

Secretory otitis media (Glue Ear)

This condition is characterised by the presence of a non-inflammatory exudate in the middle ear. The exudate is thick and glue or gum-like — hence the popular name "glue ear". It usually affects children of primary school age.

Again treatment is aimed at clearing the exudate and establishing adequate drainage in the area. Persistent oedema and obstruction of the eustachian tubes with inadequate aeration of the middle ear is commonly found in this disease.

Medical teatment should be tried first, including ***nasal decongestants*** (as previously described); ***antihistamines*** (where allergy plays a role in nasal bockage, the use of antihistamines is appropriate); other anti-allergy treatment (as allergy of the nose or upper respiratory tract is often associated with secretory otitis media, other suitable anti-allergy treatment should be considered, for example, avoidance of allergen, desensitisation, ***sodium cromoglycate nasal, beclomethasone nasal*** — see page 339 for further details); ***corticosteroids*** (these agents have a strong anti-allergy and anti-inflammatory effect and can be used either orally or by IM injection in severe cases for a short period); and ***bromhexine*** (*Bisolvon*). Bromhexine is an oral mucolytic agent which reduces the viscosity of mucus in chronic chest disease. It has recently been tried in secretory otitis media with encouraging results.

Persistent fluid behind the ear drum should be treated by myringotomy followed by aspiration of exudate with or without insertion of ventilatory tubes (grommets).

MASTOIDITIS

Mastoiditis, which may be associated with either acute or chronic otitis media, occurs when the infection spreads beyond the middle ear mucosa to involve the bone of the posterior middle ear and mastoid region.

Once the diagnosis is made, treatment is started with IV antibiotics followed by several weeks of oral therapy. If the results of culture are unknown, ampicillin or amoxycillin should be started. Adequate middle ear drainage must also be established. Surgical intervention may be required in chronic mastoiditis.

IMPACTED WAX

Wax (cerumen) consists of a mixture of the secretions from the ceruminous and pilosebaceous glands of the outer ear canal. It is normally expelled from the external ear canal in flakes, aided by movements of the jaw. Some patients, due to excessive secretion or deficient elimination, develop wax impaction.

This condition is normally treated by curettage or syringing of the ears. Occasionally wax must be softened before removal. In this instance such solutions as ***warm olive oil, saturated sodium bicarbonate solution, hydrogen peroxide*** or a proprietary preparation such as *Cerumol* or *Waxsol* can be used. In less severe cases application of the drops for a few days can lead to the wax being ejected naturally.

As with all ear drops it is important to warm the drops to body temperature before instillation. Any extreme temperature can precipitate vertigo in the patient.

NURSING IMPLICATIONS

Assessment

Before the administration of local applications to the ear, always ensure that the ear is clean. Aural cleaning should be meticulous in that all moisture, pus, mucus and debris are removed.

If the patient is in pain, the application of local heat may be helpful and can often obviate the need for continual use of analgesics.

Assess for known allergies to the medication to be used, plus concurrent use of any other drugs which may potentiate its effects (for example, antihistamines and alcohol).

Where antibiotics such as aminoglycosides are to be used, assessment of eighth cranial-nerve function and renal function may need to be done.

Ensure that the ears are kept dry during the course of treatment. Cotton wool or gauze ear plugs coated with soft paraffin should be used to prevent water entering the ear being treated.

Administration

Correctly identify the patient, drug, dosage time and route of administration to minimize the risk of drug errors. Perform aural toilet before administering all local applications.

Evaluate

Observe the patient for relief of symptoms. Watch for signs of allergy or irritation where local applications are used. Where aminoglycoside antibiotic ear drops are used, be alert for complaints of dizziness, vertigo or hearing impairment, as these drugs are ototoxic.

Patient teaching

Advise patients (or their parents) how to keep ears clean and dry and to clean ears before medication is instilled. Discourage patients from swimming. Advise patients to wear cotton wool or gauze ear plugs when showering or washing their hair. Instruct the patient not to scratch or rub ears and if the ears are itchy, see that he is prescribed an antipruritic such as crotamiton (*Eurax*) lotion or cream.

Patients with otitis media should be encouraged to breathe through the nose, and it should be stressed why this is important (see pages 345, 346). These patients should also be advised on how to blow their nose correctly. If the nose is blown too hard or pinched or blocked while being blown, a back pressure is created which could force mucus back into the eustachian tubes. Sneezing with the mouth shut can have similar results. Sniffing should also be discouraged as it may also force mucus into the eustachian tubes.

COMMON DISORDERS OF THE THROAT AND MOUTH

The following common diseases of the throat and mouth are discussed in this section: **acute pharyngitis, tonsillitis and laryngitis, mouth ulcers, fungal infections** and **herpes-simplex infections.**

ACUTE PHARYNGITIS, TONSILLITIS AND LARYNGITIS

The acute sore throat is a frequent complaint. Associated symptoms include dysphagia (difficulty in swallowing), general malaise and fever. Earache and headache can accompany pharyngitis and tonsillitis, whereas involvement of the larynx leads to aphonia (total loss of voice) or dysphonia (croaking voice). All these diseases are commonly associated with acute upper respiratory tract infection.

Treatment of acute pharyngitis

Mild attacks without fever or malaise generally resolve spontaneously in a few days. Symptomatic relief of the sore throat may be obtained in adults with the use of ***soluble aspirin*** which can be gargled before swallowing. Warm ***saline gargles*** may also be helpful.

Less than 50% of acute pharyngeal infections will be due to penicillin-sensitive bacteria; the rest are predominantly viral in origin. In severe cases, where general malaise and fever are prominent, and where bacterial culture is positive, a 10 to 14 day course of an appropriate antibiotic (usually phenoxymethylpenicillin) may be necessary. There is no curative treatment for viral infections. They do not benefit from antibiotic therapy and supportive therapy is all that is available.

Treatment of tonsillitis

Mild cases of sore throat associated with tonsillitis are best treated in adults with ***soluble aspirin*** and rest.

If despite these general measures the temperature remains high or the tonsils are markedly swollen or exudative, antibiotics should be administered. Antibiotics should also be given if previous attacks of tonsillitis have been associated with complications. A swab should be taken for culture, but prior to return of the laboratory result, a course of a penicillin is usually begun (on the assumption that the most likely pathogen will be a *Streptococcus*). Typically an immediate injection of ***benzylpenicillin*** is followed by oral ***phenoxymethylpenicillin*** for five to seven days.

Some individuals, particularly children, are subject to recurrent attacks of acute tonsillitis. In such instances, especially when complications such as otitis media are involved, tonsillectomy should be considered.

Treatment of laryngitis

In mild cases the most effective treatment is for the patient to keep quiet and treat the sore throat with soluble aspirin. More severe cases with fever, toxaemia and purulent expectoration are treated with an appropriate antibiotic.

MOUTH ULCERS

Oral ulceration may be a result of local irritation or trauma, infection or a manifestation of various systemic diseases.

The most common type of recurrent oral ulcers are called aphthous ulcers, and the typical symptom is of painful ulceration generally on non-keratinised oral mucosal membrane. Size and severity of tissue damage can vary markedly. The aetiology of these ulcers is unknown.

Table 47
Preparations Used to Treat Mouth Ulcers

Trade Name	Contains		
	Anaesthetic	Analgesic	Antiseptic
Bonjela	—	Choline salicylate	Cetalkonium chloride
Difflam	Benzydamine	—	—
Oral-B	Lignocaine	—	Cetylpyridinium chloride
Dequacaine	Benzocaine	—	Dequalinium

Less common forms of recurrent ulceration are found in association with generalised disease states such as erythema multiforma, lichen planus and pemphigus.

Most of the treatment of mouth ulcers is symptomatic. Irritant or hot food should be avoided. Oral hygiene should be emphasised. Teeth should be brushed regularly and throughly, but carefully, and with a soft-bristled brush. Mouthwashes of ***warm saline, 3% hydrogen peroxide*** solution or mild alkaline (for example, sodium bicarbonate) solutions are cleansing and soothing. Topically applied protectants such as ***compound benzoin tincture,*** *Orabase* (containing carboxymethylcellulose, gelatin, pectin and emollients), or even denture adhesive powders and pastes may be quite effective in alleviating pain. In particularly painful ulcerations, topically applied local anaesthetics, usually ***lignocaine*** or ***benzocaine*** may be necessary. Many proprietary preparations combine a local anaesthetic or analgesic (for example, a salicylate) with antiseptic agents. (See Table 47).

Carbenoxolone sodium (*Bioral*), has a protective action, as well as a direct healing action on mucosal ulcers. It is available as a gel, which should be placed on or near the lesion and allowed to dissolve.

In more severe recurrent ulcerations ***topical corticosteroids,*** used at first warning of imminent ulceration, will sometimes abort the episode, but will more frequently reduce its duration. Topical corticosteroids available include ***hydrocortisone*** and ***triamcinolone.*** Hydrocortisone 2.5 mg pellets (*Corlan*) should not be sucked but should be kept in the mouth in close proximity to the ulcer and allowed to dissolve slowly. Pellets are of less value when the lesion is mobile, that is, on cheek or tongue. ***Triamcinolone paste*** *(Adcortyl in Orabase)* is applied directly to the lesion.

In the presence of bacterial, fungal or viral infections in the mouth, topical steroids should not be used unless in conjunction with specific chemotherapy. If deep ulceration with tissue necrosis is present (major aphthous ulceration), topical therapy is often of no use and intermittent systemic corticosteroids may need to be used. Intralesional corticosteroid injections may also be tried to aid resolution of long-standing ulcers. If secondary bacterial infection is present, a ***chlorhexidine 0.2%*** mouthwash or ***tetracycline*** mouthwash may be used.

FUNGAL INFECTIONS

Candidiasis is the most common fungal infection of the mouth. *Candida albicans* is a natural inhabitant of the oral cavity but in certain conditions overgrowth of the fungus occurs. Oral candidiasis is treated by topical application of antifungal suspension or lozenges. Typical medications are nystatin *(Nystan)*, natamycin *(Pimafucin* in suspension) and amphotericin B *(Fungilin* in solution or as lozenges).

When using a suspension, the required volume of solution is swished around in the mouth for one or two minutes before being swallowed. The lozenges should be sucked and allowed to dissolve slowly. Treatment is usually given four times daily after each meal and at bedtime. Ten to 14 days of therapy is often required. In infants the local application of a 2% gentian-violet solution can be used.

ORAL HERPES SIMPLEX INFECTIONS

This is the well known lesion popularly called a "cold sore".

Idoxuridine (0.1% paint) applied as soon as symptoms are noticed can attenuate the tissue damage and decrease the duration of the ulcer. Application of alcoholic solutions can also aid recovery. Use of sunscreen preparations to avoid sunburn, and minimising chemical and physical trauma, may decrease recurrence.

NURSING IMPLICATIONS

Assessment

When patients present with a sore throat or mouth, the underlying cause should always be assessed where possible. Many sore throats are due to viral infections which are unresponsive to antibiotic treatment and will resolve spontaneously with rest and symptomatic treatment.

Some patients are at particular risk of oral diseases. These patients include those with a systemic disease which can cause oral ulceration; patients with a disease which modifies the normal healing response; patients on drugs which are toxic to oral mucosal cells, for example; cytotoxic drugs; and patients on drugs which cause immunodeficiency, for example, corticosteroids. Patients receiving radiotherapy to the head and neck region may also manifest inflammatory changes to mouth and throat mucosa. Special care should be taken with all of these patients, as they are especially prone to infections of the mouth and throat due to their compromised local and general immunological defence systems.

It should also be remembered that the appearance of a sore mouth or throat may be the first warning of drug-induced bone-marrow depression. Drugs likely to cause this reaction include phenylbutazone, gold, chloramphenicol and carbimazole, but there are many other drugs which can have this side effect.

Patient teaching

Many patients with a sore throat expect to be prescribed an antibiotic. The nurse has a role to play in educating the patient not to automatically demand an antibiotic and the reasons why unnecessary exposure to antibiotics is unwise.

All patients who are prescribed any of the drugs mentioned above, which may induce bone-marrow depression, should be warned to report the first sign of a sore throat or mouth to their doctor without delay.

SELF-EVALUATION TEST

1. Sodium cromoglycate (*Rynacrom*) should be administered:
   (a) at first sign of hay fever
   (b) p.r.n.
   (c) for no longer than one week
   (d) on a regular basis.
2. Topical decongestants should be administered:
   (a) whenever nose is obstructed
   (b) on a regular basis
   (c) no more frequently than prescribed
   (d) for no longer than seven days.
3. A drug which is *not* used in oral candidiasis is:
   (a) gentian violet
   (b) chlorhexidine
   (c) nystatin
   (d) natamycin.
4. The drug of choice in herpes simplex infection of the lips is:
   (a) idoxuridine
   (b) tetracycline mouthwash
   (c) chlorhexidine 0.02%
   (d) gentian violet 2%.
5. The drug of choice in acute otitis externa is:
   (a) ampicillin
   (b) phenoxymethylpenicillin
   (c) cloxacillin
   (d) erythromycin.
6. The drug of choice in acute otitis media is:
   (a) oral phenoxymethylpenicillin
   (b) oral amoxycillin
   (c) ampicillin ear drops
   (d) sulphonamide ear drops.

7. Prolonged use of antibiotic ear drops such as framycetin, gentamicin and neomycin should be avoided due to:
   (a) development of resistant bacteria
   (b) development of skin sensitisation
   (c) supra-infection with fungi
   (d) all of the above.
8. To prevent a relapse of chronic otitis externa the patient should be advised to:
   (a) avoid scratching or poking ears
   (b) wear ear plugs at all times
   (c) avoid sneezing with mouth shut
   (d) avoid getting water into ears.

Table 48
Drug Treatment of Common Diseases of the Ear, Nose, Throat and Mouth

Drug Group	Drug Name	Use	Action	Adverse Reactions	Nursing Implications
Sympathomimetic nasal decongestants	Nasal: Phenylephrine Oxymetazoline Xylometazoline Oral: Ephedrine Pseudoephedrine	Nasal decongestant in allergic, infective and vasomotor rhinitis	Sympathomimetic	Nasal preparations: rebound oedema of the nasal mucosa Oral preparations: hypertension, tachycardia, palpitations, nervousness, insomnia, urinary retention, sweating, flushing, tremor	***Assess:*** correct patient, dose and time, and route of administration; how long the patient has been taking the drug; if drug is to be given systemically, establish baseline BP and pulse rate; check for history of hypertension, prostatomegaly. ***Administer:*** correct dose, as ordered, for no longer than prescribed. ***Evaluate:*** for relief of symptoms and for signs of systemic absorption and side effects, such as nervousness, raised BP, tachycardia, urinary retention, insomnia, palpitations. ***Teach:*** correct administration techniques and dosage regime. Warn against continued use and that these drugs should be taken only as prescribed and for no longer than five to seven days, and to report any systemic side effects.
Mast-cell stabilizer	Sodium cromoglycate	Prophylaxis against allergic rhinitis	Inhibits release of histamine from mast cells	Irritation of nasal mucosa	***Assess:*** patient's understanding of action and use of drug. ***Administer:*** regularly, as ordered, using correct technique for administration. ***Evaluate:*** for drug effectiveness; complaints of irritation to nasal

					mucosa. ***Teach:*** correct administration technique; explain the action of the drug so that the patient understands that the drug must be used regularly as ordered and not just when symptoms occur.
Intranasal corticosteroids	Dexamethasone Beclomethasone Flunisolide	Severe rhinitis	Decrease inflammation and oedema in nasal mucosa	Burning, stinging, sneezing, haemorrhagic secretions, increased incidence of nasal and sinus infections, capillary fragility and mucosal atrophy after longterm use; little risk of systemic absorption, but possibility should not be overlooked	***Assess:*** presence of existing nasal or sinus infection; patient's understanding of administration technique (if he is to administer drug to himself). ***Administer:*** regularly, as ordered, using correct technique; ensure no more than 1mg per day (20 puffs) of beclomethasone or 0.4 mg (8 sprays) of flunisolide is given per day. ***Evaluate:*** for drug effectiveness; watch for signs of local side effects such as mucosal atrophy, haemorrhagic nasal discharges. ***Teach:*** correct method of administration; advise that drug may sting mucosa or cause sneezing in some people; ensure patient understands there is a three to seven-day time lag before drug's effects are noticed and not to think that the drug is ineffective and therefore discontinue use; ensure that he understands the reason for regular use as prescribed and not to take it "when required" for symptomatic relief.

20
ANTIHISTAMINES

Ross W. Holland and Vicky J. Grattan

OBJECTIVES

At the conclusion of this chapter the reader should be able to:

1. describe how antihistamine drugs are thought to act;
2. list common adverse reactions to antihistamines;
3. list the conditions for which antihistamines are effective;
4. identify antihistamines from a list of drugs.

PREREQUISITE KNOWLEDGE

1. The role and action of mast cells in the body.
2. Current theories on allergic reactions and associated medical conditions.

DEFINITIONS

Antihistamines — substances which block the action of histamine at the H_1 histamine receptor sites within the body.

INTRODUCTION

The body produces a range of substances that can, under some circumstances, produce allergic-type reactions. These substances include ***histamine*** and ***serotonin.*** Histamine and serotonin have important normal physiological functions. For histamine these include a role in tissue growth and repair and the control of gastric secretion, while serotonin is implicated in the control of microcirculation.

In addition to these functions, histamine is stored in mast cells in the body. When these cells are damaged by chemicals, drugs, heat or trauma, large amounts of histamine are released causing either localised or widespread allergic response.

A typical reaction would be to an insect bite resulting in a characteristic "triple response". First, a localised red spot develops due to local dilation of capillaries in direct response to histamine release. Secondly, a brighter red flare develops extending about 1 cm beyond the original spot as a result of more widespread dilation of neighbouring arterioles. Thirdly, localised oedema forms a wheal at the site of the original spot.

It is proposed that histamine, once released, acts at specific receptor sites in the various tissues, whether smooth muscle, capillary walls or gastric glands. These are further subdivided into H_1 and H_2 types. The H_2 receptors appear to be confined to the control of gastric secretions. Drugs that act on the H_2 receptors are called H_2 receptor antagonists. (Because their action is on gastric secretion these drugs are discussed in Chapter 31.)

Principles of action

Drugs that block the action of histamine at the H_1 receptors are called antihistamines. They do not prevent the release of histamine that occurs in response to injury, drugs or antigens, but appear to occupy receptor sites to the exclusion of histamine. Thus they antagonise most of the effects of histamine, reducing the intensity of allergic and anaphylactic (allergic shock) reactions. They have no action on the gastric H_2 receptors.

Antihistamines antagonise the important vasodilator effects of histamine, reduce capillary permeability and the consequent formation of oedema. They greatly diminish the itching that accompanies allergic reactions. Other effects include depression of the central nervous system; sedation; suppression of nausea and vomiting and in some cases with anti-Parkinsonian effects. Most antihistamines have an atropine-like activity which accounts for the dryness of the mouth experienced by some patients. In addition, a local anaesthetic effect has been noted in all such drugs.

Uses

Antihistamines have a place in the treatment of allergic reactions where histamine is the mediator. They are most useful for urticaria and pruritus, insect bites and stings, allergic rhinitis (hay fever), and in sinusitis for their drying effect. They are sometimes used for treatment of drug reactions and in anaphylactic shock.

Use in the treatment of bronchial asthma is limited, as this reaction is likely to be caused by substances other than histamine. Antihistamines are often used in cough mixtures for their antitussive effect. However this use is undesirable due to their atropine-like drying effect which can produce thickening of mucus within the lungs, leading to an unproductive cough.

The sedative effects are often used to advantage, although tolerance usually develops after a few days. For this purpose, short-term use only is advocated, particularly with children. Occasionally, the sedative effect is put to use as premedication, either alone or in conjunction with narcotics.

Those antihistamines which effectively suppress nausea and vomiting may be used to prevent motion sickness and are present in several commercial preparations. Some have been used to prevent morning sickness. This latter use has declined over the past few years with increasing awareness of the adverse effects of drugs on the developing foetus.

Adverse Drug Reactions

Adverse reactions to this group of substances are closely related to the pharmacological effects. Most prominent among these are drowsiness and dry mouth. Other effects include dizziness, blurred or double vision, loss of appetite, muscle weakness, lassitude and, when given by the intravenous route, hypotension. A paradoxical CNS stimulation sometimes occurs, resulting in wakefulness and hyperactivity, particularly in children when high doses are given. When antihistamines are applied topically, an allergic dermatitis is not uncommon.

Because of the potential to cause drowsiness, which occurs to some extent with all antihistamines, care should be taken not to consume alcohol, drive motor vehicles or operate machinery while taking these medications. Concurrent administration of some other medications, for example tranquillisers, anti-anxiety drugs and hypnotics, may lead to an additive anticholinergic and sedative action. Also, it should be remembered that many over-the-counter cold and hay-fever remedies contain antihistamines. Concurrent use may lead to an additive effect, particularly with regard to drowsiness.

Astemizole and ***terfenadine*** have much reduced CNS effects and cause less drowsiness.

Some examples of antihistamines

Antihistamines come from several different classes of chemical compounds. Consequently, if a particular substance is not effective, one from another class can be chosen.

Table 49 lists some of the more common antihistamines. Strengths are not included because of the multiplicity of dose forms available. It should be noted that many types of oral antihistamines are available in both normal and sustained or time-release formulations. These have completely different time-related effects and consequently cannot be substituted for each other. As with all drugs, strengths should be checked before administration.

Table 49
Some Common Antihistamines

Generic Name	Trade Name
Astemizole	*Hismanal*
Azatadine	*Optimine*
Cyproheptadine	*Periactin*
Diphenhydramine	*Benadryl*
Chlorpheniramine	*Piriton*
Mebhydrolin	*Fabahistin*
Promethazine	*Phenergan*
Terfenadine	*Triludan*

NURSING IMPLICATIONS

Assessment

Because of the frequent occurrence of sedation with antihistamine therapy, the patient's need to be fully alert should be assessed. Interactions with other drugs and alcohol in particular (which may be taken inadvertently, in cough medicine) are common, potentially dangerous and should be avoided. It should be remembered that the anticholinergic effect of antihistamines can cause respiratory secretions to become thick and sticky, and this could lead to respiratory problems in situations where a productive loose cough is desirable. Some antihistamines belong in the phenothiazine group of drugs, and therefore there is the faint possibility of extrapyramidal side effects occurring.

Administration

A large number of doses and forms are available, so orders for antihistamines should be checked carefully against container labels. Lower doses may be given to avoid sedation. Sustained-release tablets should be swallowed whole and not crushed. Crushing will alter the anticipated long-acting slow-release effect. The exact form and strength of tablet ordered should always be given. Tablets of a different form should not be substituted to "make up" a dose.

Evaluation

The effectiveness of the drug in reducing allergic response, producing sedation and causing unwanted effects should be evaluated. Allergic reactions to antihistamines can develop. Allergic dermatitis can occur with topical use. Any change in blood pressure after intravenous injection should be reported immediately. Acute poisoning may occur, especially in children, because of the common usage of antihistamine drugs.

Acute poisoning

The signs of acute toxicity include central nervous system effects, such as excitement, lack of coordination and convulsions. The pupils may become dilated and fixed, the face flushed, and fever may occur. Cardiorespiratory collapse and subsequent death can occur within 24 hours after the ingestion of 20 to 30 tablets by a young child. The treatment is symptomatic since there is no specific antidote.

Patient teaching

Patients must be made aware of the possibility of drowsiness, and the dangers when driving or operating machinery, and of the possible potentiation of sedation effects when taken with other drugs, particularly tranquillisers and alcohol.

Patients taking antihistamines should be instructed to inform their doctor, dentist or pharmacist that they are having these medications before taking other medications which may be prescribed or purchased at a pharmacy. Parents should be aware of the toxic effects, and the need to keep antihistamines out of the reach of children.

SELF-EVALUATION TEST

1. Describe how antihistamine drugs are thought to act.
2. Which of the following drugs are antihistamines?
   (a) Chlorpropamide *(Diabenese)*
   (b) Diphenhydramine *(Benadryl)*
   (c) Promethazine *(Phenergan)*
   (d) Phenytoin *(Epanutin)*
   (e) Chlorpheniramine *(Piriton)*
   (f) Dextropropoxyphene *(Doloxene)*†
3. List four conditions for which antihistamines may be used.
4. (a) What are the two most prominent adverse reactions to antihistamines?
   (b) List two others.

Table 50
Antihistamines

Drug Group	Use	Action	Adverse Reactions	Nursing Implications
Antihistamines (H_1 receptor antagonists)	Allergic reactions mediated by histamine, e.g. urticaria, pruritus, insect bites, allergic rhinitis, drug reactions, anaphylaxis	Block action of histamine at H_1 receptors	Drowsiness, dry mouth, dizziness, visual blurring, loss of appetite, muscle weakness, lassitude, hypotension	***Assess:*** for known hypersensitivity, establish baseline blood pressure (IV use); concurrent use of other anticholinergic-like drugs and CNS depressants, including alcohol. ***Administer:*** check labels carefully; lower doses to avoid sedation where necessary; give oral doses with food. ***Evaluate:*** reduction of signs of allergy, sedative effects; allergic dermatitis with topical application; blood pressure changes with intravenous use; signs of toxicity, especially in children. ***Teach:*** warn that drowsiness and dry mouth may occur and advise of potential dangers when driving and operating machinery and of the potentiating of sedative effects with other sedative-type drugs.

21
DRUGS USED IN DERMATOLOGY

Marie Thérèse Rosenburg

OBJECTIVES

At the conclusion of this chapter, the reader should be able to:

1. state the difference between creams, ointments and lotions;
2. describe the conditions under which these different types of external preparations are used;
3. be able to identify the various classes of drugs used for topical application;
4. list those drugs which are given systemically for the treatment of certain skin diseases;
5. list the untoward effects of some topical applications, particularly the corticosteroids.

PREREQUISITE KNOWLEDGE

1. Structure and functions of the skin.
2. Basic theory of emulsions.
3. Basic understanding of ultraviolet light.
4. Physiological basis of absorption mechanisms of the skin.
5. Pathogenesis of common skin diseases such as:
   (a) inflammatory responses to injury, for example, blisters;
   (b) acceleration, slowing or failure of normal function, for example, virus growth, lesions of acne.

DEFINITIONS

Topical — pertaining to a particular surface area.
Topical application — an application to be applied directly to a particular area of the skin for local action.
Skin — the outer covering of the body, consisting of the dermis and the epidermis and resting upon the subcutaneous tissues.
Topical corticosteroids — agents with a cortisone-like action, varying in potency, which, when applied locally act as anti-inflammatory agents, with little or no systemic effect.

Throughout the history of dermatology a large number of therapeutic agents have been tried in the treatment of skin diseases. The text from a fragment of papyrus dating from about the time of Rameses II, 1250 BC, directs the physician to take the talons of a falcon and the shell of a tortoise, and after pronouncing a magic incantation over them, to boil them in oil and apply the oil to the site of a wound. This was claimed to be a reliable remedy, proven a million times over.

The *Ebers Papyrus* described the benefits of the castor oil plant; the husk crushed in water and applied to the head cures headache; the plant, crushed and worked into a mass with lard and applied to the scalp promotes the growth of hair; the oil from the seeds, incorporated into an ointment and applied early in the morning for 10 days will heal wounds that have an evil-smelling discharge.

Galen, a Greek physician who lived in the second century, invented cold cream, a mixture of oils, wax and water. When applied to the skin the water evaporated, producing a cooling sensation, hence the name "cold" cream. This is still used today.

The discovery that hydrocortisone acetate had an anti-inflammatory action when applied to areas of eczema and dermatitis completely altered the management of non-infective skin disorders. In 1960 triamcinolone acetonide was discovered and found to be 10 times more potent than hydrocortisone. Since then, hundreds of corticosteroids have been synthesised, and they are the most commonly used and misused topical skin preparations available.

Skin ailments may be caused by trauma (cuts, blisters, burns); inflammatory reactions to contact with irritant substances; allergic reactions; alteration of normal function (for example, acceleration of growth leads to thickened skin and scaling); or by reactions to drugs.

TYPES OF PREPARATION

Just as a drug to be taken orally is incorporated into a suitable dosage form, such as a mixture, a tablet, an enteric-coated tablet, or a delayed-release tablet, so a drug to be applied to the skin is usually incorporated into a vehicle, the type dependent on the effect desired. The vehicles applied to the skin consist of three basic elements in varying proportions, that is water, oil or grease, and powder.

LIQUIDS

Water is used in the form of wet compresses as a means of heating or cooling the skin. The effect depends on the degree of exposure of the dressing to the air. Closed moist dressings (such as those covered with a sheet of plastic and sealed round the edges with adhesive tape) heat up rapidly, even if applied cold. They remain moist and may be left undisturbed for many hours. Thick, crusted lesions, such as those of psoriasis, are sometimes treated in this way. Open wet dressings are used when a cooling effect is desired, such as in treatment of superficial inflammation.

OILS AND GREASES

Oils and greases are used to soften rough, dry skin. Oils are frequently applied by putting a quantity of oil into the bath. A "solubilising" agent is used to disperse the oil in the water. This leaves a fine film of oil all over the body, an effect which is extremely difficult to achieve by applying an ointment by hand. Grease has a softening, protective action on the skin, retaining heat and moisture. The most frequently used grease is soft paraffin, sometimes called *Petroleum Jelly* or *Vaseline.* A grease is used on dry and scaling areas. It should not be used on weeping areas as it does not absorb moisture and keeps the area warm, leading to maceration of the skin. It is usually difficult to apply on a wet area, as it slides off. Grease and grease-based preparations are called ointments.

POWDERS

Dusting powders form a loose thin layer on the skin, so that active medicaments contained in them have a limited action. Fine powders provide lubrication between opposing skin surfaces, thus preventing irritation caused by friction. Powders should not be used on any badly weeping surface as they absorb moisture, and the exudate may cement the powder into coarse granules which irritate the skin.

WATER PLUS POWDER

These preparations are called shake lotions, because the powder, being in suspension, settles on the bottom of the bottle which must be shaken before use. After application, the water evaporates rapidly with a cooling effect, and the powder is left as a film on the skin. This is really only a modified version of the application of a dusting powder. Lotions are used for superficial inflammatory reactions and for slightly oozing conditions. They tend to dry the skin unless the environment has a high humidity. They are unsuitable for use in hairy areas.

GREASE PLUS POWDER

Ointments usually contain one or more powders mixed with grease. They are not readily absorbed into the skin, and their function is mainly protective. They usually have the consistency of butter. Pastes are mixtures of grease and a high concentration of powder, say 50% or more. They are very stiff, and difficult to apply, particularly in cold weather. Pastes do absorb moisture because of their high powder content, while the grease base helps to keep the skin from being dried out.

WATER PLUS OIL OR GREASE

By the use of an emulsifying agent, grease (or oil) and aqueous liquid can be made to form a stable emulsion called a cream. A cream may be a suspension of oil globules in an aqueous medium (an aqueous cream) or a suspension of water globules in an oily medium (an oily cream). Creams mix readily with the skin secretions, and a high degree of absorption of their active medicament may be expected. Powders may be mixed in with them but not in high concentration, as creams are relatively unstable; high concentrations of medicaments cause the emulsion to "crack", that is, revert to its original two layers of grease and aqueous liquid.

Creams are the most widely used dermatological preparations. They are useful in inflammatory conditions and may be used on weeping areas and on hairy areas. They are simple to apply and are easily removed by washing with water, in contrast to ointments, which are difficult to remove by washing. Creams are not suitable for chronic scaling skin disease where a protective effect is required.

Creams are subject to contamination by moulds, and to dehydration if stored for any length of time. A dehydrated cream should not be used, as the concentration of medicament may have risen, and this may cause damage to the skin.

SOOTHING AND PROTECTIVE PREPARATIONS

Calamine Lotion is a suspension of calamine and zinc oxide in water containing 0.5% phenol. The calamine and zinc oxide protect the skin, and the evaporation of the water cools it. Phenol in this low concentration acts as a local anaesthetic to relieve itching and as a mild antiseptic.

Coal Tar Solution (still frequently referred to by its abbreviated Latin name, Liq. Picis Carb.) is sometimes used to relieve generalised itch: 30 mL is added to 90 litres (about half a bath full) of tepid water (37°C); the patient soaks in it for 10 to 15 minutes and is then patted dry with a soft towel.

Aqueous creams are soothing to dry skin, and if they have a high water content, can replace much of the moisture which has been lost. *Cetomacrogol Cream* and *Aqueous Cream* consist of a mixture of waxes and fats emulsified in water.

Talcum powder is used to lubricate surfaces which rub together and so prevent chafing. Talc is purified native magnesium silicate and contains spores, so it is sterilised before use. Some commercial talcum powders contain boric acid. These should not be used lavishly on raw surfaces, for example a baby's nappy area, as enough boric acid may be absorbed to cause systemic poisoning.

Soft paraffin (*Vaseline, Petroleum Jelly*), hard paraffin (paraffin wax) and liquid paraffin are often used together with beeswax in varying proportions to produce an ointment of a desired consistency. Soft paraffin may also be used on its own. All of these are bland, non-sensitising and protective, but also occlusive.

Wool fat (from the wool of sheep) absorbs water to produce ***lanolin***, a form in which it is often used as a moisturising agent and to protect skin from drying.

Alpha-Keri Oil contains an extract from wool fat, liquid paraffin and dispersing agents, and is an example of a preparation used for excessively dry skin. It is usually added to the bath, or applied to the wet skin, the skin then being patted dry. In this way a film of oil can be applied easily to the whole body.

Oily Glycerin Cream is another product used for excessively dry skin as in the treatment of ichthyosis.

CLEANSERS AND KERATOLYTICS

CLEANSERS

Soap: The modern practice of hygiene encourages the frequent use of soap. This may be quite damaging to the skin, as soap is caustic, causing swelling and disintegration of the keratin layer. Unless there is considerable exudate, it is unnecessary to wash off a previous application of cream or ointment before applying another.

Medicated soaps may be useful in some conditions, for example *Gamophen Soap†* and *Phisohex,* containing ***hexachlorophane.*** If used regularly these products leave a residue of hexachlorophane on the skin which reduces the skin count of staphylococci; they are used in the treatment of boils and infected lesions and as an adjunct in the treatment of acne. Hexachlorophane can be absorbed through the skin, and its widespread use in nurseries for washing neonates (as a prophylactic against staphylococcal infections) resulted in several deaths from spongy lesions of the brain. At the time of writing, there is some suspicion that its prolonged use for hand-washing by pregnant women may be the cause of some congenital malformations.

Cleansing creams are cosmetically acceptable alternatives to soap for cleansing the face.

Hydrogen peroxide is used to cleanse open wounds and ulcers. The solution releases oxygen on contact, and the effervescent action loosens debris.

Benzoyl peroxide 10% in a lotion or cream base is used in the treatment of acne. The benzoyl peroxide, when applied to the skin, releases oxygen which penetrates into the sebaceous follicle and suppresses the organism *Corynebacterium acnes.* Benzoyl peroxide is potentially a contact sensitiser, and it may also bleach coloured garments if in contact with them. Care should be taken to avoid contact with eyes, lips and mouth.

KERATOLYTICS

The use of keratolytic agents is sometimes desirable when accumulation of keratinised cells causes flaking and scaling.

Salicylic acid is used in varying concentrations and in different vehicles. For mild scaling, 1% to 2% in soft paraffin keeps the skin warm and moist, which assists in the scaling (ex-foliating) process; 2% to 5% in cream can be used for more advanced lesions; up to 20% may be used for removal of warts, usually in *Collodion*, which forms a skin on drying. Care must be taken that the skin surrounding the wart is protected. This can be done by smearing *Vaseline* on the skin up to the edge of the wart. An occlusive dressing over the wart, by causing maceration of the keratin layer, will increase the effect of the salicylic acid. The dressing should be removed and the paint reapplied twice a day.

Resorcinol is frequently added to salicylic acid in hair lotions. It aids in removing scaling skin and is therefore useful in treatment of dandruff. It is also antipruritic. It causes darkening of the hair, a process which is intensified in the presence of alkali.

Podophyllum resin dissolved in alcohol, usually in the form of compound benzoin tincture, is used in the topical treatment of condylomata acuminata (soft venereal warts) and other warts. Podophyllum is very irritating to normal skin, which should always be protected during application of the paint. Any unusual symptoms occurring in a patient who has been treated with podophyllum should be reported to the medical officer immediately, as absorption of podophyllum has led to severe neurological complications, even death. *Posalfilin* is an ointment containing 20% podophyllum resin and 25% salicylic acid. It should be used strictly in accordance with the directions, and discontinued at the first sign of inflammation.

A Buf-Puf is an abrasive pad made of inert polyester fibres. It contains no medication and achieves its effect by removing dead skin cells by abrasion.

Urea (10% in a cream base) is frequently used to increase hydration of the skin. If an extemporaneous urea cream is used, it should be freshly prepared as it darkens on storage. Some commercially prepared creams are claimed to be more stable because of a special process used in manufacture, for example *Aquadrate*.

Vitamin A (*Retinol*) has long been believed to be involved in differentiation of epithelial tissue, as a deficiency of the vitamin gives rise to hyperkeratotic skin changes. It is therefore used, in the form of ***tretinoin*** (Vitamin A acid), in the topical treatment of some skin disorders, including severe acne, certain keratoses and psoriasis. Results in psoriasis have been disappointing. Acne may appear to worsen at the commencement of treatment and it may be eight to twelve weeks before improvement becomes obvious. *Retin-A* is a proprietary preparation of tretinoin, available as liquid, cream or gel. Topical application of tretinoin increases the susceptibility of the skin to sunlight, therefore exposure should be avoided during treatment. If exposure cannot be avoided, protective clothing should be worn, or a suitable sunscreen product used to cover the treated area. Derivatives of tretinoin, for example ***etretinate*** *(Tigason)*, may be administered orally. It is suggested for use in the treatment of dermatoses characterised by severe disorders of keratinisation, such as psoriasis, ichthyosis and lichen planus. Side effects are frequent but generally reversible and include cheilitis, mucosal dryness, palmoplantar desquamation, pruritus, thinning of the skin, partial or total alopecia, headache (occasionally) and elevation of liver enzymes. Etretinate in therapeutic doses is embryotoxic and teratogenic and is therefore contraindicated during pregnancy; it should be used with great caution in women of child-bearing potential.

NURSING IMPLICATIONS

Assessment

Nurses caring for patients with skin disorders should ensure that they understand the different functions of the products to be used. For example, do not substitute an ointment for a cream or vice versa. Assess the area to be treated as to extent and type of lesion and whether skin is dry, cracked, moist, weeping or hairy. Document baseline observations of condition of skin.

Application

Baths: ensure that the correct strength of preparation is used. Check the temperature to avoid burning or hypothermia. Assist elderly and debilitated patients.

Lotions: use sparingly. Overuse leads to drying and cracking of skin.

Wet dressings: ensure that open wet dressings are kept moist. Renew or remoisten regularly.

Powders: use sparingly. Do not use on weeping or hairy areas.

Ointments: these do not penetrate but are soothing and protective. Use only a thin smear. It is not necessary to wash off ointment before making a new application. Ointments should not be applied to oozing lesions where drainage is required but are valuable in acute and chronic lesions where there are crusts to soften. Application to hairy areas causes matting, and prolonged application to hairy areas may cause folliculitis.

Creams: exudates are absorbed freely with creams, and drainage is not inhibited. Creams are comparable with wet dressings but require changing less frequently. They are not suitable for chronic, scaling skin diseases where a protective effect is required. They may be used on hairy or weeping areas. Do not use a dehydrated cream as concentration of medication may have risen.

Keratolytics and cleansers: ensure these are used only where indicated. They soften horny layers and reduce thickening in conditions like psoriasis.

Apply podophyllum and salicylic preparations correctly, and protect healthy skin. When using resorcinol, ensure hair is free of soap.

Evaluation

Observe for signs of improvement in skin condition. Where powders, lotions and baths are used, check skin for drying or cracking. Watch for hypothermia in elderly or debilitated patients during baths or if large areas are being treated with wet dressings.

Patient teaching

If the patient is to apply the medication, teach him or her the correct procedure and any precautions to observe during application, plus any adverse effects to watch for. Most patients with skin problems should be advised against the use of soap and it should be stressed that excessive washing of the skin may be harmful. Soap has a keratolytic effect and may damage the protective horny layers of the dermis.

Patients using resorcinol need to be advised to wash their hair free of soap before application to reduce the possibility of hair darkening.

All patients with peripheral vascular disease or diabetes mellitus should be warned against the use of keratolytic agents lest skin irritation result in an ulcer. Patients being treated with topical applications of retinoids should be warned to avoid direct exposure to sunlight.

Both nurses and patients should ensure that all applications to skin are applied gently, as energetic application could aggravate the existing condition. Advise patients concerning any product which may stain the skin or clothing so that appropriate precautions can be taken.

Finally, it should be borne in mind by the nurse that conditions of the skin are often accompanied by disfigurement, feelings of rejection and a poor self-image. Emotional support of the patient is therefore important. The nurse should be careful to avoid showing any signs of rejecting a patient with a skin condition and should not react negatively to the skin lesion or the treatment involved.

ANTI-INFECTIVE PREPARATIONS

Most bacterial skin infections are caused by staphylococci or streptococci. Antibiotics which are used systemically in the treatment of bacterial infection should not as a general rule be applied topically, as it has been found that this practice encourages the development of resistant bacterial strains (because of the low antibiotic plasma concentration which results). Moreover, topical use of antibiotics, especially penicillins and streptomycin, frequently causes contact dermatitis. However, skin infections are often superficial and respond to treatment within a few days, so that both risks are lessened to a degree.

TOPICAL TREATMENT OF BACTERIAL SKIN INFECTIONS

Hexachlorophane (*Phisohex*)

As previously mentioned, topical preparations containing hexachlorophane may be used to reduce the skin count of staphylococci.

Antibiotics

The antibiotics neomycin, bacitracin and polymyxin are frequently used in combination in an ointment base for superficial infections such as impetigo. There are a number of commercial preparations of this type, for example: *Dispray Antibiotic,* powder spray. This combination has the advantage that all these antibiotics are rarely used systemically. Neomycin and bacitracin, however, can cause sensitivity reactions following prolonged application. Extensive impetigo not responding readily to topical therapy may need systemic antibiotics (see below).

Neomycin Solution 0.5% is often used for irrigation of infected wounds. If the lesion is large or the treatment prolonged, sufficient neomycin can be absorbed to cause ototoxicity. Loss of hearing may progress even after the neomycin irrigation has been ceased. Such treatment should certainly be reviewed after a week, and the risks involved in continuing therapy weighed against the expected benefit.

Persistence of or recurrence of inflammation in spite of, or following treatment with ointments containing neomycin or bacitracin, should arouse the suspicion that a sensitivity reaction has occurred, and the circumstances should be drawn to the attention of the doctor. A combination of neomycin 0.5% and chlorhexidine 0.1% is often prescribed as a nasal cream in the case of recurrent staphylococcal infections, since the offending organism frequently resides in the nose. *Naseptin* is one such cream.

Framycetin, with a similar action to that of neomycin, is used as *Soframycin Ointment,* which contains 1.5% framycetin plus 0.005% gramicidin, another antibiotic. It is available also as *Sofra-Tulle,* a sterile paraffin-gauze dressing impregnated with 1% framycetin, which is used for burns, ulcers and as a plastic-surgery dressing. Like neomycin, framycetin is rarely used systemically, and so is particularly suitable for topical use. Unfortunately it, too, often causes a sensitivity reaction. Staphylococcal infections respond well also to gentamicin which is usually applied as a 0.1% cream or ointment. However, because of its frequent systemic use, it should not be used as drug of first choice.

SYSTEMIC TREATMENT OF BACTERIAL SKIN INFECTIONS

Infected skin conditions frequently require systemic treatment with antibiotics to combat the infection, followed or accompanied by the specific treatment for the underlying condition. Another reason systemic antibiotics may be required in hospitalised patients is that hospital organisms, because of constant exposure to antibiotics, may be resistant to them in the concentrations used for topical application.

Since the commonest organisms involved are staphylococci and streptococci, one of the oral penicillins is usually adequate, but any systemic antibiotic may be used, depending on the sensitivity of the organism. Tetracycline is frequently used in the long-term treatment of acne, being given once or twice daily, often for several years. Other systemic agents used in the treatment of skin infections will be found under Antiviral Agents (below) and Antifungal Agents (Chapter 24).

ANTIPARASITICS

Gamma benzene hexachloride *(Quelleda)* is a treatment for scabies. The 1% lotion is applied to the skin, from the chin to the feet, after a hot bath. It is then left on the skin for 24 hours, after which it is washed off thoroughly.

For pediculosis capitis (infection with head lice), the use of gamma benzene hydrochloride has been superseded as lice are resistant to it. ***Carbaryl*** is now used instead.

Carbaryl *(Carylderm)* lotion should be applied to the hair, which is then allowed to dry naturally. After 12 hours, the hair can be washed with an ordinary shampoo, then combed through with a fine-toothed comb to remove dead nits from each strand of hair.

Dicophane (DDT) is also effective against lice and scabies, but is rarely used nowadays because of its persistence and its effect on the environment. If it is used, it is generally applied as a dusting powder.

ANTIVIRAL AGENTS

Idoxuridine, an antiviral agent that interferes with viral DNA synthesis, is used for the treatment of dendritic keratitis and, at times, for *Herpes* infections of the skin and mucous membranes. It is available in 5% liquid and 0.5% ointment forms *(Herpid, Kerecid)*. ***Vidarabine,*** available as 3% ointment *(Vira-A),* is also an antiviral agent active against *Herpes simplex* virus types 1 and 2.

NURSING IMPLICATIONS

Assessment

The patient's history should be reviewed for any previous episodes of allergic reaction to the substance to be used. Assess the area to be treated, and document observations concerning the appearance and extent of skin lesions.

Administration

To avoid sensitisation, antibiotic preparations should be applied for as short a time as is reasonable and, to minimise further trouble if sensitisation does occur, the drug used should, wherever possible, be one that is unlikely to be needed for systemic administration in the future.

Evaluation

Observe skin for signs of lessening of the infection. Where antibiotic preparations have been used, watch closely for signs of persistence or recurrence of inflammation which could indicate a sensitivity reaction. When neomycin is used for large lesions or for a prolonged period of time, be alert for complaints of tinnitus, dizziness or deafness, which could indicate ototoxic effects.

Patient teaching

Patients should be advised to discontinue treatment and seek medical advice if inflammation persists or recurs when using topical antibiotic preparations. The nurse also has a responsibility to educate people against the indiscriminate use of topical antibiotics due to the risk of sensitivity and the development of resistant strains of bacteria. The use of hexachlorophane to routinely wash neonates and as a hand-washing agent by pregnant women should be discouraged.

ANTIFUNGAL PREPARATIONS

Just as there are a great many bacteria, each group reacting differently to various antibiotics, so too there are many fungi, and we need several different kinds of antifungal preparations. Some of these are used systemically, such as ***griseofulvin*** and ***flucytosine.*** Some are used only topically, such as ***undecylenic acid.*** Some may be used both systemically and topically, such as ***nystatin.***

Amphotericin B (*Fungizone, Fungilin*) is used topically in the treatment of superficial *Candida albicans* infection and is one of the drugs of choice for the systemic fungal infections, the other being ***flucytosine*** *(Alcobon)* which is available as tablets and IV injection. Amphotericin B is available as lozenges for oral thrush caused by *Candida* species and as vaginal cream and pessaries for vaginal candida infection.

Adverse Drug Reactions

Side effects to systemic administration include fever, nausea, vomiting, anorexia, rash, joint pains and occasionally blurred vision, convulsions, hypotension and hypertension. Care should be exercised where renal function is impaired.

Zinc undecanoate (also undecanoic acid) has antifungal properties and is mainly applied topically in the prophylaxis and treatment of tinea pedis. It is available in ointment and powder form under the brands *Tineafax, Mycota†* and *Phytocil.*

Dithranol, a parasiticide, is used as a 0.1% and 1% ointment or paste (usually *Lassar's Paste* — zinc and salicylic acid paste BP) in the treatment of psoriasis. Since some patients are hypersensitive to dithranol, a preliminary test for sensitivity should be carried out on a small area of skin. Dithranol commonly causes discoloration of the skin and is very irritant to eyes, lips and mucous membranes.

Natamycin *(Pimafucin)* is effective against infections caused by *Candida* species and also in acute tinea and tinea versicolor. It is available as a cream — 2% for topical use in paronychia, tinea and other superficial fungal infections.

Nystatin *(Nystan)* is effective against yeast and yeast-like fungi, including *Candida albicans.* It is available in the following forms: cream and ointment for use on the skin; vaginal tablets and cream for local treatment of vulvo-vaginal candidiasis; oral tablets and capsules for treatment of candidiasis of the gastrointestinal tract, and oral drops and pastilles for thrush and other *Candida* infections of mouth, throat and tongue.

Griseofulvin (*Grisovin, Fulcin*) has revolutionised the treatment of tinea infections of the skin, hair and nails. It is administered orally and is taken up by the cells destined to become keratin, these being the cells on which the fungus lives. Absorption from the gastrointestinal tract is aided by taking the tablets with a fatty meal. In infections of the nails, an extended course of treatment is necessary, six months or more.

Tolnaftate *(Timoped)* is used as a 1% solution or cream in the treatment of various forms of tinea.

Whitfield's Ointment (benzoic acid compound BPC). Benzoic acid has antimycotic properties, and this ointment is used for treatment of fungal infections of the skin, such as ringworm and tinea pedis (athlete's foot).

Castellani's Magenta Paint should be painted on twice a day and is effective in treatment of paronychia and superficial dermatophytosis, especially when eczematous dermatitis is present.

Sodium thiosulphate solution 20% is the treatment of choice for tinea or pityriasis versicolor. It should be applied to the whole upper trunk and upper arms every day for three weeks.

Miconazole, econazole and ***clotrimazole*** are closely related antifungal agents used for topical treatment of dermal infections such as tinea pedis, tinea cruris and tinea corporis. They are effective also against candidiasis infections including paronychia, cutaneous candidiasis and external genital candidiasis. Side effects include burning, stinging, pruritus, urticaria and general irritation, particularly in children. Miconazole is available as *Daktarin Cream 2%* in a 20 g tube for topical use and as *Gyno-Daktarin-Combi-pack* for vaginal use.

Econazole is marketed as *Ecostatin* and as *Pevaryl,* both brands as a 1% cream. It is claimed to be effective in vaginal candidiasis in a three-day course.

Clotrimazole is the active ingredient of *Canesten 1% cream* and *Canesten Vaginal Tablets*. Refer also to Chapter 24.

BURNS

Treatment of burns has had a varied career. ***Tannic acid*** was long used as it formed a "skin" over the burned area, hopefully sealing in serum and sealing out germs. ***Silver nitrate*** compresses were popular for some years and still have a place in the treatment of burns. The first real breakthrough in the treatment of burns was a cream of ***mafenide acetate***, marketed in the UK as *Sulfamylon Cream*. This was effective in preventing infection by *Pseudomonas* organisms, but was painful for the patient and sometimes caused electrolyte imbalance. It has been replaced by ***silver sulphadiazine cream*** *(Flamazine)* which is equally effective against *Pseudomonas* and is painless for large areas. ***Chlorhexidine 0.2%*** is usually added to the cream as a prophylactic against staphylococcal infection. The nurse scrubs up, dons cap, sterile gown and gloves and applies the cream thickly with her gloved hand. There have been reports of sensitivity reactions to the cream.

Sunburn is of frequent occurrence in the tropical and subtropical areas of the world. It is treated in a similar way to any other burn. Frequent and prolonged exposure to the sun causes premature ageing of the skin and skin cancer. The ultraviolet (UV) "B" band causes the most damage. Many cosmetically acceptable products which filter out UV light are available, and their use should be encouraged. The Department of Health periodically publishes a classification of sunscreen products according to their ability to filter out UV light.

TOPICAL CORTICOSTEROIDS

Corticosteroids applied topically suppress inflammation and allergic reactions, produce a prolonged vasoconstriction and have a preventative effect in cell division. It is suggested that they decrease membrane permeability and inhibit release of toxic substances by attaching themselves to tissue receptors. In addition, their vasoconstrictive action decreases serum extravasation, swelling and discomfort, including itching. They are also immunosuppressive and may inhibit allergic reactions by preventing the production of antigen-antibody complexes.

Penetration is through the hair follicles and transepidermal routes with hydrocortisone and betamethasone valerate. Most others follow the transfollicular route. They are effective only when absorbed deeply into the epidermis, and the less potent steroids were formerly often covered by an occlusive polythene dressing wrap sealed by taping the edges to the skin.

Using this method of treatment, an increase of 75% to 100% in potency was achieved. Since the availability of more potent derivatives, the method is now rarely necessary. The effectiveness of topical corticosteroids appears to be related to the potency of the drug and to the concentration achieved in the cutaneous tissues. Percutaneous absorption or penetration depends on the extent of skin damage, the relative concentration of the corticosteroid preparation, the vehicle, the type of dressing and possibly the characteristics of the specific steroids. Those preparations listed as potent in Table 52 have about 360 times the activity of hydrocortisone 1%.

Table 52
Some Topical Corticosteroids

Potency	**Generic Name**		**Trade Name**
Very potent	Fluocinolone acetonide	0.2%	*Synalar Forte*
Potent	Betamethasone valerate	0.1%	*Betnovate*
	Fluocinolone acetonide	0.025%	*Synalar*
	Betamethasone dipropionate	0.05%	*Diprosone*
	Triamcinolone acetonide	0.1%	*Adcortyl* *Ledercort*
	Fluocortolone	0.5%	*Ultralanum*
Moderately potent	Hydrocortisone butyrate	0.1%	*Locoid*
	Clobetasone butyrate	0.05%	*Eumovate*
Weak	Hydrocortisone	1%	*Efcortelan* *Hydrocortistab*
	Fluocortolone	0.2%	*Ultradil Plain*

Topical corticosteroids are recommended as a supplement to, and not as a substitute for, preparations used conventionally in the management of dermatoses. It is most important to realise that dermatoses are controlled but not healed by these agents. Most dermatoses, particularly the eczematous group, respond to topical or systemic administration of corticosteroids. Other skin conditions such as those associated with systemic collagen disease, pemphigus, sarcoidosis, drug-induced eruptions and urticaria may respond to systemic but not to topical therapy.

Topical corticosteroids are recommended in the treatment of acute and chronic dermatoses, including atopic, seborrhoeic, contact and some types of chronic eczematous dermatitis, and in infantile eczema, neurodermatitis, intertriginous dermatitis and anogenital pruritus. In the treatment of contact dermatitis, the use of topical ointment is advised, due to serous exudates washing away all water-miscible preparations.

Topical corticosteroids are ineffective in the treatment of sunburn or other burns. Potent corticosteroids appear to clear partially lesions of solar malignancies (sunspots) on the face while being applied, but in reality they produce epidermal atrophy with a diffuse spread of the malignant lesion into the surrounding tissues, which is ill defined, and leaves the skin very fragile should future surgery be necessary.

Sodium retention and transient inhibition of pituitary-adrenal function have been reported when large areas have been treated for prolonged periods of time with topical corticosteroids. Prolonged facial application in adult women may result in rosacea-like dermatitis, diffuse erythema, perioral dermatitis or acne.

There are several contraindications to the use of topical corticosteroids. The stronger, more potent fluorinated preparations are associated with a higher incidence of side effects. Local complications include atrophy of the epidermis and dermis with striae and secondary haemorrhage into the tissues. Tachyphylaxis is a recognised problem, that is corticosteroids are less effective the greater their strength and the longer and more frequent their usage. Skin malignancies should not be treated with topical corticosteroids. The use of corticosteroids topically also produces a masking of bacterial and fungal infections. Particular care should be taken with children having large areas treated, or having occlusive dressings, as absorption of corticosteroids may occur, giving rise to unwanted systemic effects.

NURSING IMPLICATIONS

Assessment

Before applying a topical corticosteroid, the nurse should assess the skin condition and designated site of application. If the skin shows signs of infection, malignancy or atrophy, do not apply the corticosteroid and seek medical advice.

Application

It is important that the nurse checks the type of corticosteroid and the strength, before applying. Fluorinated corticosteroids are extremely potent, with a greater risk of systemic absorption. It could therefore be dangerous to substitute a fluorinated corticosteroid for a non-fluorinated one. Apply with an applicator, or use gloves to avoid the risk of cutaneous atrophy of finger tips. Ensure a non-touch technique is used, and take the appropriate precautions to avoid cross infection.

Evaluation

Observe for improvement in skin condition. Children having large areas treated and patients with occlusive dressings should be closely observed for signs of systemic absorption and overlying infection. Take and record temperature every four hours for these patients. Observe skin for evidence of infection or atrophy of the dermis.

Patient teaching

This should emphasise the proper application of topical corticosteroids. Patients should be advised to taper off use of topical corticosteroids gradually, as sudden cessation may cause a rebound exacerbation of the skin condition. They should also be taught self-evaluation for local and systemic adverse effects, such as atrophy of the skin, infection or oedema. It is important that patients and the general public be warned against the indiscriminate use of these preparations without first seeking medical advice or the advice of their pharmacist.

NON-STEROIDAL ANTIPRURITICS

Pruritus is a symptom, not a disease, but the intense discomfort it can produce should not be underestimated. Antipruritics are applied to relieve irritation in general diseases such as diabetes, jaundice, urticaria, the infectious fevers and following drug intoxication. They are also used in certain skin diseases. All wet dressings and shake lotions have some antipruritic effect, but certain substances have a specific action.

Calamine lotion is a suspension of calamine and zinc oxide in water. It contains phenol which acts as a mild antiseptic and antipruritic. The phenol decreases itch by anaesthetising the cutaneous nerve endings. There are various commercial preparations of calamine in ointments, creams and lotions mixed with local anaesthetics and/or antihistamines.

Camphor, when applied in 1% to 3% concentration, has mild antipruritic effects through its anaesthetic properties. It is often added to calamine lotion, as is menthol 0.25% to 2% which relieves itching by substituting a cool sensation.

Coal tar solution 3% to 10% (often in calamine lotion) is also used for the relief of itch. It is sometimes added to the bath.

Crotamiton is an antipruritic agent and local application gives rapid relief from itching. It is available as crotamiton 10% ointment or lotion (*Eurax*).

Creams and lotions containing topical antihistamines are available. However, as these often cause sensitisation to the sun and to the preparations themselves, they are not recommended.

Local anaesthetics are often used to allay pruritus by blocking nerve impulses at sensory nerve endings, but sensitisation has been reported. Lignocaine is the most commonly used local anaesthetic and is available as 5% ointment, 2% jelly, 4% solution and 10% spray under the brand name *Xylocaine.*

NURSING IMPLICATIONS

Assessment of the patient with pruritus involves firstly establishing the underlying cause, so that appropriate therapy can be initiated. Where local applications are to be used for symptomatic relief, assess the history for previous allergy to the substance and inspect the skin for signs of excessive dryness, cracking, weeping or broken areas.

Application
Observe any precautions specific to the substance being used. For example, do not apply crotamiton to mucosal areas such as the vulva or anus.

Evaluation
The patient should be evaluated for relief of the pruritus and any adverse effects, especially hypersensitivity, drying and cracking of the skin.

Patient teaching
Include instruction on correct method of application and advice to refrain from scratching or rubbing. This destroys the epidermis and sets up a vicious circle of lesion, more scratching and further damage.

PIGMENTATION DISORDERS

VITILIGO

Methoxsalen and ***trioxsalen*** are used in the treatment of vitiligo and other pigmentation deficiencies of the skin. They may be administered orally or topically, and occasionally both methods are employed. These drugs are inactive in themselves but sensitise the skin to sunlight (or artificial ultra-violet light) so that formation of melanin pigments is increased following exposure. The photosensitivity is apparent about one hour after a dose, peaks at about two hours and then gradually decreases until it is completely lost in about eight hours.

Over-exposure to sunlight or UV light after taking these drugs may result in serious burning, with blistering of the skin. In this case the photosensitivity may persist for several days. The eyes must be protected, and glasses which filter out UV light should be worn for 24 hours after ingestion of the drugs. Lips also should be protected with a sunscreen.

Topical application of these drugs is more severe in its effects than oral administration. They may need to be diluted before application to prevent excessive reactions. The lotion is applied once daily to the vitiliginous area and exposed to sunlight or UV light for 30 seconds to one minute, this time being increased if necessary on subsequent days with great caution. Should the skin blister, local treatment must be ceased immediately.

Photosensitivity reactions are of two types: phototoxic and photoallergic. Phototoxic reactions are usually dependent on the dose of the drug given and affect only the area of skin exposed to the light. Photoallergic reactions bear no relationship to the dose of the drug and may be generalised.

Foods such as carrots, celery, parsley, parsnips and mustard contain substances known as psoralens which are photosensitisers. These foods can cause phototoxic reactions. Some drugs (such as tetracyclines, phenothiazines, sulphonamides, nalidixic acid and topically applied antihistamines, sulphonamides and hexachlorophane) may cause phototoxic reactions. Photoallergic reactions can result from sulphonamides, thiazides, griseofulvin and phenothiazines. All of these drugs should be avoided during therapy with methoxsalen or trioxsalen.

NURSING IMPLICATIONS

Administration of methoxsalen and trioxsalen should always be done under close supervision. Topical preparations should not be given to patients to take home.

During treatment with these substances, evaluation is mainly concerned with observing the patient's skin for signs of burning. If this occurs the patient must be removed from the source of light immediately.

Patients receiving this treatment must be warned of the possibility of sunburn and of the need to protect the eyes and lips.

PSORIASIS

Psoriasis is a skin disease of unknown aetiology, characterised by silvery, scaly patches. When the scale is removed, erythematous papules are revealed, usually showing several bleeding points. The disease follows an unpredictable course, with spontaneous remissions and acute exacerbations. Topical therapy is the mainstay in treatment of psoriasis, and keratolytics and softening agents such as oily glycerin cream are extensively used.

In severe cases, ***corticosteroids*** are used systemically and topically. There is a high rate of relapse following treatment with systemic steroids, and it should be used only for short periods. Contemporary therapy includes the careful use of topical and systemic ***antimitotic drugs.***

Dithranol combines with deoxyribonucleic acid, thus inhibiting the synthesis of nucleoprotein and so diminishing cellular proliferation. It is applied as an 0.01% to 2% ointment or paste. Dithranol may cause a burning sensation when applied to the skin or to lesions and is irritant to the eyes. It stains the skin. Some patients are hypersensitive to dithranol.

Methotrexate, a folic-acid antagonist, also inhibits cellular proliferation. In severe, disabling psoriasis, it is given orally as well as being applied as weak soaks (0.015%). Many oral dosage regimens are used. Some of these are 25 to 37.5 mg once weekly; 5 to 15 mg per square metre of body surface once weekly; 12.5 mg daily for 12 days, stop therapy for one week, then repeat. The side effects of methotrexate include blood dyscrasias, gastrointestinal-tract ulceration and liver toxicity, and the intermittent dosage is an attempt to prevent these effects. The drug is excreted mainly through the kidney.

Vitamin A derivatives are also used in the treatment of psoriasis. (See under keratolytics page 367). Promising results have been reported in the treatment of psoriasis following a regimen of oral ***methoxsalen*** and long-range UV light. The regimen is known as PUVA: P for psoralen (the class of drug to which methoxsalen and trioxsalen belong, other names for them being methoxypsoralen and trimethylpsoralen) and UVA for UV-A light, that is UV light in the wavelength range 320 to 390 Å. The mechanism of action is inhibition of DNA synthesis. The treatment must be closely supervised to prevent serious burns.

NURSING IMPLICATIONS

Administration of dithranol should be preceded by a preliminary test for sensitivity on a small area of skin. Avoid contact with eyes.

Evaluation of patients receiving treatment for psoriasis will include observing the skin for improvement in the condition. Where dithranol is used, watch for allergic reactions. Observe for signs of burning when retinoids are used. When oral retinoids are used, observe patient for signs of adverse effects such as mucosal dryness, palmo-plantar desquamation, pruritus, thinning of the skin and alopecia.

Teach patients receiving dithranol treatment that the skin and hair may darken in colour. Patients receiving retinoid therapy should avoid direct exposure to sunlight.

HEPARINOID PREPARATIONS

A heparinoid, as its name suggests, is a substance with heparin-like activity. Heparinoids possess anticoagulant and anti-inflammatory properties, and promote fibrinolysis. They therefore increase local blood and lymph flow and accelerate reabsorption of local oedema and infiltrations. Heparinoids appear to be effectively absorbed through the skin. *Hirudoid* is a cream containing in each 100 g heparinoid equivalent to 25 000 units of heparin. *Lasonil,* an ointment, contains in each 100 g heparinoid equivalent to 5000 units of heparin plus 15 000 international units of hyaluronidase, which assists absorption and dispersion by breaking down hyaluronic acid. *Movelat* is a cream which contains, in addition to a heparinoid, an adrenal extract (corticosteroid) and salicylic acid 2%. These products are used in the treatment of sprains, contusions and haematomata, and for superficial thromboses and varicose ulcers. They are also effective in softening scar tissue. Bruising after venepuncture is dissipated more rapidly by their use.

The earlier that treatment is begun, the better the results that may be expected. Depending on the extent of the lesion, 3 to 5 cm of the cream or ointment should be applied two or three times daily. In certain cases more may be necessary. In thrombosis and thrombophlebitis it should be applied on gauze to the affected area, but in varicose ulcer it should be massaged into the skin around the ulcer in the direction of the venous return, from below the ulcer upwards. For the treatment of haematomata and scars, the cream may be massaged into the skin.

Heparinoid preparations should not be applied to bleeding areas. In suppurative processes they should not come in contact with the infected area.

NURSING IMPLICATIONS

1. Treatment should be commenced as soon as possible.
2. Avoid contact of these preparations with broken skin.

SELF-EVALUATION TEST

1. A cream consists of:
   (a) an oily substance dispersed in water
   (b) an aqueous substance dispersed in oil
   (c) a white powder evenly suspended in an aqueous vehicle
   (d) (a) and (b)
   (e) (a), (b) and (c).
2. Photosensitivity is:
   (a) an abnormal fear of being photographed
   (b) a burn caused by contact with photographic chemicals
   (c) damage to the skin as a result of exposure to sunlight or artificial light.
3. The doctor has ordered betamethasone cream to be applied to a small weeping lesion on the patient's arm. You are unable to obtain cream, but can obtain betamethasone ointment. What is likely to be the effect on the lesion if you use it?
4. Your friend asks for advice about the "tinea" lesion between her toes. The lesion is red and weeping and the skin is cracked. Would it be better to apply an antifungal powder or cream? Why?
5. The doctor has ordered salicylic acid 20% paint for a young woman with several warts on her hand. What vehicle is likely to be used and what instructions would you give the patient for its use?
6. You have been applying neomycin soaks to a large infected area on the back. The lesion is healing rapidly, then for no apparent reason it again becomes inflamed, and this inflammation persists in spite of continuing treatment. What would you suspect has happened?
7. An extensive infected leg ulcer has been irrigated with a solution of neomycin 0.5% for 10 days and, while the infection seems to be clearing, there is as yet little evidence of healing. The appropriate action for a nurse is to:
   (a) continue the treatment;
   (b) change to another treatment to speed up the healing process;
   (c) draw to the attention of the attending medical officer that prolonged treatment with neomycin may have serious side effects.

Table 53
Drugs Used in Dermatology

Drug Group	Drug Name	Use	Action	Adverse Reactions	Nursing Implications
Vitamin A derivatives	Tretinoin (topical)	Severe acne, keratosis, psoriasis	Affects differentiation of epithelial tissue	Increased susceptibility of skin to sunlight	***Assess:*** history for previous adverse effects; document baseline observations of lesions and general condition of skin. ***Administer:*** local application. ***Evaluate:*** for improvement in skin condition; observe skin for signs of photosensitivity. ***Teach:*** to avoid direct exposure to sunlight during treatment and to protect treated area with clothing or a suitable sunscreen.
	Etretinate (oral)	Disorders of keratinisation, e.g. psoriasis, ichthyosis, lichen planus	Affects differentiation of epithelial tissue	Cheilitis, mucosal dryness, palmo-plantar desquamation, pruritus, thinning of skin, alopecia, headache, elevated liver enzymes; embryotoxic and teratogenic	
Anti-infective preparations	For information about anti-infective preparations, see Chapters 22, 23, 24.				***Assess:*** age — as should be used with caution in women of childbearing potential; pregnancy; history for

					previous adverse effects to drug; document baseline observations of lesions and general condition of skin. ***Administer:*** oral as ordered. ***Evaluate:*** for signs of improvement in skin condition; for adverse effects such as mucosal dryness, palmo-plantar desquamation, pruritus, thinning of skin and alopecia.
Topical corticosteroids	Fluocinolone acetonide Betamethasone dipropionate Triamcinolone acetonide Fluorocortolone caproate Hydrocortisone Hydrocortisone pivalate Hydrocortisone butyrate Clobetasone butyrate	Control of acute and chronic dermatoses	Suppression of inflammation and allergy, production of vasoconstriction, prevention of cell division; penetrate through hair follicles and/or transepidermal routes	Epidermal atrophy, spreading of malignant lesions, rosacea-like facial dermatitis, erythema and acne; systemic absorption is a distinct possibility, leading to systemic side effects - see Chapter 11	***Assess:*** skin condition and designated site of application; skin for signs of infection, malignancy or atrophy. ***Administer:*** use sterile technique; use applicator or gloves to minimize risk of atrophy to skin. ***Evaluate:*** efficacy of medication; for evidence of development of overlying infection; temperature; for dermal atrophy, striae, thinning of epidermis, rebound effect; for evidence of systemic absorption. ***Teach:*** proper application; self-evaluation for efficacy, and local and systemic side effects; to taper off use gradually; to avoid indiscriminate use and seek medical advice.

continued

Drug Group	Drug Name	Use	Action	Adverse Reactions	Nursing Implications
Preparations used in pigmentation disorders	Methoxsalen Trioxsalen	Vitiligo and other pigmentation disorders	Sensitise skin to UV light, so formation of melanin pigments is increased	Burning, blistering of skin and eyes	***Assess:*** area to be treated (local applications); Document baseline observations of skin lesions. ***Administer:*** vitiligo — topical or oral followed by exposure of skin to sunlight or artificial UV light; Psoriasis — usually oral regime followed by exposure to UV light. Topical treatment must always be under close supervision, and the lotion should never be given to the patient to take home. ***Evaluate:*** for improvement and signs of burning; if burning occurs the patient must be removed from the source of light immediately. ***Teach:*** warn of the possibility of sunburn; protect lips with sunscreen.
Preparations used in psoriasis	Dithranol	Psoriasis	Combines with DNA and diminishes cell proliferation	Burning sensation, irritant to eyes, skin staining	***Assess:*** for previous hypersensitivity; document baseline description of skin lesions. ***Administer:*** perform a preliminary test on a small area of skin first; check for sensitivity before applying treatment; keep away from eyes. ***Evaluate:*** for allergic response, for improvement in lesions. ***Teach:*** advise that patient may feel a burning when dithranol is first applied; skin and hair may darken.

SECTION 7

22
ANTI-INFECTIVE THERAPY — GENERAL PRINCIPLES

Christine L. Odgers

The following three chapters (22, 23 and 24) deal with the topic of anti-infective therapy. These three chapters should be studied as a single entity, rather than three discrete sections. A combined table of Nursing Implications and the self-evaluation questions for all three chapters are listed at the conclusion of Chapter 24. Chapter 22 is an overview of principles and problems of anti-infective therapy. Specific drugs and classes are discussed in Chapters 23 and 24.

OBJECTIVES

As a result of studying this chapter, the reader should be able to:

1. describe the parameters on which the selection of an anti-infective agent is based;
2. describe, in general terms, the mode of action of the various groups of anti-infective agents;
3. list those anti-infective agents used to treat infections due to gram-positive organisms, gram-negative organisms, fungi, malarial parasites, trichomonads, tubercle bacilli, helminths and viruses;
4. differentiate between the various anti-infective agents in each group with respect to dosage, route of administration, major side effects and uses;
5. list the anti-infective agents that must be given by deep intramuscular injection to avoid or reduce pain, those that should be administered slowly intravenously, or in dilute solution to minimize venous irritation and thrombophlebitis, and those that should be administered orally on an empty stomach;
6. state the recommended solution(s) to be used for administering intravenously the more common anti-infective agents.

PREREQUISITE KNOWLEDGE

It is assumed that the reader has a knowledge of:

1. the basic cellular structure of bacteria and other microorganisms;
2. methods of multiplication and replication of microorganisms;
3. classification of microorganisms;
4. the more common microorganisms causing diseases in humans.

DEFINITIONS

Antibiotics — substances produced by microorganisms that, in high dilution, are antagonistic to the growth of other microorganisms. Some antibiotics are made synthetically.
Antibacterial — a drug used to combat an infection caused by bacteria.
Antifungal — a drug used to combat an infection caused by fungi.
Antiviral — a drug used to combat an infection caused by viruses.
Chemotherapy — the drug treatment of infections caused by bacteria, fungi, protozoa, viruses or worms in which the causative agent is destroyed or removed with minimal harm to the host.
Gram-negative organisms — those organisms that are decolourised by acetone applied to the smear after methyl violet in the Gram's staining test. These organisms take up the counterstain, for example, basic fuchsin, and appear pink on microscopic examination. Some examples of gram-negative organisms are *Haemophilus influenzae, Escherichia coli, Klebsiella pneumoniae* and *Proteus mirabilis*.
Gram-positive organisms — those organisms that retain the primary dye complex of the Gram's staining technique (methyl violet) and appear dark purple on microscopic examination. Some examples are *Steptococcus viridans*, *Streptococcus pneumoniae*, *Staphylococcus aureus* and *Streptococcus epidermidis*.
Non-pathogenic organisms or commensals — organisms that coexist harmlessly with host cells.
Pathogenic organisms — organisms that damage the host cells or host organism in some way.
Spectrum — the range of activity of a drug against microorganisms.
Broad spectrum — this term denotes a wide range of antimicrobial activity against gram-positive and gram-negative organisms.
Narrow spectrum — this term denotes a more restricted range of antimicrobial activity. For example, erythromycin has a range of activity restricted to gram-positive organisms, and the polymyxins are active solely against gram-negative organisms.

The goal of drug therapy in the treatment of infectious disease is to assist the body in ridding itself of the infecting organism. This is accomplished by use of an anti-infective agent which, while not seriously impairing the normal biochemical functions of the patient, is "selectively toxic" to the causative organism.

The term "anti-infective" is used in this chapter to mean all chemotherapeutic agents used against microorganisms.

HISTORY

Since ancient times people have used agents empirically for the treatment of infections. The ancient Greeks used male fern as an intestinal anthelmintic, the ancient Hindus treated leprosy with chaulmoogra. The history of modern anti-infective therapy does not begin until the late nineteenth century when salvarsan was discovered.

The present anti-infective era dates from the demonstration by Florey, Chain and others in 1940 that penicillin, discovered by Fleming in 1929, exerts a powerful systemic therapeutic effect. The success of this drug led to a search for other similar substances, and now a wide range of naturally occurring and synthetic anti-infective agents is available.

GENERAL PRINCIPLES

For the treatment of each infection there is generally one drug, or occasionally a combination of drugs, that is likely to be a better choice than other drugs or drug combinations. When an infection does not respond to a first-choice drug or the patient cannot tolerate it, there is usually a preferred order of choice among alternative drugs.
Handbook of Antimicrobial Therapy. *Medical Letter*, January 1974.

In choosing an anti-infective agent, the physician must identify, at least tentatively, the organism responsible for the infection. Often the experienced physician can correctly identify or classify the organism on the basis of the clinical evidence.

To identify the organism, a specimen is obtained. Microscopy is usually the first step. The organism is allocated to one or other of the major groups when its morphology (shape, size, grouping of cells) and staining reactions (gram-positive or gram-negative) are observed. The organism is then grown (cultured) and its susceptibility to various anti-infective agents determined. Biochemical reactions of the organism are also evaluated.

The physician must give consideration to a number of patient/host factors when selecting the anti-infective agent, the dose, the route and the frequency of administration. For example, anti-infective agents must often be administered to patients with renal dysfunction. Most antibiotics are excreted by the kidneys either as the unchanged drug or as a metabolite. Renal dysfunction *per se* is not a contraindication to the use of particular antibiotics; rather, dosage schedules should be altered to prevent toxicity.

The dosage regimens for antibiotics excreted primarily by the kidneys will be decided according to the toxicity of the drug and the type of infection to be treated. Toxic drugs, such as the aminoglycosides, should have their dose adjusted according to renal function. Serum assays are also required so that the dose can be titrated according to the serum concentration of the drug.

One of the most important factors in determining the effectiveness of anti-infective therapy is the functional state of the patient's immune system (host defence mechanisms). Patients suffering from immune system deficiencies or suppression secondary to disease or drug therapy may not respond favourably to appropriate anti-infective therapy, even when large doses are employed. The patient's immune system may not be able to mount a defence response to the invading organism. Treatment of infections in these patients requires special consideration.

Other patient factors to be considered are age, history of hypersensitivity or allergic reactions to anti-infective agents, hepatic disease and the site of infection.

Consideration must also be given to the ability of the anti-infective agent to penetrate to the site of infection. The more barriers the drug has to pass from the site of administration, the less chance it has of reaching its site of action and achieving satisfactory concentrations to inhibit growth of the organism. For example, if the drug is administered by mouth, it must be able to survive passage from the gut to the circulation. Many antibiotics are inactivated during their transit through the gut and hence can only be administered parenterally. Anti-infective agents that are administered parenterally must be absorbed from the site of injection if administered intramuscularly. If the drug is administered intravenously, it must be compatible with the fluid used as the vehicle for injection, and must be able to pass from the blood stream to the site of infection.

Once the drug reaches the site of infection it must be able to penetrate the cell wall of the bacteria to reach its site of action, or, in the case of penicillins and cephalosporins, it must be able to reach its site of action on the cell wall.

It is fundamental to the successful treatment of an infectious disease process that the correct drug, dose, route and frequency of administration are selected for the particular patient. Inadequate dosage may lead to the development of bacterial resistance, and inadequate length of treatment may lead to relapse. Systemic anti-infective agents should not be used to treat trivial, self-limiting infections.

In summary, the choice of appropriate anti-infective agent is based on:

1. the clinical diagnosis;
2. the identification of the infecting organism;
3. the results of in-vitro sensitivity tests indicating those drugs that are active against the organism isolated from the specimen;
4. drug characteristics — ability of the drug to penetrate to the site of infection, toxicity, interaction or incompatibility with other drug therapy and cost;
5. patient factors — age, hepatic and renal function, history of drug sensitivity and the status of the patient's immune response.

SELECTIVE TOXICITY

An anti-infective agent may damage the invading organism while sparing the host. This selective toxicity may be explained as follows:

1. A reaction vital to the microorganism but not to the host may be blocked. For example, the reaction may not occur in the host — penicillin blocks the manufacture of the bacterial cell wall, a structure that host cells do not possess; or the reaction may follow a different route in the host — sulphonamides block the use of para-aminobenzoic acid (PABA) in the bacterial formation of folic acid. Host cells do not synthesise their own folic acid but rather, rely on the absorption of pre-formed folic acid.
2. A reaction vital to the host may be blocked, but the sensitive site in the host may be inaccessible or more resistant, or binding to it by the drug may not be feasible; or the host may inactivate the drug, thus preventing it from being used against the invading organism.

MODE OF ACTION

Anti-infective drugs depend for their effect on an ability to inhibit a biochemical process or disrupt a vital cell structure in an invading organism without having a significant effect on the host. The five principal sites of action, illustrated in Figure 6, are as follows.

1. **The cell wall** — agents such as the penicillins, cephalosporins and vancomycin interfere with the osmotic defences of the cell wall so that the cell absorbs water and bursts.
2. **The lipoprotein cell membrane** (inside the cell wall) — disorientation of the molecules of the cell membrane, similar to the action of a detergent at an oil-water interface, results in the membrane becoming permeable and vital components escape. Amphotericin, colistin and polymyxin interfere with the integrity of the cell membrane.
3. **Ribosomes and nucleic acid metabolism** — aminoglycosides, chloramphenicol, erythromycin, lincomycin/clindamycin and the tetracyclines interfere with protein synthesis controlled by the ribosomes.
4. **DNA (deoxyribonucleic acid)** — griseofulvin and nalidixic acid interfere with the synthesis of the major nucleic acid, DNA, in the nucleus.
5. **Intermediary metabolism** — interference with the synthesis of essential components (antimetabolite action). For example, folic acid is required for growth in bacterial cells, and its metabolism is inhibited by sulphonamides, trimethoprim and pyrimethamine.

The mode of action of antibacterial agents may be described as bactericidal or bacteriostatic. *Bactericidal action* is defined as one in which the drug kills the active bacteria. *Bacteriostatic action* is the inhibition of growth, but not the killing, of bacteria; the growth of the bacteria recurs after

FIG. 6: PRINCIPAL SITES OF ACTION OF ANTI-INFECTIVE AGENTS

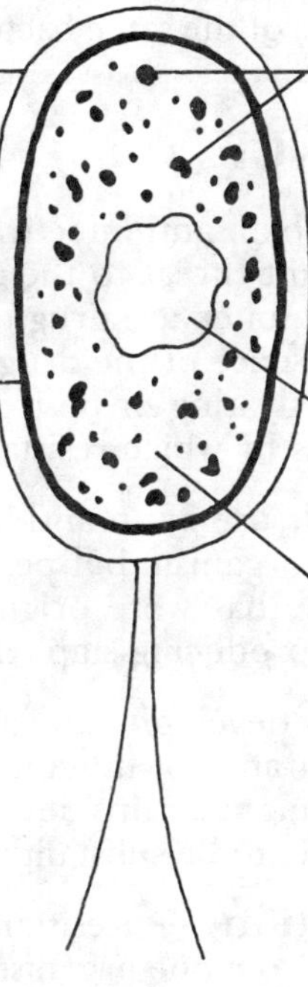

the antibacterial agent is withdrawn. Most bacteriostatic drugs become bactericidal at very high concentrations or after long periods of exposure to the organism. Similarly, the mode of action of anti-fungal agents may be described as *fungicidal* or *fungistatic*.

The action of an anti-infective drug against an organism may be significantly enhanced when it is administered simultaneously with another agent. This is known as *synergism* or *potentiation*. One example of this effect, achieved with combined therapy but unobtainable with a single antibiotic, is the total bactericidal effect exerted by pencillin and streptomycin against *Streptococcus faecalis*.

Jawetz and Gunnison[1] have proposed that the combination of two bactericidal anti-infective agents may exert a synergistic effect, whereas two bacteriostatic antibiotics will only have an *additive* effect. The additive effect is equivalent to that produced by increasing the concentration of one drug and omitting the other drug.

Certain combinations may result in a decreased rate of early bactericidal action and a reduction in the early rate of cure of infection, below that observed with a single drug. This is described as *antagonism* and may occur when a bactericidal agent, for example penicillin, is combined with a bacteriostatic agent such as tetracycline.

There are only two important indications for prescribing anti-infective

1. Jawetz, E. & Gunnison, J. B. *Antibiot. & Chemother.*, Vol. 2, 1952, p.243.

agents in combination. The first is to prevent the development of bacterial resistance, and the second is to achieve synergy as illustrated above and by, for example, the combined action of trimethoprim and sulphamethoxazole on successive stages of the same bacterial metabolic process.

BACTERIAL RESISTANCE

Bacteria may become resistant to an anti-infective agent, and the development of resistance is a constant threat to the usefulness of the drug. The types of drug resistance exhibited are drug tolerance (the organism is capable of growing in the presence of the drug) and drug destruction (the organism is capable of inactivating or destroying the drug). There are several different mechanisms by which resistance may emerge.

Selection — The therapeutic use of an anti-infective agent tends to eliminate sensitive strains of an organism but permits the multiplication and spread of a small minority that were originally resistant, such as penicillin-resistant penicillinase-producing staphylococci.

Mutation — Resistance may develop to the anti-infective agent as a result of the spontaneous appearance of mutants during the process of cell division. Whether or not mutant strains develop as a result of adaptation to the environment has yet to be substantiated.

Transduction or conjugation — Resistance may be acquired by the transfer of genetic material from one organism to another. This may be achieved by *transduction* (involving the transfer by bacteriophage of DNA carrying a gene for resistance) or by *conjugation* (involving the transfer of circular particles of genetic material, known as plasmids, while bacteria are in direct physical contact with one another).

Transduction is of particular importance in the transfer of antibiotic resistance among strains of *Staphylococcus aureus*. The transfer of resistance by the process of conjugation occurs predominantly among gram-negative bacilli. Resistance to one antibiotic is accompanied by resistance to other antibiotics closely related to it and this may be seen with penicillins. There are a few instances of cross-resistance among anti-infective agents less closely related. For example, an organism resistant to erythromycin may also be resistant to lincomycin and clindamycin, that is, the organism displays multiple-drug resistance. Measures aimed at preventing the development of resistance are important in the use of anti-infective agents. These include avoidance of unnecessary use, particularly in prophylaxis, adequate dosage for a limited time and combined treatment when using any anti-infective agent to which resistance can develop readily.

Today, many hospitals in Great Britain have adopted antibiotic policies and guidelines which are aimed at reducing the induction of resistance through restricting the overall use of anti-infective agents, restricting their use for trivial infections, and reducing unnecessary or prolonged use in prophylaxis.

HAZARDS OF ANTI-INFECTIVE THERAPY

The administration of anti-infective agents entails risks of three different types: toxic effects, sensitisation reactions and superinfection.

Toxic effects

Most anti-infective agents cause damage at one or more of four sites; liver, kidney, bone marrow and eighth cranial nerve.

Sensitisation reactions (hypersensitivity or allergic reactions)

Contact with penicillin from therapy or other causes may lead to sensitisation. A subsequent exposure to the drug may then cause immediate anaphylactic shock or death. Alternatively, a hypersensitivity reaction may not occur for some days after the first dose.

Superinfection

Superinfection may occur as a result of the substitution of a resistant microorganism for the original sensitive microorganism at the site of infection. Superinfection may also occur as the result of the proliferation of a resistant organism in the alimentary tract as a consequence of suppression of the normal flora by anti-infective therapy. Superinfection has been reported with the tetracyclines.

In fact, the more "broad" the effect of an anti-infective agent on microorganisms, then the greater is the alteration in the normal microflora and the greater is the possibility of superinfection developing. Superinfection also occurs with drugs that interfere with the response of the body to infections (the immune response), such as corticosteroids and other immunosuppressive agents.

Anti-infective agents have been, and are, subject to inappropriate use. The prescriber must consider carefully all the factors discussed in this section and others, such as the appropriate duration of treatment, before exposing the patient to the hazards associated with anti-infective therapy.

ALLERGIC REACTIONS

The occurrence of allergic reactions to anti-infective agents is probably the primary factor limiting their effective use. It has been estimated that allergic reactions to penicillins occur in 2% to 5% of the general population, and approximately 10% of those who have been previously exposed to penicillin will experience an allergic reaction. Patients with a history of hives, asthma, hayfever and eczema and other drug sensitivities are more likely to experience severe, anaphylactoid reactions to the penicillins.

The importance of accurately determining a patient's history of previous allergic reactions or exposures to the pencillins cannot be overemphasised. The nurse should report all comments the patient may make to her regarding previous adverse or allergic experiences with anti-infective agents.

The nurse should understand the different types of allergic reactions. These are categorised as immediate, accelerated and delayed reactions.

Immediate allergic reactions develop within 20 minutes following administration of the drug. The patient generally experiences itching of the palms or axilla, apprehension, weakness, coughing, sneezing, shortness of breath, or a sudden rise in body temperature. The allergic reaction may be manifested only as flushing, generalised pruritus or urticaria. It may also be anaphylactoid in nature and involve vascular collapse, shock, cardiac arrest, bronchospasm, laryngeal oedema, respiratory depression or arrest.

Accelerated allergic reactions develop within 30 minutes to 48 hours after the administration of an anti-infective agent. Urticaria and erythema, with or without fever, are the most common manifestations.

Delayed allergic reactions develop some days, and occasionally weeks, after the use of the causative agent. Skin rashes including erythema, urticaria, bullous eruptions, exfoliative dermatitis, contact dermatitis and Stevens-Johnson syndrome may develop. Other reactions may include haematological abnormalities and nephropathy. A "serum-like" sickness may occur with penicillins.

The treatment of these allergic reactions will depend on the type of reaction. Immediate anaphylactic reactions are life-threatening and must be treated promptly. If anti-infective therapy is to be continued in a patient who has experienced an allergic reaction, an agent from a different chemical group and, preferably one to which cross-sensitivity with the original drug has not been demonstrated, should be selected.

DURATION OF THERAPY

The duration of the period of therapy is important to the success of appropriately prescribed anti-infective agents. If treatment is not continued for long enough, for example for a minimum of five days in infections of moderate severity, or for 48 hours after the patient's temperature has returned to normal, relapse may occur. Prolonged periods of therapy are, in most instances, an extravagance. Anti-infective agents used for prophylaxis should not be administered for a period greater than three days. Some prophylactic regimens require only one or two doses of the appropriate anti-infective agent.

STORAGE OF ANTI-INFECTIVE AGENTS

Anti-infective agents are often susceptible to varying temperatures, with rapid deterioration occurring when the product is stored under unfavourable conditions.

The nurse should check the outer container carefully and ensure that the drug is stored at the recommended temperature. She should also check the expiry date on the container. The activity of these agents decreases with time, and some, such as the tetracyclines, break down to toxic by-products on prolonged storage.

PREPARATION FOR ADMINISTRATION

In the hospital environment, anti-infective agents are commonly administered by the parenteral route. Many of these agents are presented as a sterile powder requiring reconstitution prior to administration. The nurse should refer to the manufacturer's product insert and also any parenteral drug reconstitution guides available within the hospital prior to reconstituting the drug with the correct diluent and the correct volume of diluent. She should ensure that strict aseptic techniques are followed when reconstituting the drug.

Frequently, the dose required for administration will be different from that contained in the reconstituted solution. The nurse should check carefully the dose prescribed, calculate the number of millilitres of solution containing the required amount of the drug, and then request a second nurse to check the calculations *prior* to drawing up the solution aseptically into a sterile syringe. The incorrect dose may result in inadequate concentration of the anti-infective agent reaching the site of infection or may result in toxic effects if too much of the drug is administered.

Although the manufacturer's package insert contains directions for the storage (usually refrigeration) and life of the reconstituted solution, it is advisable to discard any remaining solution after the initial dose has been withdrawn to avoid possible contamination or deterioration of the remaining solution.

ADMINISTRATION

The nurse should follow carefully the directions for administration given by the prescriber. She should also check the directions for administration in the manufacturer's package insert and refer to any parenteral drug administration guides available in the hospital.

Anti-infective agents administered intramuscularly are often painful and may cause abscess formation. These agents are generally administered deep into the muscle mass. Some anti-infective agents may be given by rapid intravenous injections, but some should be injected slowly, often over 5 to 10 minutes into a running intravenous fluid to minimise side effects. Other anti-infective agents must be diluted in a large volume of intravenous fluid and infused very slowly. Again the nurse should refer to available information to ensure that the correct route and rate of administration are used. She must also check that the intravenous fluid and any other drugs it may contain are compatible with the anti-infective agent. Guidelines for the intravenous administration of a number of the anti-infective agents discussed in this chapter are included in Appendix C. The nurse should check with the pharmacy department of the hospital if she is uncertain of the correct method of administration of a drug.

The nurse should be aware that a number of anti-infective agents are recommended to be administered orally on an empty stomach to avoid interactions with food and to promote absorption of the drug. If the medication container does not carry any specific directions regarding the administration of the anti-infective agent with respect to food or other medications, the nurse should check with the pharmacy department and also available literature to ascertain the appropriate time to administer the drug.

NURSING IMPLICATIONS

Assessment

An accurate record of previous allergies is essential before anti-infective drugs are administered. This should include the drug provoking the response and the type of reaction experienced. Because of the frequency of potential drug interactions with anti-infective drugs, the nurse needs to be aware of the current and recent drug regimens, and to check for incompatibilities. When anti-infectives are given intravenously, compatibility between the drug and infusion fluid should be checked (see Appendix C). The prescriber should be aware of any signs of renal or hepatic impairment, in case doses need to be reduced, or therapy ceased.

Baseline temperature and other signs of infection need to be assessed before commencement of therapy. Any specimens required for culture and sensitivity testing must be collected before anti-infective therapy is initiated.

Evaluation

The patient's response to anti-infective drugs is evaluated with reference to combating the infection and any adverse effects that might occur. The signs and symptoms of infection should be monitored throughout the course of anti-infective therapy. The specific toxic effects of anti-infective drugs must be looked for, for example, hearing or renal impairment in patients receiving aminoglycosides.

Many anti-infective agents can cause phlebitis and thrombophlebitis on intravenous administration. The nurse should monitor the patient's veins carefully for any signs of phlebitis (temperature, redness, swelling, pain) and report these immediately to the medical practitioner so that the intravenous cannula may be removed.

It is important that prescribed dosing times be adhered to. Blood samples for determination of plasma concentrations of drug should be drawn at appropriate times in relation to doses of the drug. Times of drug administration and drawing of blood samples should be recorded accurately on the drug-level request form, so that maximum and minimum drug concentrations during the dosing interval can be accurately estimated.

Patient teaching

Patients should be encouraged to report any adverse effects which might be attributable to anti-infective drugs. Instruction should be given regarding which drugs to take with food and which to take on an empty stomach. The importance of completing a prescribed course, and keeping to dosage schedules, should be emphasised. Patients should be warned not to keep unused antiinfectives for future use, and not to pass them on to others for self-administration.

23

ANTI-INFECTIVE THERAPY—AGENTS Part 1

Christine L. Odgers

This chapter includes specific information relating to those groups of anti-infective agents most commonly encountered in clinical practice. The objectives, prerequisite knowledge and definitions relevant to this chapter are listed at the beginning of Chapter 22. The combined table of Nursing Implications and the self-evaluation questions may be found at the end of Chapter 24.

THE PENICILLINS

The action of penicillin obtained from *Penicillium notatum* was noted by Fleming in 1929. Penicillin was used as an anti-infective agent by Chain and Florey in 1940. The early penicillin was an amorphous compound containing impurities. It was also a mixture of several penicillin compounds. Penicillin G (benzylpenicillin) was found to be the most satisfactory.

Today a wide range of penicillins is available — these are broadly classified as natural penicillins and semi-synthetic penicillins. The semi-synthetic penicillins are prepared by adding different side chains to the penicillin nucleus (6-aminopenicillanic acid, 6-APA) and they have differing properties and antibacterial activity.

The penicillins are bactericidal and act on the bacterial cell wall. At low concentrations they may be bacteriostatic. The cell wall may be regarded as one giant molecule of mucopeptide which confers shape on the organism and permits maintenance of osmotic pressure differences between the bacterial cell and the environment. When cell-wall growth proceeds, the mucopeptide lattice is broken so that new cell-wall material can be inserted. The penicillins interfere with cell-wall synthesis in growing and dividing bacteria. Organisms with defective cell walls, spheroblasts, are produced and these are susceptible to osmotic injury under most conditions.

Bactericidal drugs like the penicillins exert their action most effectively during the growing phase of bacteria. The penicillins may be less effective when cell metabolism has been slowed down by bacteriostatic drugs.

NATURAL PENICILLINS

The two so-called natural penicillins are produced biosynthetically by fermentation from *Penicillium chrysogenum.* They are benzylpenicillin (penicillin G) and phenoxymethylpenicillin (penicillin V).

Benzylpenicillin is unstable at low (acid) pH and is readily inactivated by acidic gastric juice (hence termed acid-labile) thus generally precluding effective therapy by oral administration. Benzylpenicillin is usually administered intramuscularly, but its highly soluble potassium and sodium salts may be given intravenously.

Phenoxymethylpenicillin is not destroyed in the stomach and is quickly, though incompletely, absorbed from the small intestine. Absorption of the oral penicillins, and hence serum concentrations, are superior when these agents are administered on an empty stomach — one hour before or three hours after a meal.

Benzylpenicillin and ***phenoxymethylpenicillin*** reach their peak serum concentrations rapidly following administration and are quickly excreted in the urine. The rate of excretion may be slowed by administering probenecid approximately 30 minutes before the penicillin. Probenecid actively competes with penicillin for the same secretory sites in the renal tubules.

Benzylpenicillin is often administered in normal doses to patients with renal failure because there is no great risk of toxicity due to accumulation. Moderately large doses may result in toxic concentrations, necessitating dosage reduction. When benzylpenicillin is administered parenterally to uraemic patients, the interval between doses should be increased.

These penicillins are widely distributed throughout the body except to the bone and nervous tissue. Penetration into the cerebrospinal fluid is poor when the meninges are not inflamed. Both drugs cross the placenta.

Benzylpenicillin may be combined with procaine or benzathine to produce the salts ***procaine penicillin*** and ***benzathine penicillin*** which have low solubility, resulting in delayed absorption and prolonged action. These salts are administered parenterally only by the intramuscular route.

Oral and parenteral preparations of benzylpenicillin and phenoxymethylpenicillin, strengths available, some brand names, their dosage ranges, onset of peak serum concentrations and frequency of dosing are listed in Tables 54 and 55.

Table 54
Some Injectable Forms of Natural Penicillins

Approved Name	Brand Name(s)	Strength(s)	Dose Range (Normal Renal Function, Adult)	Onset of Peak Serum Levels	Frequency of Dosing
Benzylpenicillin	*Crystapen*	300 mg, 600 mg, 3 g, 6 g	300 mg–3 g IV	Within 15–30 min	4–6 hourly
Benzathine penicillin	*Penidural-LA*	229 mg/mL	229–916 mg	Slow	Every 5–7 days
Procaine penicillin	*Depocillin*	3 g	Gonorrhoea men: 2.4 g women: 4.8 g	Within 1–3 hours	Single dose
			Syphilis 1.2 g		Daily for 10 days
Procaine penicillin fortified (Procaine and benzyl penicillins)	*Bicillin*	3 g procaine, 600 mg benzyl penicillins	300 mg procaine and 60 mg benzyl	Biphasic	12–24 hourly

Table 55
Some Oral Forms of Natural Penicillins

Approved Name	Brand Name(s)	Strength(s)	Dose Range	Onset of Peak Serum Levels	Frequency of Dosing
Phenoxymethylpenicillin (Penicillin V)	*Apsin VK* *Crystapen V* *Distaquine V-K* *Econocil VK* *Stabillin V-K* *V-Cil-K*	125 mg, 250 mg, tabs/caps 125 mg/5 mL 250 mg/5 mL suspension	250–500 mg	Within 30–60 min	6 hourly
Phenethicillin	*Broxil*	250 mg tabs/caps 125 mg/5 mL syrup	250 mg	Within 30–60 min	6 hourly

The natural penicillins remain the most effective antibiotics against sensitive gram-positive bacteria and, relatively, the least toxic of the antibiotics. Their antibacterial spectrum includes mainly gram-positive organisms and some gram-negative cocci such as gonococci and meningococci. Gram-negative bacilli are generally resistant to benzylpenicillin and phenoxymethylpenicillin.

These penicillins are used clinically to treat streptococcal infections, respiratory tract infections in adults, childhood respiratory tract infections such as croup, bronchitis and pneumonia, and otitis media. Bacterial meningitis, bacterial endocarditis, puerperal infections and *Clostridium perfringens (welchii)* infections due to susceptible bacteria are also treated with these penicillins. Other uses of benzylpenicillin and phenoxymethylpenicillin include tetanus, anthrax, diphtheria, gonorrhoea, syphilis and prophylaxis in rheumatic fever.

Adverse Drug Reactions

Penicillin is one of the least toxic of the antibiotics, but hypersensitivity reactions commonly occur. These may be immediate reactions occurring within 20 minutes of administration and varying from pruritus and urticaria to laryngospasm, hypotension and death. A second type of allergic reaction (accelerated allergic reaction) may occur between 20 minutes and 48 hours after administration, including fever, pruritus and urticaria. Delayed reactions take the form of skin rashes or a serum sickness-like illness.

Other possible reactions are neurotoxicity, with high concentrations of penicillin in the cerebrospinal fluid, nephritis (a rare complication), and haemolysis.

Phenoxymethylpenicillin is usually well tolerated in standard dosages, but may cause gastrointestinal upsets with high dosages, especially when given on an empty stomach to promote absorption and to increase serum concentrations. Occasionally severe reactions and even death occur during or shortly after an injection of procaine penicillin. These reactions may result from the accidental intravenous administration of the drug. Some of the toxic reactions may be due to the toxic effects of procaine, ie convulsions, respiratory paralysis and abrupt hypotension.

THE SEMI-SYNTHETIC PENICILLINS

Some organisms appear to owe their resistance to penicillin, at least in part, to their ability to produce the enzyme penicillinase (a beta-lactamase) that destroys penicillin. In 1960, the first penicillinase-resistant penicillin was introduced and today a range of penicillinase-resistant penicillins is available for the treatment of staphylococcal infections where resistant organisms are particularly common.

Penicillinase-resistant semi-synthetic penicillins

Methicillin was the first penicillinase-resistant penicillin to be introduced. It has the disadvantage of being acid-labile and must be given parenterally to achieve good therapeutic concentrations. The isoxazolyl penicillins (***cloxacillin, flucloxacillin***) combine the property of penicillinase-resistance with resistance to gastric acid. They may be administered parenterally or orally.

Methicillin resistance occurs in staphylococcal strains. This is due not to the destruction of the antibiotic by a bacterial enzyme but to cell tolerance. Methicillin-resistant staphylococci are always resistant to benzylpenicillin, cephalosporins and to the other penicillinase-resistant penicillins. In addition, methicillin-resistant strains demonstrate a high level of resistance to streptomycin and are resistant to tetracycline and sulphonamides. A combination of two effective antibiotics has been advocated for the treatment of methicillin-resistant staphylococcal infections to prevent the emergence of resistance to other antibiotics.

The penicillins in this group should be injected slowly, directly into the intravenous tubing when this route is used. Concentrated solutions of methicillin can cause thrombophlebitis. In the presence of severe renal impairment the dose should be reduced.

Table 56 lists some of the penicillinase-resistant semi-synthetic penicillins, strengths available, some brands, dosage ranges, onset of peak concentrations and frequency of dosing.

Methicillin and the ***isoxazolyl penicillins*** should be reserved for the management of severe infections due to penicillinase-producing staphylococci, such as septicaemia, endocarditis, pneumonia, meningitis and osteomyelitis. These drugs should not be used for the treatment of infections caused by organisms susceptible to benzylpenicillin because benzylpenicillin is more effective and less expensive.

Disadvantages of methicillin are that it must be given parenterally and that it occasionally causes bone-marrow depression or nephritis. The main advantage of methicillin is the greater availability of unbound antibiotic compared with the isoxazolyl penicillins. The isoxazolyl penicillins, when administered orally, should be given 30 minutes to one hour before meals to obtain maximum absorption and serum concentrations.

Adverse Drug Reactions

Methicillin and the isoxazolyl penicillins suffer from the same disadvantages as the other penicillins with respect to toxicity, but hypersensitivity nephritis is less common with the isoxazolyl penicillins than after prolonged methicillin therapy. Intramuscular injections of methicillin are quite painful, and thrombophlebitis may occur following intravenous administration.

BROAD SPECTRUM SEMI-SYNTHETIC PENICILLINS

A range of semi-synthetic penicillins with a wider antibacterial spectrum (broad spectrum) has been developed. These penicillins are active against both gram-positive and gram-negative organisms. The broad-spectrum penicillins include ampicillin, amoxycillin, carbenicillin, carfecillin (carbenicillin phenyl sodium), ticarcillin, and the more recently developed agents azlocillin, mezlocillin and piperacillin.

Ampicillin is active against most of the bacteria sensitive to benzylpenicillin and is also active against some gram-negative bacilli that are resistant to benzylpenicillin. It is not penicillinase-stable and hence is ineffective against both gram-positive penicillinase-producing organisms such as staphylococci, and gram-negative penicillinase-producing organisms such as certain *Proteus* and *Klebsiella* species. Most strains of *Pseudomonas* are resistant. Ampicillin is acid-stable and can be administered by mouth, preferably on an empty stomach to enhance absorption.

Amoxycillin is closely related to ampicillin in its antibacterial spectrum, but it is more active against *Streptococcus faecalis* and *Salmonella* than ampicillin. It is sensitive to the action of penicillinase. Like ampicillin, amoxycillin is acid-stable and is administered both orally and parenterally. It is better absorbed than ampicillin and may, according to some researchers, be administered with food.

Carbenicillin and ticarcillin are unique among the semi-synthetic penicillins in their activity against *Pseudomonas* organisms, indole-positive *Proteus* species, *Enterobacter* species and some *Serratia* species. These drugs are acid-labile and must be administered parenterally. They are not active against penicillinase-producing strains of bacteria. Carfecillin is an ester of carbenicillin that is absorbed after oral administration and converted *in vivo* to carbenicillin. It is approved for use in urinary tract infections.

Piperacillin, together with ***azlocillin*** and ***mezlocillin,*** are sometimes referred to as the "fourth generation" penicillins. Their development resulted from a search for beta-lactam agents with a wider antibacterial spectrum, more anti-*Pseudomonas* activity, and less toxicity than the aminoglycosides. Their unique structure allows greater penetration of the cell wall and selected affinities for penicillin-binding proteins, thus enhancing their activity. These penicillins, also known as "ureidopenicillins", have a lower sodium content per gram (about one-third) than the disodium salts of carbenicillin and ticarcillin. Their major advantage is their enhanced activity against *Pseudomonas aeruginosa* and *Klebsiella.* However, they are more susceptible than the other beta-lactam penicillins to beta-lactamase degradation. The ureidopenicillins are not absorbed orally and hence are administered only parenterally.

The broad spectrum semi-synthetic penicillins presently available in the UK are summarised in Table 57. The dosage range given assumes normal renal function. The dose of these antibiotics must be reduced in severe renal failure.

Ampicillin and ***amoxycillin*** are used to treat urinary tract infections, bronchitis, exacerbations of chronic bronchitis, otitis media in young children and venereal disease. Urethritis due to *Neisseria gonorrhoea* can be treated using amoxycillin in a single oral dose of three grams. Ampicillin is also considered the drug of first choice in the treatment of non-penicillinase-producing *Haemophilus influenzae* meningitis when chloramphenicol is unsuitable, in group D streptococcol bacteraemia and endocarditis and typhoid fever where chloramphenicol and sulphamethoxazole-trimethoprim are contraindicated. Ampicillin may also be used in septicaemia due to gram-negative bacilli.

Carbenicillin, ticarcillin and ***piperacillin*** are mainly used in the treatment of serious infections due to sensitive *Pseudomonas aeruginosa* and with ampicillin-resistant *Proteus* species. They may be useful for the treatment of other gram-negative infections as indicated by sensitivity testing, such as *Escherichia coli* and, in some cases, *Serratia marcescens*.

Adverse Drug Reactions

Ampicillin shares with the natural penicillins the same problems of hypersensitivity due to the penicillin nucleus, 6-APA, but it is also less toxic. Delayed rashes of the maculopapular erythematous type are, however, common. Nausea and diarrhoea may occur, but they are rarely serious. Amoxycillin may be "cross-allergenic" with other penicillins and similarly is contraindicated in penicillin-allergic patients. Drug rashes, nausea and diarrhoea occur.

Carbenicillin, ticarcillin and piperacillin may provoke any of the reactions that occur with the natural penicillins in penicillin-sensitive patients, hence they are contraindicated in patients with a history of penicillin hypersensitivity. Neurotoxicity may occur with high dosages and may be partly attributed to the amount of sodium administered per one gram of the antibiotic. One gram of carbenicillin contains 5.4 millimoles of sodium ion, one gram of ticarcillin contains 5.2 to 6.5 millimoles of sodium ion and one gram of piperacillin contains 1.85 millimoles of sodium ion. Because of its lower sodium content, piperacillin may be preferred for the treatment of serious susceptible infections in patients with considerable renal impairment. Pain on intramuscular injection is often troublesome. Intravenous administration may cause thrombophlebitis and venous irritation, and these antibiotics should be administered slowly to allow adequate dilution in the vein.

THE CEPHALOSPORINS

The cephalosporins were first obtained from a mould cultured from the sea near a Sardinian sewage outfall in 1945. The cephalosporins are related to the penicillins — both have a beta-lactam ring which confers on them a similar mode of action.

The term "cephalosporins" is used in a broad sense as some of the agents discussed in this section are, chemically, cephamycins (for example, cefoxitin) or oxa-beta-lactams (latamoxef). However, all are semisynthetic derivatives of cephalosporin C, a compound elaborated by the fungus *Cephalosporium*. The cephalosporins are primarily bactericidal in action. They act by inhibiting bacterial cell-wall synthesis, like the penicillins, with resultant defective cell walls so that the protoplasts are osmotically unstable.

Cephalosporins are more effective against young, rapidly dividing organisms than against mature, resting cells that are not in the process of

Table 56
Some Penicillinase-resistant Semisynthetic Penicillins

Approved Name	Brand Name	Strength	Dose Range (Normal Renal Function, Adult)	Onset of Peak Serum Levels	Frequency of Dosing
Methcillin	*Celbenin*	1 g	1 to 2 g IM, IV	Within 30 to 60 min for IM	4 to 6 hourly
Cloxacillin	*Orbenin*	250 mg, 500 mg capsule; 125 mg/5 mL syrup; 250 mg, 500 mg, 1 g injection	250 mg to 500 mg oral 500 mg to 1 g IM, IV	Within 30 to 60 min for IM or oral	4 to 6 hourly
Flucloxacillin	*Floxapen*	250 mg, 500 mg capsule; 125 mg/5 mL syrup; 250 mg/5 mL syrup; 250 mg, 500 mg, 1 g injection	250 mg to 500 mg IM, IV, oral	Within 30 to 60 min for IM or oral	6 hourly

Table 57
Broad Spectrum Semisynthetic Penicillins

Approved Name	Brand Name	Strength	Dose Range (Normal Renal Function, Adult)	Onset of Peak Serum Levels	Frequency of Dosing
Ampicillin	*Penbritin*	250 mg, 500 mg capsule; 125 mg/5 mL, 250 mg/5 mL syrup; 250 mg, 500 mg injection	250 mg to 500 mg oral; 250 mg to 1 g IM, IV	1 to 2 hours, oral; within 30 minutes for IM	6 hourly
Amoxycillin	*Amoxil*	250 mg, 500 mg capsule; 3 g sachet; 125 mg/5 mL, 250 mg/5 mL syrup; 250 mg, 500 mg, 1 g injection	250 mg to 500 mg oral; 250 mg to 500 mg IM, IV	Within 2 hours, oral; within 1 hour for IM	8 hourly, oral; 6 to 8 hourly; IV, IM
Carbenicillin	*Pyopen*	1 g, 5 g injection	2.5 g to 5 g, IM, IV	Within 1 hour for IM	4 to 6 hourly
Carfecillin	*Uticillin*	500 mg tablets	500 mg–1 g	Within 1 hour	8 hourly
Piperacillin sodium	*Pipril*	2 g, 4 g, injection	1 g to 2 g, IM; 2 g to 4 g, IV	Within 30 min for IM	4 to 6 hourly
Ticarcillin disodiurn	*Ticar*	1 g, 3 g injection	1.5 g to 3 g, IM, IV	Within 1 hour for IM	4 to 6 hourly

cell-wall formation. In general, gram-negative bacteria are less sensitive to the cephalosporins because they contain less mucopeptide in the cell wall than gram-positive organisms. The cephalosporins, are, in general, broad spectrum antibiotics and demonstrate activity against most gram-positive organisms and some gram-negative organisms.

Bacterial resistance to the cephalosporins may be natural or acquired. Some bacteria are not affected by concentrations of cephalosporins which are lethal to other organisms because their cell surfaces are not permeable to cephalosporins or their metabolic pathways are not inhibited. Some bacteria such as *Escherichia coli, Enterobacter* species, indole-positive *Proteus, Serratia* and *Pseudomonas* are resistant because they inactivate the cephalosporins by producing beta-lactamases (cephalosporinases). Although cephalosporins are highly resistant to the penicillinase beta-lactamases, cross-resistance between penicillinase-resistant penicillins and cephalosporins occurs.

TYPES OF CEPHALOSPORINS

The cephalosporins are classified traditionally into "generations". The first generation includes ***cephalothin, cephaloridine, cephradine*** and ***cephazolin*** for parenteral use and ***cephalexin*** and ***cephradine*** for oral use. All drugs in this group lack stability to beta-lactamases elaborated by gram-negative organisms, and they are inactive against *Pseudomonas aeruginosa*. They have good activity against most gram-positive cocci. The second-generation cephalosporins differ from the first generation agents in that they have an expanded spectrum of activity which includes many gram-negative organisms, and they are stable to beta-lactamases. However, they are all ineffective against *Pseudomonas* and enterococci. This group includes the parenteral cephalosporins, ***cefoxitin*** and ***cephamandole*** and the oral agent ***cefaclor***. The third-generation cephalosporins ***cefotaxime, latamoxef, cefoperazone, ceftazidime*** and ***ceftriaxone*** have a significantly increased resistance to gram-negative microorganisms. They are active against *Pseudomonas aeruginosa*.

CEPHAZOLIN SODIUM, CEPHALORIDINE, CEPHALOTHIN SODIUM, CEPHRADINE (First generation)

Cephazolin sodium, cephaloridine and ***cephalothin sodium*** are not absorbed significantly from the gastrointestinal tract and must be given parenterally. ***Cephradine*** is absorbed well following oral administration and is administered both orally and parenterally. Therapy with the cephalosporins results in high blood concentrations that decline rapidly in patients with normal renal function. The cephalosporins are generally widely distributed to most tissues and fluids, but only small amounts diffuse into the cerebrospinal fluid even when the meninges are inflamed. Cephalosporins readily cross the placenta. They are rapidly excreted by the kidneys and as with the penicillins, the oral administration of probenecid prior to the cephalosporin usually slows the rate of excretion and produces higher and more prolonged serum concentrations.

Preparations of cephazolin, cephaloridine, cephalothin sodium and cephradine, strengths available, some brand names, dosage range in adults with normal renal function and frequency of dosing are summarised in Table 58.

Local reactions are quite common with parenteral cephalosporins. Pain and induration, occasionally accompanied by sterile abscess formation, occur frequently after intramuscular administration of cephalothin. These side effects occur to a lesser degree with cephazolin, cephaloridine and cephradine. It is recommended that the cephalosporins be administered by deep intramuscular injection or intravenously. Phlebitis and thrombophlebitis have frequently occurred following intravenous cephalothin and to a lesser degree with cephazolin, cephaloridine and cephradine.

Cephalosporins are usually not considered to be the drugs of first choice for any infection unless other antibiotics are unsuitable because of toxicity or allergy to penicillins. Parenteral cephalosporins are used in the treatment of streptococcal, and pneumococcal infections, staphylococcal infections, urinary tract infections, septicaemia due to gram-negative bacilli, *Haemophilus influenzae* infections and *Klebsiella* pneumonia due to susceptible organisms.

Adverse Drug Reactions

Cephalosporins are contraindicated in patients with a history of allergic reactions to cephalosporins. They should be avoided in patients who have had an immediate-type (anaphylactic) hypersensitivity reaction to penicillins and should be administered with caution to patients who have had delayed-type reactions (rash, fever, eosinophilia) to penicillins or other drugs. Hypersensitivity reactions have been reported to occur, ranging from mild urticaria, pruritus, maculopapular or erythematous skin rash to eosinophilia and rarely, anaphylaxis. Joint pains, oedema, genital and anal pruritus and angio-neurotic oedema have been reported with the cephalosporins.

Nephrotoxicity may occur, usually with cephaloridine. All cephalosporins should be administered with caution and in reduced dosage in the presence of markedly impaired renal function. Haematological abnormalities have been reported.

ORAL CEPHALOSPORINS (First and Second Generation)

Cephalexin was first semisynthetic cephalosporin-C derivative that was shown to be absorbed from the upper gastrointestinal tract following oral administration. ***Cephalexin***, ***cephradine*** and ***cefaclor*** are acid-stable and are well absorbed from the gastrointestinal tract, although the presence of food delays oral absorption as with the oral penicillins. The total amount of drug absorbed is not affected when these cephalosporins are administered with food. Following absorption from the gastrointestinal tract they are widely distributed to most tissues and fluids. Cephalexin, cephradine and cefaclor are excreted unchanged in the urine. The dose and/or the frequency of administration must be modified in response to the degree of renal impairment.

Table 58
Some Injectable Cephalosporins

Approved Name	Brand Name	Strength	Dose Range (Normal Renal Function, Adult)	Onset of Peak Serum Levels	Frequency of Dosing
Cephaloridine	*Ceporin*	250 mg, 500 mg injection	250 mg to 1 g IM, IV	Within 30 to 60 min for IM	8 to 12 hourly
Cephalothin sodium	*Keflin*	1 g	1 g	Within 15 to 30 min for IM	4 hourly
Cephazolin sodium	*Kefzol*	500 mg, 1 g injection	250 mg to 1 g IM, IV	Within 1 hour for IM	8 hourly
Cephradine	*Velosef*	500 mg, 1 g injection	500 mg to 1 g IM, IV	Within 30 min for IM	6 hourly
Cefotaxime sodium	*Claforan*	500 mg, 1 g, 2 g injection	500 mg to 2 g IM, IV	30 min for IM	6 to 8 hourly
Cefoxitin sodium	*Mefoxin*	1 g, 2 g injection	1 to 2 g IM, IV	Within 30 min for IM	6 to 8 hourly
Cephamandole nafate	*Kefadol*	500 mg, 1 g, 2 g injection	500 mg to 1 g IM, IV	Within 1 hour for IM	4 to 8 hourly
Latamoxef disodium	*Moxalactam*	500 mg, 1 g, 2 g injection	500 mg to 2 g IM, IV	Within 1 to 2 hours for IM	8 to 12 hourly

Table 59
Oral Cephalosporins

Approved Name	Brand Name	Strength	Dose Range (Normal Renal Function, Adult)	Onset of Peak Serum Levels	Frequency of Dosing
Cefaclor	*Distaclor*	250 mg capsule; 125 mg/5 mL syrup; 250 mg/5 mL suspension	250 mg, oral	Within 30 to 60 min	8 hourly
Cephalexin	*Ceporex* *Keflex*	250 mg, 500 mg capsule; 125 mg/ 5 mL, 250 mg/5 mL suspension	250 mg to 1 g, oral	Within 1 hour	6 hourly
Cephradine	*Velosef*	250 mg, 500 mg capsule/tablet; 125 mg/5 mL, 250 mg/5 mL suspension	250 mg to 500 mg oral	Within 1 hour	6 hourly

Dosage information for patients with normal renal function and the products available are summarized in Table 59.

Cephalexin, cephradine and cefaclor are used for the treatment of otitis media, infections of the respiratory tract, skin and soft-tissue infections and genitourinary-tract infections due to susceptible organisms. There is no evidence that these drugs are more effective than penicillins or erythromycin in infections due to mutually susceptible organisms. Their primary value appears to be as follow-up therapy to parenteral cephalosporin therapy and in the treatment of urinary-tract infections due to *Klebsiella* organisms that are resistant to other antibacterials.

Cefaclor, because of its activity against *Haemophilus influenzae*, including beta-lactamase producing strains, is favoured over cephalexin and cephradine in the treatment of otitis media and infections of the respiratory tract caused by this organism. Ampicillin is preferred, however, for the treatment of infections due to *Haemophilus influenzae* because it normally has greater in-vitro activity against this organism.

Adverse Drug Reactions

The most frequent adverse reactions are nausea, vomiting, diarrhoea, vulval irritation and discharge. Other gastrointestinal effects may occur including abdominal cramps, dyspepsia, glossitis and heartburn. Occasionally, skin rashes have been reported.

These drugs share the toxic potentials of the parenteral cephalosporins and the usual precautions of cephalosporin therapy should be observed.

CEPHAMANDOLE, CEFOXITIN (Second Generation)

Cephamandole and ***cefoxitin*** are inactive orally and must be administered parenterally. They are generally more active against gram-negative organisms than the first generation cephalosporins. However, they are inactive against enterococci and *Pseudomonas aeruginosa*.

Cephamandole exhibits high activity against *Enterobacter*, indole-positive *Proteus* species and *Haemophilus influenzae*. In fact, because of its wider spectrum of activity, some clinicians consider cephamandole the preferred cephalosporin in the treatment of nosocomial and other non-pneumococcal bacterial pneumonias, as well as for biliary-tract infections.

Cefoxitin, chemically, is a cephamycin and thus is not susceptible to degradation by beta-lactamases produced by gram-negative organisms. It is less active than cephalothin against gram-positive organisms but has greater activity against certain gram-negative strains, including indole-positive *Proteus* species, *Escherichia coli* and anaerobes including *Bacteroides fragilis*. (Cephamandole does not have good activity against the anaerobes). Cefoxitin has been used perioperatively to reduce the incidence of infections in patients undergoing large-bowel surgery or genitourinary surgery. Other more active and specific agents such as metronidazole and clindamycin/lincomycin are preferred for the treatment of proven anaerobic infection.

Dosing information for adult patients with normal renal function and the products available are included in Table 58.

CEFOTAXIME, CEFTAZIDIME AND LATAMOXEF — (Third Generation)

These new cephalosporins, like the earlier agents, have a wide therapeutic index, are relatively free from significant toxicity and lack activity against the enterococcus. Thus, superinfection with this organism may occur during therapy. They differ from the earlier cephalosporins in a number of important aspects including a markedly increased resistance to gram-negative beta-lactamases. Thus, they possess a broader spectrum of activity against gram-negative organisms including *Pseudomonas aeruginosa.* Because of their somewhat longer half-lives, they retain a high degree of activity even at low serum concentrations. In addition, they have a limited ability to penetrate inflamed meninges. Their main disadvantages include their low activity against some organisms (which at times necessitates combination therapy with other anti-infective agents) and their relatively high cost.

The third generation cephalosporins are available only for parenteral administration. They may be administered intramuscularly or intravenously, the intravenous route being the preferred route, particularly for serious infections. Cefotaxime, ceftazidime and latamoxef are excreted primarily by the renal route, therefore dosage adjustment should be made in patients with renal dysfunction. The investigational agent cefoperazone is excreted unchanged primarily by the biliary route and accumulation may occur in patients with hepatic dysfunction. Cefoperazone appears to have greater antipseudomonal activity than cefotaxime and latamoxef and is moderately active against enterococci.

The primary indication for the use of ***cefotaxime*** is in the treatment of infections due to serious sepsis where the organism has not yet been identified and a gram-negative bacillus and/or *Staplylococcus aureus* is potentially involved, and in high doses in gram-negative bacillary meningitis (however, latamoxef appears to be more effective). It is a potentially useful drug in the treatment of infection in the neutropenic patient, especially when combined with an aminoglycoside.

Latamoxef (known as moxalactam in the US and Europe), because of its enhanced gram-negative activity, is indicated for the treatment of multiple drug-resistant gram-negative infections due, in particular, to *Escherichia coli* and *Klebsiella* which demonstrate sensitivity to latamoxef. Latamoxef is indicated in the treatment of severe sepsis where the organism has not yet been identified and the suspected organisms are generally susceptible to the drug (for example, *Staphylococcus aureus, Escherichia coli, Haemophilus influenzae* and many *Proteus* species). Similarly to cefotaxime, it is potentially useful in the neutropenic patient. When used in high dosage, it is superior to cefotaxime in the treatment of gram-negative meningitis. Like cefoxitin, latamoxef has activity against beta-lactamase producing *Bacteroides fragilis* and may be used prophylactically in abdominal and pelvic surgery. Not all *B. fragilis* organisms are susceptible, however; a combination of an aminoglycoside with an anti-infective drug with activity against *Bacteroides fragilis* appears preferable in serious anaerobic abdominal and pelvic infections. Although latamoxef has moderate activity against *Pseudomonas aeruginosa* isolates, *in-vitro* susceptibility should be demonstrated before it is administered.

Several side effects have been described which are specific to, or more common with, latamoxef therapy. These include mild reversible hepatic dysfunction, elevation of prothrombin time (sometimes in association with clinical haemorrhage which may be prevented or treated by administering vitamin K), abnormal platelet adherence and a disulfiram-like reaction following the ingestion of alcohol (for example, as contained in some oral liquid medicines).

Ceftazidime is used in the treatment of infections due to serious sepsis and where the organism has not been identified or in infections due to *Pseudomonas aeruginosa.* It is useful in the treatment of infection in the neutropenic patient, especially when combined with an aminoglycoside.

Dosing information for adult patients and details of available preparations are included in Table 58.

A variety of third-generation cephalosporins are being investigated, and some of these will be available soon for clinical use. Most of these agents, however, are less active than the first-generation cephalosporins against streptococcal and staphylococcal isolates. Of these, cefsulodin and thienamycin are active against *Pseudomonas aeruginosa;* ceftizoxime, cefoperazone and thienamycin are active against *Bacteroides fragilis;* ceftizoxime is active against the Enterobacteriaceae; cefsulodin and thienamycin are active against *Staphylococcus aureus;* and thienamycin, cefoperazone and ceftriaxone appear to be active against multiple drug-resistant gram-negative organisms.

THE TETRACYCLINES

The tetracyclines are a family of closely related antibiotics. The first tetracycline, chlortetracycline, was discovered in 1948 from *Streptomyces aureofaciens,* the organism forming it. Oxytetracycline was introduced in 1950, and in 1953 tetracycline was introduced. Since then a number of other tetracyclines have been added to the range.

The tetracyclines generally are bacteriostatic rather than bactericidal in action. They appear to inhibit protein synthesis in susceptible organisms by binding to ribosomes and inhibiting binding of the transfer RNA complexes to the ribosomes, thus preventing production of polypeptides (precursors of proteins). In higher concentrations, tetracyclines also inhibit mammalian protein synthesis.

Tetracyclines have a broad antimicrobial spectrum and demonstrate activity against most gram-positive organisms that are sensitive to the penicillins and also against gram-negative organisms that are not susceptible to the penicillins. They are active against mycoplasma, rickettsiae, and spirochaetes. They show little activity against most strains of *Proteus* species and *Pseudomonas aeruginosa.*

The widespread and often indiscriminate use of this group of antiinfective agents has resulted in resistant strains of staphylococci and various coliform bacilli emerging. This has led to a decrease in their usefulness, particularly in the hospital environment. Organisms made resistant to one tetracycline are usually cross-resistant to the other tetracyclines.

TETRACYCLINES IN USE

The most commonly used members of the tetracycline family are ***tetracycline*** (the parent compound), ***doxycycline, minocycline*** and ***oxytetracycline.***

Tetracyclines are incompletely absorbed from the gastrointestinal tract; however, absorption may be increased if they are administered during the fasting state. The concomitant administration of milk, food or agents such as antacids (containing aluminium, magnesium or calcium), sodium bicarbonate and iron salts decreases the absorption from the gastrointestinal tract due to the formation of inactive complexes. Absorption of doxycycline and minocycline is affected to a lesser degree when these agents are administered with milk or food. Generally tetracyclines should be administered to patients on an empty stomach, although it may be necessary to advise some patients to take them with a light meal to help overcome the serious gastric distress that may be experienced.

Following absorption, the tetracyclines penetrate fairly well into various body fluids and tissues. The tetracyclines are concentrated in bone, especially growing bone and teeth during the early stages of calcification, causing yellow fluorescence. The deposition of tetracyclines in the teeth and bone of foetuses of pregnant women who have received tetracyclines and of infants receiving one of these agents during the first six to eight years of life has been associated with permanent discolouration and enamel defects in the teeth, and also with slowing of bone growth.

The tetracyclines are concentrated in the liver and excreted in the bile. They are partially excreted in the urine, primarily as the unchanged drug. In the presence of renal failure, accumulation of the tetracyclines occurs (except doxycycline) resulting in toxicity. The administration of outdated and deteriorated tetracycline may also result in nephrotoxicity (the Fanconi syndrome). Doxycycline is eliminated mainly by metabolism and its excretion in renal failure generally is not impaired. Its dosage does not need to be modified in these patients, however it may aggravate azotaemia.

Commercial preparations containing tetracycline and nystatin have been manufactured and promoted on the assumption that monilial bowel superinfection is the main cause of tetracycline gastrointestinal side effects. This antifungal agent prevents monilial overgrowth, but there is little evidence that this has any bearing on the gastrointestinal side effects of tetracycline therapy. The gastrointestinal effects are due to the irritant effect of the tetracycline.

Minocycline, unlike the other tetracyclines, inhibits *Candida albicans* growth *in vitro.* It is possible that use of this drug may result in fewer bowel superinfections than with the other compounds. This has yet to be confirmed by clinical studies.

Tetracyclines may be administered parenterally as well as orally. The products in general use are summarised in Table 60.

The major indications for using tetracyclines are acute exacerbations of chronic bronchitis (ampicillin and trimethoprim with sulphamethoxazole are superior), non-specific urethritis, pneumonia due to *Mycoplasma pneumoniae*, Q-fever, psittacosis, acne vulgaris, brucellosis, lymphogranuloma venereum, typhus fever and gonorrhoea (in penicillin-allergic patients). The tetracyclines may be alternated with ampicillin and other broad-spectrum anti-infective agents for long-term, intermittent suppressive therapy in patients with chronic bronchopulmonary infections. Demeclocycline is indicated in the treatment of chronic hyponatraemia associated with the syndrome of inappropriate secretion of antidiuretic hormone (SIADH), where water restriction or conventional diuretic therapy is ineffective.

Adverse Drug Reactions

The most common side effect with tetracycline therapy is looseness of the stools. Gastrointestinal symptoms such as nausea, heartburn, epigastric distress and diarrhoea are more common with tetracyclines than with most other oral antibiotics. These symptoms appear to be dose dependent. Other adverse effects include superinfection (particularly with *Candida albicans)*, hypersensitivity reactions (uncommon, but usually occurring as urticaria, asthma or facial oedema), photosensitivity, teeth pigmentation and effects on bones. Nephrotoxicity, hepatotoxicity and haematological disturbances may also occur.

Intramuscular injections of tetracycline are painful, and a local anaesthetic is included in the preparation to reduce the pain. The intravenous preparations of tetracycline should be infused slowly in dilute solutions to avoid thrombophlebitis.

THE AMINOGLYCOSIDES

Following the demonstration of the clinical efficacy of penicillin, a deliberate search for other anti-infective agents resulted in the discovery in 1944 of ***streptomycin. Neomycin*** was isolated in 1949, ***framycetin*** and ***kanamycin*** were isolated in the fifties. ***Gentamicin*** was discovered in 1964 and ***tobramycin*** in 1971. ***Amikacin, sissomicin*** and ***netilmicin*** are the most recently isolated aminoglycosides, and they appear to be more resistant to degradation by some, but not all, of the enzymes that have mediated the transferable drug resistance reported in recent years with kanamycin, gentamicin and tobramycin.

The suffix "mycin" is used to distinguish those aminoglycosides produced by a *Streptomyces* species from those produced by a *Micromonospora*, the names of which end in "micin".

The aminoglycosides are bactericidal in action, and they appear to exert their effect on sensitive bacteria by interfering with bacterial protein synthesis. This action is dependent on their ability to bind to a

Table 60
The Tetracyclines

Approved Name	Brand Name	Strength	Dose Range (Normal Renal Function, Adult)	Onset of Peak Serum Levels	Frequency of Dosing
Tetracycline	*Achromycin* (V)	250 mg capsule/ tablets 125 mg/5mL syrup 250 mg, 500 mg IV 100 mg IM	250 mg to 500 mg oral 500 mg IV 100 mg IM	Within 2 to 4 hours	6 hourly 12 hourly 4-12 hourly
	Tetrex	250 mg	250, 500 mg	Within 2 to 4 hours	6-12 hourly
Nystatin	*Mysteclin*	250 mg and 250 000 units tablets/capsules	250 mg oral	Within 2 to 4 hours	6 hourly
Demeclocycline	*Ledermycin*	150 mg capsule 300 mg tablet	150 mg to 300 mg	Within 3 to 4 hours	6 to 12 hourly to daily
Doxycycline	*Vibramycin*	100 mg, tablet/capsule 50 mg/5mL syrup	100 mg, oral	Within 2 to 4 hours	Daily
Minocycline	*Minocin*	100 mg capsule	100 mg, oral, IV	Within 2 to 3 hours, oral	12 hourly
Oxytetracycline	*Terramycin*	250 mg capsule/ tablet	250 mg to 500 mg, oral	Within 2 to 4 hours	6 hourly

particular protein or proteins of the bacterial ribosomes. The precise mechanism of action is considered to be the formation of an aberrant ribosome-messenger RNA complex that cannot be used in further protein synthesis.

The spectra of activity of the aminoglycosides are broadly similar, with exception of the activity exhibited against *Pseudomonas aeruginosa* by gentamicin, tobramycin, amikacin, sissomicin and netilmicin. This activity is not shared by the earlier members of the group. The aminoglycosides are used in serious systemic infections, and they must be administered parenterally as they are poorly absorbed from the gastrointestinal tract. Some, e.g. neomycin and framycetin, may be administered orally for bowel sterilisation before bowel surgery.

Parenterally administered aminoglycosides are excreted almost entirely by the kidneys. These anti-infective drugs have toxic effects on the vestibular branch (streptomycin, gentamicin and tobramycin) and auditory branch (kanamycin and amikacin) of the eighth nerve, and on the kidneys (neomycin being the most nephrotoxic and streptomycin the least nephrotoxic). If renal function is impaired, the blood concentrations of these drugs will rise rapidly with a consequent increased risk of toxic effects. To prevent a toxic reaction occurring, it is important that the dose is reduced when renal impairment is present.

GENTAMICIN

Gentamicin is used in the treatment of septicaemia and severe infections of the skin and soft tissues including burns, respiratory-tract infections and urinary-tract infections due to susceptible gram-negative bacteria. Gentamicin may be used in the treatment of meningitis, but the diffusion of the drug into the CSF is variable. It is of proven value in infections due to *Serratia marcescens*, but the emergence in some centres of significant levels of resistance among these organisms and others may dictate the use of amikacin.

The synergistic combination of gentamicin with benzylpenicillin or semisynthetic penicillins is utilised in the management of serious staphylococcal infections. These drugs should not, however, be mixed in solution as the penicillin will inactivate gentamicin. Other clinical settings in which gentamicin may be used in combination with other anti-infective agents include the treatment of enterococcal endocarditis (for example, with penicillin, ampicillin or vancomycin); in the empiric treatment of the febrile neutropenic host (for example, with carbenicillin, ticarcillin or piperacillin); in the treatment of pelvic and abdominal sepsis in combination with agents that are effective against *Bacteroides fragilis* (for example, metronidazole, clindamycin or lincomycin); or in combination with a cephalosporin in empiric therapy of nosocomial pneumonias.

Gentamicin is only slightly absorbed from the gastrointestinal tract. It is rapidly absorbed following intramuscular injection. The intravenous route is frequently used in patients receiving intravenous fluids. Because of the drug's potential toxicity, its use should be limited to the treatment of severe infections only, and careful consideration should be given to the patient's renal function to avoid toxic effects.

Adverse drug reactions occurring with gentamicin include ototoxicity, nephrotoxicity, allergic skin rashes and sensitisation from topical use, and less frequently, neuromuscular blockade resulting in muscle weakness and respiratory depression. The dose should be reduced in patients with impaired renal function, the very young and the elderly; dosage frequency may also be altered. The patient's renal function should be closely monitored and serum gentamicin concentrations determined in these groups of patients. Mild and transient pain may occur at the intramuscular injection site and local phlebitis may occur with intravenous administration. Other side effects include rare occurrences of urticaria, maculopapular rash, drug fever, generalised burning, headache, nausea, vomiting and diarrhoea.

TOBRAMYCIN

The spectrum of activity of ***tobramycin*** is quite similar to that of gentamicin. *Pseudomonas aeruginosa* is quite sensitive to tobramycin, and this is one of the most important features of this drug.

Resistance to tobramycin may be acquired by gram-negative organisms. Some cross-resistance has been reported between tobramycin and the other aminoglycosides; however, strains of some organisms that are resistant to other aminoglycosides may be sensitive to tobramycin.

Tobramycin is not appreciably absorbed from the gastrointestinal tract and must be given parenterally. As with the other aminoglycosides, the dose should be reduced or the frequency of administration adjusted in patients with renal failure, the very young and the elderly.

The primary indication for the use of tobramycin is in infections due to *Pseudomonas aeruginosa*. The drug is also indicated in severe mixed gram-negative infections in which *Staphylococcus aureus* is involved.

Ototoxicity is a problem with high doses of tobramycin, although this appears to be less than that attributable to the other aminoglycosides. Nephrotoxicity is another adverse effect. The use of tobramycin in conjunction with other nephrotoxic drugs should be avoided in patients with impaired renal function. Other side effects occasionally reported include pain and thrombophlebitis at the injection site, urticaria, maculopapular rash, hives, pruritus and fever. Nausea, vomiting, fatigue, headache and lethargy have also occurred.

It is common practice in hospitals to make either tobramycin or gentamicin available for routine use but not both.

AMIKACIN

Amikacin is related to kanamycin, and it is resistant to many of the aminoglycoside-inactivating enzymes, including those responsible for gentamicin-resistance. Amikacin has been used successfully in serious gram-negative infections in adults and children and appears to be a suitable alternative for gentamicin-resistant infections. The drug is generally restricted by hospitals for use in these infections. It is the drug of first choice for the gentamicin-resistant *Pseudomonas* and Enterobacteriacaeae infections. Amikacin is administered parenterally, usually by intramuscular injection, although it may be given intravenously.

Toxicity is similar to that of other later aminoglycosides, with ototoxicity and nephrotoxicity being the most serious side effects. The dosage interval should be extended for patients with renal dysfunction, and the drug should not be administered with other drugs that may add to or potentiate ototoxicity or nephrotoxicity. The use of amikacin may result in overgrowth by non-susceptible organisms.

STREPTOMYCIN

The original wide spectrum of activity of ***streptomycin*** against gram-positive and gram-negative bacteria has narrowed greatly due to the emergence of resistance. It is still a first-line drug in the treatment of tuberculosis and is used in combination with other drugs to prevent resistant tubercle bacilli from emerging. Partial to complete cross-resistance exists between streptomycin, neomycin and kanamycin, but organisms resistant to streptomycin may retain sensitivity to the other aminoglycosides.

Streptomycin diffuses fairly rapidly into body fluids and tissues after intramuscular injection. It also enters ascitic and pleural fluids. The drug does not enter the cerebrospinal fluid unless the meninges are inflamed. Streptomycin crosses the placental barrier.

Streptomycin is administered intramuscularly into a large muscle mass, and injection sites should be alternated to minimise irritation. Intravenous administration is not recommended as it produces high serum concentrations and increases the risk of neurotoxicity.

Tuberculosis is the main indication for the use of streptomycin. Combined with benzylpenicillin, it may, in rare instances, be used for the treatment of subacute bacterial endocarditis caused by *Steptococcus faecalis*.

Severe vestibular disturbance with vertigo is the most serious toxic effect associated with streptomycin therapy. Deafness may occur. Other adverse effects include hypersensitivity reactions, commonly manifested as rash and fever, neurotoxicity, neuromuscular blockade and nephrotoxicity with large doses.

NEOMYCIN AND FRAMYCETIN

Neomycin and ***framycetin*** are more toxic than streptomycin and now are not used systemically. They are not significantly absorbed following oral administration and may be used for bowel sterilisation or the treatment of intestinal infections. Neomycin and kanamycin are administered orally in the treatment of portal-systemic encephalopathy. Their ability to reduce intestinal ammonia production by decreasing the numbers of ureolytic and proteolytic bacteria in the colonic lumen is thought to be associated with a reduction in arterial blood-ammonia concentration.

Vomiting or diarrhoea may accompany the administration of large oral doses. Neomycin and framycetin are used topically for the treatment of superficial infections due to staphylococci and many gram-negative bacilli. Prolonged application to skin lesions is frequently associated with skin hypersensitivity. Ototoxicity and nephrotoxicity have been reported following oral and topical use. There appears to be little justification for their use.

KANAMYCIN

Parenteral ***kanamycin*** is used in the treatment of gram-negative staphylococcal urinary tract, respiratory tract and soft-tissue infections. Its use has been limited in recent years by the widespread acceptance of gentamicin which has greater activity against *Pseudomonas* species, and to which resistance of gram-negative organisms is less common.

Kanamycin is generally administered intramuscularly, and pain of moderate intensity may occur at the injection site. The use of the intravenous route may predispose the patient to toxicity, and thrombophlebitis may occur. Kanamycin, administered orally, has been used for bowel sterilisation.

Some aminoglycoside preparations available for use, their dosage forms, strengths, dose ranges for adults with normal renal function and dosing frequency are summarised in Table 61.

NETILMICIN

The spectrum of activity of ***netilmicin***, one of the newer aminoglycosides, is similar to that of gentamicin. However, netilmicin is more active against some strains of Enterobacteriaceae and less active against *Pseudomonas aeruginosa*. It appears to be resistant to some of the bacterial enzymes which inactivate gentamicin, and it has been shown to be active against some gentamicin-resistant isolates.

Netilmicin is not absorbed orally and must be administered by intramuscular or intravenous injection. Dosage adjustment should be made in renal impairment because, like the other aminoglycosides, the half-life is prolonged in renal impairment, resulting in increased serum drug concentrations and increased toxicity.

Netilmicin has a profile of adverse effects similar to that of gentamicin. It has been suggested from animal studies that netilmicin may be less nephrotoxic and ototoxic than gentamicin. The degree of toxicity in humans, however, remains to be established.

Serum aminoglycoside concentration monitoring

Because the margin between efficacy and toxicity is narrow with the aminoglycosides, serum concentrations must be monitored, and the peak

Table 61
Aminoglycosides

Approved Name	**Brand Name**	**Strength**	**Dose Range (Normal Renal Function, Adult)**	**Onset of Peak Serum Levels**	**Frequency of Dosing**
Framycetin	*Soframycin*	250 mg tablets 500 mg sterile powder for local use	2-4 g orally, divided doses		
Kanamycin	*Kantrex*	250 mg 1 g injection	15 mg/kg/day (deep) IM, IV	Within 1 hour after IM	8-12 hourly
Neomycin	*Nivemycin*	500 mg tablet	6 to 12 orally, divided doses		24 to 48 hours for bowel sterilisation
Amikacin	*Amikin*	500 mg injection	15 mg/kg day IM, IV	Within 1 hour after IM	12 hourly
Gentamicin	*Cidomycin* *Garamycin*	10 mg, 20 mg, 40 mg, 80 mg injection	2 to 5 mg/kg/day IM, IV	30 to 90 min after IM	8 hourly
Netilmicin	*Netillin*	15 mg, 50 mg, 100 mg, 150 mg injection	4 to 6 mg/kg/day IM, IV	30 to 60 min after IM	8 to 12 hourly
Streptomycin			1 g (deep) IM	30 min to 2 hours after IM	Daily
Tobramycin	*Nebcin*	20 mg, 40 mg, 80 mg injection	3 to 5 mg/kg/day IM, IV	30 to 90 min after IM	8 hourly

and trough concentrations must be maintained within suggested guidelines. The timing of the administration of the drug and the collection of serum samples for aminoglycoside determination is critical. Samples for "peak" concentration determinations should be taken within 30 minutes of administering an intravenous dose or within 60 minutes of an intramuscular dose.

A sample for the "trough" concentration determination should be taken immediately before the subsequent dose. Serum concentrations should be measured frequently in critically ill patients and those with variable renal function, the very young, the elderly and the obese. The dose or the dosing interval may then be adjusted on the basis of the results of these assays to ensure efficacy and safety of therapy.

ERYTHROMYCIN

Erythromycin is a macrolide antibiotic produced by *Streptomyces erythreus*. It was originally found in soil in the Philippines and subsequently purified and used clinically in 1952. There are approximately 37 antibiotics in this group, but erythromycin is the only one remaining in clinical use.

Erythromycin is classified as a bacteriostatic drug, but it may be bactericidal in high concentrations or against highly suceptible organisms. Erythromycin inhibits protein synthesis in susceptible organisms by binding to ribosomes and inhibiting polypeptide synthesis.

Erythromycin exerts its effect only against multiplying organisms. The drug generally penetrates the cell wall of gram-positive organisms more readily than that of gram-negative organisms. Gram-positive organisms may accumulate 100 times more erythromycin than gram-negative organisms.

Resistance to erythromycin develops stepwise at a rate less than or equal to that occurring to the penicillins. Resistance is rarely observed during successful short-term treatment but may occur when the drug is used over long periods to treat infections. Cross-resistance may occur with lincomycin and clindamycin, but staphylococci resistant to erythromycin are not always resistant to these antibiotics. The fear of resistance developing has been one of the factors responsible for the under-use of this drug. The pattern of resistance seems to develop from a very few organisms that are resistant in a very few patients. When erythromycin is widely used in hospital practice, these resistant organisms may multiply and spread, but in general practice this risk appears to be negligible.

Erythromycin has a similar antibacterial sprectrum to benzylpenicillin and is used in the management of patients with streptococcal infections who are suspected of being hypersensitive to penicillin (lower respiratory-tract infections, skin and soft tissue infections). Erythromycin is also used to treat chronic bronchitis and otitis media caused by *Haemophilus influenzae*, primary atypical pneumonia due to *Mycoplasma pneumoniae*, pneumonia caused by *Legionella* species, *Camphylobacter jejuni* gastroenteritis, and staphylococcal infections such as boils, carbuncles and wound infections. However, resistance may develop with prolonged treatment. Eryth-

Table 62
Erythromycins

Approved Name	Brand Name	Strength	Dose Range (Normal Renal Function, Adult)	Onset of Peak Serum Levels	Frequency of Dosing
Erythromycin base		250 mg, 500 mg tablets, capsules	250 mg to 500 mg, oral	1 to 4 hours	6 hourly or 12 hourly
Erythromycin stearate	*Erythrocin*	250 mg, 500 mg tablets	250 mg to 500 mg, oral	1 to 4 hours	6 hourly
Erythromycin estolate	*Ilosone*	125 mg/5 mL suspension 250 mg capsules 500 mg tablets 250 mg/5 mL suspension	30 to 50 mg/kg/day, oral	1 to 4 hours	6 to 8 hourly
Erythromycin ethylsuccinate		500 mg tablets 125 mg/5 mL suspension 250 mg/5 mL suspension 500 mg/5 mL suspension	50 mg/kg/day, oral	1 to 4 hours	6 to 8 hourly
Erythromycin lactobionate	*Erythrocin IV*	1 g injection	250 mg to 1 g, IV over one hour	1 hour	6 hourly

romycin may be administered in high doses during early syphilis in penicillin-allergic patients.

Erythromycin may be administered orally or parenterally. Oral formulations containing the erythromycin base must be enteric (acid-resistant) coated, as the base is inactivated by gastric acid. These preparations release the drug in the duodenum to permit absorption. Erythromycin stearate is less readily destroyed in the stomach, and it dissociates in the duodenum, liberating active erythromycin which is absorbed. The estolate and the ethylsuccinate are also available as oral formulations. Erythromycin estolate is acid-stable, but it has the disadvantage of potential hepatotoxicity.

Food usually reduces the absorption of orally administered erythromycin compounds. Following absorption, erythromycin is widely distributed in the tissues and is concentrated in the liver and the spleen. it penetrates the meninges only when they are inflamed. Erythromycin crosses the placenta. The drug is excreted primarily in the bile. Only small amounts are excreted in the urine, and there is no significant accumulation in uraemic patients.

Erythromycin may be administered parenterally as the lactobionate for intravenous injection. The intravenous injection causes venous irritation and thrombophlebitis, and it is recommended that the drug should be well diluted and infused slowly over 20 to 60 minutes to minimise these effects.

A number of the preparations of erythromycin are listed in Table 62.

Adverse Drug Reactions

Erythromycin base is one of the safest and least toxic of the antibiotics. The most common side effects of the oral erythromycins are gastrointestinal and are dose related. These include abdominal pain and cramping due to increased gastrointestinal motility, nausea, vomiting and diarrhoea. Occasionally stomatitis, heartburn, anorexia and pruritus ani have occurred.

Mild allergic reactions including urticaria, skin eruptions and rashes occur less frequently. Serious allergic reactions including anaphylaxis have been reported. Following prolonged or repeated therapy, overgrowth with non-susceptible bacteria or fungi may occur. Erythromycin estolate may produce hepatotoxicity in the form of reversible cholestatic hepatitis. This does not often occur after the administration of other erythromycins. Erythromycin estolate is contraindicated in patients with hepatic dysfunction or pre-existing liver disease. The other erythromycins should be used with caution in patients with impaired liver function or biliary excretion, and dosage reduction should be considered.

LINCOMYCIN AND CLINDAMYCIN

Lincomycin derives its name from Lincoln, Nebraska. The antibiotic was isolated from a strain of *Steptomyces lincolnensis* and was first introduced in 1963. Several chemical modifications of the lincomycin molecule have been developed in an attempt to produce an improved antibiotic, and one of these, clindamycin, is available.

Lincomycin and clindamycin appear to inhibit protein synthesis in susceptible organisms. The mode of action of lincomycin and clindamycin is similar to that of erythromycin and chloramphenicol — these antibiotics show competitive interaction in binding to their receptor on the ribosome. Lincomycin and clindamycin have a similar spectrum of activity to erythromycin and are effective against a variety of gram-positive organisms, particularly staphylococci, streptococci and pneumococci. Most of the aerobic gram-negative bacteria are resistant to lincomycin and clindamycin, however, the anaerobic organisms of the *Bacteroides* species are relatively sensitive.

The activity of clindamycin may be either bacteriostatic or bactericidal, depending on the sensitivity of the organism and the concentration of the drug. The primary activity of lincomycin appears to be bacteriostatic. Some organisms resistant to lincomycin also have shown cross-resistance to clindamycin.

Lincomycin and clindamycin are effective in the management of respiratory tract and skin and soft tissue infections caused by susceptible gram-positive organisms, particularly streptococci, pneumococci and staphylococci. They are not considered as the drugs of first choice in these infections. Both lincomycin and clindamycin are particularly effective against staphylococcal osteomyelitis.

Lincomycin and clindamycin are particularly effective against severe anaerobic infections caused by *Bacteroides fragilis* associated with appendicitis, other lower abdominal infections, post-partum infections, septic abortions and pelvic inflammatory disease. The combination of gentamicin with either lincomycin or clindamycin is used in the treatment of *Bacteroides* infections. The role of gentamicin is to cover aerobic gram-negative enteric bacteria.

Lincomycin and clindamycin are well absorbed from the gastrointestinal tract, but the presence of food in the stomach delays and reduces the extent of absorption of lincomycin. Both drugs are widely distributed in body fluids and tissues. They cross the placenta readily and also appear in breast milk. They appear to be concentrated in bone and are indicated in the management of acute staphylococcal osteomyelitis only after due consideration to their toxic effects. Concentrations in the normal cerebrospinal fluid are small.

Both drugs are excreted in the urine, bile and faeces. In patients with renal disease dosage reduction is necessary only if renal failure is severe. The dose should be reduced in liver disease.

Lincomycin and clindamycin are administered orally and also parenterally by the intramuscular and intravenous routes. Prior to intravenous administration both drugs should be well diluted and infused slowly. Lincomycin 600mg should be diluted to a minimum of 60 mL with dextrose solution (the manufacturer recommends 250 mL) and infused over 30 to 60 minutes. Clindamycin 600mg should also be diluted to 100 mL with dextrose and infused over 30 minutes.

Table 63
Lincomycin and Clindamycin

Approved Name	Brand Name	Strength	Dose Range (Normal Renal Function, Adult)	Onset of Peak Serum Levels	Frequency of Dosing
Lincomycin	*Lincocin*	500 mg capsule; 600 mg injection; 250 mg/5mL syrup	500 mg oral, 600 mg IM, IV	Within 4 hours 30 to 60 min after IM	6 to 8 hourly 12 to 24 hourly IM, 8 to 12 hourly IV
Clindamycin	*Dalacin C*	75 mg, 150 mg capsule; 75 mg/5 mL syrup; 300 mg, 600 mg injection	150 mg to 450 mg oral 300 mg to 600 mg IM, 600 mg to 900 mg IV	Within 1 hour (oral) Within 3 hours after IM	6 hourly 8 to 12 hourly IM, IV

Preparations of lincomycin and clindamycin and some dosage information are summarised in Table 63.

Adverse Drug Reactions

Gastrointestinal effects, nausea, vomiting, abdominal cramps and diarrhoea may necessitate discontinuation of therapy with oral and parenteral lincomycin and, to a lesser degree, oral clindamycin. Diarrhoea may persist for several days after discontinuation of therapy, and pseudomembranous colitis has been reported following both oral and parenteral lincomycin and clindamycin therapy. This most serious side effect may result in death. Thus these drugs should not be used for trivial infections or if other antibiotics are likely to be equally effective. Oral vancomycin, 0.5 to 2 grams per day, has proved to be effective against the causative agent in pseudomembranous colitis, *Clostridium difficile*. Alternative treatments that have been demonstrated to be effective against *Clostridium difficile* are oral metronidazole in a dose of 1.2 grams per day, or bacitracin administered in a dose of 25 000 units four times a day.

Intramuscular injections may cause pain at the injection site. If large doses of lincomycin or clindamycin are injected rapidly via the intravenous route, transient flushing, a feeling of warmth, syncope or even cardiopulmonary arrest may occur. Thrombophlebitis, erythema and swelling have been reported with high doses administered intravenously.

CHLORAMPHENCIOL

Chloramphenicol was the first broad-spectrum antibotic discovered. It was originally isolated from *Streptomyces venezuelae* in 1947. It is now produced synthetically. The drug enjoyed wide popularity because of its wide spectrum of activity and reliable absorption from the gastrointestinal tract. Its use in trivial infections became widespread, and a number of fatalities due to aplastic anaemia were reported. More recently, chloramphenicol-resistance has become a matter of concern in countries other than Japan where chloramphenicol-resistant *Shigella* have been common for many years.

Chloramphenicol is usually classified as a bacteriostatic drug because, *in vitro*, it arrests the multiplication of bacteria but does not reduce the number of living organisms. In high concentrations it may be bactericidal to some organisms, and in lower concentrations it is bactericidal to *Haemophilus influenzae*. Chloramphenicol appears to inhibit protein synthesis in susceptible, multiplying bacteria by binding to bacterial ribosomes. The effect of chloramphenicol on rapidly proliferating mammalian cells, including haemopoietic toxicity, may be related to the inhibition of protein synthesis. Chloramphenicol is active against a wide range of gram-positive and gram-negative organisms including *Salmonella* species, *Haemophilus influenzae, Vibrio cholera*, rickettsiae and mycoplasma. The drug is generally less active against streptococci, pneumococci and staphylococci than are the penicillins, erythromycin and tetracyclines.

Resistance to chloramphenicol may occur even among salmonellae and shigellae normally sensitive to chloramphenicol.

Chloramphenicol should only be used for the treatment of serious infections caused by susceptible organisms when potentially less toxic drugs are ineffective or contraindicated. It is the drug of choice for the treatment of acute infections caused by susceptible strains of *Salmonella typhi*. Chloramphenicol may be used as an alternative to ampicillin for the management of *Haemophilus influenzae* meningitis in young children and as an alternative to the tetracyclines in rickettsial diseases such as epidemic typhus fever or Rocky Mountain spotted fever.

Chloramphenicol therapy may be initiated in life-threatening infections such as septicaemia and fulminating pneumonia after specimens have been collected and results of susceptibility tests are pending. The antibiotic should be discontinued if susceptibility tests show the organism to be resistant to chloramphenicol or sensitive to a potentially less toxic drug.

Chloramphenicol is well absorbed from the gastrointestinal tract, and the usual oral dose for children is 50 – 100 mg/kg daily in divided doses every 6 hours; for adults, oral dose is 500 mg every 6 hours. The drug diffuses into many body fluids and tissues, crosses the placenta, penetrates into the eye and into the cerebrospinal fluid, even in the absence of inflamed meninges.

Following oral administration of chloramphenicol, peak serum levels are attained within two hours. The drug is inactivated primarily in the liver and is excreted predominantly in the urine. In patients with impaired renal and/or hepatic function, the dose must be reduced accordingly. Chloramphenicol may be administered parenterally by either the intramuscular or intravenous route. Rapid intravenous injection should be avoided as this may cause thrombophlebitis, and the patient may experience an intensely bitter taste, lasting a few minutes. The drug is available as a 1-gram injection (equal to 1.2g of chloramphenicol sodium succinate, brand name *Chloromycetin*). Oral therapy should replace intravenous therapy for the patient as soon as practicable.

Adverse Drug Reactions

Bone-marrow depression is the most important toxic effect of chloramphenicol and may occur as aplastic anaemia with pancytopenia (a rare complication having a high mortality rate) or haemopoietic toxicity, which is more common and appears to be dose related and reversible. Chloramphenicol therapy should be discontinued if erythropoietic depression, increased serum iron concentrations, or increased saturation of serum iron-binding globulin occur. Blood studies should be performed prior to initiation of therapy with chloramphenicol and approximately every five days during therapy. Concomitant administration of chloramphenicol and other drugs that may cause bone-marrow depression should be avoided.

The Grey syndrome, a type of circulatory collapse, can occur in premature and newborn infants receiving large doses of chloramphenicol. This syndrome is characterised by abdominal distension, vomiting, pallor, cyanosis and circulatory collapse and may result in death. The Grey syndrome has been clearly related to high toxic concentrations of the active drug in babies less than four weeks of age who have a defective capacity for inactivating the drug in the liver.

Other adverse effects include optic neuritis, nausea, vomiting, glossitis and stomatitis, sometimes associated with thrush. Hypersensitivity reactions are rare, but contact dermatitis, rashes and drug fever and occasionally anaphylaxis and angioneurotic oedema have been reported. Bleeding due to an increased prothrombin time may occur with prolonged oral administration of the drug. This is due to interference with vitamin-K production by the intestinal bacteria.

NURSING IMPLICATIONS

General nursing implications of anti-infective therapy are outlined in Chapter 22. Here, those implications for penicillins, cephalosporins, tetracyclines, aminoglycosides, erythromycin, lincomycin, clindamycin and chloramphenicol are discussed in particular.

Assessment

Previous history of hypersensitivity must be elicited before any of the antibiotics are used. Reactions to penicillins are the most likely to have occurred, and careful questioning of the patient should be performed to determine whether he or she has had previous exposure to penicillins.

Renal function must be assessed in patients prescribed aminoglycosides and cephalosporins. Baseline hearing and balance facility should be assessed in patients having aminoglycoside therapy. Assessment of liver function should be made in patients prescribed erythromycin and chloramphenicol. Tetracyclines should not be prescribed for pregnant women, young children or older children with growth impairment.

Administration

Regular, around-the-clock administration of antibacterial antibiotics is necessary to maintain therapeutic serum concentrations and to prevent the development of resistance.

Oral doses of the following groups should be timed to promote absorption from an empty upper gastrointestinal tract: penicillins, cephalosporins, erythromycin, clindamycin, and tetracyclines. Administration at least one hour before food or three hours after food is recommended. Tetracycline must not be administered with milk, antacids or iron compounds because it may be inactivated. If gastric irritation is a problem with oral administration, a careful check should be made with a pharmacist, or the manufacturer, about which foods may be safely given with each type of antibiotic, without loss of effectiveness.

Antibiotics should be given into large muscles, by deep injection when the intramuscular route is prescribed. If slow absorption is required, the site should not be massaged. Prevention of accidental intravenous administration, by aspiration of the needle, is essential. Slow injection is recommended to reduce tissue damage and pain. Slow injection or infusion via the intravenous route will prevent irritation of the veins. Mixing of drugs of different groups for intravenous infusion is not advised. Interactions can inactivate both drugs, and precipitates can obstruct intravenous lines.

Evaluation

Clinical improvement, especially reduction of body temperature, provides the basis for evaluation. At the same time, observation for allergic reactions and signs of superinfection, especially of the gastrointestinal tract, is essential.

Renal and liver functions will be assessed frequently in patients having those drugs which are known to cause nephrotoxicity, hepatotoxicity, and requiring optimal liver function for metabolism. Accurate fluid-balance records, regular urinalysis specific-gravity estimation and blood-chemistry tests are used to evaluate renal function. The urine should be inspected for the presence of blood, mucus threads and crystals.

Continual monitoring of hearing ability and balance are necessary for patients on aminoglycosides. The specific toxic effects of each drug should be checked and considered in evaluating the patient's response to antibiotic therapy.

Peripheral cannulae sites need to be inspected regularly for signs of phlebitis and extravasation. When serum concentrations are being monitored, as in aminoglycoside therapy, samples are taken at specific times in relation to doses, to estimate peak and trough concentrations.

OTHER ANTIBIOTICS

POLYMYXINS

The polymyxin group of antibiotics was first isolated in 1947 from a spore-bearing soil bacillus. Only two agents from this group have been found to be clinically useful, namely ***polymyxin B sulphate*** and ***colistin (polymyxin E).*** The other polymyxins are too toxic for clinical use.

Polymyxin B sulphate and colistin are bactericidal in action. They appear to bind to and damage, by a type of detergent action, the bacterial plasma membrane which is situated just inside the bacterial cell wall, causing leakage of intracellular components. The toxic effects of polymyxins may result from similar binding of these drugs to membranes of mammalian cells. The polymyxins are highly active against most of the important gram-negative bacteria that are normal inhabitants of the human bowel, including *Escherichia coli, Klebsiella* species and *Pseudomonas aeruginosa.* Gram-positive bacteria are all resistant to the polymyxins. There is complete cross-sensitivity and cross-resistance between polymyxin and colistin but not with other drugs. The bacteria that are usually sensitive to these drugs do not readily acquire resistance.

The polymyxins are not absorbed from the gastrointestinal tract so must be administered intramuscularly or intravenously for the treatment of systemic infections. Polymyxin B is used topically, particularly for ophthalmic infections, and as an irrigation to clear infected wounds of *Pseudomonas aeruginosa.*

Colistin *(Colomycin)* is available as an injection for intramuscular or intravenous administration. It is used primarily in the treatment of urinary tract infections caused by susceptible strains of *Pseudomonas aeruginosa.* It should not be used for the treatment of minor infections or infections that can be treated with less toxic antibiotics.

Nephrotoxicity is one of the most serious side effects of colistin. Neurotoxicity, leucopenia and hepatotoxicity and allergic manifestations such as rashes, pruritus and drug fever occur less frequently. Pain may occur at the injection site.

BACITRACIN AND GRAMICIDIN

Bacitracin and ***gramicidin*** are peptide antibiotics isolated from *Bacillus subtilis* and *Bacillus brevis* respectively. They are highly active against gram-positive bacteria, but the gram-negative bacilli are resistant. Bacitracin appears to interfere with cell-wall synthesis and probably damages the bacterial plasma membrane. Gramicidin acts on bacteria by altering the function of their plasma membrane.

Both drugs are toxic when administered systemically, nephrotoxicity being the main toxic effect. They seldom cause side effects when applied topically and are used in various topical antibiotic preparations such as creams, ointments, sprays, powders and eye and ear drops. They are often combined with neomycin and polymyxin B in these preparations. Bacitracin may also be used in solution for wound irrigation or bladder instillation. Recent studies have suggested that oral bacitracin may be a suitable alternative therapy to vancomycin in the treatment of *Clostridium difficile*-induced pseudomembranous colitis.

SPECTINOMYCIN

Spectinomycin is an antibiotic unrelated to any others and was isolated from *Streptomyces spectabilis.* It is active against a wide range of gram-positive and gram-negative organisms by inhibiting protein synthesis.

Spectinomycin is not absorbed from the gastrointestinal tract. It is available as 2 g injections *(Trobicin)* for deep intramuscular injection. It is used as an alternative to penicillin in the treatment of acute gonorrhoeal urethritis and proctitis in men and acute gonorrhoeal cervicitis and proctitis in women, when the organism is resistant to penicillin or the patient is allergic to penicillins. It is not effective in the treatment of syphilis.

Spectinomycin appears to be a relatively non-toxic antibiotic when administered as a single dose. Side effects include soreness at the site of injection, urticaria, dizziness, nausea, chills, fever and insomnia.

FUSIDIC ACID (SODIUM FUSIDATE)

Fusidic acid, obtained from the fungus *Fusidium coccineum,* has a steroid structure and is chemically related to cephalosporin P. The sodium salt, ***sodium fusidate,*** is used clinically and is marketed under the name of

Fucidin as a suspension (250 mg/5 mL), enteric coated tablets (250 mg) and as an intravenous infusion (500 mg). It is administered well diluted, to 250 or 500 mL with sodium chloride, into a large vein to avoid venospasm and thrombosis. The usual adult dose is 500 mg (oral, IV) administered every eight hours. The dose for children is 20 mg per kilogram body weight.

In contrast to the cephalosporins which inhibit bacterial cell-wall synthesis, sodium fusidate interferes with bacterial protein synthesis. This different mode of action probably explains the lack of cross-resistance between sodium fusidate and the penicillinase-resistant penicillins and cephalosporins. Methicillin-resistant staphylococci are usually sensitive to sodium fusidate. Other gram-positive organisms are much more resistant and the gram-negative bacteria are resistant, probably because the drug cannot penetrate their cell walls.

Sodium fusidate is indicated only for the treatment of severe staphylococcal infections. It is relatively non-toxic and appears to be safe in penicillin-allergic patients. Mild gastrointestinal disturbances and skin rashes may occur with the administration of the drug. As the drug is excreted primarily in the bile, it should be used cautiously in patients with impaired liver function.

VANCOMYCIN

Vancomycin was isolated from *Streptomyces orientalis* and appears to be unrelated to other commercial antibiotics. Vancomycin is bactericidal and appears to bind rapidly and irreversibly to the cell walls of sensitive bacteria, thereby inhibiting cell-wall synthesis. Vancomycin is active against many gram-positive organisms, but it is not effective against gram-negative organisms, fungi or yeasts. Resistance to vancomycin does not appear to develop during therapy, and no cross-resistance with other antibiotics has been demonstrated.

The drug is not readily absorbed from the gastrointestinal tract and may be given orally for the treatment of staphylococcal enterocolitis. An oral dose of 125 to 500 mg is administered six hourly for the treatment of pseudomembranous colitis, thought to be caused by the organism *Clostridium difficile.* To treat potentially life-threatening systemic staphylococcal infections caused by susceptible methicillin-resistant and cephalosporin-resistant bacteria that cannot be treated with other less toxic drugs, vancomycin is administered parenterally. Vancomycin is the drug of choice, in combination with an aminoglycoside, in the treatment of those patients with *Streptococcus faecalis* endocarditis who are allergic to penicillins.

Following intravenous administration, vancomycin is widely distributed in the body tissues and diffuses readily into pericardial, pleural, ascitic and synovial fluids. Vancomycin is excreted by the kidneys. The drug accumulates in renal failure necessitating a modified dosing schedule with serum concentration monitoring.

Ototoxicity and nephrotoxicity are the most serious side effects of vancomycin therapy and are most likely to occur in patients with impaired renal function. Vancomycin is irritating to tissue and causes necrosis when given intramuscularly, therefore it must be administered intravenously, and care should be taken to avoid extravasation. Pain and thrombophlebitis occur after intravenous administration and may be severe. Other side effects include nausea, fever, chills, macular rash, a shock-like state, anaphylaxis and occasionally vascular collapse. The use of vancomycin may result in the overgrowth of non-susceptible organisms.

Vancomycin is available as a 500 mg injection (brand name *Vancocin*). The usual adult dose is 500 mg diluted to 100 or 200 mL of sodium chloride 0.9% or dextrose 5% injection and administered over 20 to 30 minutes every six hours.

THE SULPHONAMIDES

In 1935, the first sulphonamide of clinical importance as an anti-infective agent, ***prontosil rubrum,*** was used, initiating a new era in the treatment of infectious diseases. Since then, many sulphonamides have been synthesised and some of these have been used for the treatment of conditions other than infections. Some examples are the oral hypoglycaemic agent tolbutamide, and the diuretic agent acetazolamide.

The antibacterial sulphonamides have been superseded to a large degree by the antibiotics and the combination antibacterial trimethoprim with sulphamethoxazole, because of the emergence of sulphonamide resistance, toxicity and the greater efficacy of the alternatives.

The sulphonamides are usually bacteriostatic in action and exert their effect by inhibiting the formation of folic acid in bacteria and parasites. Humans absorb pre-formed folic acid from the diet, but bacteria and parasites appear to be impermeable to folic acid and synthesise it from para-aminobenzoic acid. The sulphonamides act by competitively blocking the enzyme responsible for converting para-aminobenzoic acid to dihydrofolic acid.

In the early years, sulphonamides had a broad antibacterial spectrum against gram-positive and gram-negative organisms. However, the increasing incidence of resistance in organisms formerly susceptible to the sulphonamides has decreased their usefulness. Sulphonamide resistance probably occurs because mutant organisms arise which are either capable of over-production of para-aminobenzoic acid, or develop a structural change in the enzyme giving it a lower affinity for sulphonamides.

Individual sulphonamides differ markedly in their absorption, distribution and excretion, and they may be classified according to these differences into three main groups:

1. Absorbable, rapidly excreted (short acting) sulphonamides including ***sulphadiazine***, ***sulphadimidine***, ***sulphafurazole*** and ***sulphamethizole.***
2. Absorbable, more slowly excreted (medium acting) sulphonamides including ***sulphamethoxazole*** and the more slowly excreted (long acting) sulphonamides such as ***sulphamethoxypyridazine.***
3. Non-absorbable or very poorly absorbed sulphonamides such as ***phthalylsulphathiazole.***

Absorbable sulphonamides are widely distributed in the body and are excreted primarily by the kidneys. Their rates of excretion vary widely, as do their solubility characteristics at various urinary pH values. Alkalinisation of the urine and high fluid intake result in increased renal excretion.

Sulphonamides are indicated for use in only a few infections including acute, non-obstructive urinary tract infections caused by susceptible organisms such as *Escherichia coli, Klebsiella* and *Proteus mirabilis.* Chronic or recurrent urinary-tract infections usually respond only temporarily to sulphonamide therapy. Sulphonamides are of some benefit in chancroid, trachoma, nocardiosis, toxoplasmosis and resistant malaria. Certain sulphonamides applied topically are of benefit in the management of burns. A commonly used preparation is silver sulphadiazine cream. Mafenide is used topically for the treatment of burns.

The usefulness of non-absorbable sulphonamides for the suppression of bacteria in the intestinal tract prior to gastrointestinal surgery has not been established.

Sodium sulphadiazine is available as a parenteral injection for deep intramuscular or slow intravenous injection in acute infections due to susceptible organisms.

The more commonly prescribed sulphonamides are listed in Table 64.

Adverse Drug Reactions

The side effects of the sulphonamides are numerous and may involve nearly all the organs of the body. Many of the side effects appear to be hypersensitivity reactions, their incidence increasing with increased dosage. These hypersensitivity reactions include allergic rashes, for example, maculopapular or urticarial rashes, erythema nodosum, exfoliative dermatitis, or rarely, Stevens-Johnson syndrome may occur. Photosensitivity can also result. Blood dyscrasias are important complications of sulphonamide therapy, including acute agranulocytosis, thrombocytopenia, aplastic anaemia and haemolytic anaemia.

Hepatic changes may appear within three to five days of commencing therapy, possibly causing jaundice. Jaundice and kernicterus occur in the newborn or premature infants treated with sulphonamides. To avoid this complication, sulphonamides should not be given to pregnant women near term nor to newborn or premature infants.

Renal damage may occur due to precipitation of the drug in the renal tubules, known as crystalluria. This was not uncommon with the earlier sulphonamides of low solubility. Crystalluria may cause pain and haematuria, and anuria can occur if the renal pelvis or the ureters become completely occluded. A high intake of fluid (approximately 600 mL per gram of sulphonamide) and alkalinisation of the urine minimise this side effect. The most common toxic effects are headache, mental depression and general malaise. Nausea and vomiting may occur.

Table 64
Some Frequently Prescribed Sulphonamides

Approved Name	Brand Name	Strength	Dose Range (Normal Renal Function, Adult)	Onset of Peak Serum Levels	Frequency of Dosing
Sulphadiazine		1 g injection	1 to 1.5 g	Within 3 hours	4 hourly, IV
Sulphadimidine	*Sulphamezathine*	500 mg tablet	1 to 2 g, oral	2 to 3 hours	6 hourly
Sulphafurazole	*Gantrisin*	500 mg tablet; 500 mg/5 mL suspension	1 to 2 g, oral	2 to 4 hours	4 to 6 hourly
Sulphamethizole	*Urolucosil*	100 mg tablets 100 mg/5 mL suspension	200 mg	2 hours	4 to 6 hourly
Phthalylsulphathiazole	*Thalazole*	500 mg tablet	2 to 12 g daily, divided	Poorly absorbed	

TRIMETHOPRIM AND SULPHAMETHOXAZOLE

Trimethoprim is a synthetic compound related to the antimalarial, pyrimethamine, and it has both antibacterial and antimalarial activity. Trimethoprim blocks bacterial folic acid synthesis at the stage immediately following that blocked by the sulphonamides (see Figure 7).

FIGURE 7: MODE OF ACTION OF TRIMETHOPRIM AND SULPHAMETHOXAZOLE

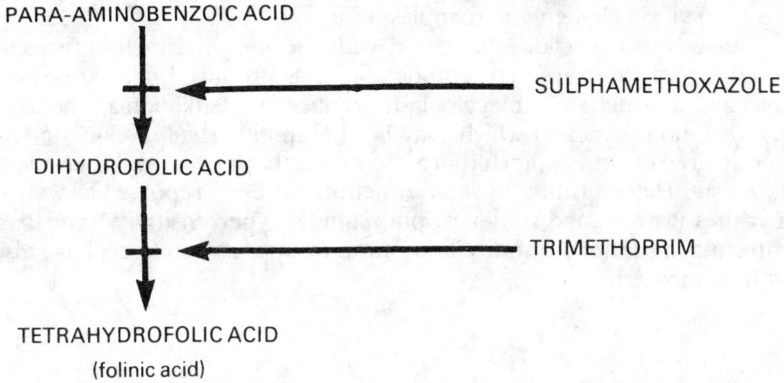

The combination of trimethoprim with sulphamethoxazole in a weight ratio of 1:5 is marketed for oral and parenteral administration as *Bactrim* and *Septrin.* For oral administration a suspension may be used containing 40 mg of trimethoprim and 200 mg of sulphamethoxazole per 5 mL dose, or tablets containing 80 mg: 400 mg or 160 mg: 800 mg of the anti-infective agents. The usual adult dose is 160 mg of trimethoprim with 800 mg of sulphamethoxazole administered every 12 hours. The dose should be reduced for patients with renal failure or poor hepatic function.

The parenteral formulation contains 80 mg of trimethoprim and 400 mg of sulphamethoxazole per 5 mL of solution. It should be diluted to 125 mL and infused slowly over 60 to 90 minutes as the solution is highly alkaline.

Trimethoprim-sulphamethoxazole is indicated for the treatment of chronic and recurrent urinary-tract infections caused by susceptible bacteria including *Escherichia coli, Klebsiella, Enterobacter* and certain species of *Proteus.* The combination also is effective in the treatment of cystitis. It is an effective alternative therapy for certain venereal diseases such as urethritis and cervicitis due to *Neisseria gonorrhoea,* granuloma inguinale and infections due to *Chlamydia trachomatis.* Trimethoprim-sulphamethoxazole now may be considered the treatment of choice for infections caused by ampicillin-resistant strains of *Shigella.* It is an excellent alternative to chloramphenicol and amoxycillin in the treatment of enteric fever due to *Salmonella typhi* and *paratyphi,* especially when chloramphenicol-resistant strains are isolated. Because of the combination's good activity against *Streptococcus* *pneumoniae* and *Haemophilus influenzae*, it is very useful in the treatment of acute otitis media and acute bronchitis and may be used for prophylaxis of chronic bronchitis. Trimethoprim-sulphamethoxazole is the therapy of choice in the treatment of *Pneumocystis carinii* pneumonia, a life-threatening infection in the immunosuppressed patient. It is also of value in the treatment of *Nocardia asteroides* infections. Other possible indications for the use of trimethoprim-sulphamethoxazole include as a prophylactic agent against potential Enterobacteriaceae infections in neutropenic patients, as an alternative treatment in some gram-negative infections such as brucellosis and in vibrio cholera and toxoplasmosis.

Serious adverse reactions associated with the use of trimethoprim-sulphamethoxazole are rare. The combination has produced haematological abnormalities (such as megaloblastic anaemia, leukopenia, neutropenia, thrombocytopenia) which may be due to either sulphonamide hypersensitivity or the interference of trimethoprim with folic acid metabolism. Deterioration in renal function has been reported as well as skin rashes (as outlined under sulphonamide hypersensitivity) and gastrointestinal irritation; jaundice and immunosuppressive effects have also been documented.

TRIMETHOPRIM

Trimethoprim *(Ipral)* is marketed as a single-agent product for the treatment of acute urinary-tract infections caused by sensitive organisms. Following oral administration, 200–400 mg daily, trimethoprim is readily absorbed, and high concentrations are detected in the kidneys and urine.

It was initially considered that the use of trimethoprim alone would result in the rapid development of resistant organisms. These fears, however, have been largely unjustified. In fact, some workers have argued that the use of trimethoprim alone in the treatment of acute infections is superior to the combination because the problems of sensitivity to sulphamethoxazole and its toxic side effects are avoided.

NURSING IMPLICATIONS

Assessment

Before treatment with sulphonamides or trimethoprim, the patient's history should be reviewed by the nurse for evidence of blood dyscrasias, renal impairment or liver disease. Evidence of any of these conditions could influence the decision to prescribe these drugs. They should not be used in pregnant women near term or in lactating patients. The nurse should also check for known hypersensitivity to any of the sulphonamides and related compounds such as the thiazide diuretics, chlorthalidone, acetazolamide and the sulphonylurea hypoglycaemic agents.

Obstetric and neonatal nursing staff should be aware that these drugs can precipitate jaundice and kernicterus in the newborn or premature infant, and they should not be given during pregnancy or to the neonate. The clinical manifestations of the infection should also be recorded to establish a baseline for observations.

Administration
It is advisable to give these drugs with food or after meals to help eliminate nausea and gastrointestinal side effects. Ensure the patient takes plenty of fluids during the day to minimise the risk of crystalluria, if the more insoluble sulphonamides are being used.

Evaluation
Once treatment has started, the nurse should evaluate the patient for clinical improvement and adverse effects. With respect to the latter, nurses must be alert for the development of blood dyscrasias. Signs and symptoms of these include reports of a sore throat, fever, prostration, ulcerations of the mouth or rectum or vagina, bleeding gums, nose bleeds and unexplained bruising.

Observe the skin for signs of hypersensitivity and photosensitive reactions. Watch urine for signs of haematuria, and monitor the pH of the urine. Administer a urinary alkaliniser if ordered.

Patient teaching
Patients should be advised to take the drug with food or after meals and to increase their fluid intake. With some drugs, their urine may become orange coloured, and if fair skinned, they should avoid exposure to sunlight. They should be advised of the signs of adverse effects, including hypersensitivity reactions, and to report these if they occur. As with all anti-infective therapy, they should be advised of the importance of completing the prescribed course.

24
ANTI-INFECTIVE THERAPY—AGENTS
Part 2

Christine L. Odgers

This chapter examines a wide variety of anti-infective agents. Some may be less frequently encountered than those discussed in Chapter 23 but nonetheless have a significant role in the clinical arena. Objectives, prerequisite knowledge and definitions relevant to this chapter are listed at the beginning of Chapter 22. (*Note:* Anthelminthic agents are discussed in Chapter 31.)

URINARY ANTISEPTICS AND pH MODIFIERS

NALIDIXIC ACID

Nalidixic acid is unrelated to other antibacterial drugs and has been regarded as a urinary antiseptic, because initially it was thought that therapeutic concentrations of the drug were achieved in the urine only. More recently it has been shown that therapeutic serum concentrations are also obtained.

Nalidixic acid is believed to inhibit bacterial synthesis of DNA. The antibacterial spectrum of the drug includes most gram-negative organisms except *Pseudomonas aeruginosa* and *Bacteroides* species. Gram-positive organisms are largely resistant to nalidixic acid. The drug is bactericidal *in vitro* to a number of the susceptible gram-negative organisms, and its bactericidal activity is not significantly affected by changes in urinary pH. Bacterial resistance has been reported to occur in up to 25% of patients receiving nalidixic acid.

Nalidixic acid is well absorbed following oral administration and excreted mainly in the urine. It is used in the treatment of acute and chronic urinary-tract infections caused by susceptible gram-negative organisms. Its usefulness may be limited by the development of resistance and by side effects.

The usual oral dose of nalidixic acid (*Negram,* 500 mg tablets) is 1 gram administered six-hourly for 7 to 10 days. Urine should be cultured and the isolated organisms tested for susceptibility before administration of the drug. Urine culture and sensitivity testing should be conducted during treatment to determine if resistance has developed to the drug. Nalidixic acid should not be administered to patients with impaired renal or hepatic function or to patients with cerebral damage.

Adverse Drug Reactions

Side effects of nalidixic acid most commonly involve the central nervous system — headache, malaise, drowsiness, dizziness, vertigo, syncope, sensory changes, visual disturbances, excitement, depression, confusion, and even grand mal attacks have been described. If these reactions occur, nalidixic acid should be discontinued and other appropriate therapy instituted.

Because these neurologic side effects have been observed in infants and young children following therapeutic doses and in patients with a history of a seizure disorder, the use of nalidixic acid in these groups is not recommended. Gastrointestinal side effects including nausea and vomiting (and less frequently diarrhoea and abdominal pain) may occur. Allergic reactions to nalidixic acid include rash and urticaria. Photosensitivity reactions consisting of erythema and bullae on exposed skin surfaces may occur.

NITROFURANTOIN

Nitrofurantoin is a synthetic nitrofuran compound used solely for the treatment of urinary-tract infections such as *Escherichia coli* and some strains of *Proteus* and *Klebsiella* species. *Pseudomonas* organisms are usually resistant. The drug is active against those gram-positive cocci that sometimes cause urinary-tract infections, including *Streptococcus faecalis, Staphylococcus aureus* and *S. epidermidis.*

The drug is reported to be bactericidal in high concentrations and bacteriostatic in low concentrations. An important property of nitrofurantoin is that the sensitive microorganisms do not readily become resistant to the drug.

Nitrofurantoin is rapidly and well absorbed following oral administration. The dosage is usually 50 to 100 mg administered four times a day — both for the crystalline form (*Furadantin,* 50 mg and 100 mg tablet) and the macrocrystalline form (*Macrodantin,* 50 mg and 100 mg capsule). The drug is rapidly excreted in the urine; although alkalinisation of the urine increases the urinary concentration, the antibacterial effect of the drug decreases in alkaline urine. Acidification of the urine results in enhanced reabsorption of the drug with increased renal tissue concentrations which may be of value when treating pyelonephritis.

Nitrofurantoin is useful only in the treatment of urinary-tract infections — acute uncomplicated infections localised in the urinary tract such as urethritis, prostatitis and pyelonephritis, and chronic bacteruria. Nitrofurantoin is contraindicated in all patients with any degree of renal function impairment as a therapeutic concentration of the drug is unlikely to be obtained in the urine.

Adverse Drug Reactions

The side effects of nitrofurantoin are mainly gastrointestinal disturbances including nausea and vomiting. These side effects may be controlled by reducing the dose, or by administration of the drug with food or milk. It has been claimed that the macrocystalline form of nitrofurantoin (*Macrodantin*) is less irritating to the gastrointestinal tract, and this has been attributed to its relatively slower absorption. Headache, dizziness, malaise and nystagmus have also been reported. Peripheral neuritis is a serious toxic effect of nitrofurantoin and most often occurs in patients who develop high blood concentrations with renal failure. Acute allergic reactions manifested by sudden, severe dyspnoea, chills, fever and skin eruptions, as well as pulmonary infiltration, pulmonary oedema and pulmonary effusion have been reported during therapy with nitrofurantoin. Three types of blood disorders may occur: haemolytic anaemia, megaloblastic anaemia and bone marrow depression.

Metabolites of nitrofurantoin may impart a brown colour to the urine of patients receiving the drug. Yellow discolouration of the teeth in infants is thought to be due to repeated direct contact of the drug with erupting teeth.

HEXAMINE HIPPURATE AND HEXAMINE MANDELATE

Hexamine (methenamine) was introduced as a urinary antiseptic agent in 1894. The antibacterial effect of hexamine and its salts is dependent upon the release of formaldehyde in an acid medium. Formaldehyde is a nonspecific antibacterial agent effective against most gram-negative bacilli including *Pseudomonas.* Gram-positive cocci are relatively resistant. The development of resistance to hexamine has not been reported because bacteria and fungi do not become resistant to formaldehyde.

Hexamine mandelate is a combination of hexamine and mandelic acid. Mandelic acid, in addition to its antibacterial activity, potentiates that of hexamine by making the urine more acid. However, many patients treated with hexamine mandelate still require supplementary acidifying agents to keep the urine pH as low as 5.0. Hexamine mandelate is available for oral administration as 250 mg and 500 mg tablets (*Mandelamine*).

Hexamine hippurate is a combination of hexamine and hippuric acid. It is claimed that it is effective in lower daily doses than hexamine mandelate (1 gram twice a day compared with 1 gram four times a day for hexamine mandelate). It is also claimed that additional urinary acidification is unnecessary. The hippurate salt may give higher urinary formaldehyde concentrations. Hexamine hippurate is available as 1 gram tablets (*Hiprex*).

Hexamine mandelate and hexamine hippurate are administered orally, usually as enteric-coated tablets to prevent the release of formaldehyde in the acid contents of the stomach. They have been used for the treatment of urinary-tract infections caused by susceptible organisms, including pyelonephritis, cystitis and infections accompanying a neurogenic bladder. Today they are infrequently used due to the availability of many other anti-infective agents. Urinary pH should be monitored during therapy and supplementary acidification provided. These hexamine salts do not achieve a therapeutic concentration of formaldehyde in the urine in the presence of renal failure due to impaired renal excretion.

Adverse Drug Reactions

Both hexamine salts are generally well tolerated, although some patients develop gastrointestinal side effects such as nausea, vomiting and diarrhoea. These effects possibly are due to the local irritant effects of free formaldehyde. Dermatological reactions manifested as skin rashes, urticaria and pruritus may occur. High doses or prolonged administration may lead to urinary-tract irritation due to the liberated formaldehyde. This may result in frequency, dysuria, albuminuria and haematuria.

Hexamine salts are contraindicated in patients with renal insufficiency, hepatic insufficiency or severe dehydration.

ANTIFUNGAL AGENTS

Most of the major antibiotics are produced by fungi, and therefore it is not surprising that fungi should be resistant to them. There are, however, some highly specialised antibiotics and synthetic compounds that are effective as antifungal agents and in general have little or no antibacterial activity.

AMPHOTERICIN

Amphotericin is a member of the polyene group of antifungal agents and was isolated in 1956 from *Streptomyces nodosus* found in soil. There are two forms of amphotericin, A and B, the latter being more effective and used clinically.

Amphotericin and the other polyene antifungal agents such as nystatin and natamycin probably act on sensitive fungi by binding to sterols (ergosterol) in the fungal cell membrane and thus interfere with cell permeability. These drugs are not active against organisms such as bacteria which do not contain sterols in their cell membranes. Some mammalian cells such as certain kidney cells and erythrocytes contain sterols (cholesterol) and thus are subject to alterations in cellular permeability when exposed to amphotericin. Amphotericin has a higher affinity for ergosterol than cholesterol.

Amphotericin is fungistatic in concentrations obtained clinically. The drug is active against pathogenic yeasts, for example, *Cryptococcus neoformans,* and pathogenic yeast-like fungi such as *Candida albicans (Monilia)* and *Torulopsis glabrata*. Moulds or filamentous fungi such as *Aspergillus* and the *Cladosporium* species are usually sensitive to amphotericin, but the dermatophytes or ringworm fungi are usually resistant. The dimorphic fungi, *Histoplasma capsulatum* and *Coccidioides immitis*, are sensitive. Fungi resistant to amphotericin are frequently resistant to other polyene antibiotics. Acquired resistance to amphotericin has not been a problem in clinical practice. Amphotericin and flucytosine are used together, if possible in full dosage, to inhibit infections caused by strains of *Cryptococcus neoformans, Candida albicans* and *Candida tropicalis*. It was thought that this combination was synergistic and that the binding of amphotericin to sterols in the fungal cell membranes increased the permeability of the cytoplasmic membrane, thus allowing greater penetration of flucytosine into the fungal cell. Recent evidence disputes that synergism occurs. Amphotericin is used in combination with flucytosine to prevent the development of resistance when the latter drug is used alone.

Amphotericin is poorly absorbed from the gastrointestinal tract and may be administered orally in suspension, or as tablets or lozenges for the treatment of superficial *Candida* infections. The drug may be administered as a bladder irrigation for the treatment of bladder *Candida* (monilial) infections.

Amphotericin must be administered parenterally to treat systemic infections. It is administered by slow intravenous infusion in dextrose over four to six hours under close medical supervision for the treatment of aspergillosis, disseminated candidiasis, pulmonary, disseminated or meningeal coccidioidomycosis, pulmonary or disseminated cryptococcus and pulmonary or disseminated histoplasmosis. The intrathecal and intraventricular routes are occasionally indicated in patients who are dangerously ill with meningitis and who are not responding to intravenous therapy.

The colloidal amphotericin is precipitated from solution if it is mixed with solutions containing anions and cations such as sodium chloride or potassium chloride and dextrose solutions of low pH (pH below 5). Preparations of amphotericin, strengths and dosing information for adult patients with normal renal function are summarised in Table 65.

Adverse Drug Reactions

The incidence of adverse reactions with parenterally administered amphotericin is high. These reactions include side effects that may occur during intravenous infusion, for example, fever, chills, headache, anorexia, nausea and vomiting. These side effects are considered to be dose related and are usually less severe when the drug is infused slowly or on alternate days. Thrombophlebitis is a common problem, and pain at the injection site and extravasation causing local irritation may occur. Anaphylactic reactions are rare.

Nephrotoxicity is the most common and the most important side effect of intravenous therapy with amphotericin. Some degree of renal impairment occurs in almost all patients treated with the drug. Renal toxicity may be minimised by adequate alkalinisation of the urine, by giving a small initial dose of the drug, and by slowly increasing the dose to the least amount that is effective against the organisms. The daily dose should not be increased above 1 mg per kilogram body weight. The recommended total cumulative dose of amphotericin, which varies with the type of infection, ranges from 1.5 to 2.5 grams. Hypokalaemia develops in most patients receiving intravenous amphotericin due to excessive renal losses. Potassium supplementation is necessary for most patients.

Haematological side effects occur—a normochromic normocytic anaemia which generally is reversible on removal of the drug. Liver function abnormalities are rarely detected. Cardiac arrest has been reported with rapid intravenous administration of amphotericin. Intrathecal administration has resulted in headaches, nausea, vomiting, urinary retention, pain along lumbar nerves, paraesthesias, visual changes and arachnoiditis. Because of its numerous and serious side effects, parenteral amphotericin should be used only by physicians who have experience with this form of therapy and the following parameters should be monitored prior to commencing therapy and then at regular (twice weekly) intervals: haematocrit, serum potassium, magnesium, bicarbonate, creatinine and BUN.

NYSTATIN AND NATAMYCIN

Nystatin and ***natamycin*** are polyene antifungal agents, like amphotericin, and were isolated from *Streptomyces* in 1950 and 1955 respectively. They are unsuitable for parenteral administration and are only used for the treatment of superficial infections.

Many preparations of nystatin are available for the treatment of topical *Candida* infections—skin infections, oral candidiasis ("thrush"), vaginal candidiasis and candidiasis of the intestinal tract. A nystatin aerosol has been used to treat pulmonary aspergillosis.

Natamycin, like nystatin, is poorly absorbed from the gastrointestinal tract and is available for the treatment of topical *Candida* infections. Unlike the other antifungals, natamycin is active against *Trichomonas vaginalis,* although metronidazole is more effective for this condition. Some preparations of nystatin and natamycin are listed in Table 65.

Adverse Drug Reactions

There are virtually no side effects related to the topical use of nystatin or natamycin. Nausea and vomiting may occur following large oral doses of nystatin. These drugs do not cause irritation or allergic reactions when applied to skin or mucous membranes.

IMIDAZOLES

The imidazoles currently available for clinical use include ***clotrimazole, econazole, isoconazole, ketoconazole*** and ***miconazole.*** Others are under development. They have activity against a broad range of microorga-

Table 65
Antifungal drugs

Approved Name	Brand Name	Strength(s)	Dose Range (Normal Renal Function, Adult)	Frequency of Dosing
Amphotericin	Fungizone	50 mg injection	0.25 mg to 1 mg/kg daily by slow IV	Daily
	Fungilin	10 mg lozenge	10 mg	6 hourly
		100 mg tablet	100 mg to 200 mg, oral	6 hourly
		100 mg/mL suspension, topical cream and ointment	100 mg (1 mL)	6 hourly
Nystatin	Nystan	500 000 units tablet;	500 000 to 1 000 000 u oral	6 hourly
		100 000 units pastilles		
		100 000 units/mL suspension;	100 000 u (1 mL), oral	6 hourly
		100 000 units vaginal tablets, vaginal cream, topical cream, ointment and gel	100 000 u vaginally	Daily
Natamycin	Pimafucin	10 mg/mL suspension	10 drops, oral	8 hourly
		2.5% sterile suspension	0.1 mL in aerosol	8 hourly
		25 mg vaginal tablets	25 mg vaginally	12 hourly
	Pimafucin and Pimafucort	Topical cream and ointment		

Flucytosine	Alcobon	500 mg tablet; 2.5 g/250 mL injection	100 to 200 mg/kg/day, oral, IV; peak serum level in 2 to 4 hours, oral	6 hourly
Griseofulvin	Fulcin Grisovin	125 mg, 500 mg tablet	500 mg to 1g, oral	Daily
Clotrimazole	Canesten	100 mg, 200 mg, 500 mg vaginal tablets Vaginal cream, topical cream	Vaginally	100 mg daily, 500 mg single dose
Econazole	Ecostatin Pevaryl	150 mg vaginal pessaries, vaginal cream, topical cream	Vaginally	Daily
Isoconazole	Travogen	300 mg vaginal tablet Topical cream	600 mg vaginally	Single dose
Ketoconazole	Nizoral	200 mg tablet	200 mg to 400 mg oral, peak serum level in 2 h	Daily
Miconazole	Daktarin Gyno-Daktarin Monistat	200 mg/20 mL injection, 100 mg vaginal tablet, vaginal cream, topical cream, oral gel	200 mg to 1200 mg IV over 30 to 60 min, vaginally	8 hourly daily Daily

nisms, including fungi and bacteria and appear to interact with sterol or fatty-acid metabolism resulting in disruption of the cell membrane and leakage of cytoplasmic contents. They also interfere with oxidative enzymes. They are related to the antiprotozoal and anti-anaerobic agent, metronidazole, and to the antithyroid agents, carbimazole and methimazole.

Clotrimazole, econazole, isoconazole and miconazole are poorly absorbed from the gastrointestinal tract and are poorly soluble in water. They are used topically and vaginally for the treatment of *Candida* infections and superficial dermatophyte infections.

Miconazole is available as a parenteral formulation for the treatment of systemic candidiasis, histoplasmosis and other fungal infections. Adverse effects related to its parenteral use include phlebitis, aggregation of erythrocytes, anaemia, thrombocytosis, skin rashes, hyperlipidaemia (due to the vehicle) and hyponatraemia. Rapid infusion may lead to tachycardia and other cardiac arrhythmias.

Ketoconazole has the advantage that it can be administered orally to treat a wide range of superficial and systemic fungal infections. However, it is poorly absorbed from the gastrointestinal tract when gastric acidity is insufficient, for example in achlorhydria, or if the patient is receiving antacids or histamine-2 antagonists such as cimetidine. Concomitant administration with these drugs should be avoided. Side effects that have been reported with oral ketoconazole therapy include nausea, vomiting, abdominal pain, diarrhoea, skin rash, gynaecomastia and severe hepatotoxicity.

FLUCYTOSINE

Flucytosine (5-Fluorocytosine, 5-FC) was synthesised in 1957 for the treatment of leukaemia. The drug proved ineffective for this purpose as it had no cytotoxic acitivity, but it was found to have selective antifungal activity against *Cryptococcus neoformans* and the yeast-like fungus *Candida albicans.* Other *Candida* species and *Torulopsis glabrata* appear to be susceptible to flucytosine.

Flucytosine appears to penetrate fungal cells where it is converted to fluorouracil, a known antimetabolite. This may act as a false substrate within the fungal cell, interfering ultimately with nucleic acid and protein synthesis.

Flucytosine is well absorbed from the gastrointestinal tract and is widely distributed in body tissues and fluids including the cerebrospinal fluid. The drug is used only in the treatment of serious infections caused by susceptible strains of *Candida* and *Cryptococcus* organisms. Fungaemia, endocarditis and urinary tract infections caused by *Candida* and meningitis and pulmonary infections caused by *Cryptococcus* have been effectively treated with this agent.

There is an increasing emergence of organisms resistant to flucytosine when long-term therapy is used. Combination therapy with amphotericin is recommended in meningeal cryptococcus infections to prevent or delay the emergence of resistant organisms.

Flucytosine is available as 500 mg tablets, with a brand name of *Alcobon.* An intravenous formulation is also available (refer Table 65).

Adverse Drug Reactions

Although flucytosine appears to have a low order of toxicity compared with amphotericin, toxic effects of the drug are elicited on rapidly proliferating cells, particularly the bone marrow and lining of the gastrointestinal tract. Moderate hypoplasia of bone marrow (resulting in anaemia, leukopenia, pancytopenia, thrombocytopenia or rarely, agranulocytosis) may occur. Gastrointestinal effects include nausea, vomiting, anorexia, abdominal bloating and diarrhoea. The incidence of severity of vomiting may be decreased or eliminated if the oral dose is given over a 15-minute period.

Transient liver enlargement has been noted in some patients, together with altered hepatic function tests. Nephrotoxicity has not been ascribed to flucytosine, although the dose should be reduced and renal function monitored in patients with renal impairment. Frequent serum concentration assays of the drug should be performed in patients with impaired renal function.

GRISEOFULVIN

Although ***griseofulvin*** was isolated from *Penicillium griseofulvium* in 1939, it was not until 1947 that its potential for the treatment of human infections was realised.

Griseofulvin exerts its fungistatic action primarily by disrupting the cell's nuclear division process. This results in abnormal DNA production which may arrest cellular division. Griseofulvin is deposited in keratin precursor cells rendering them an unfavourable environment for fungal invasion. Infected skin, hair or nails are then replaced with tissue not affected by the dermatophyte.

Griseofulvin inhibits the dermatophytes or ringworm fungi, but has no activity against other filamentous fungi, yeasts or yeast-like fungi.

Absorption of griseofulvin following oral administration is variable and occurs mainly in the duodenum. The absorption of micro-sized griseofulvin particles is enhanced by concomitant administration with a high fat meal. Following absorption, the drug is concentrated in skin, hair, nails, liver, fat and skeletal muscles.

Griseofulvin is used in the treatment of mycoses of the skin, hair and nails — tinea corporis, tinea pedis, tinea cruris, tinea capitis and tinea unguium — caused by susceptible species of *Trichophyton, Microsporum* and *Epidermophyton.* Because the drug is not effective against other fungal infections, the infecting organism should be identified as a dermatophyte before initiating therapy.

Response to therapy depends upon the rate of keratinisation and time necessary for desquamation of infected keratinised structures. Soles, palms and nails respond more slowly than less keratinised skin, and toe nails repond at the slowest rate.

Refer to Table 65 for products available and dosing information.

Adverse Drug Reactions

Griseofulvin is a relatively non-toxic drug and there are no reports of renal, haemopoietic or liver toxicity. Headache is a frequent side effect of griseofulvin therapy, occurring in the early states of treatment. Epigastric distress, nausea and vomiting, excessive thirst, diarrhoea, flatulence and oral thrush due to monilial overgrowth may occur. Hypersensitivity rashes, maculopapular or urticarial rashes may occur in some patients but disappear when the drug is discontinued. Photosensitivity rashes have also been reported.

Griseofulvin is contraindicated in patients with porphyria due to its effect on porphyrin metabolism. The drug is contraindicated in hepatocellular failure, and in patients with a history of hypersensitivity to the drug.

NURSING IMPLICATIONS

Assessment

Amphotericin

This is a toxic drug and all patients should be carefully assessed prior to its administration. The patient's history should be reviewed for previously undisclosed allergy to the drug, renal or haemopoietic disorders. Results of laboratory tests such as blood urea, creatinine and serum potassium should be at hand before administration commences. When a systemic infection is to be treated with parenteral amphotericin, the nurse should establish baseline observations of vital signs before therapy is commenced.

Administration

Intravenous administration is by slow infusion in dextrose which has been buffered to the correct pH. Do not infuse amphotericin in saline or ward stock dextrose solutions. Administer urinary alkaliniser as ordered.

Evaluation

During intravenous administration, the patient's vital signs should be monitored regularly due to the high incidence of adverse reactions associated with this agent. Watch for signs of thrombophlebitis such as redness and pain along the vein. Prevent extravasation of the solution as skin irritation can occur.

Patients receiving either oral or parenteral amphotericin should be evaluated for signs of nephrotoxicity and hypokalaemia. Monitor urine output, as oliguria or haematuria could indicate nephrotoxicity. Muscle weakness is a sign of hypokalaemia.

Nystatin and Natamycin

These substances are administered either orally or applied locally. They are generally well tolerated. Patients should be instructed in the correct method of application and dosage regimen and the importance of completing the entire course of therapy in order to ensure eradication of the infection.

Imidazoles

Patients who are to receive ketoconazole should be assessed for concurrent use of antacids or histamine-2 antagonists as the absorption of this drug is reduced when there is insufficient stomach acid. Their history should also be reviewed to exclude any previous allergy to the drug or liver disease.

Those patients who are receiving oral ketoconazole should be observed for signs of adverse reactions such as allergic response, gastro-intestinal upsets and hepatotoxicity.

When patients are to receive parenteral miconazole, the nurse should establish baseline recording of vital signs, ensure there is no history of previous allergy to the preparation, and ensure that any laboratory results concerning the patient's haemopoietic function are at hand.

Intravenous infusion of miconazole should be slow, over a one-hour period. As the fluid can cause severe irritation to the skin, it is important to prevent extravasation at the infusion site during administration.

Nursing evaluation for patients receiving miconazole intravenously will include frequent recording of vital signs in order to detect early signs of cardiac arrhythmias or allergic reaction. Observe for signs of phlebitis and skin irritation at the infusion site.

Flucytosine

Nursing assessment of patients who are to receive flucytosine should aim to identify any previously undisclosed history of liver, renal or haemopoietic disorders. Patients who are especially at risk include those who have recently had (or are receiving) chemotherapy or radiotherapy for malignancy, as these therapies can cause bone-marrow depression.

To decrease the incidence of nausea which can occur with this drug, the administration of oral doses may be spaced 15 minutes apart.

Blood counts should be done frequently during the course of therapy, and the nurse should evaluate the patient for signs of bone-marrow depression, such as bruising, bleeding, haematuria or sore throat. The nurse should also observe for and report any adverse gastro-intestinal effects or signs of CNS toxicity such as confusion, headache, vertigo and jaundice, the latter being indicative of hepatotoxicity.

Griseofulvin

Patients who are to receive this drug should be assessed for any previous undisclosed history of hypersensitivity to the drug, hepatic disease or porphyria.

Griseofulvin is usually self-administered, and patients should be advised that taking it with a high-fat meal will enhance its absorption. They should also be told that completion of the whole course is required in order to avoid recurrence of the fungal infection. As the drug can cause photosensitivity, patients should be advised to avoid excessive exposure to ultraviolet light. Patients should be taught the side effects of the drug and advised to consult their physician should these occur.

METRONIDAZOLE AND ANTITRICHOMONAL AGENTS

METRONIDAZOLE

Metronidazole has been used since 1959 to treat protozoal infestations due to *Trichomonas vaginalis* and also amoebiasis. In recent years the drug's activity against the obligate anaerobes, including *Bacteroides fragilis*, has been recognised, and metronidazole is included among the drugs of first choice for these infections.

The exact mechanism of action of metronidazole is not known. It has been postulated that within the cells of microorganisms possessing nitro-reductase enzymes, the nitro-group of metronidazole is reduced, thereby generating extremely reactive intermediate derivatives which bind to the oganism's DNA, inhibiting its synthesis and thus causing cell death. The lack of bactericidal activity of metronidazole against aerobic organisms has been rationalised on the basis that these organisms do not possess nitro-reductase activity.

Metronidazole is usually well absorbed after oral administration, primarily from the small intestine. Following a therapeutic oral dose effective serum concentrations of the drug are reached in one to three hours and maintained for at least 12 hours. The drug is excreted mainly in the urine. Metronidazole readily crosses the placental barrier and appears in the milk of nursing mothers.

For the treatment of trichomoniasis, the usual adult dose is 200 mg administered orally three times a day for seven days. The drug should be administered with food. To treat giardiasis, 2 grams is administered orally each day in divided doses with meals for three days. Amoebiasis is treated by administering 400 to 800 mg three times a day for 5 to 10 days. Acute ulcerative gingivitis is treated by administering 200 mg of metronidazole orally for three days. Metronidazole has been used to treat *Clostridium difficile*-induced pseudomembranous colitis.

Metronidazole may be given alone or concurrently with other appropriate antibacterial agents to treat anaerobic infections, particularly *Bacteroides fragilis.* The drug may be administered intravenously at a rate of 7.5 mg per kilogram or, for an adult, in a dose of 500 mg in 100 mL of fluid infused at the rate of 5 mL per minute. Oral metronidazole should be substituted as soon as possible and the oral dose is 400 mg three times a day. Alternatively, metronidazole may be administered rectally in a dose of 500 mg to 1 g (adult dose) at eight-hour-intervals. Preparations of metronidazole available are *Flagyl* 200 mg and 400 mg tablets. A suspension of benzoylmetronidazole (equivalent to 200 mg of metronidazole, 5 mL), is available for oral administration. The intravenous infusion of metronidazole contains 500 mg of metronidazole in 100 mL of fluid.
The paediatric parenteral preparation contains 100 mg per 20 mL, 5mL is available for oral administration. The intravenous infusion of metronidazole contains 500 mg of metronidazole in 100 mL of fluid.

The paediatric parenteral preparation contains 100 mg 20 mL, and the recommended administration rate is 5 mL per minute. Suppositories containing either 500 mg or 1 g are available and are used to prevent postoperative infections due to anaerobic bacteria following gynaecological surgery and colonic surgery.

Adverse Drug Reactions

Toxic effects are not common and are usually mild. The most common reactions to metronidazole therapy are dermatological (rash, pruritus, urticaria); gastrointestinal (nausea, anorexia, furry tongue, dry mouth, abdominal discomfort, a metallic taste in the mouth); headache and dizziness. Transient leucopenia, darkening of the urine and dysuria have been reported less frequently. Metronidazole taken in combination with alcohol may produce abdominal cramps, nausea, vomiting, headaches and flushing. Patients are advised to avoid taking alcohol when receiving metronidazole.

Metronidazole has been shown to be mutagenic and carcinogenic in bacteria and some animal species, therefore the drug should not be given to pregnant women unless the benefits outweigh the risks. Caution should be exercised in administering the drug to nursing mothers as the drug is excreted in the breast milk.

TINIDAZOLE

Tinidazole *(Fasigyn)* is similar to metronidazole and is administered orally to treat protozoal infections — trichomoniasis, giardiasis and amoebiasis. It is active against gram-negative anaerobic bacilli, including *Bacteroides fragilis.* A single two-gram dose has been found to be effective therapy in vaginal trichomoniasis and in urogenital trichomoniasis in males. It is effective against giardiasis.

Side effects are generally mild and self-limiting. The most common side effects are gastrointestinal – nausea, vomiting, anorexia and a metallic or bitter taste in the mouth. Other reactions include headache, tiredness, furry tongue, itching and skin rashes. The urine may be darker in colour. Alcohol should be avoided when the patient is receiving tinidazole. Administration of tinidazole is contraindicated in the first three months of pregnancy.

NATAMYCIN

Natamycin (*Pimafucin,* 25 mg) is available as pessaries for the treatment of trichomoniasis.

NURSING IMPLICATIONS

Nursing assessment prior to the administration of metronidazole should aim to identify current alcohol use and the presence of haemopoietic disorders. As the drug is mutagenic and can be excreted in mother's milk, the presence of a pregnancy should be excluded. Caution should be exercised if it is necessary to administer the drug to nursing mothers. The mother should be advised to cease breast feeding during the course of treatment.

The administration of metronidazole with food may minimise the risk of gastro-intestinal upsets. When evaluating patients taking this drug, watch for and report signs of allergy, such as rash or pruritus. Numbness, tremor, ataxia, or paraesthesia may indicate CNS toxicity. Sore throat, fatigue and increased bleeding tendencies are indicative of leucopenia.

Patient teaching should stress the avoidance of alcohol during the course of therapy as metronidazole exerts a disulfiram-like (*Antabuse*) effect which can cause distressing symptoms such as flushing, tachycardia, nausea, vomiting and even circulatory collapse. Patients should be advised that the drug may cause a metallic taste in the mouth and that the urine may become discoloured. All patients who are self-administering the drug should be counselled regarding these adverse effects.

ANTITUBERCULAR AGENTS

The advent of effective antitubercular drugs, notably ***streptomycin*** (1944), ***para-aminosalicylic acid*** (1946) and ***isoniazid*** (1952) completely revolutionised the treatment of all forms of tuberculosis. However, the emergence of strains resistant to these and newer drugs has dominated the management of tuberculosis. The guiding principle in the management of tuberculosis is prolonged, concurrent use of two or more drugs to which the organisms are susceptible.

The usual duration of chemotherapy for tuberculosis is 18 to 24 months. However, short-course regimens of nine months duration, using at least two first-line drugs (such as isoniazid and rifampicin) may be considered for the treatment of uncomplicated pulmonary tuberculosis.

ISONIAZID

Isoniazid (isonicotinic acid hydrazide) is highly active against *Mycobacterium tuberculosis* and other organisms of the genus *Mycobacterium,* although most strains of *Mycobacterium avium, Mycobacterium fortuitum* and *Mycobacterium marinum* are resistant. The drug is ineffective against all other microorganisms.

The exact mode of action of isoniazid is not known, although several mechanisms including interference with bacterial proteins, nucleic acids, carbohydrates and lipids have been proposed. Recent investigations have suggested that isoniazid inhibits the synthesis of mycolic acids (important constituents of the mycobacterial cell wall) by interfering with the enzyme mycolase synthetase (an enzyme which appears to be unique to mycobacteria). Isoniazid is active only against rapidly growing sensitive tubercle bacilli and does not affect these bacilli when they are in a metabolic resting state. Resistant strains of initially sensitive organisms develop rapidly when isoniazid is used alone in the treatment of active tuberculosis.

Isoniazid is readily absorbed from the gastrointestinal tract. Following administration, peak isoniazid blood concentrations are achieved within one to two hours. Although a proportion of the population acetylate (metabolise) the drug rapidly, the rate of acetylation does not alter the efficacy of the drug when it is administered daily. A relationship has been noted between rapid inactivation of isoniazid by those patients who are "fast acetylators" and poor therapeutic response in some intermittent regimens.

The drug is widely distributed in the body tissues, organs and fluids including cerebrospinal fluid, pleural fluid and ascitic fluid. Isoniazid crosses the placental barrier and appears in the milk of nursing mothers. The drug and its metabolites are excreted primarily in the urine.

The usual dose of isoniazid in the treatment of active pulmonary tuberculosis is 4 to 8 mg per kilogram body weight daily, administered in a single daily dose or as divided doses, in conjunction with other tuberculostatic drugs. The drug may also be administered in a dose of 300 mg daily for preventive therapy. Isoniazid is available as 50 mg and 100 mg tablets for oral administration, 50 mg/5 mL elixir and 25 mg/mL injection.

The side effects of isoniazid are generally dose related and appear to occur more frequently in slow isoniazid inactivators, the elderly and malnourished patients. These side effects include vertigo, twitching of the limbs, increased reflexes and retention of urine. Psychosis, confusion, coma and convulsions may occur if toxic serum concentrations of the drug are attained. Peripheral neuritis may develop and presents in the form of burning hands and feet. This is a more common complication. Adult patients receiving isoniazid excrete large amounts of pyridoxine, and it has been postulated that this neuritis may be due to pyridoxine deficiency. Pyridoxine therapy may prevent this neuritis from developing.

The most serious adverse effect associated with isoniazid therapy is a drug-induced hepatitis. The mechanism of hepatotoxicity has not been fully elucidated. However, it is thought that the hepatitis may be secondary to conversion of isoniazid to acetylhydrazine or related hepatotoxic derivatives which are capable of inducing hepatic necrosis. The incidence of hepatitis is increased in patients who are older, who take rifampicin and who consume alcohol daily. Whether or not the incidence is higher in those patients who are rapid acetylators of isoniazid awaits resolution.

Isoniazid therapy has been associated with arthritic symptoms (arthralgias of knees, elbows and wrists) and systemic lupus erythematosus.

RIFAMPICIN

Rifampicin is active against many bacteria, gram-positive and gram-negative, and its range of activity includes *Mycobacterium tuberculosis.* The drug is marketed as *Rifadin* and *Rimactane* (150 mg and 300 mg capsules) for the treatment of tuberculosis and leprosy. Rifampicin is active against the *Legionella* species and is used, in combination with erythromycin, to treat *Legionella* pneumonia.

Rifampicin inhibits RNA synthesis in susceptible cells. The drug appears to be bactericidal as well as bacteriostatic in action. Resistant strains of initially sensitive organisms develop rapidly when rifampicin is used alone in the treatment of tuberculosis and other infections.

The drug is well absorbed orally and the usual adult dose for the treatment of tuberculosis is 450 mg to 600 mg administered daily as a single dose one hour before breakfast.

The main toxic effect of rifampicin has been on the liver with the production of hepatocellular damage or of jaundice from cholestasis. Hypersensitivity reactions are relatively rare. Thrombocytopenia and other haematological changes have also been reported. Patients receiving the drug intermittently may experience abdominal, flu-like and respiratory side effects. Rifampicin stains the urine reddish brown.

Rifampicin has the ability to induce the action of liver enzymes with the result that the metabolism of it and various other drugs is altered. For example, the metabolism of oral contraceptives, corticosteroids, warfarin, orally administered hypoglycaemics, methadone and digoxin is increased, resulting in decreased serum concentrations of these drugs and hence decreased efficacy.

ETHAMBUTOL

Ethambutol (*Myambutol,* 100 mg and 400 mg tablets) is active only against mycobacteria. The exact mode of action of ethambutol is not completely known, but the drug diffuses rapidly into and is firmly bound by actively growing, sensitive tubercle bacilli. It inhibits cell metabolism and arrests multiplication.

Resistant strains develop rapidly when ethambutol is used alone in the treatment of tuberculosis. Combination therapy with other tuberculostatic drugs delays the emergence of resistance. There is no evidence of cross-resistance between ethambutol and other tuberculostatic drugs and strains of *Mycobacterium tuberculosis* resistant *in vitro* to isoniazid and streptomycin are usually susceptible to ethambutol.

Ethambutol is readily absorbed after oral administration, and there is no gastrointestinal intolerance. The recommended dose for adults is 15 mg per kilogram body weight administered as a single daily dose. The dose should be reduced in renal failure.

The most frequent side effects of ethambutol therapy are ocular toxicities (including decreased visual acuity and loss of green colour vision) which appear to be related to the dose of the drug and the duration of therapy. Patients treated with ethambutol should be advised to report all ocular symptoms. Peripheral neuritis occurs rarely. Hepatic and renal function tests should be performed regularly during therapy with this drug.

PYRAZINAMIDE

Pyrazinamide (*Zinamide,* 500 mg tablets), a derivative of nicotinamide, has a relatively low activity against *Mycobacterium tuberculosis.* The drug is relatively toxic and is not used as a first-line drug for the treatment of tuberculosis. Resistance develops rapidly if the drug is used alone.

The drug is sometimes included in the therapeutic regimens for retreatment of patients whose tubercle bacilli have become resistant to one or more of the first line drugs. The recommended oral dose of pyrazinamide is 20–35 mg/kg up to a maximum of 3 g daily, administered orally in divided doses.

Pyrazinamide interferes with the excretion of urate and, as a result, gout may be clinically manifested. Nausea, vomiting, arthralgias and drug-induced fever may occur, and the drug has ability to induce hepatitis.

PARA-AMINOSALICYLIC ACID

Para-aminosalicylic acid (PAS) was regarded for many years as one of the front-line drugs for the treatment of tuberculosis. Today it has been replaced in regimens by either rifampicin or ethambutol. These drugs are more effective and produce fewer side effects.

CAPREOMYCIN AND CYCLOSERINE

Capreomycin and ***cycloserine*** are regarded as reserve drugs in the treatment of tuberculosis because of their toxicity. Both drugs should be used only as an adjuvant in the treatment of pulmonary tuberculosis and should be combined with two other drugs. Nephrotoxicity and ototoxicity are the most important toxic effects of capreomycin therapy. Neurotoxicity is the most important toxic effect of cycloserine.

NURSING IMPLICATIONS

Assessment

The patient's general physical condition, history of liver or kidney disease or alcohol abuse should be assessed before isoniazid therapy is begun. A history of previous liver damage may contraindicate the use of rifampicin. Dose levels of ethambutol and cycloserine need to be reduced for patients with poor renal function. Baseline visual function should be established before ethambutol therapy is commenced.

Administration

A daily dosage schedule is recommended for rifampicin. Gastrointestinal irritation caused by ethambutol can be reduced by giving the drug with food. Drug therapy may need to be closely supervised to ensure compliance.

Evaluation

Patients' responses to antitubercular drugs should be evaluated with close attention to adverse effects on the liver, kidneys and central nervous system.

Patient teaching

It is essential that patients understand the importance of complying with dose schedules, multiple drug treatment and the duration of treatment. They should be warned not to take rifampicin intermittently, that it can reduce the effectiveness of oral contraceptives, and that body secretions (including urine) may take on a reddish tinge. Patients taking ethambutol should be instructed to report any visual disturbance.

ANTILEPROTIC AGENTS

The treatment of leprosy is specific, the drug of choice for all types and stages being dapsone. In cases of intolerance to dapsone (early polyneuritis, acute reaction or psychosis), another drug should be substituted such as clofazimine or thiacetazone.

Recent evidence has suggested that rifampicin may be as effective as, or superior to, dapsone in treating leprosy. However, because almost all bacteria develop resistance to rifampicin, it should be used in combination with dapsone (see below).

DAPSONE

Dapsone is known as the "parent sulfone" of a group of compounds, sulfones, that have antileprotic activity. Dapsone is used in the treatment of both lepromatous and tuberculoid types of leprosy.

The drug is bacteriostatic rather than bactericidal in action. It has been suggested that dapsone acts by limiting the utilisation of a metabolite essential to the organism's growth.

Dapsone is almost completely absorbed from the gastrointestinal tract following oral administration. The drug is distributed in body tissues and is found in high concentrations in the liver and kidneys. Dapsone is excreted slowly in the urine.

Dapsone is used as part of a multi-drug chemotherapeutic regimen, as recommended by the WHO Group on Leprosy (1982). Rifampicin is given 450–600 mg daily (preferably before breakfast) for at least 4 weeks. Clofazimine is given 100 mg 3 times a week for one year to previously untreated people. Dapsone is given 25–50 mg twice weekly, gradually increasing to 400 mg twice weekly for life.

Adverse Drug Reactions

The most common toxic effect of dapsone is anaemia. Sensitivity to dapsone may be manifested as dermatitis. The slow introduction of therapy will reduce the incidence and severity of these side effects. Liver damage occurs as an acute toxic effect of excessive dosage. The erythema nodosum leprosum type of "lepra reaction" is a common occurrence during treatment of lepromatous leprosy.

Patients who have chronic liver, kidney or cardiovascular disease, or refractory types of anaemia or albuminuria should be observed closely for at least six months following the introduction of dapsone therapy. Dosage reduction may be indicated.

CLOFAZIMINE

Clofazimine (*Lamprene,* 100 mg capsule) is the drug of choice in cases where there is resistance to dapsone. The dose ranges from 100 mg three times a week to 100 mg daily. Treatment should be continued for at least six months. This drug imparts a red discoloration to the skin and urine.

ANTIMALARIALS

The choice of a drug or a combination of drugs for the chemotherapy or chemosuppression of malaria depends on the following factors:

1. The prevalence of drug-resistant strains of plasmodia.
2. The species of infecting parasite.
3. The stage of parasitisation — different antimalarial drugs exert their effects at different stages of the parasite's life cycle. Therapy or suppression may be aimed at: the pre-erythrocytic stages (or "tissue" stages) that take place in the liver; the erythrocytic stage in which the parasites multiply rapidly in erythrocytes; or the exo-erythrocytic or secondary tissue stages of the relapsing malarias that also take place in the liver.
4. Other factors, including the frequency of administration, the race of the recipient, the degree of host immunity and epidemiologic factors must be considered.

Drug resistance is a growing problem with the antimalarials, and combination products are being developed and used to treat infections due to drug-resistant strains.

CHLOROQUINE

Chloroquine is a synthetic antimalarial drug used for the treatment of chloroquine-sensitive pathological *Plasmodium* infections.

The precise mechanism of antimalarial activity has not been determined, but it has been postulated that chloroquine's activity is based on its ability to form complexes with DNA. Chloroquine is effective only against asexual erythrocytic forms of plasmodia and is not capable of exerting true causal prophylaxis, nor can it effect a radical cure, except in falciparum malaria.

Chloroquine is rapidly and almost completely absorbed from the gastrointestinal tract. The drug is used in a dose of 300 mg (chloroquine base) once or twice a week for prophylaxis in countries where there is no chloroquine resistant *Plasmodium falciparum* infection. For the treatment of acute malarial attacks, adults may receive 600 mg of chloroquine base initially, followed by 300 mg after six to eight hours and 300 mg on each of two successive days.

Preparations of chloroquine include:

Avloclor 250 mg (as phosphate) = 150mg chloroquine base;
Nivaquine 200 mg (as sulphate) = 150 mg chloroquine base.

There is also a parenteral formulation, *Nivaquine,* containing 40 mg chloroquine base per 1 mL. This is administered by IV infusion in acute malarial attacks.

Adverse Drug Reactions

The side effects of chloroquine in the doses used for the treatment of malaria are usually mild and reversible. Following prolonged therapy, serious and sometimes irreversible toxicity occurs including ocular changes (retinopathy is the most serious effect), gastrointestinal disturbances, dermatological reactions, neurologic reactions and blood dyscrasias. The drug accumulates in the liver and should be administered with caution to patients with liver disease, alcoholism and those who are receiving hepatotoxic drugs.

PYRIMETHAMINE

Pyrimethamine is a synthetic antimalarial drug which also has antitoxoplasmic activity.

The drug is a folic-acid antagonist, and its antimalarial activity probably results from the greater need for nucleic-acid precursors by the parasite than by the host. The erythrocytic stage is the most vulnerable stage to pyrimethamine. The drug may also arrest exo-erythrocytic nuclear division.

Pyrimethamine arrests sporogeny in the mosquito and thus is useful in preventing transmission of the disease. Pyrimethamine is a true causal prophylactic agent — it prevents the causal organism from becoming established in the liver (that is, the liver phase of the organism's life cycle) — for falciparum malaria.

Pyrimethamine is effective for suppressive prophylaxis of primary attacks of malaria and relapses, preventing completion of the asexual blood phase. It usually produces a radical cure of falciparum malaria, providing eradication of tissue parasites as well as relief of malarial symptoms.

Pyrimethamine resistance develops rapidly when it is used as a single agent, particularly with *Plasmodium falciparum.* Therefore it is used mostly in combination with a sulphonamide to sequentially block two steps in the metabolic conversion of para-aminobenzoic acid (PABA) to tetrahydrofolic acid (refer Figure 7).

The adult oral dose for suppressive prophylaxis, true causal prophylaxis of falciparum malaria and for transmission control is 25 mg once per week. Pyrimethamine is available as a 25 mg tablet (*Daraprim*) for oral administration. It is available in combination with dapsone (*Maloprim*) for prophylaxis against chloroquine-resistant falciparum malaria. The combination with sulfadoxine, *Fansidar,* although indicated both for the prophylaxis and short-term treatment of chloroquine-resistant falciparum malaria, is reserved by a number of clinical microbiologists for treatment only.

Adverse Drug Reactions

Pyrimethamine has a low order of toxicity in the recommended suppressive or therapeutic dosage for malaria. Dermatoses have been noted in some patients. Toxic effects may be those of folic acid deficiency.

PROGUANIL

Proguanil hydrochloride is an antimalarial drug and folic acid antagonist effective against the exo-erythrocytic forms of some strains of *Plasmodium falciparum.* It acts as a causal prophylactic for these sensitive organisms.

The drug is marketed under the brand name of *Paludrine* and is available as 100 mg tablets.

PRIMAQUINE PHOSPHATE

Primaquine phosphate is effective against the fixed tissue (liver) stage of the plasmodium. The important clinical use of this drug is to produce a radical cure of relapsing vivax malaria. In the treatment of acute attacks of vivax malaria or if *Plasmodium falciparum* is associated with the *P. vivax* infection, the drug should be given in conjunction with a fast-acting blood schizonticide such as chloroquine.

The drug is available as a tablet containing 7.5 mg of primaquine base. The usual adult dose for producing a cure of vivax malaria is 15 mg of the base daily for 14 to 21 days.

At usual therapeutic doses, primaquine shows low toxicity. Abdominal cramps and epigastric distress occur with the oral administration of the drug, effects which may be relieved by administering primaquine with meals or antacids. Haematological disturbances have been reported and occasionally urticarial reactions.

QUININE

Quinine is a more toxic and less effective antimalarial than chloroquine and other new synthetic agents. It is unreliable in the suppression of falciparum malaria. A valid use is its administration in combination with primaquine for the radical cure of relapsing vivax malaria. Quinine is only active against the erythrocytic phases of plasmodial infections.

Quinine salts are readily absorbed following oral administration, and many brands of tablets are available. In the treatment of chloroquine-resistant *Plasmodium falciparum* infection, 800 mg of quinine may be administered orally or parenterally every eight hours for 14 days, supplemented with a dose of sulfadoxine-pyrimethamine or one of the other antimalarials.

Quinine dihydrochloride, 5–10 mg/kg up to 500 mg, may be administered by slow intravenous infusion over 4 hours for emergency treatment of acute attacks. A marked fall in blood pressure often accompanies the intravenous dose. The oral administration of quinine is well tolerated, although therapeutic doses may produce tinnitus, impairment of hearing, dizziness, tremor and palpitation.

NURSING IMPLICATIONS

Assessment

When antimalarial drugs are to be administered either prophylactically or to treat an acute attack, the nurse should be familiar with the type of drug to be used, its dosage regimen, and adverse effects. Bearing in mind which drug has been ordered, the nurse's history-taking will include such aspects as previous history of cardiac, hepatic or renal impairment, haematological disorders, visual disturbances or previous history of convulsive disorders. Observations will include race of patient, vital signs and overall clinical appearance of the patient.

Evaluation

If therapy is short term, evaluation will include observations for signs of gastrointestinal upsets (which can usually be remedied by giving the drug with meals) and allergic skin reactions.

During long-term therapy, the nurse may need to evaluate for such adverse effects as visual impairment, blood dyscrasias, cardiac, neurological, hepatic or renal problems, depending on the drug being used.

Patient teaching

This will include advising the patient of the importance of taking the medication strictly at the specified times, educating him or her concerning the signs of adverse effects and the importance of seeking medical advice if the latter occur.

VIRUSES

The term "virus" (toxin of animal origin) was first used to describe any microorganisms that could pass through filters impermeable to bacteria and that could not be grown on the usual cell-free culture media. The progress of molecular biology in recent years has led to a stricter definition based mainly on chemical criteria. Thus, entities that become infectious at any stage of their life cycle are called viruses if they possess *only one* of the two classes of nucleic acids as carriers of their genetic information, either ribonucleic acid (RNA), or deoxyribonucleic acid (DNA). This possession of only one kind of nucleic acid is now the primary classification criterion of a virus and implies that these organisms have no enzymes of their own such as are necessary for internal metabolism. It also explains their resistance to all antibiotics, the action of which is based on their ability to block some stage of microbial metabolism.

Infectious viral particles (virions) consist of a strand or strands of either DNA or RNA, but not both, surrounded by a protein coat (capsid). They do not possess ribosomes and are dependent on those of host cells to provide for their reproduction.

FIGURE 8: EXAMPLES OF THREE RECOGNIZED FORMS OF VIRAL STRUCTURES

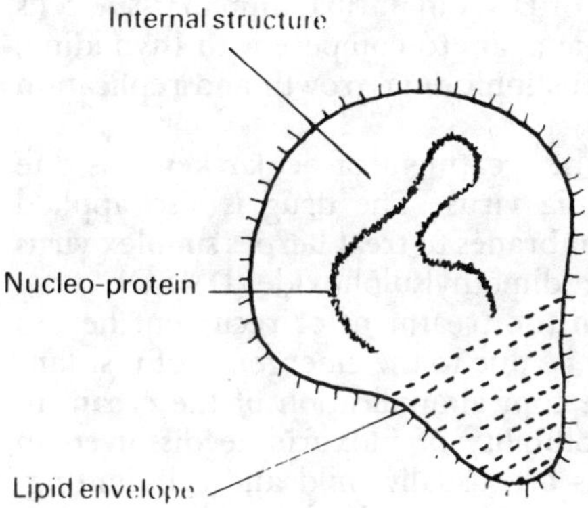

INFLUENZA VIRUS

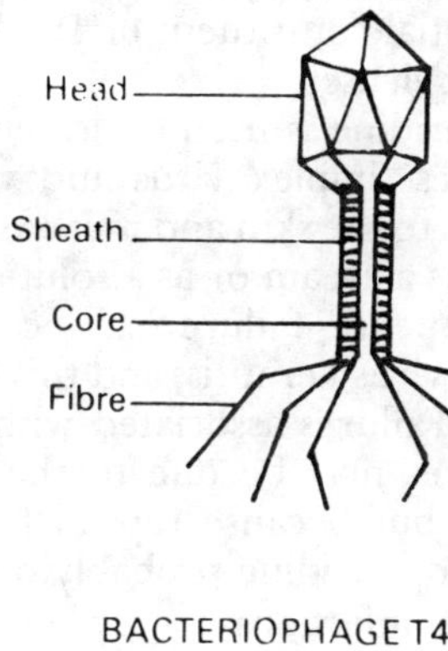

BACTERIOPHAGE T4 VIRUS

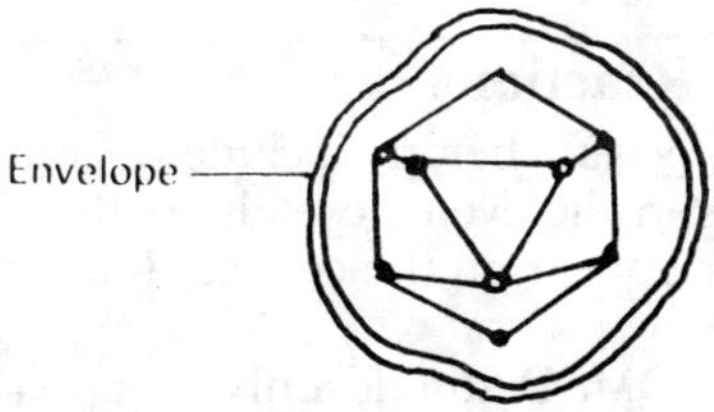

HERPES VIRUS

ANTIVIRAL AGENTS

Viruses are intracellular parasites that take part in metabolism of the host cells and thus present a more difficult problem of chemotherapy than do bacteria. They can be attacked before they enter cells or during passage from cell to cell or else prevented from entering cells, and now it is possible to interfere with them within the cell. The main difficulty with treating viral infections is that virus multiplication has often passed its peak before symptoms occur.

The true viruses are not affected by antibacterial drugs, hence these agents should not be used to treat viral infections. The fact that new proteins not present in the normal cell are synthesised in virus-infected cells offers the possibility of a selective inhibition of viral replication by chemical agents. Many substances are known to inhibit replication *in vitro* without damage to the cell cultures, but *in vivo* most fail because the required concentration is high and/or the side effects are too severe.

IDOXURIDINE

Idoxuridine, synthesised in 1959 as a possible antitumour agent, was later shown to inhibit the growth of *Herpes virus hominis keratitis* in humans.

Idoxuridine inhibits the synthesis of DNA in normal human tissue cells and in viruses containing DNA. It appears to compete with thymidine, an essential constituent of DNA, thus inhibiting growth and replication of DNA viruses.

Idoxuridine is used topically in the treatment of ocular keratitis due to herpes simplex virus and vaccinia virus. The drug is also applied topically to the skin and mucous membranes to treat herpes simplex virus lesions as a cream or as a solution in dimethylsulphoxide (DMSO).

Therapeutic failure may occur in the treatment of recurrent herpes simplex virus keratitis, and this may be due to the emergence of resistant strains. Failures associated with the topical application of the cream to cold sores may be due to the insolubility of idoxuridine dissolved in DMSO, but because topical lesions are usually mild and self-limiting, topical idoxuridine probably only has a place in the treatment of severe recurrent infections.

Idoxuridine is marketed under various brand names for topical and ophthalmic application.

Adverse Drug Reactions

Side effects from ocular therapy include occasional allergy with resultant pain and pruritus in the eye or eyelids. With frequent ocular instillation, small defects may appear on the cornea. Idoxuridine in DMSO must not be applied to the eye.

Idoxuridine in DMSO should only be applied topically for three or four days, otherwise the skin may become macerated and secondary bacterial infection may intervene. Rarely, patients may develop skin irritation with oedema and urticarial vesicles as a result of DMSO application.

VIDARABINE

Vidarabine (adenine arabinoside or ***ara-A)*** was originally synthesised as a potential antitumour drug. The drug has a broad antiviral spectrum, but it is primarily active against the herpes and pox viruses. Topical vidarabine, however, has not been shown to be effective in the treatment of cutaneous or genital herpes simplex virus infections. Vidarabine inhibits intracellular viral multiplication by inhibiting the host cell's DNA polymerase.

The drug is available as an ophthalmic ointment (*Vira-A, 3%*) for the treatment of human viral kerato-conjunctivitis due to *Herpes simplex virus, Types 1 and 2.* Vidarabine is also available as a parenteral suspension for the treatment of severe herpes virus infections, including herpes simplex encephalitis. It is indicated in the treatment of herpes zoster varicella infections in immunosuppressed patients.

This drug has very low solubility, the upper limit being 450 mg per one litre of infusion fluid. The total daily dose of 10 mg per kilogram body weight should be infused over 12 to 24 hours.

Adverse Drug Reactions

The drug is relatively non-toxic in low doses, although haematological changes may occur with higher doses and also neurotoxicity. Hypokalaemia, hypophosphataemia and hypocalcaemia have been reported with high intravenous doses.

AMANTADINE

Amantadine (*Symmetrel* 100 mg capsules) is a useful chemoprophylactic agent against *Influenza A* virus infections in humans. Its routine use for this purpose is not recommended because of its side effects. Amantadine is used also in the treatment of Parkinson's disease.

Amantadine is not virucidal at the concentrations needed for inhibition, and it does not affect the adsorption of viruses to cells. It has been suggested that the drug acts by interfering with the penetration of the virus into susceptible cells.

For prophylactic use, it is recommended that amantadine therapy should be commenced immediately Influenza A2 virus is known to be epidemic in the community, or after the patient has come into contact with the disease. Amantadine is only effective during the period of its administration. The usual adult dose is 200 mg daily given orally in two divided doses for 10 days after a single exposure, or for four weeks or more if repeated exposures occur during an epidemic.

Amantadine may produce amphetamine-like side effects and symptoms such as nervousness, difficulty in concentration, dizziness, light-headedness, slurred speech, ataxia, drowsiness and insomnia. Atropine-like side effects consisting of blurred vision, dry mouth and palpitations may also occur.

ACYCLOVIR

Acyclovir is converted by a herpes-specific enzyme (thymidine kinase) to the active triphosphate compound acyclovir triphosphate, which appears to selectively inhibit herpes virus DNA polymerase. Cellular thymidine kinase in uninfected host cells does not effectively utilize acyclovir as a substrate. *In vitro,* it is the most active drug against herpes viruses and is far more active than vidarabine, the only other systemic antiviral available. Resistance to acyclovir has been reported, the commonest mechanism of resistance being a failure of the virus to produce the enzyme thymidine kinase.

Acyclovir *(Zovirax)* is available as 200 mg tablets, 200 mg/5 mL suspension, 250 mg powder for IV infusion, 5% cream and 3% eye ointment.

Topical and oral preparations are used in the treatment of herpes simplex infections of the skin and mucous membranes. Intravenous injection is used to treat severe herpes simplex infections and to treat varicella and zoster infections in the immunocompromised patient.

Oral dose: 200 mg five times a day at approximately 4 hourly intervals. Topical preparations are applied five times a day. IV infusion: 5 mg/kg 8 hourly, or 10 mg/kg in varicella zoster in immunosuppressed patients.

Few adverse effects have been associated with intravenous administration. These include phlebitis, rash, anaemia or leucopenia, and possibly neurotoxicity. Transient stinging may be experienced following its ophthalmic use. Skin inflammation may result if extravasation occurs with intravenous administration. Increased liver enzymes have been reported and also raised blood urea concentrations.

CYTARABINE

Cytarabine or cytosine arabinoside (*Cytosar*) is used for the treatment of leukaemia and has a potential use in the treatment of DNA virus infections. Its antiviral spectrum is similar to that of idoxuridine.

VACCINES

Vaccines are indicated in the primary prevention of certain viral infections such as poliomyelitis, measles, rubella, mumps, hepatitis B and influenza. Vaccines are preparations of antigenic material which are administered with the object of inducing in the recipient a specific active immunity to infection by the corresponding infecting agent. The vaccines may contain living or dead microorganisms.

IMMUNOGLOBULINS

Immunoglobulins, which constitute the antibody proteins of the plasma, are used to provide passive protection against certain viral infections. ***Normal (human) immunoglobulin*** has been successfully used to modify or prevent hepatitis A in people who have been in contact with the disease. Specific immunoglobulins (purified forms of normal immunoglobulin which have a specific action against a particular viral disease) have been prepared, for example, hepatitis B, tetanus, varicella and herpes zoster.

INTERFERONS

Interferons are proteins produced in human or animal cells following their exposure to viruses. They have the capacity to exert, at least in homologous cells, virus non-specific antiviral activity by inducing production of enzymes which have the capacity to inhibit cellular RNA and protein synthesis and block viral reproduction. Thus they are potentially useful in the treatment of viral infections.

Current investigations into antiviral therapy with interferons have concentrated on the efficacy of human leucocyte interferon (IFNα). It has been administered parenterally to cancer patients with segmental herpes zoster, to renal transplant recipients as a prophylactic to delay the shedding of cytomegalovirus and to decrease the incidence of viraemia, and to treat chronic HBsAg-positive hepatitis. It has been evaluated also as a topical application in the treatment of herpes keratitis.

No appreciable adverse effects have been associated with the topical application of human leucocyte interferon. The adverse effects associated with its parenteral administration include pyrexia, shivering, malaise, nausea, vomiting, fatigue, pain and erythema at the site of injection. Transient hypotension has been reported with rapid intravenous administration. Other adverse effects include myelosuppression with leucopenia and thrombocytopenia. It is not clear whether these adverse effects are due to interferon or to contaminating proteins in the preparations.

Further research is required before the clinical usefulness of the interferons is confirmed.

Table 66
Anti-infective Therapy

Drug Group	Drug Name	Use	Action	Adverse Reactions	Nursing Implications
Anti-infective agents (general)	All drugs listed in Chapters 23 and 24	See Chapters 23 and 24 and in this table	See Chapters 23 and 24 and in this table	See Chapters 23 and 24 and in this table	***Assess:*** history of reaction, allergy; possible interactions with other drugs, food, IV fluids; kidney and liver function. ***Administer:*** store and reconstitute according to manufacturer's instructions; check whether oral doses to be given with or without food; for IV doses, check compatibility with fluid, recommended dilution, rate of administration; adhere to time schedules to maintain serum concentration at therapeutic level; ensure prescribed course is completed, but not exceeded. ***Evaluate:*** signs of infection abating, superinfection occurring; toxic effects, gastrointestinal disturbances; allergic reactions immediate, accelerated or delayed; blood samples for drug concentrations, to determine trough and peak levels. ***Teach:*** adverse effects, signs of allergy; food, drug interactions; dose schedules; importance of prescribed course.
Antibacterial antibiotics	Penicillins	A wide variety of gram-positive and gram-negative infections	Bactericidal inhibition of bacterial cell-wall synthesis	Very low toxicity; hypersensitivity reactions are common; rarely: neurotoxicity, nephritis, haemolysis	***Assess:*** history of hypersensitivity, previous penicillin use, baseline temperature, signs of specific infection. ***Administer:*** around the clock; oral on an empty stomach; IM deep into large muscle, slowly, do not massage; IV slowly, at correct dilution, in compatible fluid. ***Evaluate:*** improvement in signs of infection, for hypersensitivity, for superinfection.

Cephalosporins	A wide variety of gram-positive and gram-negative infections	Bactericidal inhibition of bacterial cell-wall synthesis	Hypersensitivity reactions may occur; nephrotoxicity, haematological abnormalities	***Assess:*** as for penicillins; renal function. ***Administer:*** as for penicillins. ***Evaluate:*** as for penicillins; urine output.
Tetracyclines	A wide variety of gram-positive and gram-negative organisms, especially those "gram-negatives" not susceptible to penicillin	Bacteriostatic; inhibit protein synthesis by binding to bacterial ribosomes	Diarrhoea, nausea, heartburn, epigastric distress, superinfection with *Candida albicans*, hypersensitivity is uncommon, nephrotoxicity, hepatotoxicity, haematological abnormalities, thrombophlebitis with IV administration	***Assess:*** as for penicillins; pregnancy; age — not given to children under 8 or with growth impairment; liver disease; renal function. ***Administer:*** as for penicillins; do not give with milk, iron or antacids. ***Evaluate:*** as for penicillins; urine output, uraemia; jaundice.
Aminoglycosides	Oral: presurgical bowel sterilisation; parenteral: serious gram-negative infections	Bactericidal, interfere with bacterial protein synthesis in ribosomes	Ototoxicity, nephrotoxicity, neuromuscular blockade	***Assess:*** as for penicillins; renal function; baseline hearing and balance. ***Administer:*** as for penicillins; reduced doses in renal impairment; high fluid intake. ***Evaluate:*** as for penicillins; ototoxicity — hearing loss, dizziness, vertigo; nephrotoxicity — urine output, uraemia; neuromuscular blockade — respiratory depression, decreased pulse rate, ataxia.
Erythromycin	Most effective in gram-positive infection, but some gram-negative activity	Bacteriostatic in normal concentrations bactericidal in high concentrations; inhibits protein synthesis in ribosomes	Abdominal cramps, nausea, vomiting, diarrhoea, stomatitis, heartburn, anorexia, pruritus ani, occasional skin rash, anaphylaxis; erythromycin estolate is hepatotoxic	***Assess:*** as for penicillins; liver function. ***Administer:*** as for penicillins. ***Evaluate:*** as for penicillins; liver impairment — jaundice, hepatomegaly, pale stools, dark urine.

continued

Drug Group	Drug Name	Use	Action	Adverse Reactions	Nursing Implications
	Lincomycin Clindamycin	Gram-positive infections, gram-negative anaerobic infections	As for erythromycin	Nausea, vomiting, diarrhoea, cramping, pseudomembranous colitis; IV use: transient flushing, syncope, cardiopulmonary arrest, thrombophlebitis	***Assess:*** as for erythromycin. ***Administer:*** as for erythromycin. ***Evaluate:*** as for erythromycin; for diarrhoea containing blood or mucus; abdominal pain.
	Chloramphenicol	Active against a wide range of gram-negative and gram-positive organisms including *Salmonella, Haemophilus influenzae, Vibrio cholerae,* rickettsiae and *Mycoplasma;* reserved for serious infections due to toxicity	Bacteriostatic in low concentrations; bactericidal in high concentrations; bactericidal to *Haemophilus* in low concentrations, inhibits bacterial protein synthesis	Aplastic anaemia, pancytopenia, haemopoietic toxicity, circulatory collapse in newborn (Grey syndrome), optic neuritis, nausea, vomiting, glossitis, stomatitis, hypersensitivity reactions, anaphylaxis, angioneurotic oedema, increased prothrombin time	***Assess:*** as for penicillins; renal function, liver function. ***Administer:*** as for penicillins. ***Evaluate:*** as for penicillins; bone-marrow depression, Grey syndrome in newborns; bleeding; optic neuritis, gastrointestinal inflammation.
Sulphonamides	Sulphadiazine Sulphadimidine Sulphafurazole Sulphamethizole Sulphameth-	Urinary tract infections, chancroid, trachoma, nocardiosis,	Bacteriostatic; inhibit folic acid synthesis in bacteria and parasites	Hypersensitivity and allergic reactions, photosensitivity, agranulocytosis, thrombocytopenia,	***Assess:*** for previous hypersensitivity to sulpha or related drugs, liver or kidney disease, blood dyscrasias, pregnancy or lactation; concurrent use of anticoagulants, methotrexate,

	oxazole Sulphamethoxy-pyridazine Phthaiylsulph-athiazole	toxoplasmosis, malaria		aplastic and haemolytic anaemias, jaundice, renal damage, headache, mental depression, malaise, nausea, vomiting	sulphonylurea hypoglycaemics, thiazides, uricosuric drugs; establish baseline observations of clinical signs of infection. ***Administer:*** with food or following meals at equal intervals during the day. ***Evaluate:*** for abating signs of infection, for hypersensitivity reactions, blood dyscrasias (high fever, prostration, mucosal ulceration, lassitude, fatigue, dizziness, headache, unexplained bleeding, bruising); Stevens-Johnson syndrome (fever, headache, erythematous rash, rhinitis, conjunctivitis, stomatitis); renal dysfunction (decreased urinary output, proteinuria, blood in urine, renal colic); maintain sufficient fluid intake to ensure at least 1500 mL output daily. ***Teach:*** importance of adequate fluid intake to produce at least 1500 mL daily; indicators of adverse effects — see above; importance of completing course of therapy; that urine might turn an orange colour and to avoid excessive exposure to ultraviolet light.
Trimethoprim	Trimethoprim	Often used in combination with sulphamethoxazole for urinary-tract and other infections	Antibacterial, inhibits bacterial folic acid synthesis	Very few adverse reactions; haematologic abnormalities are possible	***Assess:*** history of blood dyscrasis, renal impairment, liver disease, pregnancy, or lactation; document clinical signs of infection. ***Evaluate:*** for reduction in or absence of clinical manifestations of infection; for blood dyscrasias, see above; observe skin for signs of hypersensitivity reactions. ***Teach:*** correct dosage regimen and to report adverse effects if they occur.

continued

Drug Group	Drug Name	Use	Action	Adverse Reactions	Nursing Implications
Urinary antiseptics	Nalidixic acid	Gram-negative urinary-tract infections	Inhibits bacterial DNA synthesis, urinary antiseptic	Headache, malaise, drowsiness, dizziness, vertigo, syncope, sensory changes, visual disturbances, excitement, depression, confusion, seizures, nausea, vomiting, abdominal pain, diarrhoea, rash, urticaria, photosensitivty reactions	***Assess:*** for known hypersensitivty to drug; history of convulsive disorders, weight, age, pregnancy, lactation, hepatic and renal disease. ***Administer:*** correct dose, orally, usually 1 g 6-hourly during 24 h for 7 to 10 days; best to give with food to help eliminate risk of GIT upsets. ***Evaluate:*** for reduction of clinical manifestations of infection; for side effects, especially visual disturbances and CNS; observe skin for signs of photosensitivity and hypersensitivity reactions; for signs of GIT disturbances. ***Teach:*** correct dosage regimen, signs of adverse reactions and to avoid exposure to sunlight.
	Nitrofurantoin	Gram-positive and gram-negative urinary-tract infections	Bactericidal, action enhanced in acidic urine	GIT disturbances, headache, dizziness, malaise, nystagmus, peripheral neuritis, acute allergic reactions, pulmonary toxicity, bone-marrow depression, haemolytic and megaloblastic anaemias, brown urine	***Assess:*** for impaired renal function, age, weight, pregnancy, blood dyscrasias, known hypersensitivity to drug. ***Administer:*** orally with food at equal intervals during 24 hour. Evaluate; for reduction of clinical manifestations of infection; pH of urine; administer urinary acidifier if ordered where reabsorption of drug is indicated in pyelonephritis; watch for adverse effects, including GIT disturbances, CNS (headache, dizziness, nystagmus) disturbances, blood dyscrasias, and allergic reactions. ***Teach:*** to expect urine to become brown; correct dosage regimen.

	Hexamine hippurate Hexamine mandelate	Gram-negative urinary-tract infections	Release of antibacterial formaldehyde in acid urine; ensure adequate acidification of urine	GIT disturbances, rash, urticaria, pruritus, high doses and prolonged therapy lead to irritation of urinary tract	***Assess:*** hepatic and renal function, age, weight, fluid balance, pregnancy, pH of urine. ***Administer:*** orally with food at equal intervals during 24 hr. ***Evaluate:*** pH of urine; maintain at or below 5.0; administer urinary acidifier as ordered; watch urinary output; if prolonged administration, test urine for protein and blood; observe for rash, complaints of painful urination and gastric upsets. ***Teach:*** adverse effects and to report if they occur; ensure patient understands correct dosage regimen.
Antifungal agents	Amphotericin	Superficial and systemic fungal infections	Fungistatic, binds to sterols in fungal cell membrane and interferes with fungal cell permeability	Topical use: ADRs are rare; parenteral use: high incidence of ADRs, fever, chills, anorexia, nausea, vomiting, thrombophlebitis, nephrotoxicity, hypokalaemia; reversible normochromic, normocytic anaemia, occasional liver function abnormalities, cardiac arrest after too-rapid infusion	***Assess:*** for previous allergy to drug, pregnancy, lactation, haemopoietic disorders, renal function, serum potassium; establish baseline observations of vital signs prior to parenteral administration. ***Administer:*** IV by slow infusion in dextrose buffered to correct pH. ***Evaluate:*** for redness, swelling, pain at infusion site, muscle weakness (hypokalaemia), oliguria, haematuria; monitor vital signs frequently during administration; monitor for signs of allergy and other adverse effects.
	Nystatin Natamycin	Topical and vaginal fungal infections	Fungistatic, as above	Virtually no ADRs from topical application	***Teach:*** the importance of proper application and completion of prescribed course of therapy.
	Ketoconazole	Orally for superficial and systemic fungal infections	Interacts with sterol or fatty acid metabolism in fungal cell; interferes with oxidative enzymes	Nausea, vomiting, diarrhoea, abdominal pain, rash, gynaecomastia, severe hepatotoxicity	***Assess:*** history for previous allergy, liver disease, concurrent use of antacids or H2 antagonists. ***Evaluate:*** for nausea, vomiting, abdominal pain, diarrhoea, skin rashes, gynaecomastia and jaundice.

continued

Drug Group	Drug Name	Use	Action	Adverse Reactions	Nursing Implications
	Miconazole	Topical and vaginal fungal infections; used IV for systemic candidiasis, histoplasmosis and other fungal; infections	As for ketoconazole	Topical use: ADRs are rare; IV use: phlebitis, pruritus, nausea, vomiting, fever, chills, drowsiness, erythrocyte aggregation, anaemia, thrombocytosis, rash, hyperlipidaemia, hyponatraemia, too-rapid infusion leads to cardiac arrhythmias	***Assess:*** history for previous allergy, haemopoietic disorders; prior to parenteral administration establish baseline observations of vital signs; ensure laboratory results of any blood tests or electrolyte studies to hand. ***Administer:*** IV by slow infusion over one hour; prevent extravasation; administer topically or vaginally as ordered using correct administration procedure. ***Evaluate:*** IV administration monitor vital signs frequently; watch for cardiac effects and signs of allergic reaction; for signs of phlebitis and skin irritation at infusion site; local applications — observe for oedema, pruritus, irritation at site of application.
	Flucytosine	Serious systemic infections caused by *Candida* and *Cryptococcus*	Penetrates fungal cells where it is converted to fluorouracil which interferes with protein synthesis	Much less toxic than amphotericin; hypoplasia of bone marrow; nausea, vomiting, anorexia, abdominal bloating, diarrhoea, transient liver enlargement and alteration in liver function tests	***Assess:*** history for liver, renal or haemopoietic disorders, previous or concurrent radiotherapy or chemotherapy for malignancy. ***Administer:*** oral dose, space at 15-min intervals to reduce nausea. ***Evaluate:*** initiate regular blood counts; watch for confusion, headache, vertigo, bruising, bleeding, sore throat, GIT upsets, jaundice; report elevated blood urea, creatinine.
	Griseofulvin	Usually administered orally, for mycoses of skin, hair and nails caused by *Trichophyton, Microsporum* and *Epidermophyton*	Fungistatic disrupts division of cell nucleus; is best absorbed from the gut in the presence of fat	Relatively non-toxic; headache, epigastric pain, nausea, vomiting, diarrhoea, thirst, flatulence, oral thrush, hypersensitivity rashes.	***Assess:*** history for hypersensitivity, hepatic disease or porphyria. ***Administer:*** with high-fat foods. ***Evaluate:*** for effectiveness of drug; for adverse effects. ***Teach:*** to take drug with high-fat food; to avoid excessive exposure to ultraviolet light; the importance of completing prescribed

				photosensitivity rashes	course, self-evaluation for adverse effects.
Antitrichomonal agents	Metronidazole	Protozoal infections, serious anaerobic bacterial infections administered orally, rectally, IV	Inhibition of DNA synthesis in susceptible microorganisms	Rash, pruritus, urticaria, nausea, anorexia, furry tongue, dry mouth, abdominal discomfort, metallic taste, headache, dizziness, leucopenia, darkening of urine, dysuria; Note: interaction with alcohol	***Assess:*** pregnancy, lactation, current alcohol use, history for haemopoietic disorders. ***Administer:*** with food to minimize GIT upsets. ***Evaluate:*** for signs of allergy, GIT upsets, signs of CNS toxicity and leucopenia. ***Teach:*** to expect metallic taste and discolouration of urine, to avoid use of alcohol, self-evaluation for adverse effects.
Antitubercular agents	Isoniazid	Tuberculosis; concomitant administration of pyridoxine is advisable	Active only against rapidly growing tubercle bacilli	Resistance develops rapidly when drug is used alone; vertigo, twitching of limbs, increased reflexes, urinary retention; psychoses, confusion, coma, convulsions if serum concentrations too high; peripheral neuritis is common and may be prevented by administration of pyridoxine	***Assess:*** physical condition, liver, kidney function, alcohol use, CNS function. ***Administer:*** according to schedule. ***Evaluate:*** for adverse effects on kidney, liver, CNS. ***Teach:*** need for compliance, multiple drugs, long-term therapy.
	Rifampicin	Tuberculosis, leprosy	Bactericidal and bacteriostatic	Hepatocellular damage, jaundice, rare hypersensitivity reactions, haematological changes, respiratory effects, reddish-brown urine	***Assess:*** liver damage. ***Administer:*** in daily doses. ***Evaluate:*** for liver damage. ***Teach:*** as for isoniazid; daily doses essential; interaction with oral contraceptives; urine may be reddish.

continued

Drug Group	Drug Name	Use	Action	Adverse Reactions	Nursing Implications
	Ethambutol	Tuberculosis (mycobacteria only)	Inhibition of cellular metabolism	Resistance develops rapidly when used alone; ocular toxicity, rare peripheral neuritis	***Assess:*** as for isoniazid; visual function. ***Administer:*** as for isoniazid; with food. ***Evaluate:*** visual function. ***Teach:*** as for isoniazid; need for eye testing.
Antimalarials	Chloroquine	*Plasmodium* infections	Complexes with DNA	Retinopathy, GIT disturbances, dermatologic reactions, neurologic reactions, blood dyscrasias, chloroquine accumulates in the liver	***Assess:*** for history of renal or hepatic disease, retinal or visual field defects, concurrent use of other drugs which are hepatotoxic including alcohol. ***Administer:*** prophylactic oral doses — as ordered with meals; in acute attacks, oral or parenteral doses as ordered. ***Evaluate:*** ophthalmic examinations at regular intervals during long-term therapy, be alert for reports of blurred vision, blind spots, night blindness; also evaluate for gastrointestinal disturbances, skin reactions, neurological reactions and blood dyscrasias. ***Teach:*** correct dosage regimen; self-evaluation for adverse effects.
	Pyrimethamine	Antimalarial Antitoxoplasmic	Folic acid antagonist arrests sporogeny in mosquito and prevents liver-phase infection in humans	Dermatoses, folic acid deficiencies	***Assess:*** if high doses to be used, for history of convulsive disorders and folic acid deficiency. ***Administer:*** with meals on same day each week when used as antimalarial, or at same time each day when used to treat toxoplasmosis. ***Evaluate:*** for signs of folic acid deficiency, for example, fever, sore

					tongue, rash, diarrhoea; initiate bi-weekly haematology studies during treatment of toxoplasmosis.
	Primaquine	Antimalarial	Effective against fixed tissue liver stage of plasmodia	Abdominal cramps, epigastric distress, urticaria, haematological abnormalities	***Assess:*** for history of renal or haemopoietic disorders; document race of patient — some dark-skinned people demonstrate a primaquine sensitivity which can result in an acute anaemia. ***Administer:*** with meals or antacids. ***Evaluate:*** for gastrointestinal disturbances, evidence of haemolysis in dark patients such as decreased urinary output, dark or red urine, chills or fever. ***Teach:*** self-evaluation for adverse effects, importance of regular blood tests.
	Quinine	Antimalarial	Active against erythrocytic phases of plasmodial infections	IV use: marked hypotension; oral use: tinnitus, hearing impairment, dizziness, tremor, palpitations	***Assess:*** for history of cardiac or renal disease; establish baseline blood pressure if being administered parenterally. ***Administer:*** oral doses — with meals as ordered; parenteral doses — in acute attacks, as ordered. ***Evaluate:*** for nausea, vomiting, diarrhoea, sweating, blurred vision, tinnitus, hearing deficiency; monitor blood pressure during parenteral doses. ***Teach:*** correct dosage regimen; self-evaluation for adverse effects.
Antiviral agents	Idoxuridine	Ocular keratitis due to viral infections, herpes simplex skin lesions	Inhibits growth and replication of viral DNA	Ocular therapy: allergy with pain and pruritus in eye or eyelids, corneal defects; skin therapy: skin	***Assess:*** previous history of allergy to this drug. ***Administer:*** use correct technique for instilling eye drops; avoid contact of dropper with eyelids or lashes; observe correct storage

continued

Drug Group	Drug Name	Use	Action	Adverse Reactions	Nursing Implications
				maceration with DMSO base and secondary bacterial infection, skin irritation, oedema	precautions. ***Evaluate:*** for drug effectiveness; for signs of allergic reaction such as pain, pruritus in eye or lids. ***Teach:*** proper administration procedure; importance of completing prescribed course.
	Vidarabine	Antiviral eye ointment: viral keratoconjunctivitis IV: severe herpes virus infections	Inhibits host cell DNA polymerase and so prevents intracellular viral multiplication	IV: haematological changes, neurotoxicity hypokalaemia, hypophosphataemia, hypocalcaemia	***Assess:*** for previous allergy to this drug, pregnancy, renal or hepatic disease, weight of patient; possibly serum potassium levels; establish baseline observations of clinical signs of infection. ***Administer:*** ophthalmic ointment — dose as ordered, use correct administration technique; IV: dose ordered according to body weight — no more than 450 mg per L of infusion fluid, due to low solubility of drug; ensure drug is well mixed in infusion fluid before administration; infuse over 12 to 24 h as ordered. ***Evaluate:*** ophthalmic use — for drug effectiveness and for local adverse effects such as burning, irritation, pain and photophobia; intravenous use — for drug effectiveness and adverse reactions such as neurotoxicity, nausea, vomiting. ***Teach:*** for ophthalmic self-administration — correct administration techniques, importance of completing prescribed course.

Amantadine	Prophylaxis against influenza A viral infections; Parkinson's disease (see Chapter 29)	Interferes with viral penetration into susceptible cells	Nervousness, lack of concentration, dizziness, light headedness, slurred speech, ataxia, drowsiness, insomnia, blurred vision, dry mouth, palpitations	***Assess:*** previous history of psychiatric disorders, cardiac, hepatic or renal disorders; hypertension, concurrent use of anticholinergic drugs, MAO inhibitors, tricyclic antidepressants and other antipsychotic drugs; establish baseline blood pressure and pulse rate. ***Administer:*** with food. ***Evaluate:*** for signs of sympathomimetic and atropine-like side effects; — blood pressure (lying and standing), pulse rate, urinary output, changes in behaviour, slurred speech, drowsiness, insomnia, palpitations, blurred vision, dry mouth. ***Teach:*** that the drug is for prophylactic use only (when used as antiviral agent); that skin pigmentation may occur; to evaluate for side effects and to report them if they occur.
Acyclovir	Herpes infections (topical and systemic)	Inhibits herpes virus DNA polymerase	IV use: phlebitis, rash, anaemia, leucopenia, neurotoxicity, raised liver enzymes, raised blood urea; ophthalmic use: transient stinging	***Assess:*** document clinical signs of the viral infection; in systemic use assess hepatic and renal function. ***Administer:*** topically as ordered; use correct administration technique; intravenously — as ordered; prevent extravasation of fluid into skin. ***Evaluate:*** for drug effectiveness; in topical use for signs of local stinging or irritation; with IV use, behavioural changes, signs of phlebitis (redness, swelling, pain at infusion site). ***Teach:*** for topical self administration, correct administration technique and importance of completing prescribed course.

SELF-EVALUATION TEST

1. Selection of an appropriate anti-infective agent should be based on a number of factors. What are these factors?
2. Combination therapy with anti-infective agents is indicated in certain circumstances. Which of the following statements is (are) specific justification(s) for combination therapy?
   (a) To delay the emergence of microbial mutants resistant to one drug through the use of a second drug.
   (b) To achieve prompt treatment of a desperately ill patient suspected of having a serious infection.
   (c) To allow for a reduction in the dosage of one or both drugs.
   (d) To achieve bactericidal synergism.
   (e) To cover a mixed infection.

   Give two examples to illustrate statement (a) and the conditions for which these combinations are indicated.
3. Which of the following statements correctly describes some of the properties of penicillins?
   (a) Patients who are allergic to benzylpenicillin are allergic to the other penicillins.
   (b) The penicillins are bactericidal and act by disrupting the permeability of the cell membrane.
   (c) Oral penicillins should be administered 60 minutes before meals and at bedtime to achieve higher serum antibacterial activity.
   (d) Ampicillin is active against some gram-negative bacteria resistant to benzylpenicillin.
   (e) Semi-synthetic penicillins can be administered in a mixed solution with gentamicin to treat serious staphylococcal infections.
4. List five indications for the use of each of the following agents.
   (a) Benzylpenicillin
   (b) Ampicillin
   (c) Cloxacillin
5. Complete the following statements describing the administration and absorption of cephalosporins.
   (a) .... and .... frequently occur after the intravenous administration of cephalothin.
   (b) .... and .... are well absorbed from the gastrointestinal tract. These cephalosporins are acid ....
   (c) Cephalosporins administered by the intramuscular route cause .... and .... and occasionally sterile .... formation.
   (d) The intravenous dose of cephamandole for an adult, in mild to moderate infections, is .... administered every .... hours.
6. Adverse effects to cephalosporins are similar to those encountered with the penicillins. Nevertheless:
   (a) patients with a history of delayed penicillin hypersensitivity can be

treated with cephalosporins.
(b) the use of diuretic agents or aminoglycosides may add to nephrotoxicity when used with the cephalosporins.
(c) the cephalosporins appear to cause less immediate hypersensitivity reactions than the penicillins.
(d) patients with hepatic dysfunction are at special risk of drug accumulation or toxic serum concentrations when receiving cephalosporins.

7. Tetracyclines are incompletely absorbed from the gastrointestinal tract because of:
(a) poor solubility in acid and neutral solutions.
(b) enzymatic degradation.
(c) complex formation with co-administered food, milk or antacids.
(d) poor solubility in alkaline or neutral solutions.

8. The following adverse effects may be experienced with tetracycline therapy, *except:*
(a) ototoxicity
(b) thrombophlebitis
(c) photosensitivity
(d) nausea, heartburn and diarrhoea
(e) hepatotoxicity

9 (a) Gentamicin is used in the treatment of ...., ... and ....
(b) Aminoglycosides are excreted almost entirely by the ....
(c) High blood concentrations of the aminoglycosides may cause .... due to damage to the .... cranial nerve and also ....
(d) In the presence of renal dysfunction the parenteral dose of the aminoglycoside should be .... or the dosage interval ....
(e) Topical application of the aminoglycosides is frequently associated with ....

10. (a) List some of the indications for the use of erythromycin.
(b) What is the dose range, route and frequency of administration of erythromycin base for an adult with a staphylococcal skin infection?

11. (a) .... is a serious side effect associated with lincomycin and clindamycin therapy.
(b) This side effect is due to the organism ....
(c) .... in a dose of 125–500 mg orally every six hours is used to treat this side effect.
(d) This drug (c) is generally administered intravenously to treat potentially life-threatening systemic .... infections.

12. Chloramphenicol is active against a wide variety of gram-positive and gram-negative organisms. Why is it not more widely used?

13. (a) Sulphonamides are used to treat non-obstructive urinary tract infections caused by the following gram-negative organisms: ...., ..., and ....
    (b) .... was a common side effect with the early sulphonamides and its incidence could be reduced by .... of the urine and .... fluid intake.
    (c) The usual dose of trimethoprim-sulphamethoxazole to treat a mild to moderate urinary-tract infection due to a susceptible organism is .... orally .... a day.
    (d) Photosensitivity rashes are associated with the use of sulphonamides and the urinary antiseptic ....
14. Which of the following criteria must be observed in the preparation and administration of amphotericin?
    (a) The lyophilised powder must be reconstituted with at least 10 mL of water for injections.
    (b) The reconstituted drug is diluted with sodium chloride for administration.
    (c) The reconstituted drug is diluted with dextrose for administration.
    (d) The dilute solution of amphotericin should be administered slowly (intravenously) over four to six hours.
    (e) The patient's renal function should be monitored closely.
    (f) The patient's serum potassium level should be monitored closely.
    (g) Supplemental potassium may be added as the chloride to the amphotericin infusion.
15. (a) Metronidazole is one of the drugs of first choice for the treatment of ...., particularly *Bacteroides fragilis*.
    (b) This drug has been used for many years to treat ...., ... and ....
    (c) The usual adult dose of metronidazole for intravenous infusion is .... mg in .... mL administered .... times a day.
    (d) Metronidazole in combination with .... may produce abdominal cramps, nausea, vomiting, headaches and flushing.
16. The following statements relating to viral infections and their treatment are correct, *except:*
    (a) viral multiplication has often passed its peak before symptoms of the infection occur.
    (b) antibacterial agents may be used to treat viral infections.
    (c) idoxuridine is used to treat herpes simplex virus lesions on the skin and in the eye.
    (d) hypokalaemia, hypophosphataemia and hypocalcaemia may occur with high dose parenteral vidarabine therapy.
    (e) amantadine is recommended for prophylactic therapy against Influenza A and B viruses.

25
IMMUNIZATION

Brian J. Feery

OBJECTIVES

At the conclusion of this chapter the reader should be able to:

1. define the terms vaccine, active immunization, passive immunization, antigen, antibody, antitoxin, immunoglobulin;
2. describe the method of active and passive immunization;
3. name the vaccines and sera in normal use;
4. list the contraindications for vaccination;
5. list the major side effects of vaccination.

PREREQUISITE KNOWLEDGE

1. Basic immunology.
2. Major infectious diseases.

DEFINITIONS

Antigen — substance which induces the production of antibodies. It is usually a protein or a polysaccharide.
Antibody — a specific globulin produced by a host in response to antigenic stimulation.
Immunity — resistance to infection.
Active immunity — immunity induced by infection or immunization which results in the production of antibodies and cell-mediated responses.
Passive immunity — immunity conferred by giving preformed antibodies (sera, antitoxin, immunoglobulin, antivenom).
Exotoxin — a toxin excreted by intact organisms, for example, tetanus or diphtheria toxins.
Homologous serum — serum obtained from the same species.
Heterologous serum — serum obtained from a different species.
Vaccine — a preparation of antigens administered to induce active immunity to an infecting agent. A vaccine may contain live organisms, killed organisms, cell fragments or modified toxins called toxoids.

IMMUNITY TO DISEASE

Immunization depends on the presence of an adequate immune response to natural infection. Immunity in its broadest sense covers all the mechanisms which enable the host to resist the entry, multiplication and harmful effects of pathogenic organisms. Immunity to infection is not an absolute entity. It may be modified by age, nutrition, infection, and by therapy.

Immunity may be naturally or artificially acquired. Naturally acquired active immunity results from past infection. Passive immunity is transferred across the placenta by maternal antibodies.

Artifical immunity results from active immunization with vaccines and passive immunization with antiserum or immunoglobulin.

FIGURE 9: CLASSIFICATION OF ACQUIRED IMMUNITY

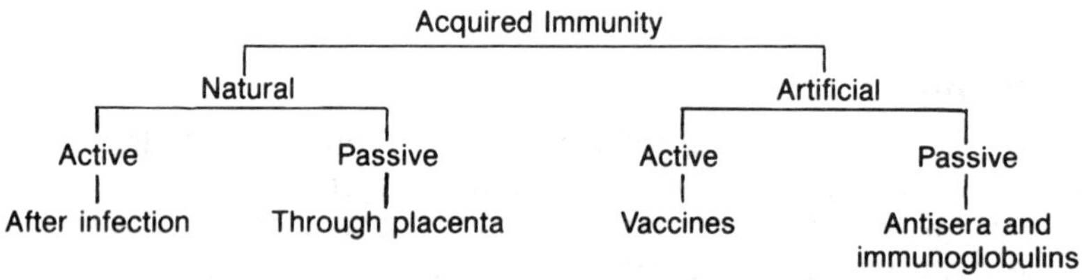

GENERAL PRINCIPLES OF IMMUNIZATION

The aim of immunization is to produce immunity sufficient to protect an individual against a clinical attack of disease. It is the purpose of immunization to induce a lasting artificial immunity to infection, but passive short-term protection may be conferred by giving heterologous or homologous antisera or immunoglobulin.

By using vaccines it is possible to provide substantial if not complete protection against many infectious diseases. The degree of protection varies from almost absolute long-term protection against disease such as tetanus and diphtheria, to short-term protection against diseases such as influenza or cholera. Viral vaccines for poliomyelitis, measles and rubella produce protection rates of about 95%, and this protection may be boosted subsequently by subclinical infections.

PASSIVE IMMUNIZATION

Passive immunization is used in people who are at risk of disease, yet are known to be (or suspected of being) non-immune or insufficiently immune. In passive immunization, preformed antibodies are given to the patient who requires protection against the disease. These antibodies may be homologous (that is, from the same animal species) or heterologous, that is, from a foreign or different animal species.

Heterologous antisera, as far as humans are concerned, are those produced in other mammals. In most cases the horse is used since it has a large blood volume and is an efficient producer of antibodies, but cattle, sheep, goats and rabbits have been used.

Vaccines or ***toxins*** are given to animals as in active artificial immunization. After antibody formation has reached its optimum level, serum is collected and chemically processed. The resulting product is a concentrated solution of the antibody fraction of serum. Antivenoms to snake bite, tick bite and spider bite are made by this method. Immunization of human beings with these antisera induces artificial passive immunity.

Since heterologous antiserum, even after the most careful refinement, contains protein material foreign to humans, it may cause allergic reactions of varying severity in sensitive people. Because these reactions may be severe and sometimes life threatening, as in anaphylactic shock, and because of the short duration of protection after the administration of heterologous serum, every effort should be made to protect the individual with active immunization where possible.

In passive immunization using **homologous antisera,** the principle is the same, but the source of the antisera is human. Antibody in serum is contained in the globulin fraction. As the product is of human origin, allergic or hypersensitivity reactions are uncommon. There may be local tenderness and stiffness at the site of injection and occasionally mild pyrexia, malaise and urticaria occur.

Pooled human immunoglobulin is used to protect against measles, hepatitis A, and other viral infections. Blood from donors with immunity to a particular disease is processed to produce a concentrated solution of specific human immunoglobulins. This immune globulin may be injected into susceptible non-immune patients for passive immunization. Specific human immunoglobulin may be used to protect against tetanus, diphtheria, chickenpox, hepatitis B, or Rh(D) sensitisation.

ACTIVE IMMUNIZATION

Active immunization depends on the existence of an adequate immune response. **Live attenuated vaccines** such as ***poliomyelitis vaccine, measles vaccine*** or ***rubella vaccine*** and **inactivated vaccines** such as ***tetanus*** or ***typhoid*** vaccines are used. Inactivated vaccines may contain whole organisms, modified extracts, subunit particles or toxoids.

The protective response following inactivated vaccines depends mainly on the production of specific antibodies. The magnitude and duration of immunity will depend on the nature and amount of antigen used; the number of injections (or doses) given; the time interval between doses; the age of the person being immunized and degree of interference from passively acquired antibodies (for example, maternal antibodies may interfere with measles immunization in the first year of life); and the ability of the antibody system to produce antibodies.

The response following live attenuated vaccines resembles more closely a natural infection in that local and general cell-mediated and antibody responses are induced.

Once a primary response to an antigen has been initiated, the recipient retains a specific imprint of the stimulus and will usually respond quickly to another stimulus with the same antigen either in the form of a dose of vaccine or an infection by the organism.

Primary Course with Inactivated Vaccines

The first injection of a vaccine is the primary or sensitising dose. Antigens from the vaccine induce an immune reaction in the regional lymph glands. This reaction initially involves phagocytosis and processing by macrophages, then stimultion of T and B lymphocytes which undergo blast transformation and proliferation, and finally the production of families of cells including antibody-forming plasma cells and memory cells.

FIGURE 10: ACTIVE ACQUIRED IMMUNITY

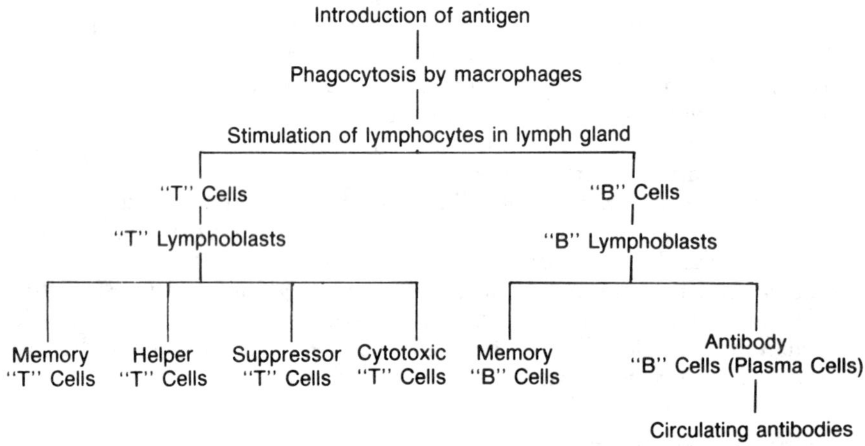

The response to the first injection or primary response is different from responses to subsequent stimuli. With the primary response there is usually a lag period of at least a week before antibody is detectable in the circulation. Antibody titres rise to reach a peak between the second and fourth week. The titre then falls over the ensuing months, eventually becoming undetectable. The duration of the antibody response will vary from antigen to antigen and will depend also on the height of the initial antibody peak. The height of this peak is related to the size of the initial dose.

Re-exposure to the same antigen weeks, months, or even years later provokes a secondary antibody response, which is usually different from the primary response. Antibody appears more rapidly, and the titre is higher, the peak being reached within 7 to 14 days. The subsequent decline in antibody is also slower than that observed after primary antigenic stimulation. Adequate immunization with inactivated vaccines usually involves a primary course of at least two doses of vaccine at intervals of not less than four weeks duration, and a booster dose after 6 to 12 months.

The type of immunoglobulin (Ig) antibody response depends on the antigens in the vaccine. Protein antigens induce an initial IgM response followed by an IgG response, but polysaccharide antigens tend to induce IgM antibody responses. Occasionally IgG-type responses are observed after polysaccharide vaccines, perhaps because of antigenic determinants on the molecule which cross-react with groups on other bacterial antigens. IgA immunoglobulin responses are also observed in the serum, but local IgA antibody is not produced when inactivated vaccines are given parenterally.

Booster Doses

Booster doses are necessary at intervals ranging from six months with cholera vaccine to 10 years with tetanus vaccine to maintain a satisfactory level of immunity. These doses will stimulate a rapid production of antibody which returns to a high level and persists in some cases for long periods.

Repeating booster doses too frequently does not induce progressively higher levels of immunity and may be harmful because each successive dose increases the risk of inducing hypersensitivity reactions in the recipient.

Interval Between Doses

Immunization with inactivated vaccines usually involves more than one dose to induce an adequate immune response. The recommended minimum interval between doses in the primary immunization course is four weeks. It has been found that this interval is necessary to achieve an optimum secondary response, but longer intervals between injections do not impair the ultimate response or necessitate the addition of extra doses. It is never necessary to repeat any of the doses of a primary course, even though the recommended interval has been exceeded by months or even years. This is because of the induction of an immunological memory response involving T and B cells with the primary dose, and this memory enables the individual to respond with a secondary response to subsequent doses.

Adjuvants are sometimes used in vaccines to enhance antibody responses. Thus toxoids (for example, tetanus toxoid) which have been adsorbed onto mineral carriers, such as aluminium hydroxide or phosphate, are more potent antigens than when used alone, and the dose required to produce immunity can be reduced. In some cases, the mixing of a bacterial vaccine with a non-adsorbed toxoid has also been found to increase the antigenicity of the toxoid, for example, in Triple Antigen, the adjuvant properties of pertussis vaccine have been used as the adjuvant for the tetanus and diphtheria toxoids. Vaccines containing adjuvants must be given by deep subcutaneous or intramuscular injection because the aluminium will act as an irritant if given superficially.

Combined Vaccines

Some individual vaccines can be combined and the combined vaccines have obvious advantages over single vaccines. For example, fewer injections are required for primary immunization. Combined vaccines are prepared in such a way as to ensure there will be no depression of anti-body responses due to competition between antigens. For example, Triple Antigen contains diphtheria, tetanus and pertussis vaccine.

Immunization with Live Vaccines

The immune response induced by live attenuated vaccines more closely resembles the response induced by natural infection. It involves not only circulating IgM, IgG and IgA antibody responses, and cell-mediated responses, but also local IgA antibody and cellular immune responses which occur when vaccine is administered by the natural route of infection. It is usually assumed that these responses will give greater protection than inactivated vaccines, but this has not always been demonstrated. Live vaccines usually induce long-term immunity after a single dose and may increase the possibility of eradication of wild-type infection. They may, however, cause clinical manifestations of illness in individuals with immune deficiencies and in a small proportion of normal individuals.

Table 67
Types of Vaccines

Bacterial			Rickettsial	Viral	
Living	**Killed**	**Toxoid**	**Killed**	**Living**	**Killed**
BCG	Cholera Typhoid Plague Pertussis	Diphtheria Tetanus	Typhus	Measles Mumps Rubella Poliomyelitis (Sabin) Yellow Fever	Influenza Hepatitis B Poliomyelitis (Salk)

PRECAUTIONS AND CONTRAINDICATIONS TO IMMUNIZATION

Modern potent purified vaccines and antisera have been associated with a low level of adverse reactions. Nevertheless, there are certain individuals in whom immunization with certain antigens is containdicated, or alternatively should be undertaken with due precautions. It is important therefore to consider the following contraindications and precautions.

THE PATIENT

Under this heading, the following factors should be considered.

Age — Children over two years should not be given pertussis vaccine because the risk of the disease is decreased at this age. Individuals over seven years of age should not be given full-strength diphtheria vaccine (use diluted toxoid) because the risk of hypersensitivity reactions increases with age. Infants under one year should not be given yellow-fever vaccines due to an increased risk of encephalitis.

State of health — Persons to be vaccinated should be in good health. Acute illness would normally be a contraindication to vaccination. Live vaccines should not be given to patients with an immunodeficiency disease nor to patients on immunosuppressive therapy. Pertussis vaccines should not be given to any child with a history (or family history) of convulsions, fits or other neurological disorders.

Previous reaction to vaccination— If a reaction has taken place previously, precautions should by taken before further doses are given. For example, if a combined vaccine (such as Triple Antigen) has been given, a change to combined diphtheria tetanus (CDT) vaccine could be considered because the pertussis component is more likely to be the cause of adverse reactions. If a single vaccine has been used and it is necessary to complete a course, fractional doses may be used in conjunction with an oral antihistamine.

Pregnancy — There is a theoretical risk of administering live viral vaccines during pregnancy. Pregnancy is a contraindication to the use of rubella vaccine, but there is inadequate information at the moment to indicate that the vaccine is likely to cause rubelliform deformities in the foetus. On the limited published data, it would appear to be unlikely.

There is no convincing data that attenuated poliomyelitis vaccine or yellow-fever vaccines have been associated with undue complications during pregnancy. If there is an established risk of infection, then the use of these vaccines is justified. There is also no convincing data that inactivated vaccines have caused complications during pregnancy.

THE IMMUNIZING AGENT

A number of components in the vaccine may cause reactions: ***the active ingredient*** — bacterial, viral or toxoid antigen in a vaccine or the globulins in an antiserum; ***the antiseptic or preservative; the adjuvant,*** for example, aluminium salts; ***remnants of the culture medium*** not completely removed during processing, for example, egg components in yellow-fever vaccine.

THE VACCINATOR

Special attention must be paid to the following;

Technique of injection, for example, strict asepsis, correct site and route of administration.

Clean and sterile equipment; avoid chemical and bacterial contamination.

Strict compliance with manufacturer's instructions for storage, administration and precautions.

The principles of immunology and allergy, for example, avoid hyperimmunization or repeated use of heterologous antiserum from the same animal species.

TYPES OF REACTIONS

Reactions may be local or general, immediate or delayed, and specific or non-specific.

Table 68
Acute Reactions

Local	General
Pain	Anaphylaxis
Itching	Vaso-vagal attack
Redness	Anaphylactoid reaction
Swelling	Toxic reaction
Urticaria	Rash

Combinations of the above may occur in varying degrees, so that reactions to vaccination may be mild and transient or more severe and persistent. Anaphylaxis can follow a parenteral injection. This type of reaction is extremely rare with purified modern vaccines and with homologous antisera (for example, human immunoglobulins), but repeated doses of heterologous antiserum causes a distinct and increasing risk of sensitization and hence anaphylaxis. Precautions must be taken before heterologous antiserum is used.

Table 69
Delayed Reactions

Local	General
Pain	Fever
Redness	Malaise
Swelling	Urticaria
Itching	Adenitis
Urticaria	Arthralgia
Vesiculation	Neurological Reactions
Induration	Non-Specific Reactions

RULES FOR AVOIDING REACTIONS

1. Make sure syringes and needles are clean and sterile, both chemically and bacteriologically.
2. Always store immunizing agents as directed by manufacturer.
3. Do not use out-of-date material.
4. Check patient history for previous reactions or allergies.

5. If a previous reaction has occurred, take steps as in "The Patient" section.
6. Select site for injection to avoid blood vessels and other important structures.
7. Use aseptic technique at all times, and always use a fresh syringe and needle for each patient.
8. After insertion of needle, always pull back on plunger (aspirate) to make sure the needle is not in a vein.
9. Have adrenaline 1:1000 IV injection available in case of anaphylaxis.
10. Make sure patient (or parent) knows what agent has been given; give a written record of immunization.

TREATMENT OF REACTIONS TO IMMUNIZING AGENTS

Most reactions are mild and self-limited, and no specific treatment is required. The most dangerous reaction is acute anaphylactic shock, and the drugs normally used in treatment are as follows.

Adrenaline — it should be emphasised that adrenaline is the fastest acting and most effective single means of controlling anaphylaxis.

Corticosteroids — valuable adjuncts to recovery after initial shock is overcome.

Antihistamines — useful in the treatment of urticaria and angioneurotic oedema.

Other drugs which have been used include aminophylline, noradrenaline and isoprenaline.

For those interested in greater depth in the subject of immunization and available vaccines, *Immunisation Against Infectious Disease* (published by the DHSS) is recommended.

NURSING IMPLICATIONS

The nurse responsible for immunization procedures will aim for effective immunization, with minimisation of the potential for adverse reactions. Careful assessment of the patient and scrupulous technique are essential. In the case of anaphylaxis, the nurse must be prepared to institute cardiopulmonary resuscitation procedures.

Assessment

The patient's age, state of health and history of allergy or previous reaction to vaccination should be determined before vaccination is commenced. It should be ascertained whether the patient is pregnant or is likely to become pregnant during the course of vaccination.

Administration

Ensure that the patient is relaxed and seated, and that he (or the parent, in the case of a child) is aware of which agent is to be given. A written record of the immunization should be given to the patient, with information about the full course of immunizations, where appropriate. Patients should know to avoid vigorous exercise and alcohol for several hours.

Immunizing agents must be stored and reconstituted as directed by the manufacturer. Agents should be used at room temperature, rather than straight from the refrigerator, and should be shaken well before use, to ensure even dispersion of contents. Expiry dates must be adhered to.

Adrenaline (1:1000) should be available for use in case of anaphylaxis, and resuscitation equipment should be nearby. Contamination of syringes and needles (both chemical and bacterial) must be avoided. The outside of the giving needle should not be coated with vaccine. Vaccine is not to be given intravenously, so it is imperative to check that the needle is not in a blood vessel by aspirating before injecting.

Mass immunization tends to increase the hazards and potential dangers. When it is necessary to immunize large numbers of people at one time, great care is required at all stages to avoid contamination and transfer of disease. The nurse should protect herself legally by administering only those vaccines which she has prepared herself. He or she must be familiar with DHSS regulations.

Evaluation

The success of immunization is judged by the protection afforded the individual or population from each disease. Individual evaluation is possible by monitoring of antibody titres or by screening techniques, such as Mantoux testing for tuberculosis immunity.

SELF-EVALUATION TEST

1. Name the types of immunity.
2. Define active immunity.
3. What is the difference between heterologous serum and homologous serum?
4. The onset of active immunity from vaccination is: (a) rapid, (b) moderate, (c) slow.
5. Name the drug of choice in the treatment of anaphylactic shock: aminophylline, corticosteroids, adrenaline, isoprenaline, noradrenaline.
6. Name the killed bacterial vaccines commonly available.
7. Which of the following viral vaccines are live viral vaccines?
   Measles, smallpox, influenza, yellow fever, rubella, Sabin poliomyelitis vaccines.
8. The recommended intervals between primary immunization doses can be lengthened but not shortened.
   (a) True
   (b) False
   (c) Intervals remain the same
9. One of the following antisera is not an homologous product (to humans): tetanus, hepatitis B, Rh(D), antivenom.
10. One of the following is not a killed bacterial vaccine: tetanus, plague, pertussis, BCG, cholera.

Table 70
Primary Immunization Schedule

Age	Disease	Vaccine	Route
3 months	Diphtheria-tetanus-pertussis	Triple Antigen	Deep subcutaneous or intramuscular
	Poliomyelitis	Sabin	Oral
4½-5 months	Diphtheria-tetanus-pertussis	Triple Antigen	Deep subcutaneous or intramuscular
	Poliomyelitis	Sabin	Oral
8½-11 months	Diphtheria-tetanus-pertussis	Triple Antigen	Deep subcutaneous or intramuscular
	Poliomyelitis	Sabin	Oral
12 months	Measles/mumps	Measles/mumps	Subcutaneous
18 months	Diphtheria-tetanus	Combined Diphtheria and Tetanus (CDT)	Deep subcutaneous or intramuscular
5 years or prior to school entry	Diphtheria-tetanus	Combined Diphtheria and Tetanus (CDT)	Deep subcutaneous or intramuscular
	Poliomyelitis	Sabin	Oral
10 to 14 years (females only)	Rubella (preferably in last year of primary school or first year of high school)	Rubella	Subcutaneous
15 years or prior to leaving school	Diphtheria-tetanus	Adsorbed Diphtheria Tetanus (ADT)	Deep subcutaneous or intramuscular

Note: Contraindications to the pertussis component. Triple Antigen should be omitted and CDT used instead for children with:

(a) a previous history of neurological disease, including seizures, convulsions or cerebral irritation in the neonatal period;
(b) a previous reaction to the vaccine other than minor reactions and/or mild fever; or
(c) a family history of neurological disease other than that due to trauma or infections.

These children should be given the CDT vaccine at 2 months, 4 months and 18 months of age.

Table 71
Immunization and Vaccines

Drug Group	Drug Name	Use	Action	Adverse Reactions	Nursing Implications
Vaccines	BCG Cholera Typhoid Plague Pertussis Diphtheria Tetanus Typhus Measles Mumps Rubella Poliomyelitis Yellow fever Influenza Hepatitis B	Protective	Promotion of artificial immunity	Acute local reactions: pain, itching, redness, swelling, urticaria General local reactions: anaphylaxis, vasovagal attack, anaphylactoid reaction, toxic reaction, rash. Delayed local reactions: pain, redness, swelling, itching, urticaria, vesiculation, induration Delayed general reactions: fever, malaise, urticaria, adenitis, arthralgia, neurological reactions, non-specific reactions	***Assess:*** Age, general state of health. Previous reaction to vaccination; pregnancy. ***Administer:*** give written record of immunization; store vaccines in refrigerator, use at room temperature; reconstitute to manufacturer's instructions; ensure patient is relaxed; strict aseptic technique; adrenaline 1:1000 available. ***Evaluate:*** observe if previous reaction has occurred; antibody titres, screening tests; incidence of disease. ***Teach:*** Immunization schedule — give written advice.

26

DISINFECTANTS, ANTISEPTICS AND INFECTION CONTROL

John Timmins

OBJECTIVES

At the conclusion of this chapter the reader should be able to:

1. define the terms "disinfectant" and "antiseptic";
2. list two limitations to the use of disinfectants;
3. list three definite uses of disinfectants and antiseptics;
4. list three possible misuses of disinfectants and antiseptics;
5. describe the actions, limitations and uses with their dilutions of the six major groups of disinfectants and antiseptics;
6. list the nursing implications of the use of an antiseptic solution on a patient's wound;
7. describe the principle of two-phase preoperative skin preparation;
8. list the principles of nurses' hand hygiene when dealing with patients' dressings;
9. answer questions on any of the previous objectives from case studies or multiple-choice questions.

PREREQUISITE KNOWLEDGE

A basic knowledge of chemistry and microbiology would be helpful in understanding the uses and actions of disinfectants and antiseptics.

DEFINITIONS

Disinfectants —may be regarded as bactericidal agents which act by combining with proteins and other components of the cell protoplasm and so prevent infection by destroying or removing pathogenic microorganisms in the non-sporing or vegetative state.

Antiseptics — (or skin disinfectants) are antimicrobial agents which may be bacteriostatic or slowly bactericidal depending on the particular chemical and its concentration, and which counter sepsis by destroying or inhibiting the growth of pathogenic microorganisms in the non-sporing or vegetative state.

These agents are not usually active against bacterial spores.

Disinfectants are non-specific in acting against both bacterial and tissue cells, while antiseptics are more selective and, in concentrations used, cause little tissue damage. Some disinfectants can be used as antiseptics in a more dilute form. Thus the term "antiseptic" is commonly applied to antimicrobial agents used on living tissues.

Bactericidal agent — one which causes death to the bacterial cell by destroying its structure.

Bacteriostatic agent — one which stops the growth, division and multiplication of a bacterial cell without necessarily causing its death. (These cells can then be removed mechanically or by natural bodily defences.) However, once this agent is removed, the cells may recommence growing.

Tuberculocidal agent — one which kills cells of *Mycobacterium tuberculosis.*

Fungicidal agent — one which kills fungi.

Virucidal agent — one which kills viruses.

Bacterial spores — thick-walled resting cells produced by certain bacteria (from soil), including those which cause tetanus and gas gangrene. They are highly resistant to heat and completely resistant to many chemical disinfectants.

Some disinfectants may, however, kill spores (*sporicides*) besides the non-sporing or vegetative state of the microorganisms, for example, formaldehyde and glutaraldehyde. When a disinfectant kills all types of microorganisms, it is termed a *biocide;* when it stops the growth of all types of microorganism, it is termed a *biostat.*

HISTORY

Antony van Leeuwenhoek first described the "little animals" he saw under his self-made microscopes in 1677. Nearly 200 years elapsed before some practical application was seen in controlling microorganisms. Louis Pasteur, in the second half of the nineteenth century, demonstrated that microbes contaminated sterile culture media, and he was able to control unwanted fermentations in beer and wine by gentle heating (pasteurisation). In the 1860s, Joseph Lister applied Pasteur's theory of airborne microbes to surgery and reasoned that infections in wounds were the result of airborne contamination. By using disinfectant dressings soaked in phenol for application to surgical wounds, especially amputations, he found a marked reduction in the incidence of serious infections. This process became known as antiseptic surgery, later to be replaced by aseptic surgery.

USES, LIMITATIONS AND MISUSES OF DISINFECTANTS AND ANTISEPTICS

USES

The ***definite usages of disinfectants and antiseptics*** can be categorised as:

1. disinfection of the hospital environment, where specified, with an agent effective in clean or dirty conditions;
2. disinfection of clean articles or surfaces;
3. skin disinfection (antisepsis).

To meet these uses, a range of different disinfectants is required, as no one disinfectant will provide the antimicrobial range, properties and uses that will be desired in meeting different circumstances.

The ***efficiency of disinfectants and antiseptics*** depends on:

1. the concentration of disinfectant or antiseptic; if concentrates are used, exact portions of the active substance and water must be measured before mixing;
2. temperature;
3. the number of organisms originally present; cleaning is a disinfecting process;
4. the presence of protective films of dried organic matter, for example, milk, blood, pus, excreta, oil; such soiling may prevent a disinfectant from working by protecting the microorganisms;
5. whether the surface to be cleaned is smooth, or rough and porous (significant in older hospitals);
6. adsorption onto suspended material, for example textiles, fibres, container surfaces;
7. inactivation by interacting with some other types of disinfectants or antiseptics; by interacting with some types of detergents; or by contamination with lipids and organic matter;
8. the pH of the medium;
9. the type of vehicle used, for example, water or alcohol.

LIMITATIONS

Disinfectants have their uses and their limitations, and should not be recommended under the following circumstances.

1. When sterilisation is required, except in an emergency.
2. When disinfection can be accomplished better by pasteurisation, that is, moist heat from 60°C to 100°C for varying lengths of time, for example, 65°C for 10 minutes. This is the process of first choice for anaesthetic equipment.
3. When it is unnecessary, as in the case of ordinary cleaning of floors, sinks and sluices. The frequency of cleaning required is not reduced by the addition of disinfectants in these areas. The value of using disinfectants is questionable when washing floor surfaces, except in special circumstances, for example, theatres, burns units, and isolation wards. Even in theatres, the use of disinfectants is giving way to strict cleaning procedures simply using detergents.
4. There is a further specific limitation: when diathermy is being performed, alcoholic solutions of disinfectants and antiseptics should never be used, either in the theatre or preoperatively in the ward where garments may absorb excess flammable liquid.

A general limitation in the use of all disinfectants and antiseptics is the life of the diluted solutions at ward level. The absolute maximum length of time an opened container of disinfectant or antiseptic should remain in use is seven days, but in practice, volumes of solutions used should be reduced to a size whereby the ward shelf-life of disinfectants and antiseptics is in effect no more than 24 hours. Solutions of disinfectants that are in open continual use should be replaced every 24 hours. It is a general misconception that disinfectants and antiseptics are effective indefinitely or against all types of organisms. In fact, dilute aqueous antiseptic solutions are prone to contamination if used and stored for any length of time. Antiseptic solutions should ideally be packaged in sterile disposable containers and used once only, then discarded.

MISUSES

The dangers of misuse must be recognised by all persons handling disinfectants and antiseptics. Some notorious causes of contamination with gram-negative bacilli are:

1. contamination of quaternary ammonium compounds (QAC) with *Pseudomonas aeruginosa* derived from bark stoppers; glass, rubber or plastic caps should be used, never cork;
2. inactivation of chlorhexidine by cork;
3. organisms trapped between caps and liners; use new caps for each refill or clean caps without liners;

4. ward stock bottles refilled without cleaning; all bottles returned from the wards for re-use must be thoroughly cleansed and preferably "pasteurised", then dried; if necessary, bottles may need to be sterilised;
5. adsorption of QACs by gauze swabs or by mophead materials.

Not only can some microorganisms survive and indeed grow in disinfectant and antiseptic preparations (particularly dilute solutions), but cases have been reported that once such preparations have become contaminated, particular organisms may then come to depend on that disinfectant or antiseptic substance for their survival. It is therefore important that consideration be given to the careful handling of disinfectants and antiseptics in the ward to prevent misuse and contamination which may result in these preparations actually spreading infection instead of helping to contain it.

CLASSES OF DISINFECTANTS AND ANTISEPTICS

ALCOHOLS

Ethanol (ethyl alcohol) and propan-2-ol or ***isopropanol*** (isopropyl alcohol) are bactericidal in combination with water and are most effective in the following dilutions: ethanol 70% to 80% v/v, and isopropanol 50% to 60% v/v.

Bacterial spores are resistant to alcohols. Alcohols can be used as bactericidal agents but are mainly used as solvents for other chemical disinfectants and to potentiate their antibacterial activity.

It is important to remember that alcohols should not be used in the theatre when diathermy is being employed due to the risk of fire; nor should they be used on humidicribs or in confined spaces where toxic amounts of vapours may be inhaled.

CHLORHEXIDINE

This diguanide compound is bactericidal while being bacteriostatic in high dilutions. Bacterial spores are resistant to it. While generally being considered incompatible with soaps, it may, however, be compatible with trace amounts. It is not affected by serum or protein nor absorbed by dressings. Chlorhexidine is suitable for disinfection of urological instruments and for bladder and vaginal irrigation.

Dilutions for various uses (as final concentrations of chlorhexidine gluconate) are given in Table 72.

Table 72
Uses and Dilutions of Chlorhexidine Gluconate

0.02%	(1 in 5000) in aqueous solution: bladder irrigation (solution must be sterile)
0.05%	(1 in 2000) in aqueous solution; used for cleaning instruments such as endoscopes
0.5%	in 70% ethanol: preoperative skin preparation; disinfection of clean instruments in emergencies and of thermometers
1%:	in creams for burns; in aqueous solutions for preoperative skin preparation near sensitive tissues
4%:	in lotion for hand disinfection (for example *Hibiscrub*)

Chlorhexidine is commonly used in combination with cetrimide (see next section) in an aqueous dilution of 1:100 from the concentrate which is supplied as *Savlon Hospital Concentrate*, and in an alcoholic dilution of 1 in 30, used for the same purposes as chlorhexidine 0.5% in 70% ethanol.

Chlorhexidine, in the higher dilutions, may be particularly prone to contamination. These solutions should not be stored for more than one week, once opened.

QUATERNARY AMMONIUM COMPOUNDS (QAC)

These compounds are bactericidal while being bacteriostatic in high dilutions. They are also surface-active, so that they concentrate on all types of surfaces giving rapid bactericidal action. They are partially inactivated by serum proteins and dressings such as gauze and chemically inactivated by soaps and phospholipids.

Cetrimide has been used for skin and wound disinfection in strengths of 0.1% to 1%. For preoperative skin disinfection, a 0.5% solution in 70% ethanol has been used after making sure the skin was free of soap.

QACs were used for environmental sanitation, but other chemicals are more desirable in this field, and their main use today is in combination with the diguanides (such as chlorhexidine), as set out previously.

Examples of QACs are: ***cetrimide*** (for example, *Cetavlon* products; combined with chlorhexidine in *Savlon Hospital Concentrate)*, ***benzalkonium chloride*** (*Roccal*), ***cetylpyridium chloride*** (for example as used in *Merocet* mouthwash).

PHENOLS

These compounds are bactericidal. Except for hexachlorophane, dilution markedly affects their activity. They are more active in acid pH. They fall into two main groups, chlorinated phenols and bisphenols, the former being mainly used as environment disinfectants, and the latter as antiseptics.

Chlorinated phenols

Dettol contains a chloroxylenol and was used as an antiseptic for skin and mucous membranes in a 5% dilution for clean situations. It is not suitable for use in heavily contaminated situations and should not be used as an environment disinfectant. More effective disinfectants have superseded its use as an antiseptic.

Hycolin is a mixture of halogenated phenols and is used in a 1.2% dilution for ward and theatre disinfection, or from a 0.5% dilution in clean situations to 1.5% to 2% in dirty situations. The only problem in its use as a disinfectant for inanimate objects is its blanching effect on perspex as in humidicribs. A 2% dilution with 0.5% sodium nitrite can be used for instrument disinfection. Rapid disinfection of endoscopic instruments should not damage lens cement, while prolonged immersion may.

Bisphenols

An example of bisphenol antiseptic is ***hexachlorophane.*** It is used in hand soap (2% to 3%) and in a detergent emulsion *(Ster-Zac DC skin cleanser)* for skin antisepsis where its value depends on a cumulative effect by repeated application. This effect is removed by alcohol. For specific uses see page 501.

CHLORINE COMPOUNDS

Chlorine compounds include the ***hypochlorites***, sodium hypochlorite (*Milton 1%*) and ***chlorinated lime*** (*Dakin's Solution, Eusol*), inorganic chloramines, and organic chloramines (for example chloramine-T, used as tablets in colostomy or ileostomy bags). These substances are bactericidal. The hypochlorite activity is related to the concentration of undissociated HOCl. Organic matter and alkaline pH reduce activity. Because they have relatively low residual toxicity, chlorine compounds are useful for the disinfection of relatively clean, impervious surfaces, such as babies' feeding bottles, baths, wash basins and food equipment.

Sodium hypochlorite is available as a 1% solution, stabilised (*Milton*). *Dakin's Solution* and *Eusol* have no antibacterial activity *in vivo*, but are useful in removing slough from granulation tissue, as in leg ulcers.

Table 73
Uses and Dilutions of Hypochlorites

125 ppm (e.g. 1 in 80 dilution of *Milton*	— baby feeding bottles and teats — food utensils — clean stainless steel surfaces — face masks
500 ppm (e.g. 1 in 20 dilution of *Milton*)	— emergency disinfection of instruments — thermometers
10 000 ppm (e.g. neat *Milton*)	— virus-contaminated equipment, e.g. with blood of hepatitis-suspected patient

IODINE COMPOUNDS (Iodine, Iodophors)

Iodine as tincture of iodine or weak iodine solution (2.5%) is used as an antiseptic for intact skin only. It stains skin where iodophors do not, and the hypersensitivity shown to iodine does not appear to be exhibited by iodophors. ***Iodophors*** are complexes of iodine, held in loose chemical combination with detergent surfactants.

Iodine is biocidal and iodophors are bactericidal while being biocidal in high concentrations. Activity is reduced in alkaline pH and in the presence of organic matter. Iodophors are used for disinfection at concentrations of 0.75% to 1.5% available iodine. Their main uses are as surgical scrubs and preoperative skin preparations where the usual strength is the 1% available iodine used as the original solution (see page 501). Examples of iodophors are *Betadine* and *Videne* and other povidone-iodine products such as an ointment used to prevent infection around the site of entry of a catheter.

ALDEHYDES (formaldehyde, glutaraldehyde)

Formaldehyde is biocidal (being sporicidal above 40°C) as a 4% aqueous solution (addition of alcohol decreases sporicidal activity). Formalin (aqueous solution of formaldehyde 34% to 38%) is used diluted two to twenty times with water, the usual strength being 10% formalin (that is about 4% formaldehyde). It is widely used in urine collection bottles to keep the urine sterile and for preservation of dead tissue specimens. It is too irritating for use on living tissue. Formaldehyde vapour from formalin can be used in fumigating rooms which have held patients with cholera, typhoid, plague or open staphylococcus infection.

Formalin in sodium chloride 0.9% solution (as used for the storage of pathology specimens) should *never* be labelled "Formal Saline" due to its obvious confusion with "Normal Saline", whose substitution with the former could be disastrous.

Glutaraldehyde has a wide range of activity, being tuberculocidal and slowly sporicidal. The biocidal activity is greatest at pH 7.5 to 8.5. It is used as a 2% solution (available as *ASEP*, *Cidex*, or *Totacide 28*) which usually needs to be activated by a liquid or powder supplement before use. This solution is an irritant to skin and mucous membranes and a severe irritant to the eye, requiring the use of goggles. It is less irritating to the skin than 4% formaldehyde and is faster acting while bacterial spores are sensitive at a much lower temperature (20°C).

MERCURY COMPOUNDS

These compounds are biostatic, so are not considered as disinfectants. They are still used as preservatives for pharmaceuticals. Mercury compounds may be inorganic or organic, for example, thiomersal, phenylmercuric nitrate (PMN), nitromersol and mercurochrome (the least active).

While being biostatic, they are slowly bactericidal and fungicidal. Thiomersal is used for preservation of antisera. PMN is used as a preservative in ophthalmic solutions.

TRIPHENYLMETHANE DYES

These dyes are not used as disinfectants and are of limited value as antiseptics because of intense staining, but they are used as bacteriostats against particular organisms. ***Crystal violet*** (or gentian violet), ***brilliant green*** and ***malachite green*** are biostatic and are not inactivated by serum, but are readily absorbed on dressings.

A 0.5% aqueous solution of crystal violet (or 1% solution containing 20% alcohol) is used topically for staphylococcal, *Candida albicans* and mycotic skin infections. Triple Dye (an aqueous solution of crystal violet 0.25%, brilliant green 0.25%, proflavine 0.12%) is used for skin and vaginal infections. Bonney's Blue (Bonney and Browning's Blue Paint) is brilliant green 500mg, crystal violet 500 mg, alcohol (90%) 50 mL, water to 100 mL. It is used as a preoperative skin preparation. Skin-marking dye, as used for radiotherapy skin marking is Compound Crystal Violet Paint (BPC 1954).

USES ON SKIN AND MUCOUS MEMBRANES

The skin cannot be sterilised by any agent that it can tolerate, so chemical antiseptics can only be used to reduce the transient exogenous bacteria and the resident endogenous bacterial flora of the skin. An antiseptic should have a rapid bactericidal action against a wide range of organisms, and its effect should last for several hours, while it should also be non-sensitising and non-irritant. Antiseptics are indicated for use in two areas: on the patient's skin and on surgeons' and nursing staffs' hands.

THE PATIENT'S SKIN

For treatment of wounds, burns and skin infections, where a general cleansing action is wanted together with antisepsis treatment, the most suitable preparation is an aqueous solution of ***cetrimide*** 0.15% with ***chlorhexidine*** 0.015% (*Savlodil, Travasept*). This affords a wide antibacterial range while the detergent action of the QAC positively cleanses the site.

For preoperative skin preparation, an initial mechanical removal of organisms is desirable by shaving and washing. This washing should be carried out using an antibacterial cleanser such as chlorhexidine detergent (*Hibiscrub*) or using ordinary washing procedures followed by an antiseptic such as *Savlodil* or the alcoholic solutions described below after all soap has been removed. Then immediately prior to the operation, an alcoholic solution of bactericide or an iodophor is usually used. This should be coloured to demarcate the area of application and should be applied twice in order to ensure mechanical removal of surface contaminants, to aid penetration into the skin, and to give sufficient time (approximately one to two minutes) for bactericidal action.

This double preoperative preparation procedure — both at ward level and in the theatre — is referred to as "two-phase skin preparation". The initial ward treatment will remove exogenous bacteria and start to reduce endogenous bacteria. The theatre treatment will reduce these endogenous bacteria to a minimum.

Examples of alcoholic solutions of bactericide include 0.5% chlorhexidine, 0.5% of a QAC, and tincture of iodine. Non-alcoholic antiseptics of similar efficacy to these solutions are iodophors containing approximately 1% available iodine.

The disadvantage of uncomplexed iodine solutions is the risk of skin reactions, while with QACs, the disadvantage is that they are inactivated by soap on the skin. Thus chlorhexidine (which is less sensitive to soap than QACs) and iodophor preparations are preferred.

Insertion of a subclavian catheter should also be regarded as an operative procedure and similar preparations, as outlined above, taken. After insertion of the catheter, the site of entry can be smeared with a povidone-iodine ointment. This iodophor product will lessen the chance of organisms entering along the catheter line.

For disinfection of sites adjacent to sensitive tissues, aqueous chlorhexidine 1% should be used. Iodophors may be irritant to conjunctival and urethral tissues due to their acidity.

In urinary-tract procedures, aqueous solutions of chlorhexidine should be used in varying strengths. Prior to catheterisation, swabbing of the external genitalia and the genito-urinary area should be carried out with aqueous chlorhexidine 1%. After insertion of the catheter, povidone-iodine ointment may be used to seal the meatus, as long as this does not prove to be too irritating to the urethra.

For skin grafting, an aqueous solution of 1% chlorhexidine or an aqueous diguanide/QAC mixture (for example, *Savlon*) may be used.

For infants' skin, the 3% hexachlorophane emulsion *Phisohex* has been used as a dry wash applied to the umbilicus and whole skin area. The cumulative effect obtained reduces staphylococcal infection in the newborn, whose skins are particularly susceptible to this gram-positive organism.

A complication of this treatment is the possibility of colonisation of the skin by gram-negative organisms. Another reported side effect is possible neurological toxicity from dermal absorption. Some authors recommend the rinsing of the skin after application of hexachlorophane. However, arguments against such CNS damage being directly attributable to hexachlorophane are put forward by other authorities.

Alcoholic versus Aqueous Antiseptics

Alcohols (ethanol 70% and isopropanol 55%) have a rapid bactericidal action, but their effect is short-lived. Combination with a chemical antiseptic is required to produce a sustained bactericidal effect on the patient's skin.

Alcoholic solutions of antiseptics are thus generally used for preoperative skin preparation except where sensitive tissues are involved, for example, conjunctiva, urethra, vulva and vagina, and for skin grafting where aqueous solutions are used.

Aqueous antiseptics are used for open wounds and burns to reduce painful irritation.

SURGEONS' AND NURSING STAFFS' HANDS

For surgeons, a surgical wash of up to five minutes in running water with soap and the use of sterile rubber gloves is not a sufficient safeguard against infection of the surgical site, due to the possibility of undetected punctures in the gloves. Hand disinfection with long-acting bactericides prior to gloving is necessary.

Hexachlorophane preparations were among the first surgical handwashes to be used regularly. This antiseptic substance improved the effectiveness of ordinary bar soap, but the liquid hexachlorophane preparations, both liquid soap and detergent emulsion, are superior to hexachlorophane bar soap. An example of the detergent emulsion type is *Ster-Zac DC skin cleanser,* containing 3% hexachlorophane.

The efficiency of hexachlorophane preparations has been questioned with respect to the varying susceptibilities of bacterial populations of the hands and the length of time taken to achieve a desired degerming action with its exclusive and frequent use.

The alternatives to the slow and cumulative effect of hexachlorophane, whose spectrum is restricted to gram-positive organisms, are either other antiseptics also formulated in hand-washing detergents, or antiseptic lotions applied after washing. The other detergent antiseptics are ***iodophors*** (for example, *Betadine Surgical Scrub*) and ***chlorhexidine*** in a concentration of 4% in detergent solution (for example *Hibiscrub*). To prevent chafing with the use of any detergent hand-washing preparation, always ensure that the hands are wet with water before applying the detergent solution.

The antiseptic lotions can be used after washing with ordinary soap and contain a rapidly acting bactericide such as chlorhexidine or iodine in alcoholic solution or iodophors. A plain alcohol hand rinse is of no value since its action is not a continuing one. With the bactericide the action is immediate and penetrating and at the same time sustained.

The hexachlorophane soap wash can be combined with the post-wash alcoholic solution, but the cumulative effect of the hexachlorophane is negated with its removal by the alcohol.

The nursing staff could follow the procedure (above) for washing surgeons' hands. For carrying out ward dressings, the methods used include the continuous use of 3% hexachlorophane soap; or emulsion on and off duty; or intermittent use on duty of the chlorhexidine 4% detergent solution (*Hibiscrub*), or detergent iodophor preparation such as *Betadine Surgical Scrub*. Some nurses have experienced hand sensitivities from the constant washing between patients. Replacement of the detergent antiseptics with plain soap has resulted, but this should be as liquid soap and not bar soap, which may foster growth of pathogens. Antiseptic washes for nurses are still preferred wherever possible.

NURSING IMPLICATIONS

Disinfection means the destruction of bacteria but not necessarily of fungi, viruses or spores. **Sterilisation** means 100% destruction of all types of micro-organisms. Thus "99% sterilised" or "partially sterilised" are self-contradictory terms. Use the correct term when referring to either disinfection or sterilisation.

Bacteria may still grow in solutions of disinfectants and antiseptics, particularly those of the weaker strengths. These solutions must be carefully handled to avoid contamination and should not be stored in a moist, warm area which might promote the growth of organisms.

The disinfectant or antiseptic should only be used in the recommended dilutions and would normally be available at ward level as ready-to-use solutions. These must not be diluted further. If concentrates have to be provided, exact quantities of the disinfectant and water must be measured before mixing.

Disinfectants and antiseptics have a maximum "life" of one week once opened for use in the ward. The use of these solutions should be reduced to 24 hours or ideally to a once-only use with disposable containers. Disinfectants and antiseptics must *never* be "topped up".

Instruments wherever possible should be sterilised. Disinfection by "pasteurisation" is the next best process. The presence of dried organic matter such as blood, pus, excreta, oil or milk on instruments will form a protective layer which will negate the effect of a disinfectant. Make sure all instruments for disinfection have been thoroughly cleaned mechanically before immersion.

Instruments and skin must have all soap removed before the use of disinfectants and antiseptics. The cumulative effect of the use of hexachlorophane (for example, *Ster-Zac DC skin cleanser* antiseptic) on the skin is destroyed by alcohol, for example methylated spirits or alcoholic hand lotions.

Alcoholic solutions of antiseptics should not be used near sensitive tissues such as conjunctiva and urethra.

INFECTION CONTROL

Development of the subspecialty

While hospitals may have monitored levels of infections in wards for many years, this was normally a function of the Department of Microbiology alone. However, in the mid 1970s, with the increasing presence in hospital wards of ***methicillin-resistant Staphylococcus aureus*** (MRSA), Infection Control committees started to appear in hospitals to set policies and procedures to control nosocomial or hospital-acquired infections.

These committees had multidisciplinary representation with the key figure being the infection-control trained nurse. The value of having a full-time trained nurse in this role soon became apparent with more precise information on the type, location and incidence of infections being obtained through regular infection surveys. Summaries of these information-gathering exercises were then disseminated to key personnel in the hospital.

This led to better preventative methods being established with the cooperation of medical, surgical, nursing, microbiology, pharmacy and cleaning staff meeting to combat a problem of mutual interest and concern. Policies on antibiotic usage, disinfectants and antiseptics, and isolation techniques were strengthened and integrated. Possible vectors for the transmission of organisms about the hospital were identified and measures taken to prevent the spread of any infection from its source.

New guidelines were laid down on staff and patient hygiene, on the handling of staff and patient infections, and on the duties of infection-control personnel. The Department of Health began issuing recommendations for infection-control policies and hospitals started to produce infection-control procedural manuals. Such a group has become more formalised as the Infection Control Nursing Association which helps coordinate and disseminate information on procedures and policies for this new subspecialty.

TERMS OF REFERENCE FOR AN INFECTION CONTROL COMMITTEE

1. To develop and periodically review written standards for hospital sanitation and medical asepsis.

2. To develop a practical system for monitoring, reporting, evaluating and keeping records of hospital associated infections amongst patients and personnel.
3. To regularly analyse data on infections, evaluate current trends and experience, and undertake such control measures as may be indicated.
4. To develop and coordinate procedures for isolation of patients.
5. To facilitate the teaching of information pertinent to Infection Control and Isolation policies to employees on all levels, including medical staff and students.
6. To provide counsel and advice on infection-control matters.
7. To assist in educational and research programmes related to infection control and epidemiology.
8. To provide assistance on the development of an employee health programme.

COMPOSITION OF THE COMMITTEE

The Committee should comprise at least the following personnel.

1. Microbiologist
2. Infection-control trained nurse
3. Physician
4. Surgeon
5. Director of pharmacy or deputy
6. Director of nursing or deputy or assistant
7. General services manager

Other departments to be represented on the committee could include central sterile supply, intensive care, theatres, ward charge nurses and nursing education. Other groups or departments could be coopted from time to time to deal with a particular situation or to offer expert advice, for example catering, engineering and so on.

QUALIFICATIONS AND QUALITIES OF AN INFECTION CONTROL TRAINED NURSE

The person appointed to this position should be a senior trained nurse with clinical experience. He or she should have experience in supervision and teaching. As the scope of the position is broad, any further qualifications or certificates would be an advantage.

Besides enthusiasm and dedication, other important qualities that this person should possess are tact and diplomacy. Interaction with groups within the hospital and with other outside infection-control staff (for example, at seminars and conferences) is important.

SELF-EVALUATION TEST

1. Define the terms "disinfectant" and "antiseptic".
2. Disinfectants are normally used:
   (a) when sterilisation is required;
   (b) on instruments that can't be autoclaved or heated;
   (c) in detergent solutions to clean ordinary floors;
   (d) after the bottle has been opened for more than one week.
3. The definite uses of disinfectants and/or antiseptics are:
   (a) general disinfection of the hospital environment (True/False);
   (b) disinfection of clean articles or surfaces (True/False);
   (c) skin antisepsis (True/False);
   (d) sterilisation of surgeons' hands and arms (True/False)
   (e) prevention of growth under storage conditions (True/False).
4. (a) Acceptable closures for disinfectants/antiseptic solutions are: (i) glass (ii) rubber (iii) cork (iv) plastic
   (b) Chlorhexidine may be inactivated by cork (True/False).
   (c) Antiseptic solutions may be topped up if more than half-full (True/False).
   (d) Empty bottles of antiseptics should be cleaned and dried before re-use (True/False).
5. Write down the class or classes of the following chemicals and their most common dilution in use, for example *Milton* — chlorine compound, 1 in 80.
   (a) ethanol
   (b) *Savlodil*
   (c) *Hycolin*
   (d) chlorhexidine
   (e) iodophors (use dilution expressed as percentage of available iodine)
6. (a) Sterilisation means at least 95% destruction of microorganisms (True/False).
   (b) Bacteria may grow in ward solutions of disinfectants and antiseptics (True/False).
   (c) Instruments wherever possible should be sterilised (True/False).
   (d) The efficacy of disinfectants is decreased by dried films of pus and excreta but not of blood or milk (True/False).
   (e) Instruments for chemical disinfection should be thoroughly cleaned and free from soap (True/False).
7. Describe the benefits of two-phase preoperative skin preparation in the ward and in the operating theatre.
8. Describe a desirable procedure to prevent cross-contamination during daily ward dressings. How does this compare to the methods of nurses' hands hygiene as laid down in the nurses' procedures of your hospital?

9. *Case Study* Mr AB returns from theatre afebrile following a vagotomy and pyloroplasty. Five days later, he is febrile and a swab of his suture line grows *Pseudomonas aeruginosa.* His wound has been dressed with an antiseptic solution usually kept in the procedure room with a couple of other such bottles on the shelf above the sink, next to a hot-water pipe. This a convenient spot because it is close to the door, and these bottles are frequently used. Nurse CD was seen pouring the remains of another bottle of the same antiseptic into this particular bottle 10 days ago so that she could obtain a replacement for the near-empty bottle from the pharmacy.

   Comment on possible sources of the infection in Mr AB's wound.

   What are some of the dangers you see in this ward's procedures, and what could you suggest to the charge sister to improve the situation?

27

ANTINEOPLASTIC AGENTS

Anne de Fraine

OBJECTIVES

At the conclusion of this unit the reader should be able to:

1. define the terms "antineoplastic", "cytotoxic", "cancer", "neoplasm";
2. describe in general terms the mechanism of action of the drugs covered, their major side effects and nursing implications;
3. classify the antineoplastic agents into their relevant group by mechanism of action;
4. list the significant individual toxicities of the more commonly used agents.

PREREQUISITE KNOWLEDGE

1. General principles of cell division and replication, with particular emphasis on the role of deoxyribonucleic acid (DNA), ribonucleic acid (RNA) and protein synthesis.
2. Definitions of the following terms: "malignant", "benign", "metastasis", "carcinoma", "sarcoma", "leukaemia", "lymphoma", "complete remission", "partial remission".
3. The place of chemotherapy in the overall treatment of cancer (that is, recognition of the other modes of therapy such as surgery and radiotherapy).

Antineoplastic agents, as the term implies, are used to treat neoplasms. Neoplasm may be defined as any new or abnormal growth, either benign or malignant. The antineoplastics are more particularly used to treat malignant neoplasms. The term "anticancer agent" is also used to describe these drugs. Cancer is not a single disease, but a large group of diseases characterised by uncontrolled growth and spread of abnormal cells. The natural course of these diseases, untreated, is usually fatal to the host. Antineoplastic drugs are cytotoxic (cause cell death) by virtue of their ability to interfere with normal cellular growth by a variety of mechanisms, preventing cell division and proliferation. They have a particular affinity for cells in the process of dividing, which is believed to have some relevance in explaining two important points:

First, the malignancies that currently respond best to chemotherapy are the more rapidly growing ones: for example, testicular carcinoma, lymphoma, acute leukaemia, small cell anaplastic carcinoma of the lung.

Second, the principal adverse reactions of these drugs involve the following normal tissues of the body, which at any given time have a large number of cells in the process of cell division — bone marrow (suppression of activity), hair follicles (alopecia), mucosal membranes (mucositis, especially of oral mucosa), and the gonads (menstrual irregularities, decreased spermatogenesis, sterility). The effects on these tissues are usually reversible. The other major adverse effect is nausea and vomiting which is related to an effect on the vomiting centre in the CNS.

The antineoplastic agents are discussed under the headings of alkylating agents, antimetabolites, antitumour antibiotics, mitotic inhibitors and miscellaneous agents. Each section contains a table listing the major therapeutic indications and the most common and/or important toxicities and adverse reactions of each drug. The drugs are then discussed in more detail in the text.

ALKYLATING AGENTS

Although the mechanism of these agents is not yet completely clear, it is known that they alkylate (form covalent linkages with) nucleic acids and hence interfere with DNA synthesis. These agents are attacked by "nucleophilic" sites on nucleic acids which result in the addition of a portion of the alkylating agent to the nucleophilic site. Cross linkage of the two DNA strands appears to play an important role in the antitumour action of these drugs.

FIGURE 11. REPRESENTATIVE ALKYLATING AGENTS

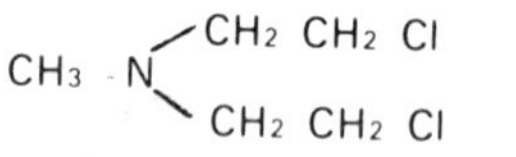

Nitrogen mustard

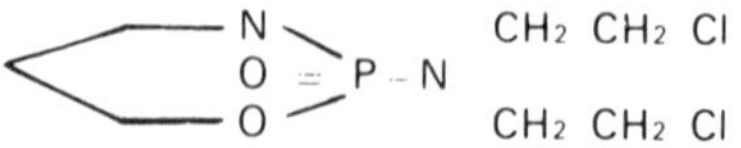

Cyclophosphamide

Reactive sites of the nitrogenous bases are:

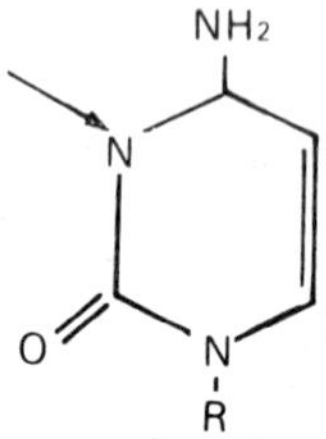

Cytosine

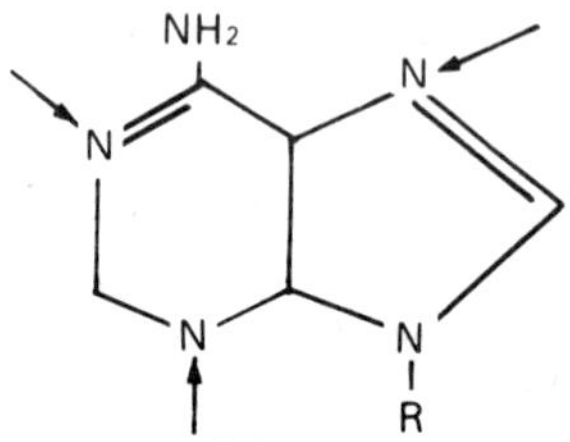

Adenosine

The alkylating agents may be subclassified into three groups, as indicated in Table 74.

Table 74
Major Alkylating Agents

Generic Name	Brand Name	Strength	Administration
1. *Nitrogen Mustards*			
Mechlorethamine Nitrogen mustard	*Mustine*	10 mg vials	Slow injection into a fast-running IV infusion
Cyclophosphamide	*Endoxana*	10-50 mg tablets	Oral
		vials: 1 g 500 mg 200 mg 100 mg	IV infusion over one-half to 1 hour in 500 mL. N/S or D/S
Chlorambucil	*Leukeran*	2 mg 5 mg	Oral
Melphalan	*Alkeran*	2 mg 5 mg	Oral
		100 mg vial	IV
2. *Alkyl Sulfonates*			
Busulphan	*Myleran*	0.5–2 mg tablets	Oral
3. *Ethylenimines*			
Triethylene thiophosphoramide	*Thiotepa*	15 mg vials	IV Intracavitary

N/S: normal saline; D/S: dextrose in normal saline

NITROGEN MUSTARDS

Sulphur mustard was used as a poisonous gas during World War 1 because of its vesicant action on the skin, eyes and respiratory tract. After the war the serious systemic complications following exposure were noted. These included leukopenia, bone-marrow aplasia and dissolution of lymphoid tissue. This led to its development as a possible antineoplastic agent and to the preparation of thousands of variants of the basic chemical structure.

Mustine

This was the first of the nitrogen mustards to be introduced into clinical use. Its major therapeutic indication is the treatment of Hodgkin's disease where it is used predominantly in combination with vincristine, procarbazine and prednisone (the so-called MOPP regimen). It is also of use against non-Hodgkin's lymphomas and mycosis fungoides. It has demonstrated some minor activity against a few solid tumours.

Mustine is rapidly acting and rapidly metabolised. It is rapidly degraded in water and body fluids and hence should be used immediately upon preparation.

Great caution should be taken in administration since extravasation of the drug causes a severe local tissue reaction. Prompt application of ice packs and administration of isotonic sodium thiosulphate will minimise this reaction. Thrombophlebitis is also a potential problem of administration. Anorexia, nausea and vomiting are common side effects but adequate antiemetic cover will usually minimise the severity. Bone-marrow depression (neutropenia and thrombocytopenia) is a dose-limiting complication. On occasion, a macropapular skin eruption or Herpes zoster skin lesion may be associated. Herpes infection is probably related to a latent viral infection not uncommonly present in lymphoma patients. Menstrual irregularities and foetal abnormalities have been reported.

Cyclophosphamide

Cyclophosphamide was developed as a result of efforts to modify the structure of mustine to achieve an agent with greater affinity for malignant cells. It is a broad spectrum antineoplastic agent, demonstrating activity against acute and chronic lymphoid leukaemias, Hodgkin's disease and non-Hodgkin's lymphomas, various bone and soft-tissue sarcomas, and carcinoma of the breast, lung, ovary and prostate. Its immunosuppressive properties have encouraged its use in the control of organ rejection after transplantation and in non-neoplastic disorders such as rheumatoid arthritis, Wegener's granulomatosis and nephrotic syndrome in children, where there is altered immune activity. The parent compound, cyclophosphamide, requires metabolic activation by the cytochrome P-450 enzyme system in the liver. The drug is well absorbed after oral or IV administration and is excreted predominantly in the urine.

None of the severe CNS problems associated with typical nitrogen mustards have been reported with cyclophosphamide. Its side effects include nausea and vomiting, bone-marrow depression (neutropenia more commonly than thrombocytopenia), alopecia, mucosal ulcerations, infertility in males, and menstrual irregularities. The major complication however is the potential for causing haemorrhagic cystitis which is attributed to irritant reactive metabolites. To ensure adequate renal function, oral fluids should be encouraged. Parenteral administration of cyclophosphamide should be as an infusion, and urine output should be greater than 2 litres/day for 48 hours after dosage. It is advisable that oral tablets should be taken before 4 pm.

Chlorambucil

This derivative of mustine is predominantly used in the treatment of chronic lymphocytic leukaemia, though it is also useful against Hodgkin's disease and related lymphomas, multiple myeloma and carcinoma of the ovary, breast and testis.

Chlorambucil is the least toxic of the nitrogen mustards. Nausea and vomiting may occur though this is usually limited to doses of greater than 20 mg orally. Bone-marrow depression is encountered, and dermatitis has been reported.

Oral absorption is adequate and reliable.

Table 75
Therapeutic Uses of and Adverse Reactions to Major Alkylating Agents

Drug	Therapeutic Indications	Toxicities and Adverse Reactions
Mustine	Hodgkin's disease Non-Hodgkin's lymphoma	Nausea and vomiting Myelosuppression Macropapular rash Tissue necrosis if extravasated
Cyclophosphamide	Leukaemia Lymphoma Bone and soft tissue sarcoma Carcinoma of breast, lung, ovary, prostate	Nausea and vomiting Myelosuppression Alopecia Oral mucositis Haemorrhagic cystitis
Chlorambucil	Chronic lymphocytic leukaemia Lymphoma Multiple myeloma Carcinoma of breast, ovary, testis	Nausea and vomiting Myelosuppression Dermatitis
Melphalan	Multiple myeloma Carcinoma of breast and ovary	Myelosuppression
Busulphan	CML (chronic myelocytic leukaemia)	Myelosuppression Nausea and vomiting Pulmonary fibrosis
Thiotepa	Lymphoma Carcinoma of breast and ovary Malignant effusions Bladder carcinoma (local instillation)	Fever Allergic skin reactions Myelosuppression

Melphalan

L-phenylalanine mustard or L-PAM has beneficial effects in the treatment of multiple myeloma and carcinoma of the breast and ovary. It is usually administered orally though an IV form is available. Melphalan has no acute toxicity. Nausea and vomiting are uncommon and bone-marrow depression tends to develop slowly. The IV form of the drug is not a vesicant.

ALKYL SULFONATES

Busulphan *(Myleran)* is a unique alkylating agent in that its pharmacological action is almost exclusively myelosuppression.

It is administered orally, the usual dose being 4 to 12 mg initially, with appropriate adjustment to clinical response. Principal toxic effects relate to its myelosuppressive properties. At total cumulative doses greater than 300 mg, white-cell counts may not recover. Thrombocytopenia may be a problem. Nausea and vomiting, diarrhoea, impotence, sterility and amenorrhoea have been reported. Hyperuricaemia has been noted, and concurrent administration of allopurinol may be indicated.

TRIETHYLENIMINES

Triethylenethiophosphoramide (*Thiotepa*) is an alkylating agent that is infrequently used. Responses have been seen in carcinoma of the ovary and breast and after local instillation for carcinoma of the bladder. Instillation of *Thiotepa* into body cavities to prevent the reaccumulation of malignant effusions is still used on occasion. Its toxic effects include bone-marrow depression, nausea and vomiting, gastrointestinal perforation, mild anaemia, allergic reaction, headache and fever.

ANTIMETABOLITES

This group of drugs exerts cytotoxic activity by virtue of structural similarity to metabolites required by the cell for normal growth and replication. They may be split into three subclassifications: ***folic acid analogues*** (methotrexate); ***purine analogues*** (6-thioguanine, 6-mercaptopurine), and ***pyrimidine analogues*** (5-fluorouracil, cytosine arabinoside, 5-azacytidine).

FOLIC ACID ANALOGUES

Folic acid is an essential dietary factor concerned with the metabolic transfer of 1-carbon units which are used in the synthesis of thymidylic acid and purine bases.

Methotrexate exerts its cytotoxic action by binding irreversibly to the enzyme dihydrofolate reductase and thereby inhibiting both DNA and RNA synthesis.

Folinic acid (*calcium leucovorin*) is a derivate of tetrahydrofolic acid which can by-pass this inhibition by supplying the end product of the reaction. This prevents much of the toxicity without reversing the antitumour effect. This is the principle behind the so-called "high dose methotrexate and folinic acid rescue" regime used in the treatment of tumours such as osteogenic sarcoma, carcinoma of the head and neck and renal carcinomas.

Methotrexate is strongly bound to plasma proteins and hence concurrent administration of salicylates is usually contraindicated. The sulphonamides interfere with the synthesis of folic acid, by inhibiting the formation of dihydrofolic acid, and hence should be used with caution in conjunction with methotrexate.

Table 76
Antimetabolites

Generic Name	Brand Name	Strength	Administration
1. Folic Acid Analogues			
Methotrexate		2.5 and 10 mg tablet	Oral
		5 mg vial	IMI
		50 mg vial	IVI
		500 mg vial	IV infusion in N/S,
		1g vial	D/S or 5% dextrose
			Intrathecal
2. Pyrimidine Analogues			
5-fluorouracil (5FU)		250 mg capsules	Oral
		250 mg/10 mL	IV bolus
Cytarabine (Cytosine arabinoside)	*Cytosar*	100 mg vial	SCI
			IMI
			IVI
			Intrathecal
			IV infusion
5-azacytidine		100 mg vial	IV infusion over 15 to 20 minutes in 50 to 300 mL N/S or dextrose
3. Purine Analogues			
6-mercaptopurine	*Puri-Nethol*	10 and 50 mg tabs	oral
6-thioguanine	*Lanvis*	40 mg tabs	oral

N/S: normal saline; D/S: dextrose in normal saline

Methotrexate is a broad-spectrum antitumour agent demonstrating activity against the acute leukaemias, choriocarcinoma, Burkitt's lymphoma, osteogenic sarcoma, rhabdomyosarcoma, and carcinoma of the head and neck, breast, lung, cervix, ovary, testis and kidney. Methotrexate is used as an immunosuppressive agent and for the treatment of psoriasis refractory to other forms of therapy.

Bone-marrow suppression is a dose-limiting toxicity; severe neutropenia and bone-marrow aplasia may occur. Mucocutaneous reactions are common, including mucosal ulceration, skin hyperpigmentation, alopecia and rash. Mucosal ulceration may be so severe as to necessitate dose reduction or temporary discontinuation of the drug. Nausea and vomiting may occur; severe diarrhoea is a frequent and dose-limiting reaction. Renal tubular damage may be caused by deposition of methotrexate crystals in the tubules. Urinary alkalinisation and adequate hydration with "high-dose" methotrexate administration will minimise the risk of this occurring. Other adverse reactions include amenorrhoea, defective spermatogenesis, fever and chills, and hepatic dysfunction.

PYRIMIDINE ANALOGUES

5-fluorouracil

This drug exerts its antineoplastic action by blocking the synthesis of thymidylic acid by inhibiting the enzyme thymidylate synthetase. 5-FU is usually administered intravenously, since absorption after oral dosage is incomplete and unpredictable. When administered orally the ampoules should be emptied into a glass of milk or water, as acidic fruit juices may chemically alter the drug. 5-FU is of use in the treatment of hepatoma, carcinomas of the breast, ovary, gastrointestinal tract, prostate, pancreas, cervix and bladder, and skin (as topical application (1%-5%) such as *Efudix* cream).

The major toxic reactions involve the action of 5-FU on the bone marrow and gastrointestinal epithelium and oral mucosa. Anorexia, nausea, vomiting, diarrhoea, stomatitis, mouth ulceration and proctitis may occur. The principal dose-limiting reaction is myelosuppression. Other adverse reactions include alopecia, darkening of veins, dermatitis, nail changes, and hyperpigmentation of the skin. Neurologic manifestations such as ataxia have been reported.

Cytarabine

This drug is a structural analogue of 2-deoxycytidine, although its precise mechanism of action is undecided. The main indications for the use of cytarabine are acute leukaemia of adults, blast crisis phase of chronic myeloid leukaemia, and Burkitt's lymphoma. It may also be administered intrathecally for the treatment of carcinomatous meningitis and meningeal leukaemia.

In addition to its antineoplastic activity it has immunosuppressive properties and has been used in the treatment of herpes keratitis and disseminated herpes zoster, though adenosine arabinoside is now the agent preferred.

Cytarabine is a potent myelosuppressive agent, producing leukopenia, thrombocytopenia and anaemia with megaloblastic changes. Other toxic reactions include nausea, vomiting, anorexia, diarrhoea, stomatitis, alopecia, fever, hepatic dysfunction, thrombophlebitis at site of injection, and dermatitis.

5-Azacytidine

This investigational agent is a structural analogue of cytidine and is incorporated into DNA and RNA, interrupting normal cell division. Its major indication is acute myeloid leukaemia, though some activity against carcinomas of the breast and ovary, lymphoma and mesothelioma has been demonstrated. Adverse reactions include bone-marrow suppression (leukopenia, thrombocytopenia and anaemia), nausea and vomiting, diarrhoea, fever, hypotension (rarely), stomatitis, neuromuscular weakness and lethargy.

Table 77
Summary of Therapeutic Uses and Adverse Reactions to Antimetabolites

Drug	Therapeutic Indications	Toxicities and Adverse Reactions
Methotrexate	Acute leukaemia Choriocarcinoma Burkitt's lymphoma Wide range of solid tumours	Myelosuppression Oral mucositis Alopecia Rash Diarrhoea Nephrotoxicity
5-fluorouracil	Carcinoma of breast, ovary, gastrointestinal tract, prostate, cervix, pancreas, bladder, skin, hepatoma	Nausea Diarrhoea Oral mucositis Myelosuppression Dermatological manifestations
Cytosine arabinoside	Adult acute leukaemia CML (blast crisis) Burkitt's lymphoma	Myelosuppression Nausea and vomiting Fever Rash
5-azacytidine	Acute granulocytic leukaemia Carcinoma of breast and ovary Lymphoma	Myelosuppression Nausea and vomiting Diarrhoea Fever Hyperglycaemia Hepatotoxicity Neurotoxicity — coma
6-mercaptopurine	Acute leukaemia CML (blast crisis)	Myelosuppression Nausea and vomiting Dermatological reactions Cholestatic jaundice
6-thioguanine	Acute leukaemia	Myelosuppression Cholestatic jaundice

PURINE ANALOGUES

6-Mercaptopurine (6-MP)

This antipurine and its immunosuppressive derivate, azathioprine, were developed during the 1950s. The precise mechanism by which they cause cell death is not clearly understood. Mercaptopurine undergoes metabolic deactivation by two main pathways, one of which is catalysed by the enzyme xanthine oxidase. Hence concurrent administration of allopurinol, a xanthine oxidase inhibitor, necessitates reduction of the dose of mercaptopurine to 25% of the normal dose.

The principal use of 6-MP is in the treatment of acute leukaemia, especially of childhood. It may cause a brief remission in the blast crisis phase of chronic granulocytic leukaemia. Some responses have been reported in the therapy of choriocarcinoma.

Bone-marrow depression occurs though this is usually gradual in onset. Anorexia, nausea and vomiting are seen quite often, stomatitis and diarrhoea rarely. Dermatologic reactions have been noted. Cholestatic jaundice has been reported in about one-third of adult patients — if this occurs, therapy should be discontinued.

6-Thioguanine (6-TG)

Again, the mechanism of action of this drug is not clearly understood. Unlike 6-MP, concurrent administration of allopurinol does not necessitate a reduction of the dose of 6-TG, suggesting alternative pathways for metabolic deactivation. Clinically 6-TG is used in the therapy of acute leukaemia, and in combination with cytarabine is most effective for induction of remission in acute granulocytic leukaemia.

Toxic reactions include myelosuppression and cholestatic jaundice necessitating withdrawal of the drug. Nausea and vomiting are encountered rarely.

ANTITUMOUR ANTIBIOTICS

Many of these agents bind selectively with DNA-forming complexes which block the formation of DNA-dependent RNA. More specific information on mechanism of action is given under each drug heading. These agents are isolated from various species of the fungus *Streptomyces*. The commonly used antitumour antibiotics are listed in Table 78.

Actinomycin D

Actinomycin D acts by binding with double-helical DNA to form a complex which inhibits rapidly proliferating cells. It is both a potent antitumour and an immunosuppressive agent.

Actinomycin D is particularly useful in treating childhood malignancies, especially Wilms' tumour and rhabdomyosarcoma. Activity has been demonstrated in neuroblastoma, Ewing's sarcoma and osteogenic sarcoma.

In adult neoplastic disease, its primary uses are in the treatment of methotrexate resistant choriocarcinoma in women and testicular tumours. Activity has been noted in soft tissue sarcomas and some lymphomas.

Toxic effects include anorexia, nausea and vomiting. Diarrhoea is commonly noted and may require administration of antidiarrhoeal agents for several days after each dose of the drug. Ulceration of the oral mucosa is common. Dermatological manifestations include alopecia, erythema and increased skin pigmentation in previously irradiated areas. Bone-marrow depression, particularly thrombocytopenia, may be seen. Care should be taken with administration, since extravasation of the drug may result in severe local cellulitis and tissue necrosis.

Table 78
Commonly Used Antitumour Antibiotics

Generic Name	Brand Name	Strength	Administration
Actinomycin D (dactinomycin)	*Cosmegen* *Lyovac*	0.5 mg vials	IV infusion in 50 mL N/S, D/S or dextrose 5% over 20 to 30 minutes
Bleomycin		15 mg (unit) ampoules	IMI IVI IV infusion
Daunorubicin		20 mg vials	Slow injection into a fast running IV infusion
Doxorubicin	*Adriamycin*	10 mg vials 50 mg vials	Slow injection into fast running IV infusion
Mithramycin	*Mithracin*	2500 mcg vials	Slow IV infusion over 4 to 6 hours
Mitomycin	*Mitomycin C* *Kyowa*	2 mg vials 10 mg vials	IV infusion in 50 mL N/S, D/S or dextrose 5% over 20 to 30 minutes

N/S: normal saline; D/S: dextrose in normal saline.

Bleomycin

Bleomycin is one of a group of antibiotics isolated from fermentation of *Streptomyces* species. Its mode of action is thought to relate to its ability to cause DNA fragmentation. It blocks the cell cycle, causing accumulation of cells at G_2 phase. Bleomycin's selective action against squamous cell carcinomas and toxicity peculiar to lung and skin relates to the absence of aminopeptidases, which detoxify bleomycin, in these tissues. Bleomycin is useful in the treatment of squamous cell carcinomas of the head, neck, oesophagus, skin and genitourinary tract. Activity against testicular tumours and lymphomas has also been demonstrated.

Unlike the majority of antineoplastic agents, bleomycin causes minimal marrow suppression. Fever and shaking chills occur commonly and concurrent administration of promethazine 25 mg IM is advisable. Nausea and vomiting may be encountered. The major toxicity of bleomycin presents as skin or pulmonary lesions. Mucocutaneous reactions include alopecia, stomatitis, hyperpigmentation, hyperkeratosis, erythema, ulceration and vesiculation of the skin, especially in pressure areas. Pulmonary toxicity is the most serious of the adverse reactions, causing occasional fatalities. "Bleomycin lung" usually presents as cough, dyspnoea and decreased pulmonary function. Progression to severe and sometimes fatal pulmonary fibrosis may occur. A total cumulative dose of 300 mg (units) is usually set as the maximum a patient should receive. Discontinuation of the drug is indicated in the case of pulmonary toxicity, and use of corticosteroids has produced beneficial effects in some reported cases.

ANTHRACYCLINES — Doxorubicin, Daunorubicin

The anthracycline antibiotics, ***daunorubicin*** and ***doxorubicin,*** though structurally similar, display marked differences in clinical antitumour activity. Daunorubicin is limited to the treatment of acute leukaemia while doxorubicin (*Adriamycin*) demonstrates a broad spectrum of activity against a wide range of solid tumours, including carcinoma of the breast, thyroid, lung, bladder, cervix, ovary and testis, bone and soft-tissue sarcomas, Hodgkin's and non-Hodgkin's lymphomas, and acute leukaemias. Although the mechanism of action of these drugs is not fully elucidated, it is proposed that they inhibit DNA synthesis by binding specifically to DNA. There is no satisfactory explanation for the differing activities of these two agents. Both drugs are metabolised in the liver and excreted primarily in the bile. Impaired liver function may necessitate reduced dosage to minimise toxicity.

The clinical toxicities of these agents are very similar, including bone-marrow depression which is a major dose-limiting complication. Neutropenia is usually more marked than thrombocytopenia. Nausea and vomiting are commonly encountered, as are alopecia and stomatitis (which may be severe). These problems are reversible. Dermatological manifestations, including hyperpigmentation of nail beds and rash, may occur with *Adriamycin.* Cardiomyopathy is a unique toxicity of the anthracycline antibiotics. This is characterised by tachycardia, arrhythmias and transient ECG changes. Progressive congestive cardiac failure may follow. A dose of 550 mg/m^2 has been set as the maximum cumulative dose which a patient should receive. The risk of cardiac problems is increased in patients receiving concomitant cyclophosphamide, so a dose of 400 to 450 mg/m^2 is suggested as the maximum in these patients.

Mithramycin

Mithramycin has been largely superseded by other drugs in the treatment of neoplastic disorders. It has been used in the past with beneficial effects against disseminated testicular carcinomas, but its use now is limited to the treatment of severe hypercalcaemia, particularly when associated with advanced or metastatic carcinoma involving bone. The recommended dose for treatment of hypercalcaemia is 25 mcg/kg per day IV. Toxicity seen at this dose level is less severe. It has also been used experimentally in the treatment of Paget's disease.

The exact mode of action is not known, but it is believed to act in similar fashion to actinomycin D. It also appears to have a direct effect on osteoclasts, resulting in lowering of plasma calcium concentrations in hypercalcaemic patients.

The major sites of toxicity are the bone marrow, liver and kidneys. It may cause a severe haemorrhagic diathesis and thrombocytopenia. Adverse gastrointestinal, cutaneous and neurological reactions have been observed.

Mitomycin C

The primary therapeutic uses of ***mitomycin C*** are in the treatment of adenocarcinomas of the gastrointestinal tract, lung, pancreas, bladder, breast and soft-tissue sarcomas.

Bone-marrow depression (thrombocytopenia and leukopenia) is usually delayed in onset – 20 to 30 days after the dose of the drug. Anorexia, nausea, vomiting and diarrhoea are commonly observed. Mucocutaneous reactions include stomatitis, alopecia and rash. Pain on injection may necessitate slowing of infusion rate, and care should be taken as a severe local tissue reaction may occur if the drug is extravasated. Hepatotoxicity has also been reported (see Table 79).

Table 79
Therapeutic Uses of and Adverse Reactions to Antitumour Antibiotics

Drug	**Therapeutic Indications**	**Toxicities and Adverse Reactions**
Actinomycin D	Childhood tumours — Wilms' tumour, Ewing's sarcoma, other sarcomas Adult tumours — choriocarcinoma, testicular tumours	Nausea and vomiting Oral mucositis Dermatological reactions — alopecia, radiation recall, erythema Myelosuppression Tissue necrosis if extravasated
Bleomycin	Squamous cell carcinoma Testicular tumours Lymphoma	Fever, shaking chills Oral mucositis Dermatological manifestation Pulmonary toxicity
Daunorubicin	Acute leukaemia	Nausea and vomiting Myelosuppression Alopecia Oral mucositis Dermatological manifestation Cardiotoxicity Tissue necrosis if extravasated
Doxorubicin	Acute leukaemia Lymphoma Wide range of solid tumours — carcinoma and sarcoma	As for daunorubicin
Mitomycin C	Carcinoma of gastrointestinal tracts, lung, pancreas and breast	Myelosuppression Nausea and vomiting Diarrhoea Dermatitis Alopecia Tissue necrosis if extravasated

MITOTIC INHIBITORS

This group of antineoplastic agents block cell mitosis (division) with metaphase (the second stage of mitosis) arrest.

The two subgroups of mitotic inhibitors are the ***vinca alkaloids*** — vincristine, vinblastine and vindesine — which are extracted from the periwinkle plant, *Vinca rosea*; and the ***epipodophyllotoxin derivatives*** — VP16-213 (etoposide) and VM-26 (teniposide).

Table 80
Mitotic Inhibitors

Generic Name	Brand Name	Strength	Administration
1. *Vinca Alkaloids*			
Vinblastine	*Velbe*	10 mg vials	Slow injection into fast running IV infusion
Vincristine	*Oncovin*	1 mg vials 2 mg vials 5 mg vials	Slow injection into fast running IV infusion
Vindesine	*Eldisine*	5 mg vials	Slow injection into fast running IV infusion
2. *Epipodophyllotoxin Derivatives*			
VP16-213 (Etoposide)	*Vepesid*	100 mg/5 mL	Slow IV infusion in 300 to 500 mL N/S over 1 hour

N/S: Normal saline

VINCA ALKALOIDS

During the 1950s crude fractions from the periwinkle plant were investigated as oral hypoglycaemic agents. The discovery that they had an effect on cells of rapidly proliferating tissue such as bone marrow led to their development as anticancer agents. Structurally, vincristine and vinblastine are very similar, but there are some differences in their clinical activity and potential toxicities. The lack of cross-resistance between these agents is an important and surprising feature. It seems likely that these drugs bind specifically with the protein tubulin which is an important component of the microtubules. Other drugs such as colchicine and podophyllotoxin act by the same mechanism.

Vincristine

Vincristine has a broad spectrum of clinical activity, producing beneficial responses in acute leukaemia, blast crisis phase of chronic leukaemia, Hodgkin's disease and non-Hodgkin's lymphomas, Wilms' tumour, brain tumours, a variety of sarcomas, and carcinomas of the breast, testis, ovary and cervix.

The major adverse reaction to vincristine is neurotoxicity. This presents primarily as a peripheral neuropathy with paraesthesias, numbness and tingling of extremities, loss of deep tendon reflex, muscular and neuritic pain, foot drop, headache, double vision and hoarseness. The more severe manifestations may be avoided by discontinuation or reduced dosage at the time of occurrence of minor symptoms. Bone-marrow suppression is rarely a problem. Severe constipation may be prevented by routine administration of laxatives such as *Dorbanex* and *Dioctyl*. Other adverse effects observed include alopecia, stomatitis, nausea and vomiting. The syndrome of inappropriate ADH secretion resulting in low serum sodium levels has been reported.

Vinblastine

Vinblastine has a spectrum of activity similar to that of vincristine. It is effective in the treatment of acute and chronic leukaemias, Hodgkin's disease and non-Hodgkin's lymphomas, neuroblastoma, as well as carcinomas of the breast, lung, oral cavity, testis and bladder.

Neurotoxicity is far less of a problem with vinblastine than with vincristine, though neurological manifestations such as temporary mental depressions, paraesthesias and loss of deep-tendon reflex may occur. Unlike vincristine, vinblastine may cause significant myelosuppression, so any indications of infection or bleeding should be reported. Gastrointestinal disturbances including nausea, vomiting, anorexia and diarrhoea may occur — administration of antiemetic and antidiarrhoeal agents may give symptomatic relief. Symptoms related to dysfunction of the autonomic nervous system such as constipation, paralytic ileus, abdominal pain and urinary retention may be encountered — the use of drugs such as *Dioctyl* and *Buscopan* (one four times daily) is often beneficial in alleviating these problems. Extravasation during administration may cause cellulitis and phlebitis. Application of ice packs may help. Other less common adverse reactions include alopecia, dermatitis, oral mucositis and rectal bleeding.

Vindesine

Vindesine is a new semisynthetic vinca alkaloid. Like vincristine and vinblastine, it causes metaphase arrest by interfering with the spindle structure of the cell. Like the other vinca alkaloids, vindesine is active against acute and chronic leukaemias, Hodgkin's and non-Hodgkin's lymphoma. There have been reports of activity against carcinoma of the breast, lung and kidney.

The major adverse reactions of vindesine are myelosuppression (particularly of white blood cells) and neurotoxicity which manifests in a manner similar to that induced by vincristine. Nausea and vomiting may occur but are usually mild. Vindesine is a potent vesicant, producing cellulitis and phlebitis on extravasation. Care should be taken with administration. Other less common effects include alopecia, stomatitis, and possible photosensitivity reactions.

EPIPODOPHYLLOTOXINS

This group of drugs is derived from the may-apple or mandrake plant. Recent studies of the mechanism of action of these agents suggest that they have a different site of action to the classic spindle poisons such as the vinca alkaloids. A two-fold mechanism of action is suggested — metaphase arrest and prevention of cells from entering mitosis by acting in the G_2 phase of the cell cycle. ***Etoposide*** *(VP 16-213)* is the epipodophyllotoxin currently in use in the UK.

This class of drugs is highly lipid soluble and has the ability to cross the blood-brain barrier. The spectrum of activity and side effects of these agents is similar. Malignancies against which they are effective include acute monocytic leukaemia, small cell anaplastic carcinoma of the lung, Hodgkin's disease and non-Hodgkin's lymphoma, carcinoma of the breast, bladder, thyroid, kidney and testis, and CNS tumour.

Some nausea may result from administration of these agents though this is usually mild when given alone. Anorexia and vomiting occur less often. Bone-marrow suppression (leukopenia and thrombocytopenia) necessitates regular (usually weekly) monitoring of blood counts. Since these agents are lipid soluble, the patient may experience fever, shaking, chills and hypotension. Slowing of the rate of infusion and administration of promethazine *(Phenergan)* 25 mg IM may help. Alopecia and stomatitis have also been reported. As a result of its derivation from podophyllotoxins, etoposide may cause vein irritation — slowing the infusion rate may decrease any stinging sensation.

MISCELLANEOUS AGENTS

Miscellaneous antitumour agents include aminoglutethimide, m-AMSA, L-asparaginase, dacarbazine, hexamethylmelamine, hydroxyurea, mitotane, the nitrosoureas (carmustine, lomustine, semustine, streptozocin), cis-platinum, procarbazine, steroids and tamoxifen.

AMINOGLUTETHIMIDE (250 mg tablet)

This agent exerts its effect on hormonally-sensitive tumours, such as breast and prostatic carcinoma, by producing a "medical adrenalectomy" by the prevention of steroid synthesis. It is used in the treatment of advanced breast cancer.

The most common side effects are gastric discomfort, drowsiness and lethargy, and adrenal insufficiency, which usually requires replacement therapy. A morbilliform rash may occur within the first week of therapy — this spontaneously settles within four to five days. Less common adverse reactions include myelosuppression, facial flushing, virilisation and respiratory depression.

Table 81
Therapeutic Uses of and Adverse Reactions to Mitotic Inhibitors

Drug	Therapeutic Indications	Toxicities and Adverse Reactions
Vinblastine	Acute leukaemia Lymphoma Neuroblastoma Carcinoma of breast, lung, oral cavity, testis, bladder	Myelosuppression Nausea and vomiting Constipation Abdominal cramps Tissue necrosis if extravasated
Vincristine	Acute leukaemia Lymphoma Wilms' tumour Brain tumours Sarcoma Carcinoma of breast, testis, ovary, cervix, lung	Nausea and vomiting Neurotoxicity Constipation Tissue necrosis if extravasated
Vindesine	Acute leukaemia Lymphoma Carcinoma of breast, lung and kidney	Myelosuppression Neurotoxicity Nausea and vomiting Tissue necrosis if extravasated
Etoposide	Acute myoblastic leukaemia Small cell carcinoma of the lung Lymphoma Carcinoma of breast, bladder, thyroid, testis, brain	Myelosuppression Fever, shaking chills Hypotension Vein irritation

m-AMSA

m-AMSA (acridinyl anisidide) is a new IV agent currently undergoing trials to determine its activity against various malignancies. It is an acridine dye (like acriflavine) that inhibits DNA synthesis and binds to DNA. It is administered as an IV infusion in 500 mL of 5% dextrose over at least one hour.

The dose-limiting toxicity is bone-marrow suppression: thrombocytopenia is less severe than leukopenia. Mild nausea and vomiting may be encountered. Thrombophlebitis has been reported; this can be avoided by slowing the rate of infusion. Other toxicities infrequently seen include alopecia, local irritation on extravasation, mucositis and cardiac arrhythmias.

L-ASPARAGINASE

This drug inhibits the enzyme asparagine synthetase and depletes cells of asparagine, which is an essential growth requirement of certain neoplastic tissues. Its primary indication is acute lymphoblastic leukaemia.

Responses have been seen in other forms of leukaemia, non-Hodgkin's lymphomas, and malignant melanoma. L-asparaginase is derived from two bacterial sources, *E. coli* and *Erwinia* species.

The drug has minimal effects on bone marrow and mucosal surfaces but severe toxicities affecting the liver, kidney, pancreas, CNS (lethargy, somnolence, depression) and clotting mechanisms are observed. Since L-asparaginase is a foreign protein, hypersensitivity reactions ranging from mild allergic type to anaphylaxis have been reported.

DACARBAZINE (100 mg, 200 mg vials)

Imidazole carboxamide (***dacarbazine*** *(DTIC)*) was initially believed to act as an antimetabolite. More recent studies, however, indicate that its mechanism of action is more likely to be by alkylation after metabolic activation by the liver. Its primary use is in the treatment of malignant melanoma, though it has shown some activity against soft-tissue sarcomas.

Nausea and vomiting and a flu-like illness may occur. Occasional myelosuppression is observed and hepatotoxicity has been reported. Alopecia, facial flushing, paraesthesia occur less frequently. DTIC is an irritant to the veins, and the rate of infusion may need to be decreased if patients complain of a "stinging" sensation. Extravasation of the drug can cause a severe cellulitis, so care should be taken with administration.

HEXAMETHYLMELAMINE (50 mg, 100 mg capsules)

This drug is an investigational agent demonstrating activity against bronchogenic, ovarian and bladder carcinomas. Its mechanism of action is unclear.

It is taken orally. Since it may cause quite severe nausea and vomiting, it is often administered with or after food to minimise these problems. Other adverse reactions include bone-marrow suppression, dermatologic manifestations (rash, pruritus, eczematous skin lesions) and neurologic manifestations (numbness, ataxia, insomnia).

HYDROXYUREA (Hydrea 500mg capsules)

The primary site of action of hydroxyurea is the enzyme ribonucleoside diphosphate reductase. Inhibition of this enzyme causes inhibition of DNA synthesis.

The principal use of this drug is in the treatment of chronic granulocytic leukaemia. Bone-marrow suppression is the major toxic effect. Other reactions include macropapular rash and megaloblastoid changes.

MITOTANE (500 mg tablets)

Mitotane ***(o,p'DDD,*** *Lysodren)* is an oral agent which causes destruction of the adrenal cortex. Its only use is in the palliative (symptomatic) treatment of adrenocortical carcinomas. The initial dose is usually 4 to 6 grams daily, increasing to the maximum tolerated dose (usually 12 to 16 grams daily).

Anorexia and nausea are common side effects. Mental depression, lethargy, visual disturbances and dermatitis are observed frequently.

NITROSOUREAS

These agents are highly lipid soluble and their ability to cross the blood-brain barrier has led to their use in the treatment of meningeal leukaemia and CNS tumours.

Carmustine or BiCNU (100 mg vials)

This was the first of the nitrosoureas to be used clinically and is effective against a range of malignancies, including Hodgkin's disease and other lymphomas, carcinoma of the breast, lung and gastrointestinal tract, meningeal leukaemia, primary brain tumours and myeloma. Tissue uptake of the drug after IV administration is rapid.

The most significant side effect is delayed bone-marrow suppression, which may not be evident until some three to four weeks after dosage. Nausea and vomiting, oesophagitis, flushing of the skin and CNS toxicity have been noted. BiCNU is not a vesicant, but local burning pain on administration is common and may necessitate slowing of the infusion. Cases of renal and hepatic toxicity have been reported.

Lomustine or CCNU (10 mg, 40 mg capsules)

Although a parenteral form of this drug is available investigationally, it is usually administered orally. Active metabolites appear in the CSF within 30 minutes of administration. Beneficial effects have been reported on its use in the treatment of Hodgkin's disease and other lymphomas, malignant gliomas, carcinoma of the breast and prostate, adenocarcinomas of the gastrointestinal tract, malignant melanoma and small-cell carcinomas of the lung.

Its toxicity is limited to nausea and vomiting, which is common, and delayed bone-marrow suppression.

Semustine or Methyl CCNU (1 mg, 50 mg, 100 mg capsules)

Methyl CCNU is usually administered orally although a parenteral form is available. Although this agent has activity against many of the same tumours as its two previously mentioned analogues, its effectiveness is mostly inferior to CCNU and BiCNU. Its primary use is in combination with 5-fluorouracil in the treatment of colorectal carcinomas.

As with CCNU, the principal dose-limiting toxicity is delayed bone-marrow suppression. Nausea and vomiting occur frequently and may be severe.

Streptozocin (1 g vials)

Streptozocin is a naturally occurring antibiotic nitrosourea which is isolated from the fungus *Streptomyces acromogones.* It demonstrates a unique cytotoxicity for beta-cells of the pancreatic islets. Its use is limited to the treatment of functional, malignant islet-cell carcinoma of the pancreas and metastatic carcinoid tumours.

Nausea and vomiting are experienced by most patients. Bone-marrow suppression (leukopenia, thrombocytopenia, anaemia) is common. Reversible renal and hepatic function abnormalities have been reported, as well as neurological manifestations, most commonly dizziness and ataxia. Rigors may occur during administration.

CIS-PLATINUM (Cis-Diamminodichloroplatinum)

Although the exact mechanism of action of this agent is uncertain, the target of the drug is DNA. Since its development in 1969, it has demonstrated activity against testicular, ovarian, genitourinary, head and neck, prostatic and osteogenic malignancies.

The dose-limiting toxicity is nephrotoxicity — a total cumulative dose of 600 mg/m^2 is rarely exceeded. This toxicity presents as renal proximal tubular damage similar to that of heavy metal poisoning. Special IV infusion regime, including pre-therapy and post-therapy hydration and concomitant administration of mannitol, is employed to minimise the risk of renal toxicity. Dose-related myelosuppression, including anaemia, is observed. Nausea and vomiting, often severe and usually resistant to antiemetics, and high-frequency hearing loss are common.

Table 82
Miscellaneous Agents

Drug	**Therapeutic Indications**	**Toxicities and Adverse Reactions**
Aminoglutethimide	Breast carcinoma	Drowsiness, lethargy Rash Adrenal insufficiency
m-AMSA		Fever Phlebitis Myelosuppression Electrolyte disturbances Cardiac arrhythmias Oral mucositis
L-asparaginase	Acute lymphocytic leukaemia	Hepatotoxicity Nephrotoxicity CNS toxicity Hypersensitivity reactions Effects on clotting mechanisms
Dacarbazine	Melanoma	Nausea and vomiting Fever Hepatotoxicity Tissue necrosis if extravasated

continued

Hexamethylmelamine	Carcinoma of ovary and lung Lymphoma	Nausea and vomiting Myelosuppression Skin reactions Neurotoxicity
Hydroxyurea	Chronic myelocytic leukaemia	Myelosuppression Rash
Mitotane	Adrenal carcinoma	Anorexia, nausea Mental depression Lethargy Visual disturbances Dermatitis
Nitrosoureas Carmustine	Lymphoma Carcinoma of breast, lung, gastrointestinal tract, brain Multiple myeloma	Nausea and vomiting Myelosuppression Pulmonary toxicity CNS toxicity Tissue necrosis if extravasated
Lomustine	Lymphoma Brain tumours Carcinoma of breast, prostate, lung, gastrointestinal tract	Nausea and vomiting Myelosuppression
Semustine	Colorectal carcinoma	Nausea and vomiting Myelosuppression
Streptozocin	Metastatic islet cell carcinoma of pancreas Carcinoid Lymphoma	Nausea and vomiting Shaking chills Hypoglycaemia Myelosuppression Nephrotoxicity
Cis-platinum	Carcinoma of testis, ovary, genitourinary tract, head and neck Osteogenic sarcoma	Nausea and vomiting Nephrotoxicity Myelosuppression, especially anaemia Ototoxicity
Procarbazine	Lymphoma CNS tumours Small cell carcinoma of lung Multiple myeloma	Nausea and vomiting Myelosuppression Dermatitis CNS disturbances Postural hypotension
Tamoxifen	Carcinoma of breast and prostate Melanoma	Hot flushes Nausea Skin rash

PROCARBAZINE (Natulan 50 mg capsules)

This oral methylhydrazine derivative is a mild monoamine oxidase inhibitor whose mechanism of cytotoxic action is uncertain. The primary indication for its use is Hodgkin's disease, though it also has some activity against oat-cell carcinoma of the lung, non-Hodgkin's lymphomas, myeloma and some brain tumours.

The most common toxicities include bone-marrow suppression, anaemia, nausea and vomiting, which may initially be severe. Dermatologic and neurologic manifestations have been reported. Neurologic reactions include lethargy, depression, drowsiness, CNS hyperexcitability and myalgia. Alcohol may cause intense warmth and reddening of the face. and an *Antabuse*-like reaction. As procarbazine is a mild monoamine oxidase inhibitor, hypertensive reactions may occur from its use concurrently with sympathomimetic agents, tricyclic antidepressants and foods high in tyramine.

STEROIDS

The pharmacology, major clinical uses and toxicities of these agents are discussed in Chapter 11.

Corticosteroids *(prednisone, prednisolone, dexamethasone, hydrocortisone)*

The mechanism of cytotoxic action of the corticosteroids is unclear but their ability to suppress mitosis in lymphocytes makes them of value in the treatment of acute and chronic lymphocytic leukaemia and malignant lymphomas. They also demonstrate activity against multiple myeloma and carcinoma of the breast.

Hormonal Steroids

Certain organs in the body are dependent upon hormones for their growth and function. Tumours arising from these organs may be treated by hormonal manipulation. These tumours are, particularly, carcinomas of the breast, prostate and endometrium, though other malignancies, such as renal carcinoma, may also benefit from this form of therapy. The agents used include ***drostanolone propionate*** *(Masteril)*, an androgen, oestrogens such as ***stilboestrol*** and progestogens such as ***medroxyprogesterone.***

TAMOXIFEN (Nolvadex)

Tamoxifen is an "anti-oestrogenic" compound which exerts its action by binding to oestrogen receptor sites on tumour cells, thereby preventing those sites from binding oestrogen which encourages the growth of certain tumours. Its principal use is in the treatment of breast carcinoma, though it has demonstrated activity against malignant melanoma and some renal carcinomas.

NURSING IMPLICATIONS

Nurses administering cytotoxic drugs must know the specific toxicities of each. The medical officer must be notified if signs of toxicity are observed, so that dosage can be reduced or ceased. Nursing interventions appropriate for the specific toxic effects of each of the large range of drugs in use is beyond the scope of this book, and reference to the extensive literature on oncological nursing is recommended.

The following discussion refers to the more generalised effects encountered in the use of drugs whose actions are cytotoxic. Trester's paper "Nursing management of patients receiving cancer chemotherapy" presents a comprehensive review of adverse reactions and appropriate nursing interventions.[1]

Assessments

The full-blood count, including differential white-cell count and platelet count, must be available before each cycle of therapy begins, since haematological toxicity is the major dose-limiting toxicity of many of these agents.

Any sign of infection (especially fever), is significant, since the patient may be neutropenic either from the effects of the neoplasm or previous drug treatment. Treatment with broad-spectrum antibiotics is indicated, to prevent a potentially fatal infection. The choice of antibiotics will vary from hospital to hospital but may include a broad-spectrum semisynthetic penicillin or a cephalosporin, and an aminoglycoside. It is imperative that, while cultures should be taken, the antibiotics must be started immediately. Non-absorbable oral antibiotics and antifungals such as neomycin and nystatin are commonly employed for prophylaxis against infection from normal body bacterial flora and fungal overgrowth in patients who are neutropenic for long periods of time, such as patients with acute leukaemia undergoing induction therapy.

The possibility of alopecia is best discussed with the patient before therapy begins. It should be stressed that hair loss is temporary, and arrangements to fit a wig or to wear some other form of head covering can be made before alopecia occurs. Alopecia need not be seen as a primary reason for refusing therapy. Contact with other patients and discussion of ways in which they have dealt with hair loss may be helpful in overcoming anxiety. Patients should know that all body hair will be affected.

Previous patterns of nausea and vomiting should be identified, so that intervention can be planned to minimize its effects in individual patients. Previous response to antiemetic drugs should also be documented.

The specific toxicities of each drug in a particular regimen or protocol should be known, so that specific baseline assessments such as cardiac and pulmonary function tests can be carried out before the beginning of each cycle.

Administration

Because some of these agents may cause severe chemical cellulitis should they be extravasated, great care must be taken to ensure that proper administration precautions are followed. Drugs having this potential include adriamycin, daunorubicin, actinomycin D, mitomycin C, DTIC, vincristine, vinblastine, BiCNU and nitrogen mustard. These drugs are administered as slow IV infusions or as slow IV push into the side arm of a fast-running IV infusion.

Although the use of chemical names incorporating numbers or letters is generally avoided, the abbreviations 5FU (5-fluorouracil), 6TG-6 thioguanine), and 6-MP (6-mercaptopurine) are still often used by prescribers, and nurses must take care to administer the correct dosage.

When high dosages of methotrexate are used, followed by folinic acid rescue, it is *imperative* that folinic acid be administered at exactly the prescribed time after the methotrexate dose, to prevent methotrexate toxicity. The distinction must be made between folinic acid and folic acid, since folic acid will have no effect, and death may occur if "rescue" is delayed. Supplies of folinic acid (calcium leucovorin) must be on hand when the methotrexate therapy is started.

Adverse reactions often require treatment with other drugs. Common examples are:

(a) *Liquifilm* tears (or similar products) may be required if the patient loses his eye lashes;

(b) frequent, regular mouthwashes with saline, or products such as *Corsodyl* and *Eludril*, are required for oral hygiene when stomatitis is a problem; *Nystatin Oral Suspension* is commonly used to prevent fungal suprainfection;

(c) allopurinol may be used to prevent hyperuricaemia caused by the increased nitrogenous wastes resulting from cell breakdown;

(d) antidiarrhoeal medications and laxatives.

The adverse reaction that is most unpleasant for the patient is the high incidence of nausea and vomiting that occurs with many cytotoxic drugs. Adequate antiemetic cover must be given, and the routine use of antiemetic drugs for 24 to 48 hours after therapy is often beneficial. Conventional agents such as metoclopramide *(Maxolon, Primperan)*, prochlorperazine *(Stemetil)*, domperidone *(Motilium)* and thiethylperazine *(Torecan)* are commonly used. Intractable vomiting may require the administration of drugs such as diazepam *(Valium)*, chlorpromazine *(Largactil)*, lorazepam *(Ativan)* or dexamethasone *(Decadron)* in an effort to control this problem. The patient's response to antiemetic drugs should be documented for future reference.

Evaluation

Nursing evaluation of cytotoxic therapy is most directly concerned with evaluation of adverse effects. Some effects may be so severe that doses need to be reduced or therapy ceased.

The medical officer must be notified of any sign of infection. Temperature and white-cell counts should be monitored, and signs of infection should be looked for. However, when the patient is neutropenic or taking steroids, inflammation may not be evident. Trauma to the skin should be avoided, by such measures as use of an electric razor, rather than a safety razor. Visitors (and staff) may need to be screened for infection. Protective isolation may become necessary if severe leucopenia develops.

The platelet count should be monitored for thrombocytopenia. Any sign of haemorrhage should be reported. Intramuscular and subcutaneous injections are best avoided, and the sites of invasive procedures need to be observed for bleeding.

Anaemia is likely, and haemoglobin levels, haematocrit and red-cell counts should be measured regularly. Nursing activities should be planned to allow adequate periods of rest. Blood transfusion may become necessary.

Evaluation of fluid and electrolyte balance is critical in patients who are vomiting or have diarrhoea, or both, and who may not be able to tolerate any oral fluids. Intravenous fluid therapy will often be necessary to maintain hydration.

Stomatitis is a common problem following administration of cytotoxic drugs, especially methotrexate, adriamycin, daunomycin, actinomycin D, 5-fluorouracil and cyclophosphamide. This reaction ranges from mild to severe mucosal ulceration necessitating a reduction in the dosage of the offending agent. The mucous membranes of the mouth should be inspected regularly, and gentle oral hygiene measures performed frequently. A bland diet, excluding hot and spicy foods, is usually most suitable. Pureed food, a fluid diet or tube feeding might become necessary. Changes in taste sensations, nausea and vomiting can diminish the appetite so that the provision of sufficient kilojoules to maintain anabolic metabolism can become a problem.

Some cytotoxic drugs are excreted more readily at alkaline pH. Each specimen of urine should be pH tested, and oral sodium bicarbonate is usually prescribed to maintain an alkaline urinary pH.

The medical officer should be notified at the first indication of any specific toxicity, such as haematuria or dysuria in patients receiving cyclophosphamide.

Patient teaching

Patients must be informed about the expected outcomes of cytotoxic treatment, its adverse effects, and ways in which they can minimise those effects. Some patients will choose not to be treated, and others may decide not to continue with treatment if the adverse effects become unacceptable.

Teaching must start before chemotherapy begins, and the information must be given at times when the patient is ready and able to receive it. Family members will usually need to be included, since their support and help is crucial.

Information should include: expected results of treatment (palliation, remission, cure); generalised adverse effects of cytotoxics; likelihood of hair loss and eventual regrowth; the need to seek attention for infection and to avoid contact with persons suffering from infections; oral hygiene measures; dietary modification; prevention of trauma; observation for bleeding; the need to take adequate rest; the need for birth-control measures during treatment to avoid the risk of teratogenesis; and signs of specific toxicities of individual drug regimes.

Several studies have shown that adequate educational programmes can help cancer patients receiving cytotoxic therapy to reduce adverse effects and to initiate self-care early and successfully.[2,3]

References

1. Trester AK. Nursing management of patients receiving cancer chemotherapy. *Cancer Nursing*, 1982; 5(3): 201-210.
2. Dodd MJ. Assessing patient self-care for side effects of cancer chemotherapy. *Cancer Nursing*, 1982; 5(6): 447-451.
3. Dodd MJ. Self-care for side effects in cancer chemotherapy: an assessment of nursing interventions, Part II. *Cancer Nursing*, 1983; 6(1): 63-67.

SELF-EVALUATION TEST

1. According to mechanism of action, place the following drugs in the correct classification.

Drugs	**Classification**
Cyclophosphamide	Alkylating agent
Doxorubicin	Antimetabolite
Melphalan	Mitotic inhibitor
Etoposide	Antitumour antibiotic
Bleomycin	
Methotrexate	
Cytosine arabinoside	
5-fluorouracil	
Cis-platinum	
Chlorambucil	

2. A patient with small-cell anaplastic cancer of the lung, being treated with cyclophosphamide, doxorubicin and vincristine, complains of a tingling sensation in his fingers and toes. Which drug, if any, is the most likely cause of this problem?
3. Name two treatment modalities other than chemotherapy for a malignancy.
4. Name the two groups of highly lipid-soluble drugs that have the ability to cross the blood-brain barrier, achieving high concentrations in the CNS.
5. A young man with an osteogenic sarcoma is to commence therapy with "high-dose methotrexate". What precautions must be taken?
6. A patient with acute lymphocytic leukaemia, being treated with 6-mercaptopurine, is found to be hyperuricaemic. The doctor wishes to commence allopurinol. What precautions must be taken and why?
7. Name the four major side effects of the cytotoxic drugs.
8. Define the terms cytotoxic, cancer, malignant, alopecia and neoplasm.

Table 83
Antineoplastic Agents

Drug Group	Drug Name	Use	Action	Adverse Reactions	Nursing Implications
Antineoplastic Agents	Mustine Nitrogen mustard Cyclophosphamide Chlorambucil Melphalan Busulphan Thiotepa Methotrexate 5-fluorouracil 5-azacytidine 6-mercaptopurine 6-thioguanine Actinomycin D Bleomycin Daunorubicin Doxorubicin Mithramycin Mitomycin Vinblastine Vincristine Vindesine Etoposide Aminoglutethimide m-AMSA L-asparaginase Dacarbazine Hexamethylmelamine Hydroxyurea Mitotane Carmustine Lomustine Semustine Streptozocin Cis-platinum Procarbazine	See previous tables in this chapter and body of chapter	See previous tables in this chapter and body of chapter	See previous tables in this chapter and body of chapter	***Assess:*** full-blood count and differential; for any sign of infection; previous history of nausea, vomiting; baseline tests for specific toxicities. ***Administer:*** slow IV infusion or slow IV push through side arm to fast IV infusion; avoid extravasation; correct dose, where numbers and letters are used in generic names; artificial tears if eye lashes lost; antiemetics before and during treatment; mouthwashes; antifungal oral suspension; allopurinol to prevent hyperuricaemia; antidiarrhoeals or laxatives; folinic acid at exactly prescribed time after high dose of methotrexate. ***Evaluate:*** general and specific adverse effects; for infection; bone-marrow response; for trauma; adequate rest; for ulceration of buccal membranes; kilojoule intake, to ensure anabolism; fluid and electrolyte balance — for dehydration or oedema; urinary pH and output; changes in body image — emotional reactions; need for emotional support. ***Teach:*** expected outcome; adverse effects; self-care measures to prevent and treat adverse effects; dietary modification; to seek medical attention for infection; need for contraception.

SECTION 8

28
PSYCHOPHARMACOLOGY

Virginia E. Richardson

OBJECTIVES

At the conclusion of this chapter the reader should be able to:

1. list the different classes of drugs used in the treatment of psychiatric disturbances;
2. list the basic pharmacological actions of each class of drugs;
3. identify which classes of drugs are used to treat the major psychiatric disorders;
4. itemise the more important adverse effects and the toxic effects of each class of drugs.

PREREQUISITE KNOWLEDGE

1. An understanding of the major categories of psychiatric disturbances.
2. A knowledge of the anatomy and physiology of the central nervous system.

Psychotherapeutic drugs are palliative, not curative. There are many drugs available for the treatment of a variety of conditions including schizophrenia or mania, depressive illness, anxiety and insomnia. Drugs must not be relied upon solely as treatment for psychiatric disturbances but should be used in conjunction with other forms of therapy such as psychotherapy, group therapy and relaxation therapy.

When commencing treatment with psychotherapeutic drugs, small doses should be used initially to minimise side effects and to enable a gradual build-up to the optimum therapeutic dose required by the individual. Treatment with psychotherapeutic agents may be chronic or intermittent depending on the type or severity of psychiatric disorder.

Patients suffering from some psychiatric disorders may have difficulty complying with complicated drug treatment regimens; many of the psychotherapeutic agents have long half-lives and may be administered as a once-daily dose which aids in improving compliance.

Many medically used drugs can induce psychiatric symptoms even when used in therapeutic doses, but more especially when they are abused. Elderly patients are particularly sensitive to such effects. The centrally acting antihypertensive agents, anticholinergic agents, anti-anxiety drugs, alcohol, caffeine and other central stimulants are particularly liable to produce such effects.

Table 84
Classification of Psychotherapeutic Agents

1. **Neuroleptics** (formerly major tranquillisers or antipsychotic drugs)
   Definition: Drugs with therapeutic effects on psychoses and other types of psychiatric disorders
   Phenothiazines, e.g. chlorpromazine
   Butyrophenones, e.g. droperidol
   Thioxanthines, e.g. flupenthixol
   Diphenylbutylpiperidines, e.g. pimozide

2. **Antimanic**
   Definition: Drugs effective in the treatment of manic states
   Lithium carbonate

3. **Anxiolytic sedatives** (formerly minor tranquillisers or sedatives)
   Definition: Substances which reduce pathological anxiety, tension and agitation without therapeutic effect on disturbed cognitive or perceptual processes
   Barbiturates, e.g. amylobarbitone
   Propanedioles, e.g. meprobamate
   Benzodiazepines, e.g. diazepam

4. **Antidepressants**
   Definition: Drugs effective in the treatment of pathological depressive states
   Tricyclics, e.g. amitriptyline
   Tetracyclics, e.g. mianserin
   Monoamine oxidase inhibitors (MAOI), e.g. tranylcypromine

5. **Psychostimulants**
   Definition: Drugs which increase the level of alertness and/or motivation
   Amphetamine
   Caffeine
   Methylphenidate
   Cocaine

6. **Hypnotics**
   Definition: Drugs which are used to induce sleep
   Barbiturates
   Benzodiazepines
   Miscellaneous

NEUROLEPTICS

Neuroleptics were formerly known as major tranquillisers or antipsychotic drugs.

The neuroleptic drugs are used to alleviate the symptoms of major psychiatric illnesses, that is, to treat the psychoses rather than the neuroses. Neuroleptic drugs are palliative, not curative. They prevent relapse and enable the patient to function within the community. Schizophrenia is the major condition in which neuroleptics are used. About 1% of the population is estimated to be suffering from some form of schizophrenia. Other conditions which respond to neuroleptic therapy include organic psychoses and the manic phase of manic depressive illness.

Chlorpromazine, the first neuroleptic drug to be introduced (1952), revolutionised the treatment of psychotic patients. Prior to its introduction, the psychotic patient was institutionalised and had very little hope of rehabilitation or recovery. Drug treatment of these patients was limited to massive doses of bromides and barbiturates.

Chlorpromazine belongs to a class of chemically related substances called phenothiazines. Following the introduction of chlorpromazine, a number of phenothiazine substances were marketed as well as a number of non-phenothiazine substances which were also discovered to possess antipsychotic activity.

Table 85
Neuroleptic Agents

Class	Generic Name	Trade Name	Daily Dose Range (mg)
Phenothiazines	Chlorpromazine	*Largactil*	50–1600
	Fluphenazine	*Moditen*	2.5–20
		Modecate	12.5–100
	Perphenazine	*Fentazin*	12–24
	Trifluoperazine	*Stelazine*	4–60
	Thioridazine	*Melleril*	30–200
	Trimeprazine	*Vallergan*	10–40
	Pericyazine	*Neulactil*	15–75
Butyrophenones	Haloperidol	*Serenace*	2–100
	Droperidol	*Droleptan*	2–100
Thioxanthines	Flupenthixol	*Depixol*	3–18
Diphenylbutyl piperidines	Pimozide	*Orap*	2–20

The neuroleptics are usually given orally as tablets, capsules or syrups. A number of them are also available in injectable form. Of particular importance is the slow-release injectable form of the phenothiazine compound, fluphenazine decanoate (*Modecate*). This is an oil-soluble depot preparation and is administered IM at 2 to 4 weekly intervals. It is gradually released over a period of time. It is of use in patients who are poor compliers with tablet therapy or those who have poor absorption of orally administered drugs.

Administration

Parenteral phenothiazine administration should be given by deep intramuscular injection, because solutions are extremely irritating. Nursing staff should take care not to spill such substances on their skin or in the event of spillage to wash the area well with water as skin irritation may ensue. In general avoid mixing injection solutions in the same syringe due to the risk of chemical and physical incompatibility.

To obtain rapid control of violent or dangerous behaviour, a technique known as "rapid neuroleptisation" may be used. This involves single or repeated intramuscular or intravenous administration of fluphenazine hydrochloride or haloperidol, alone or in combination with intravenous diazepam. Such a technique should be used only in physically healthy patients, and close clinical observation should be maintained for emergence of cardiovascular and neurological side effects. Dosage schedules will vary depending upon the clinical circumstances.

Action

All classes of neuroleptics are believed to act by blocking the action of the chemical transmitter dopamine in the mesolimbic area, globus pallidus and corpus striatum of the brain. The drugs may cause a lack of initiative, disinterest in the environment, reduced display of emotion, slowness in response to external stimuli and drowsiness. Patients are easily aroused and seem to have intact intellectual function, and are less agitated, restless and impulsive. Although some neuroleptics may cause drowsiness it must be emphasised that they do not exert their action by sedation. Sedative effects are merely secondary to antipsychotic effects. With the exception of thioridazine all the neuroleptics are powerful anti-emetics.

Adverse Drug Reactions

Because the neuroleptic drugs act on all organ systems and have many autonomic properties, a number of adverse effects may be expected. These occur to varying degrees with the different compounds available and include the following.

Sedation — particularly with chlorpromazine and thioridazine; however, tolerance can develop to this effect.

Autonomic effects — including dry mouth, blurred vision, constipation, urinary hesitation or retention — especially prevalent with thioridazine and chlorpromazine.

Endocrine effects — these effects are more common in women and include breast enlargement and lactation, also alterations in the menstrual cycle.

Dermatological effects — photosensitivity, especially in fair-skinned patients, may be a problem with chlorpromazine.

Ocular effects — with thioridazine, deposition of pigment in the retina, cornea and lens is possible. Retinopathy with loss of visual acuity may occur with thioridazine in doses exceeding 800 mg per day over a extended period.

Hepatic effects — all neuroleptics can affect liver function and cause jaundice. The problem is most common with chlorpromazine.

Haemopoietic effects — depression of white-cell count is possible although extremely rare with neuroleptics.

Cardiovascular effects — changes in ECG readings and hypotension, especially in elderly patients on high doses, may be a problem. Thioridazine and chlorpromazine have been implicated most often. Haloperidol may also cause hypotension when administered IV.

Seizures — all neuroleptics, especially in high doses, have the potential to lower the seizure threshold in epileptic and non-epileptic patients.

Extrapyramidal effects — all neuroleptics cause extrapyramidal effects to varying degrees. This is due to their ability to block dopaminergic transmission. As stated previously, the blockade of dopaminergic transmission is the main mechanism by which neuroleptics exert their antipsychotic action. Extrapyramidal effects may manifest within a few hours and up to several months after commencing therapy. The effects seen are akinesia, akathesia, acute dystonic reactions and drug-induced Parkinsonism. They may be reduced or eliminated by dose reduction of the neuroleptic or by administration of anti-Parkinsonian medications such as benzhexol (*Artane*), benztropine (*Cogentin*), procyclidine (*Kemadrin*), orphenadrine (*Disipal*), and amantadine (*Symmetrel*).

Late onset or tardive dyskinesia may occur in some patients following long-term treatment exceeding one year. It may occur with any of the currently available drugs and is more prevalent in elderly patients. In some cases tardive dyskinesia may be irreversible even on discontinuation of neuroleptics, and no effective treatment is available. All patients on long-term antipsychotic drugs should be regularly reviewed for the emergence of orofacial or limb dyskinesias, and where this occurs, medication should be discontinued if possible.

Sedation, hypotension and extrapyramidal adverse effects are the most commonly occurring and troublesome adverse effects seen with the neuroleptics. Table 86 is a guide to the relative incidence of these effects with the more commonly used neuroleptics.

Drug Interactions

The sedative effects of CNS depressant drugs and alcohol may be enhanced by neuroleptics. Phenothiazines may reverse the antihypertensive property of guanethidine, and serious rises in diastolic pressure may occur. Chlorpromazine may interfere with the metabolism of phenytoin, leading to phenytoin toxicity. Phenothiazines can impair the metabolism of tricyclic antidepressants. Antacids may interfere with the absorption of phenothiazines so doses should be spaced about two hours apart. Levodopa will not reverse the Parkinsonian symptoms induced by phenothiazines because dopamine receptor sites are already occupied by phenothiazines, and addition of more dopamine will therefore have no effect.

Precautions

Phenothiazines should be administered by deep IM injection. Staff handling phenothiazines should take care not to spill solutions onto the skin. Abrupt withdrawal of phenothiazines is often associated with nausea, vomiting, insomnia and headache. Phenothiazine drugs and any accompanying anti-Parkinsonian drugs should be withdrawn slowly.

Table 86
Adverse Effects of Neuroleptics

Drug	Extrapyramidal Effects	Sedative Effects	Hypotensive Effects
Chlorpromazine	++	+++	+++
Thioridazine	±	+++	++
Fluphenazine	+++	++	+
Perphenazine	+++	+	+
Trifluoperazine	+++	+	+
Haloperidol	+++	+	+
Pimozide	+	+	+

± minimal
\+ low
++ moderate
+++ high

Contraindications

Contraindications include known phenothiazine hypersensitivity and hypotensive states, cases of coma resulting from ingestion of CNS depressants, and in serious head injury. Use with caution in patients with a history of liver dysfunction.

NURSING IMPLICATIONS

Assessment

The following assessments are important before administering neuroleptic medication: behavioural aspects of the patient's participation in the environment; sleep patterns and the number of hours slept; motor dexterity in the performance of specific motor tasks; aspects of interpersonal relationships, especially mannerisms; the appropriateness of the conversation; the amount of motor activity; and the presence of hallucinations or delusions. The degree of insight, judgement and decision-making skills are also important.

In terms of medication, the drugs taken, alcohol intake and previous drug hypersensitivity should be assessed. Previous seizure activity should be noted. A history of diseases will be age-dependent, but previous cardiovascular disease, glaucoma, myasthenia gravis and benign prostatic hypertrophy are important. Baseline vital signs, cardiac function, weight and blood pressure (lying and standing) should be recorded.

Administration

The person administering IM or IV phenothiazines should be careful during handling as contact dermatitis can occur. Observation for non-compliance is important. Regular measurements of lying-and-standing blood pressure should reveal the presence of postural hypotension, should it occur. Abrupt withdrawal of the phenothiazines may result in nausea, vomiting, headache, and insomnia, so medications should be tapered off slowly.

Evaluation

Management and evaluation of a patient who is taking neuroleptic medication mainly involves observing for therapeutic effects and the recognition and appropriate intervention should adverse effects occur. Interactions may occur when neuroleptic drugs are taken concurrently with alcohol or other CNS depressants. Observe for seizures, and treat with the appropriate anticonvulsant. Drowsiness may occur, so activities may need to be supervised initially while in hospital. New behaviours should be evaluated carefully. The emergence of dystonias can be a major problem in the younger age group and tardive dyskinesia in the older age group may indicate the need to maintain as low a therapeutic dose as possible. Akathesia which is characterised by constant pacing movements may indicate the need to reduce the dose or withdraw the drug. Pseudo-Parkinsonism with rigidity and dyskinesia may indicate a need to lower the dose of neuroleptic drugs, although tolerance may develop in some situations.

It is especially important that the nurse be fully conversant with the signs and symptoms of extrapyramidal side effects and the fact that these effects sometimes occur after even one dose of a neuroleptic. It is important to remember that these effects can manifest when the nurse is least expecting it, for example, when the drug is being used as an antiemetic in a non-psychiatric situation.

Extrapyramidal and other side effects can be distressing for the patient, so much so that they may be reluctant to take the medication if they have had previous experience with its side effects. Remember that the patient has the right to be informed and to refuse his or her medication and it is often the nurse's role to listen to the patient and counsel appropriately.

Neuroleptics should be used with caution in glaucoma, so the presentation of blurred vision should be reported. Anticipate the sudden presentation of cardiac toxicity, and ensure that resuscitation equipment is adequate. Regular blood screening is important, and observation of bruising, bleeding, lethargy or mouth ulcers may indicate leucopenia or agranulocytosis. Darkening of the skin may occur. Frequent liver function tests are necessary as any abnormality may necessitate cessation or change of medication. Regular weighing should take place and weight gain may be managed by encouraging a balanced diet and adequate exercise. Regular gynaecological check-ups for lactation and menstrual abnormalities may be necessary for women. In men, the development of gynaecomastia may indicate the need to change or cease administration.

Teaching

Patient education is vitally important and a fundamental process for discharge protocols. The patient should be advised not to suddenly discontinue the medication and to be wary of taking concurrent over-the-counter medications, especially antihistamines. If drowsiness occurs, driving or the use of machinery should be avoided. Rising slowly from the lying position will help to avoid postural hypotension. The patient should be advised to avoid taking hot baths in situations of hypotension.

The onset of fatigue or sore throat or bruising would indicate a need to consult a medical officer. Transient decrease in libido and ejaculatory failure may occur in some male patients. The family should be involved in the patient-education programme. Information concerning adverse effects is important, and gaining cooperation of the family members may help avoid non-compliance. Patients should be advised about not becoming too cold in the winter or too hot in the summer as it may be difficult for them to control their body temperature. The patient should be advised to avoid overexposure to sunlight and to use UV-blocking sunscreens.

LITHIUM CARBONATE

Lithium carbonate is the only specific antimanic drug known. Its antimanic properties were discovered in 1949 by an Australian psychiatrist, John Cade.

Table 87
Dose Forms of Lithium Carbonate

Generic Name	Trade Names	Usual Daily Dose Range
Lithium carbonate 250 mg tablets	*Camcolit 250*	500–2000 mg
Lithium carbonate 300 mg	*Phasal*	600–2000 mg
Lithium carbonate 400 mg	*Priadel, Camcolit 400*	400–2000 mg
Lithium carbonate 450 mg	*Liskonum*	450–2000 mg
(These tablets *must* be swallowed whole and not crushed or dissolved.)		

Lithium-carbonate administration has no discernible psychotropic action in normal subjects. Lithium carbonate is used in the treatment of the manic phase of manic-depressive illness and for long-term maintenance therapy where it reduces the frequency and/or severity and duration of manic and depressive episodes.

It is specifically indicated for manic depressive illness and is of no value in other forms of psychotic illness. It is of little value in the primary treatment of the depressive phase of manic depressive illness; antidepressant drugs or electroconvulsive therapy should be employed first in this phase. Then lithium therapy should be instituted to maintain stability of mood in the patient. The duration of lithium therapy may vary from two to three years to indefinitely.

Lithium is slow to enter cells, and so there is a time lag between the commencement of therapy and signs of improvement in the patient. Therapeutic blood levels take 7 to 14 days to build up. Therapeutic blood levels required in the treatment of acute mania range from 1.0 to 1.5 mmol/L, whereas in the long-term maintenance treatment of manic depressive disorder, effective levels lie between 0.5 and 1.2 mmol/L. The patient should be maintained at the lowest level consistent with optimum therapeutic effects. Above levels of 1.5 to 2.0 mmol/L, serious toxic effects are more likely.

All patients receiving lithium therapy should have their serum lithium levels monitored frequently, at least monthly during maintenance therapy and more frequently during the initial phase of therapy. Blood samples for lithium estimations should be taken 12 hours after the administration of the last dose. Lithium should be administered in divided doses. There is no effective sustained-release formulation available.

Adverse Drug Reactions

Polydipsia (excessive thirst) resulting from polyuria (excessive urinary loss) can be troublesome initially. It is reversible on discontinuation of therapy, but this is not usually necessary as symptoms will subside within a few weeks. Patients should be reassured.

Skin reactions such as acne may appear during the first few weeks of therapy, but usually disappear spontaneously.

In a small percentage of patients, lithium may cause enlargement of the thyroid gland and some degree of hypothyroidism. These symptoms are reversed on discontinuation of lithium therapy or when thyroxine is given. Thyroid function should be assessed prior to starting lithium therapy and yearly during long-term treatment.

Lithium is eliminated primarily via the kidney, and any impairment of renal function would alter lithium clearance. Acute lithium toxicity may result in kidney damage which may in turn predispose the patient to further episodes of toxicity. A nephrogenic diabetes insipidus-like syndrome may occur in a small percentage of patients and will require a thorough renal evaluation if lithium is to be continued. From 10% to 20% of patients report persistent increase in urine volume and thirst during lithium treatment, but prospective studies of renal function in patients maintained on lithium at therapeutic plasma levels do not show evidence of progressive renal impairment.

Lithium crosses the placenta and the incidence of congenital malformations (especially cardiac) in the children of mothers on lithium is greater than in the general population. Lithium is generally contraindicated during the first trimester of pregnancy, but if discontinuation of lithium would seriously compromise the mother's health, it may be used with great caution and frequent blood level estimations. Lithium is excreted in breast milk, so mothers should be encouraged not to breast feed.

Toxicity

At blood levels above 1.5 mmol/L, the patient will begin to exhibit signs of toxicity. Acute toxicity is seen at concentrations of 2 mmol/L or greater. There is no specific antidote to lithium poisoning; treatment consists of withdrawing the drug, giving adequate fluid and electrolyte replacement and aiding renal excretion of lithium by administration of sodium bicarbonate. Haemodialysis is the treatment of choice for severe lithium poisoning. Where the plasma level exceeds 3.0 to 4.0 mmol/L, where anuria is suspected or where there is evidence of shock or coma, the patient should be dialysed. Prolonged severe toxicity may lead to irreversible neurological damage or death.

Early signs of toxicity include sluggishness, lethargy, fine tremor (particularly of the hands), nausea, vomiting, anorexia, abdominal discomfort and diarrhoea. At very high blood levels, ataxia, slurred speech and a marked tremor occur. Finally, seizures, loss of consciousness from cerebral anoxia and shock and cardiac impairment (due to electrolyte imbalance) and ultimately death will occur.

Causes of high blood levels are multiple and include: excessive dosage; reduction in lithium excretion (which occurs when renal damage is present); when sodium intake is low (from special or sometimes 'fad' diets); or when sodium loss is great (for example, after excessive sweating or diuretic therapy); drug interactions.

Drug Interactions

Drugs which increase lithium blood levels or increase toxicity are ethacrynic acid (*Edecrin*), frusemide (*Lasix*), chlorthalidone (*Hygroton*), methyldopa (*Aldomet*), thiazide diuretics (*Bendrofluazide, Chlorthalidone*), and indomethacin (*Indocid*).

Drugs which reduce lithium blood levels are sodium bicarbonate, sodium chloride, aminophylline, theophylline, and acetazolamide *(Diamox)*.

High doses of lithium and haloperidol given concomitantly have been reported to cause neurotoxicity. Lithium may prolong the neuromuscular blockade produced by suxamethonium or decamethonium. Lithium may also prolong recovery time after barbiturate anaesthetic induction, with thiopentone (*Intraval*).

Cardiac and renal disease are contraindications to lithium therapy, and possibly also pregnancy and breast feeding.

NURSING IMPLICATIONS

Assessment

Assessment of lithium levels within 12 hours of the last dose (except in situations of acute toxicity) is extremely important. Note concurrent medications, especially diuretics. A reduced-sodium diet should be noted.

Evaluation of baseline vital signs such as weight, sleep patterns and fluid balance are important. A history of cardiac or cerebrovascular disease, cerebral organic dementia, and renal or thyroid disease are relevant. Assess thyroid function.

Administration and management

The management of the patient taking lithium carbonate is mainly concerned with the maintenance of adequate blood-sodium levels. The concurrent use of drugs high in sodium should be avoided as it will result in decreased blood-lithium levels. Other drugs such as frusemide (*Lasix*) or methyldopa (*Aldomet*) will increase blood-lithium levels. An extremely low dietary sodium intake will result in increased blood-lithium levels. Adequate hydration should also be maintained.

Evaluation

It is important to observe for therapeutic effectiveness. Observation of behavioural parameters should be noted. Dietary sodium intake should be monitored, and observation for the signs of fluid and electrolyte imbalance (as characterised by polyuria and polydipsia) should be reported. Skin reactions may occur during the first few weeks of treatment. Observe thyroid function, especially in relation to the presentation of hypothyroidism.

Teaching

Patient education involves informing the patients of expected therapeutic effects and assisting them in recognising any deviation. The adverse effects of lithium carbonate should be taught and the patient encouraged to visit a medical officer should these occur. If drowsiness occurs, the patient should be discouraged from driving a vehicle or using machinery. Dietary advice should be given and regular blood screenings for lithium levels carried out. The patient should be instructed to avoid over-the-counter drugs which contain sodium.

ANXIOLYTIC SEDATIVES

Anxiolytic sedatives were formerly known as minor tranquillisers or sedatives.

"Anxiolytic" is the name given to those compounds which are effective in alleviating the symptoms of anxiety. The benzodiazepines are the most widely used anxiolytic agents, but prior to their introduction, barbiturates, bromides and meprobamate were used.

BARBITURATES

The barbiturates were first used early this century. They, along with the bromides, enjoyed wide use in the treatment of anxiety states prior to the introduction of meprobamate and then the benzodiazepines. Today they are considered unsuitable for continuing therapy in the treatment of the anxious patient because of their addiction potential, profound sedative effect and the fact that they interact with a considerable number of drugs. Their use is mainly restricted to the treatment of convulsive disorders and as anaesthetic induction agents. Dozens of barbiturates have been marketed, but those listed in Table 88 are the most commonly used.

Table 88
Commonly Used Barbiturates

Generic Name	Trade Name	Purpose	Duration of Action
Amylobarbitone	*Amytal*	Hypnotic	Intermediate
Sodium amylobarbitone	*Sodium Amytal*	Hypnotic	Intermediate
Pentobarbitone	*Nembutal*	Hypnotic	Intermediate
Quinalbarbitone	*Seconal*	Hypnotic	Intermediate
Phenobarbitone		Hypnotic, anticonvulsant	Long
Methylphenobarbitone	*Prominal*	Anticonvulsant	Long
Thiopentone	*Intraval*	Anaesthetic	Ultra short
Methohexitone	*Brietal Sodium*	Anaesthetic	Ultra short

MEPROBAMATE

Meprobamate was extremely popular for the treatment of anxiety states in the late 1950s and early 1960s. However, its antianxiety activity is variable, and tolerance and physical dependence may develop quickly, as with barbiturates. For these reasons, it has been largely replaced by the benzodiazepines.

BENZODIAZEPINES

A number of benzodiazepines are marketed. They may be divided into two broad categories as in Table 89.

The benzodiazepines are administered orally as tablets, capsules or liquids. Diazepam and clonazepam may be administered intravenously. Diazepam injection is prepared in a non-aqueous solvent and is incompatible with many IV fluids and other drugs; advice should be sought before mixing diazepam injections with other drugs or IV fluids. Diazepam is poorly absorbed when injected IM.

Both the site and mechanism of action of the benzodiazepines are unclear. Proposed sites include the reticular activating system, median forebrain bundle and hypothalamus. Benzodiazepine receptors closely located to GABA receptors have been identified in brain, and it is hypothesised that benzodiazepine actions may be mediated through this system.

The benzodiazepines are regarded as the drugs of choice in the treatment of anxiety states. They have numerous other uses including treatment of convulsive disorders, insomnia, muscle spasm, night terrors and somnambulism in children and are employed in obstetrics and in the treatment of acute alcohol withdrawal.

Table 89
Some Benzodiazepines

Generic Name	Trade Name
Long acting (with a half-life exceeding 10 hours)	
Diazepam	*Valium*
Chlordiazepoxide	*Librium*
Clorazepate	*Tranxene*
Nitrazepam	*Mogadon*
Clonazepam	*Rivotril*
Medazepam	*Nobrium*
Bromazepam	*Lexotan*
Flurazepam	*Dalmane*
Flunitrazepam	*Rohypnol*
Alprazolam	*Xanax*
Short acting (with a half-life of less than 10 hours)	
Lorazepam	*Ativan*
Oxazepam	*Serenid*
Temazepam	*Normison, Euhypnos*
Triazolam	*Halcion*

The Committee on the Review of Medicines (UK 1980) found all benzodiazepines to be efficacious in short-term treatment of anxiety and insomnia with no agent being more effective than the other. The usual division of benzodiazepines into rigid treatment categories of anxiolytic agents (for example, diazepam) and hypnotics (for example, nitrazepam) is not based on the known pharmacological and clinical properties of the group. More appropriate treatment categories are as follows.

Short-acting compounds are used to treat anxiety, insomnia and other appropriate conditions in elderly patients and those with renal or hepatic impairment. The short-acting compounds are suitable for the treatment of insomnia in patients who do not have accompanying anxiety and in whom daytime alertness is required.

Long-acting compounds are useful in the treatment of anxiety states accompanied by insomnia where the loss of a degree of daytime alertness may even be beneficial and also for the treatment of muscular spasm, acute alcohol withdrawal, seizures, night terrors and somnambulism in children. Long-acting preparations are best avoided in elderly patients and in those with renal or hepatic impairment as they will tend to accumulate in these patients.

Adverse Drug Reactions

Adverse reactions are extensions of the general pharmacology of the group and are predominant in elderly patients. They include sedation, ataxia, dizziness, vertigo, dysarthria, incoordination, muscle weakness and blurred vision. After excessive dosage or when accumulation has occurred, there may be impairment of intellectual function, motor performance, coordination and reaction. Rarely, skin reactions and paradoxical excitement may occur. Fortunately, adverse drug reactions to benzodiazepines occur remarkably rarely, but care should be exercised by patients who operate machinery or drive motor vehicles. The benzodiazepines are comparatively safe in overdose and fatalities are rare, even after gross overdosage; intensive care may be required to prevent such complications as inhaled vomitus and obstructed airways.

Addiction Potential

Recent studies have confirmed that many patients taking benzodiazepines chronically (that is, for periods longer than four months) may experience withdrawal symptoms. This physical dependency may occur even at therapeutic dose levels. Withdrawal symptoms occur earlier and are more severe with the short-acting compounds. To avoid the risks of dependency, these drugs should be used for short-term treatment only.

After abrupt withdrawal of short-acting drugs, withdrawal symptoms may appear within 24 hours, and three to 10 days after withdrawal of longer acting compounds. Symptoms include anxiety, apprehension, tremor, insomnia, nausea and vomiting. Therefore, all benzodiazepine therapy (unless given on an occasional basis only) should be withdrawn gradually.

Drug Interactions, Precautions and Contraindications

Benzodiazepines have relatively few clinically significant drug interactions except for the expected potentiation of the sedative properties of other CNS depressants, for example, alcohol, neuroleptics, antidepressants, antihistamines and other hypnotics and sedatives. It should be noted that unexpected interactions with alcohol may occur during the day or evening following the nocturnal use of long-acting benzodiazepines. Cimetidine will potentiate the sedative effects of diazepam and increase plasma diazepam levels.

Care should be exercised in the administration of benzodiazepines to the elderly and to patients with liver and kidney disease, as outlined above. These drugs are not suitable for use in disorders such as depression, tension headache and dysmenorrhoea (occurring in the absence of anxiety), nor in the treatment of psychotic disturbances. Benzodiazepines are without analgesic or antidepressant activity.

Except for myasthenia gravis, there are no absolute contraindications for the benzodiazepines. It is advisable to avoid using them in children wherever possible.

NURSING IMPLICATIONS

Barbiturates

Assessment

In the assessment of a patient taking barbiturates, it is important to consider age, as the elderly may have an increased sensitivity to the drug. Abuse potential (including suicidal tendency) should be recorded. A history of allergic states or dermatological reactions is important. Current medication and the presence of pregnancy or lactation should be noted. Renal and liver function should be assessed. Baseline vital signs such as blood pressure, pulse rate, weight and sleep patterns along with blood screening tests are necessary.

Administration

It is important to comply with legal requirements in relation to the administration and recording of these drugs.

Evaluation

If administering these drugs continuously, careful monitoring is essential. The dose should always be tapered off and never ceased abruptly as withdrawal seizures may occur. Concurrent use of barbiturates with CNS depressants should be avoided. The presentation of drowsiness or ataxia may necessitate that the patient be supervised during certain activities. Dermatological reactions should be reported as they may indicate systemic lupus erythematosus. Regular weighing, evaluation of sleep patterns, and blood pressure (lying and standing) should be recorded. Evaluation of the therapeutic effect (indicated by a relief of symptoms) will indicate an effective dose level. Dependency may be a problem in the long-term administration of these drugs.

Teaching

Patients should be taught how to identify deviations from the therapeutic response. They should also be taught to identify adverse reactions. They should avoid situations which require alertness or concentration when drowsy or dizzy. Education concerning compliance and the effects of sudden withdrawal of the drug should be stressed. Alcohol and other CNS depressants should not be used concurrently. The presentation of sore throat or mouth ulcers necessitates a visit to their medical officer. Educate patients to rise slowly from the lying position and to avoid hot baths in case of hypotension. Although it is preferable not to prescribe warfarin concomitantly with barbiturates, this may be unavoidable in some instances. Patients should be instructed to comply carefully with dosage regimens in these cases.

Benzodiazepines

Assessment

Regardless of the benzodiazepine prescribed, the implications for nursing care remain the same. However, it is important to be aware of the duration of action of the drug prescribed, as this knowledge can assist in evaluation for signs of toxicity and cumulative effects. Assessment should begin with the patient's history for any evidence of previous hypersensitivity to benzodiazepines. The patient's mode of employment and lifestyle should also be considered, as people who operate power machinery or who drive a car need to be informed of the sedative effect of the drugs. Baseline measures of vital signs and blood pressure will need to be done to form an objective measure of the anxiety state. Nursing staff should be especially aware that the elderly and those with renal and/or hepatic insufficiency will be less capable of metabolising and excreting the drugs, and therefore accumulation and toxicity can occur.

Administration

In hospital this requires the usual procedure for administration of restricted drugs. If the patient shows signs of toxicity (such as excessive sedation, ataxia and so on) withhold the drug and seek further orders.

As a general rule, parenteral preparations of diazepam should not be diluted with other solutions or mixed in the same syringe or bottle with other drugs. Intravenous injections should be given slowly and directly into the vein (not diluted), and the patient's blood pressure checked regularly. Flush the vein with normal saline after IV administration of diazepam.

The majority of benzodiazepines, however, are self-administered in the home, and the use and abuse of these drugs has reached alarming proportions. Nurses who work in general-practice surgeries should be alert for patients who frequently request renewals of prescriptions of these medications. Community health nurses should be alert for patients who have weak or inadequate coping mechanisms and who subscribe to the belief that "there's a pill to cure everything". These people may be actual or potential benzodiazepine abusers.

Evaluation

The nurse should note the patient's subjective reports of reduced anxiety. The monitoring of vital signs can give objective signs of reduced anxiety, that is, lower blood pressure, pulse and respiratory rates. Observe for adverse effects, including rashes, signs of toxicity, for example, excessive sedation and ataxia. Supervise elderly patients who may be at risk of falling, especially in bathrooms or on stairs.

Teaching

This should include instructions regarding the criteria for determining the effectiveness of therapy and identifying the adverse effects. Warnings should be given concerning the sedative effects of the drug and of the dangers of driving cars or operating machinery. Patients should be advised of the potentiating effects of alcohol and other tranquillizing drugs. Patients and the community in general should be informed concerning the addictive potential of these drugs. Such information can help prevent irresponsible use and abuse. Importantly, patients taking benzodiazepines need to be counselled concerning the fact that abrupt withdrawal following prolonged use can result in severe withdrawal effects.

It should be emphasised that these drugs, while they relieve the symptoms of anxiety, do not resolve the actual problem. Proper counselling of these patients should be employed, which may reduce or eliminate the need for this type of drug.

ANTIDEPRESSANTS

Antidepressant drugs are effective in the treatment of pathological depressive states and include four classes of compound: tricyclic antidepressants, tetracyclic antidepressants and monoamine oxidase inhibitors. Antidepressant drugs relieve depression by elevating the mood of the patient, but they are not strictly CNS stimulants.

Depression must be viewed as a distinct clinical entity. There are several types of depression, however, and each type requires different treatment.

1. Depression secondary to physical illness or organic brain disease or to the use of certain drugs. In such cases treatment of the underlying disorder or removal of the offending drug is appropriate therapy in the majority of cases.
2. Reactive secondary depression, usually triggered by some disturbing event in the patient's life, for example, loss of a parent, child or spouse. This form of depression usually resolves spontaneously and any treatment required would best be comprised of tender loving care, psychotherapy or alteration to the patient's environment.
3. Endogenous depressions respond best to antidepressant drug therapy, since they are probably caused by a genetic biochemical abnormality. As with reactive depression, a traumatic event in the patient's life may trigger the depression. In the case of a patient with reactive depression, their response to such an event is appropriate while the patient with endogenous depression exhibits an inappropriate response.

Treatment of depression may be multiple, and involve psychotherapy or electroconvulsive therapy. It must be remembered that depressive patients can be suicidal, and the risk of suicide must be taken into account when selecting therapy.

TRICYCLIC ANTIDEPRESSANTS

Tricyclic antidepressants may be administered orally in daily divided doses or as a single large daily dose at bedtime. Elderly patients often cannot tolerate a single large dose and so are best treated by divided dose regimens. The advantages of a single daily dose are threefold.

First, it optimises the sedating effects of the tricyclics, thus obviating the need for a hypnotic. (Sleep disturbances are a part of depressive illness.) Second, it encourages compliance. Third, it reduces the incidence of most of the troublesome side effects of the tricyclics, as these are most intense during the first few hours after administration, and the patient will therefore sleep through them.

The antidepressant activity of the tricyclics is postulated to be due to their ability to block neuronal uptake of amines such as noradrenaline and serotonin and thus increase the effective concentrations of these substances in the brain. The tricyclics have a number of pharmacological actions in addition to their antidepressant activity, including anticholinergic, antiserotonin, antihistamine, hypothermic and antiemetic actions.

The tricyclic antidepressants are the drugs of first choice for those forms of depression which respond to drug therapy. If a patient fails to respond to tricyclic therapy and electroconvulsive therapy is considered unsuitable, the monoamine oxidase inhibitors are usually the next choice. Treatment should be initiated with low doses and gradually built up until response is obtained. It may take seven to 21 days after initiation of therapy to obtain a response.

Table 90
Tricyclic Antidepressants

Generic name	Trade Name	Average Daily Doses (mg)
Amitriptyline	*Tryptizol, Elavil, Lentizol*	50–150
Protriptyline	*Concordin*	10–60
Nortriptyline	*Allegron, Aventyl*	50–100
Imipramine	*Tofranil, Praminil*	50–200
Trimipramine	*Surmontil*	50–300
Desipramine	*Pertofran*	25–200
Doxepin	*Sinequan*	30–300
Dothiepin	*Prothiaden*	75–150
Clomipramine	*Anafranil*	30–150

Adverse Drug Reactions

Sedation is common, especially during initial therapy.
Anticholinergic effects include dry mouth, blurred vision, constipation, urinary hesitancy or retention. Other anticholinergic drugs will potentiate these effects.
Cardiovascular effects include postural hypotension which is common particularly in elderly patients or those on high doses. AV conduction time may be prolonged. Tachycardia and extrasystoles may occur, especially at high doses. Skin rashes, blood dyscrasias, jaundice, weight gain and sweating are less common adverse effects. Manic excitement is a rare paradoxical reaction.

Toxicity is not uncommon; toxic reactions are mainly anticholinergic cerebral or cardiac.

Drug Interactions

1. Phenytoin, phenylbutazone, aspirin, hyoscine and phenothiazines displace tricyclics from plasma protein binding sites and so may potentiate tricyclic action.
2. Neuroleptics and steroid preparations (including oral contraceptives) will interfere with liver metabolism of tricyclics, thereby enhancing their effects.
3. Barbiturates and anti-epileptics will increase liver metabolism of tricyclics and so diminish their action.

4. Tricyclics enhance the effects of alcohol and other sedatives.
5. The anticholinergic effects of tricyclics are potentiated by combining them with other anticholinergic compounds such as some of the anti-Parkinsonian drugs.
6. Tricyclics will potentiate the action of biogenic amines such as noradrenaline.
7. Tricyclics prevent the action of the antihypertensive agent guanethidine.
8. The central antihypertensive effect of clonidine may be blocked by tricyclics.
9. Severe CNS toxicity leading to coma is possible when tricyclics and monoamine oxidase inhibitors are combined. However, although this is an extremely severe reaction, it is very rare.

Contraindications

Contraindications to tricyclic therapy include glaucoma and urinary retention.

TETRACYCLIC ANTIDEPRESSANTS

Mianserin (*Bolvidon*) is a tetracyclic antidepressant. Its dose range is 30 to 120 mg daily and its mechanism of action is thought to be similar to the tricyclics. However, it appears to be less cardiotoxic and to have fewer undesirable autonomic properties than tricyclics. Recent reports show it to be more toxic than was originally thought. It appears that mianserin is associated with increased risk of neutropenia and agranulocytosis.

MONOAMINE OXIDASE INHIBITORS (MAOIs)

The monoamine oxidase inhibitors were introduced in the mid 1950s after it was noticed that patients receiving the antitubercular drug iproniazid had an improvement in mood. A variety of similar substances have since been introduced. The monoamine oxidase inhibitors are not drugs of first choice in the treatment of depression but should be reserved for use in cases where other drug treatments and therapy regimens have been inadequate.

Monoamine oxidase inhibitors are only given by the oral route and are well absorbed. They begin to exert their action within five to ten days after commencement of therapy.

The drugs inhibit the enzyme monoamine oxidase (MAO). MAO is responsible for the breakdown of amines such as serotonin and noradrenaline. If MAO is inhibited then serotonin, noradrenaline and other catecholamines accumulate in the brain.

Table 91
Monoamine Oxidase Inhibitors

Generic Name	Trade Name	Average Daily Dose Range (mg)
Phenelzine	*Nardil*	15–60
Tranylcypromine	*Parnate*	10–30
Isocarboxazid	*Marplan*	10–20
Iproniazid	*Marsilid*	25–50

If tricyclic antidepressants fail and electroconvulsive therapy is unsuitable, the monoamine oxidase inhibitors may be tried. It may take several days before a response is evident.

Adverse Drug Reactions

Hypertension — transient hypertension is not uncommon and hypertensive crises may occur which are characterised by headache, palpitations, nausea and vomiting. Occasionally such crisis may lead to subarachnoid or intracranial haemorrhage. These crises may be precipitated by the ingestion of certain foods or drugs.
Liver damage — may be caused by chronic ingestion of these drugs.
Hypotension — can occur and is probably due to the ganglion blocking effects of these drugs.
Insomnia — tranylcypromine in particular has a rapid and direct CNS stimulant action in addition to its ability to inhibit MAO. In order to avoid insomnia, it should not be given in the late afternoon.

Other less common effects are gastric upsets, dizziness, dry mouth, muscle weakness, cardiac arrhythmia and disturbances in red and green colour vision.

Drug Interactions

1. Drugs which can interact with MAOIs to cause a hypertensive crisis are:
   (a) adrenaline, ephedrine, phenylephrine, methoxamine, phenylpropanolamine, metaraminol, isoprenaline, tyramine and dopamine;
   (b) (*Tenuate Dospan*), fenfluramine (*Ponderax*), amphetamine and dexamphetamine;
   (c) reserpine, methyldopa, levodopa and pethidine.
   (d) tricyclic antidepressants.
2. Foods which can cause the same reaction include cheese (especially processed and matured types); yeast extracts (Marmite and Bovril); pickled herrings; alcoholic beverages, especially home-brewed beer, chianti, red vermouth and red wine generally (spirits are safe); banana skins and broad-bean pods, also figs, plums and pineapples; caviar; chicken and beef livers; aged samples of meat, fish, poultry, offal, game, yoghurt, liver pâté, packaged soups, stock cubes, cream, high protein

concentrates; chocolates and coffee. All of these foods are rich in tyramine, serotonin and histamine.

MAOIs will inhibit the metabolism of many drugs and so potentiate their action. Some examples are CNS depressants including alcohol, barbiturates, opiates, benzodiazepines and anaesthetic agents; atropine; cocaine; antihistamines; tricyclic antidepressants; oral hypoglycaemic agents; antihypertensive drugs and muscle relaxants (for example, tubocurarine).

NURSING IMPLICATIONS

Assessment

The manifestations of the depression should be accurately assessed. Medications (especially anticholinergics) and socially acceptable drugs such as alcohol should be noted. The presence of pregnancy or lactation should be recorded. A history of cardiovascular disease, hypertension, epilepsy, diabetes mellitus, glaucoma, constipation, organic brain disease or liver disease is relevant. Baseline blood pressure, pulse rate, weight, bowel habits and sleep patterns should be noted and an ECG taken to compare with later changes, should they present.

Administration and evaluation

When administering the tricyclic antidepressants, taper off the dose and do not suddenly cease the medication as withdrawal symptoms may occur. The therapeutic effect of antidepressant drugs may take up to three weeks to manifest. As the patient's depression begins to improve, the risk of suicide may paradoxically increase, due to an increased drive and will on the patient's part to carry out an attempt. Observe for abnormal behaviour during this time. Ensure that the diet is adequate to prevent constipation. Also observe and report other anticholinergic effects such as dry mouth, blurred vision and urinary retention or hesitancy. Monitor blood pressure (lying and standing) and report any observation of tachycardia or cardiac arrhythmias.

The administration of MAOIs necessitates monitoring of (lying and standing) blood pressure, observing for postural hypotension. Hypertensive crises may occur, and this is usually indicated by the onset of headache. Atropine-like effects such as constipation may occur. Euphoria may present and should be reported. Toxic overdose may present as psychosis or coma, so changes in behaviour or consciousness should be noted and reported. Dietary considerations include the withdrawal of all tyramine-containing foods. Sympathomimetic amines should not be administered concurrently. The monitoring of liver function is essential.

Teaching

Patient education for antidepressant drugs includes teaching about the expected therapeutic effect and the recognition of deviations from this effect. Also, the recognition of adverse effects should be taught. Exercise and adequate diet should be encouraged to prevent weight gain. A list of tyramine-containing foods should be distributed and information concerning the effects of tyramine rich foods explained to patients on monoamine oxidase inhibitors. As with most other drugs which act on the CNS, situations which require alertness or concentration should be avoided if the patient is dizzy or drowsy. Patients should be educated to rise slowly from the lying position to avoid postural hypotension. With MAOIs, the patient should understand that the presentation of a headache may indicate the onset of a hypertensive crisis and should not be treated with analgesics. Generally patients should avoid taking over-the-counter medications concurrently, especially cough and cold preparations. Dry mouth caused by tricyclic antidepressants may be alleviated to some degree by sucking hard sweets or chewing gum to stimulate salivation.

PSYCHOSTIMULANTS

Psychostimulants are drugs which increase the level of alertness and/or motivation. Since many of these drugs are dependence producing, only a select few remain on the market, and these are strictly controlled by poisons legislation.

DEXAMPHETAMINE

Dexamphetamine is available as 5 mg tablets. The normal dose range is 2.5 to 5 mg administered orally three times daily.

Dexamphetamine is a powerful central nervous system stimulant. In addition to its effects on the CNS, it also elevates blood pressure, increases pulse rate and diminishes the appetite. Due to its central effects, it stimulates respiration and reverses the effect of CNS depressant drugs (for example, anaesthetics and hypnotics).

Dexamphetamine has been used over the years for a number of indications, including increasing wakefulness and diminishing fatigue, in mild cases of depression and for apathetic or withdrawn senile behaviour, for reversing the effects of anaesthetics and overdoses of hypnotic agents and to increase response to psychotherapy. It has also been employed to diminish appetite and in the treatment of narcolepsy and hyperkinetic states in children arising from minimal brain dysfunction. Strict legislative controls now restrict its use to the treatment of narcolepsy and childhood hyperkinetic states.

Adverse Drug Reactions

Central effects include restlessness, dizziness, tremor, talkativeness, tenseness, irritability, weakness, insomnia, euphoria, fever, confusion, delirium, panic and hallucinations.
Cardiovascular effects include headache, pallor or flushing, palpitations, cardiac arrhythmias, hypertension or hypotension and sweating.
Gastrointestinal effects include dry mouth, anorexia, nausea, vomiting, diarrhoea and abdominal cramping.

Precautions and Abuse Potential

Use dexamphetamine with great caution in patients with long-standing asthmatic disease or any degree of cardiac disease. It is not advisable to use dexamphetamine in patients with a history of anorexia, insomnia or psychopathic, homicidal or suicidal tendencies.

Tolerance to doses of dexamphetamine develops easily, leading to increasing doses of the drug being required to produce the desired physiological effect. True physical addiction to amphetamines can occur, and on discontinuation of therapy, the patient will experience a withdrawal syndrome characterised by prolonged sleep, lassitude and fatigue, hyperphagia and occasional profound depression. There is an amphetamine-induced toxic syndrome characterised by vivid visual, auditory and tactile hallucinations, skin excoriation and paranoia.

CAFFEINE

Caffeine is not used therapeutically in psychiatric practice. Some combined analgesic preparations contain small doses of caffeine designed to give mild CNS stimulation and mood elevation. If administered in therapeutic doses, caffeine stimulates the central nervous system and minimises drowsiness and fatigue. It produces a diuresis, stimulates cardiac muscle, relaxes the smooth muscle of the bronchioles and blood vessels causing dilatation, and it stimulates gastric secretion. It is not normally employed in the treatment of psychiatric disorders.

COCAINE

The most clinically important action of cocaine is its ability to block nerve conduction when locally applied (that is, as a local anaesthetic). However, cocaine is also a powerful CNS stimulant which has often been used to lessen the sense of fatigue and increase capacity for work. Cocaine stimulates emesis, respiration, the cardiac muscle (in moderate doses) and causes a rise in body temperature. It may be used in the eye as a local anaesthetic and is mydriatic. Due to its powerful CNS stimulant action, cocaine is frequently abused. Psychological addiction can result from its continued use.

The major clinical uses of cocaine are as a local anaesthetic particularly in ophthalmic and ENT work, and as a component of narcotic analgesic mixtures for pain alleviation in the terminally ill (for example, Brompton Cocktail). These analgesic mixtures normally contain morphine, alcohol and cocaine, the cocaine being used to counteract to some degree the central depressant actions of morphine and alcohol. However, more recent evidence suggests that cocaine does not add anything to the effectiveness of the Brompton Cocktail. Many hospitals now use a simple morphine mixture from which gin and other alcoholic products contained in the Brompton Cocktail have also been removed. This simple morphine mixture now therefore consists of morphine in a solution containing a preservative and an anti-oxidant.

NURSING IMPLICATIONS

Assessment

Psychostimulants may be used therapeutically for two reasons: in the management of narcolepsy; and hyperkinesis in children. It is therefore important to note for which condition the patient is being treated. In children it is important to assess weight, height, sleep patterns and motor activity. A history of epilepsy, psychological disorders or diabetes mellitus should be recorded. Establish baseline vital signs such as BP, pulse rate and weight. Note the presence of pregnancy or lactation.

Administration

Nurses should be aware of legislative controls which apply to stimulant drugs and should record drugs appropriately. Compatibilities should always be checked prior to mixing.

Evaluation

Regular weighing is an important feature of management. This is mainly because appetite suppression will occur, even though these drugs are no longer used to treat obesity. Psychostimulants should not be administered to people with a history of depression or alcohol abuse. During treatment, observe and report abnormal motor activity such as dyskinesia. Do not suddenly cease medication as withdrawal may occur. Note the presence of adverse effects such as skin rash, bruising, diarrhoea, constipation, visual disturbances or behavioural changes.

Teaching

Patient education involves teaching about the expected therapeutic effect and how to recognise deviations from this in terms of adverse effects. Inform the patient that if they miss a dose *not* to take an extra dose to 'catch up'. In some cases, situations which require alertness or concentration should be avoided if visual disturbances are present.

HYPNOTICS

The word hypnotic is derived from the Greek *hupnos*, meaning sleep. Hypnotics are drugs which will induce sleep. Over the years many agents have been used such as alcohol, opium, belladonna and bromides. Today a variety of compounds are used (see Table 92).

Table 92
Hypnotic Agents

1. Barbiturates
2. Benzodiazepines
3. A variety of miscellaneous compounds including the following:

Generic Name	Brand name	Usual Dose Range
Chloral hydrate	*Noctec*	500–1000 mg
Chlormethiazole	*Heminevrin*	1–2 caps
Dichloralphenazone	*Welldorm*	1.3–1.95 g

The hypnotics are usually given orally as tablets, capsules or liquids. Where a rapid hypnotic effect is desired, for example, in extreme psychiatric disturbances, some hypnotics may be administered parenterally along with a neuroleptic.

Hypnotics should be taken on retiring. They must not be taken too early as the patient may become drowsy and disoriented and have some form of accident or forget they have taken their dose and "double up" on it. Hypnotics should not be administered routinely. This practice is to be deplored as it can lead quickly to dependence. They should be taken only when really necessary and other methods tried first, for example, a hot bath, listening to soothing music, relaxation techniques, hot drinks or a small nightcap. Hypnotics should be used with great caution in the elderly as the aging brain is more sensitive to their action, and it is easy to produce a toxic confusional state resembling dementia or organic brain disease by chronic administration of hypnotics.

All hypnotics depress the central nervous system, but the different agents vary in their degree of selectivity of action on different parts of the CNS.

Workers in sleep laboratories have identified five stages of sleep during the sleep-cycle — "dreaming time" or rapid eye movement (rem) sleep followed by successive stages of deepening sleep culminating in stage 4, the deepest sleep. These stages are repeated in cycles throughout the night. There is more stage-4 sleep in the early hours of sleep and more dreaming time during the latter stages of sleep. The young have more stage-4 sleep than the old. Suppression of dreaming time can produce emotional disturbances.

While all hypnotics depress the amount of rem sleep, the barbiturates depress the rem stage of sleep rather more than the benzodiazepines. Cessation of drugs which suppress rem sleep can cause a rebound increase in dreaming time, often producing disturbing nightmares.

Hypnotics are used to relieve insomnia. There are three major types of insomnia: difficulty falling asleep; difficulty staying asleep and early-morning waking. Just as the anxiolytic agents do not relieve the cause of anxiety, the hypnotics do not relieve the cause of insomnia. No drug produces a true physiological sleep, but some hypnotics disturb the physiology of sleep to a lesser extent than others. Hypnotics should be prescribed in as low a dose as possible and for short periods only.

Adverse Drug Reactions

1. ***Barbiturates*** may cause disorientation, dizziness, ataxia, depression, sleep disturbances, altered dreaming patterns. Paradoxical excitement can occur in children and the elderly. Hangover is common due to the long duration of action of many barbiturates. A rare effect is the development of systemic lupus erythematosus (SLE).
2. ***Benzodiazepines*** may cause nightmares, confusion or rashes, but these only occur rarely. Long-acting benzodiazepines produce a hangover effect. The benzodiazepines are, however, the hypnotic agents of choice due to their low incidence of adverse reactions and low toxicity.
3. ***Chloral hydrate*** may cause gastric irritation, skin rashes, itching. It is relatively free of adverse reactions and is often considered suitable for the very young and very old.
4. ***Chlormethiazole*** occasionally may cause sneezing and rhinitis in younger patients and gastrointestinal disturbances; there have been many cases of rapidly acquired dependence especially with alcoholics and those with a history of drug abuse. Hypotension and bronchorrhoea can occur during intravenous infusion. Chlormethiazole in the treatment of alcohol withdrawal should be reserved for inpatient use.

Drug Interactions

1. The hypnotics will have additive sedating effects with other drugs possessing CNS depressant activity.
2. Barbiturates stimulate liver microsomal enzymes and therefore increase the metabolism and decrease the efficiency of a number of drugs, for example, phenytoin, warfarin, and low-dose oral contraceptives.
3. Chloral hydrate enhances the anticoagulant effect of warfarin and may lead to haemorrhage.
4. Chloral hydrate when combined with alcohol may produce an unpleasant vasodilating reaction, characterised by tachycardia, palpitations and facial flushing.

Contraindications

1. Barbiturates should never be given to patients suffering from porphyria as an acute attack may be precipitated.
2. Hypnotics should be used with great caution or not at all in patients with compromised liver function, since a prolongation of CNS depression may occur.
3. Chloral hydrate is contraindicated in patients with peptic ulcer due to its gastric-irritant properties.

NURSING IMPLICATIONS

Assessment

Hypnotics include the barbiturates and benzodiazepines which have been discussed previously. A variety of other compounds gathered together as a miscellaneous group includes chloral hydrate and chlormethiazole. The important assessment parameters are similar to groups of drugs previously discussed under psychopharmacology. It is important to assess the current medication regime for possible interactions especially with other CNS depressants. Assessment of liver function is essential as decreased function will lead to an increased length of CNS depression.

It should be stressed that an important function of the nurse is proper assessment of the reason for the patient's insomnia before resorting to the use of drugs to handle it. Often, simple nursing measures can be instituted which may avoid the need to use drugs altogether. For example, listening to the patient's anxieties and counselling appropriately may do far more to promote proper rest for the patient than a drug-induced sleep from which he wakes only to face the original anxiety once more. Simple physical measures to promote comfort (such as position change, a back rub or an extra blanket and so on) should not be overlooked.

Administration

Administration is usually oral, although hypnotics may be given parenterally. Chloral hydrate mixture may be chilled, or it may be given in capsule form to avoid the unpleasant taste. It should be given with food or milk to avoid gastric irritation, as should chlormethiazole. Hypnotics should be administered later (rather than earlier) in the evening as drowsiness during activities while preparing for sleep may lead to accidents. Care and supervision of the elderly person taking hypnotics is essential, and bedrails may be needed to protect the patient during the night.

Dependence may be a problem with routine administration. The medication must be tapered off and never stopped abruptly as severe withdrawal convulsions may occur. Care must be taken with parenteral infusion of chlormethiazole as profound hypotension and respiratory obstruction may occur. Dermatological reactions such as an irritating rash may be observed in patients taking chloral hydrate.

Evaluation

Evaluating the therapeutic effect of these drugs is essential, as they are administered to relieve insomnia. Adverse reactions should be noted, especially states resembling dementia. Note should be taken of the length of time over which the medication has been administered.

Teaching

Patient teaching, especially of the elderly, may prevent serious adverse effects and accidents. Teaching relatives about the therapeutic and adverse effects will be beneficial to the patient, for example, adverse effects of combining hypnotics with CNS depressants, especially alcohol, and of suddenly ceasing the medication.

Advise the patient to take the medication immediately on retiring and to avoid situations that require alertness and concentration having once taken the medication. Also advise the patient *not* to take extra medication if he or she misses a night dose. Supervision may be needed for the confused elderly patient.

SELF-EVALUATION TEST

1. It is advisable to recommend the use of a sunscreening agent to patients taking one of the following drugs:
   (a) methaqualone
   (b) chlorpromazine
   (c) benztropine
   (d) droperidol
   (e) temazepam
   (f) lithium carbonate
2. Tardive dyskinesia is an adverse reaction brought about by which two of the following drugs?
   (a) lithium carbonate
   (b) oxazepam
   (c) chlorpromazine
   (d) perphenazine
   (e) chlordiazepoxide
   (f) trimipramine
   (g) doxepin
   (h) amitriptyline
3. With which of the following drugs should tyramine-rich foods be avoided?
   (a) amitriptyline
   (b) tranylcypromine
   (c) phenelzine
   (d) haloperidol
   (e) thioridazine
4. A 52-year-old process worker presents with a six-month history of insomnia. There is no history of anxiety or depressive illness. The physician decides to prescribe a hypnotic drug. Which one of the following would be the most suitable drug. Give reasons.
   (a) nitrazepam
   (b) oxazepam
   (c) temazepam
   (d) chlorpromazine
   (e) chloral hydrate
5. Why is the anti-Parkinsonian agent L-dopa unsuitable for counteracting extrapyramidal side effects caused by chlorpromazine?
6. A 45-year-old manic depressive patient who has had uneventful lithium carbonate therapy for seven years develops the following symptoms: lethargy, confusion and a slight tremor of the hands. On taking a history, the psychiatrist discovers that in recent months the patient has been placed on the following therapy: glibenclamide 5 mg in the morning for mild diabetes and *Aldomet* 250 mg three times daily with *Lasix* 40 mg in the morning for hypertension. Which of the newly prescribed drugs may have caused the patient's symptoms and by what mechanism?

7. Neuroleptic agents are useful in the treatment of insomnia and anxiety states.
   (a) true
   (b) false
8. Tricyclic antidepressants are most useful in the treatment of one of the following types of depression.
   (a) depression associated with manic-depressive illness
   (b) endogenous depression
   (c) depression secondary to organic brain disease
   (d) depression secondary to personal loss
9. Describe the nursing procedures you would follow after the administration of an IV dose of diazepam.

Table 93
Psychopharmacological Agents

Drug Group	Drug Name	Use	Action	Adverse Reactions	Nursing Implications
Neuroleptics					
Phenothiazines	Chlorpromazine Fluphenazine Perphenazine Trifluoperazine Thioridazine Trimeprazine Pericyazine	Palliative treatment of psychoses, e.g. schizophrenia, organic psychoses, manic depression	Block central action of dopamine	Sedation, anticholinergic effects, breast enlargement, lactation and menstrual difficulties in women, photosensitivity reactions, pigmentation of cornea, retina and lens, jaundice, depression of white cell count, ECG changes, hypotension, lower seizure threshold, extra-pyramidal effects	***Assess:*** baseline parameters of "lying and standing" BP, pulse rate, respiration rate, temperature, weight and sleep patterns; present disease presentation; concurrent medication, alcohol use and known drug reactions; pregnancy or lactation; history of diseases especially cardiovascular, cerebrovascular, kidney, liver or glaucoma. ***Administer:*** parenteral; do *not* mix with other medications, care in preparation to avoid dermatological reactions; IVI rate must be carefully monitored if given by continuous infusion, and tissue extravasation prevented. ***Evaluate:*** therapeutic effectiveness as indicated by a reduction of present symptoms; for adverse reactions, tolerance and compliance. ***Teach:*** effective self-evaluation of therapeutic effect, adverse reactions and problems of sudden withdrawal of medication; advise not to continue activities that require alertness and concentration if drowsy; to seek medical advice if adverse reactions appear.
Butyrophenones	Haloperidol Droperidol	As above	As above	As above	As above
Thioxanthines	Flupenthixol	As above	As above	As above	As above

Diphenylbutyl piperidines	Pimozide	As above	As above	As above	As above
Anti-manic	Lithium carbonate	Manic phase of manic-depressive illness; long-term maintenance therapy	Reduces frequency and/or severity and duration of manic and depressive episodes	Polydypsia, skin rashes, hypothyroidism, nephrogenic diabetes insipidus; Toxicity: nausea, vomiting, lethargy, tremor, anorexia, abdominal discomfort, diarrhoea, ataxia, slurred speech, loss of consciousness, electrolyte imbalance, cardiac impairment	***Assess:*** baseline vital signs, weight, sleep patterns, hydrational, nutritional and electrolyte status; present disease presentation; present medications and lithium-carbonate blood levels; presence of pregnancy or lactation; history of cardiac or cerebrovascular disease, organic dementia, renal or thyroid disease. ***Administer:*** with food. ***Evaluate:*** therapeutic effect in normalisation of behavioural parameters and sleep patterns; adverse effects and conditions which may effect nutritional, hydrational and electrolyte status; monitor blood electrolytes regularly and dietary sodium intake. ***Teach:*** that it is essential to maintain adequate hydration and sodium level; to have regular blood-lithium estimations; to recognise deviations from therapeutic effectiveness, differentiating between adverse effects and representation of disease symptomatology; the importance of immediately seeking medical advice when conditions of diarrhoea or vomiting or other conditions which alter fluid and electrolytes present; not to carry out tasks which require concentration or alertness when drowsy.

continued

Drug Group	Drug Name	Use	Action	Adverse Reactions	Nursing Implications
Anxiolytic Sedatives					
Barbiturates	Amylobarbitone Sodium barbitone Pentobarbitone Methylpheno-barbitone Phenobarbitone Quinalbarbitone	Anxiety states, sedation, anticonvulsant insomnia	CNS depression	Hypotension, decreased heart rate, respiratory depression, dizziness, ataxia, rash, decreased gastric secretions, tolerance, liver enzyme induction, contraindicated in patients with porphyria.	***Assess:*** baseline vital signs, BP, temperature, respiration rate, weight, sleep patterns and age; abuse potential; previous drug reaction and alcohol intake; presence of pregnancy or lactation; past or present history of allergic states, dermatological disorders, liver disease or haematological disorders. ***Administer:*** usually orally and self-medicated but see Chapters 29 and 30 for IM and IV administration and doses. ***Evaluate:*** therapeutic effectiveness; adverse effects, particularly those involving the CNS such as drowsiness or ataxia which may indicate a need for patient supervision; BP — lying and standing; blood-screening results; dependency problems, weight gain and sleep patterns. ***Teach:*** identification of deviations from therapeutic effect especially manifestations of CNS disturbance; the importance of compliance and the serious consequence of suddenly ceasing the medication; to avoid activities requiring concentration or alertness while drowsy or dizzy; to avoid alcohol and other CNS depressants during course of treatment.

Benzodiazepines	Diazepam Chlordiazepoxide Clorazepate Nitrazepam Clonazepam Medazepam Bromazepam Flurazepam Flunitrazepam Alprazolam Lorazepam Oxazepam Temazepam Triazolam	Anxiety states, convulsive disorders, insomnia, muscle spasm, night terrors, somnambulism, alcohol withdrawal	Mechanism is unclear, action is central and probably related to GABA receptors	Habituation, tolerance, sedation, ataxia, dizziness, vertigo, dysarthria, incoordination, muscle weakness, skin rash, blurred vision	***Assess:*** **for previous hypersensitivity to drug, pregnancy, lactation, age, liver,** renal function, myasthenia gravis; concurrent use of other CNS depressant drugs including alcohol; concurrent use of cimetidine; employment, re use of power driven machinery or driving; vital signs as objective measure of anxiety. ***Administer:*** usually at home; in hospital — orally, as ordered; parenteral doses — do not dilute; IV, by slow injection into vein; flush vein with normal saline after administration; monitor blood pressure after IV administration. ***Evaluate:*** drug effectiveness, for example, reduced anxiety (subjective) or lowered blood pressure, pulse rate and respirations (objective); adverse effects, for example, rash, signs of toxicity. ***Teach:*** to evaluate for adverse effects (the patient or member of family); to avoid using power tools, industrial machinery and driving; to move from reclining to standing position slowly to avoid postural hypotension; to avoid alcohol, abrupt withdrawal and that the drug can produce dependency.

continued

Drug Group	Drug Name	Use	Action	Adverse Reactions	Nursing Implications
Antidepressants					
Tricyclics	Amitriptyline Protriptyline Nortriptyline Imipramine Trimipramine Desipramine Doxepin Dothiepin Clomipramine	Pathological depression	Mood elevation	Sedation, anticholinergic effects, postural hypotension, cardiac effects, skin rashes, blood dyscrasias, jaundice, weight gain, sweating, paradoxical manic excitement	***Assess:*** baseline vital signs of "lying and standing" BP, pulse rate, respiration rate, hydration status, weight, sleep pattern and bowel habits; previous drug reactions, concurrent medications especially alcohol intake; presenting disease symptoms pattern; history of behavioural disturbances, convulsions, glaucoma, thyroid, liver, renal disease. ***Administer:*** ensure compliance. ***Evaluate:*** therapeutic effectiveness as evidenced by normalisation of behaviour; adverse effects such as dermatological reactions, postural hypotension and a altered sleep pattern; changes in bowel habits or stool appearance, for example, clay stools: GIT irritation, weight gain; changes in pulse rate or quality, blood dyscrasias, jaundice, and urinary retention; in some cases there may be an increased risk of suicide early in treatment. ***Teach:*** expected therapeutic and adverse effects, and appropriate measures to be taken to avoid adverse effects; risk of sedation and risks associated with sudden cessation of therapy.

Tetracyclics	Mianserin	As above	As above	Similar to tricyclics, but fewer cardiac and anticholinergic effects; increased risk of agranulocytosis and neutropenia	As above
Monoamine oxidase inhibitors	Phenelzine Tranylcypromine Isocarboxazid Iproniazid	As above	Inhibit monoamine oxidase and allow accumulation of catecholamines in brain	Severe hypertension, liver damage, hypotension, insomnia, gastric upset, dizziness, dry mouth, muscle weakness, cardiac arrhythmias, disturbances of colour vision. *Note*: care with tyramine containing foods and over-the-counter medications for cough and cold	***Assess:*** baseline vital signs such as lying BP and standing BP, pulse rate, weight, and hydration status; current medications and alcohol intake; history of hypertension, glaucoma, cardiac or cerebrovascular disease, liver or renal disease; diet or any recent changes in diet. ***Administer:*** usually orally. ***Evaluate:*** therapeutic effectiveness, adverse effects, BP (lying and standing), constipation and behavioural changes. ***Teach:*** the importance of recognising deviations from the therapeutic effect and presentation of adverse effects; to avoid tyramine containing foods and over-the-counter remedies.

continued

Drug Group	Drug Name	Use	Action	Adverse Reactions	Nursing Implications
Psychostimulants	Dexamphetamine	Narcolepsy, hyperkinesia in children	CNS stimulation	Restlessness, dizziness, tremor, tenseness, irritability, euphoria, fever, confusion, panic, hallucinations, headache, pallor, flushing, cardiac arrhythmias, sweating, hypertension or hypotension, dry mouth, anorexia, nausea, vomiting, diarrhoea, abdominal cramps	***Assess:*** disease presentation, e.g. hyperkinesia in children; important parameters are weight, height, BP, pulse rate, respiration rate and motor activity; the presence of pregnancy or lactation; concurrent medication, previous drug reaction; history of epilepsy, behavioural disorders, asthma, anorexia, insomnia or cardiovascular disease. ***Administer:*** according to legal requirements; do *not* mix with alkaline drugs, e.g. barbiturates. ***Evaluate:*** therapeutic effectiveness, tolerance, dependency and withdrawal reactions including psychosis; adverse reactions involving the CNS, tremor, depression, euphoria, confusion, cardiovascular, BP, pulse change, palpitations, arrhythmia, GIT, dry mouth, anorexia, diarrhoea. ***Teach:*** therapeutic effectiveness and to recognise adverse effects, abuse potential and problems of withdrawal.

	Cocaine	Mostly as local anaesthetic in eye and ENT procedures, occasionally used in morphine-based mixtures for severe or terminal-illness pain	Blocks nerve conduction; counteracts CNS depression caused by morphine	As for other stimulant drugs	
Hypnotics					
Barbiturates	See this chapter's section on anxiolytic sedatives.				
Benzodiazepines	See this chapter's section on anxiolytic sedatives.				
Miscellaneous drugs	Chloral hydrate Chlormethiazole	Insomnia	CNS depressant	Gastric irritation, rash, hypotension, paradoxical excitement, hangover, visual blurring, confusion, toxic convulsions, delirium, habituation and tolerance, withdrawal symptoms	***Assess:*** baseline vital signs, BP, respiration rate and pattern, sleep patterns; current medications and alcohol intake; previous drug reactions; age; history of chronic respiratory disease or dermatological disorders, liver or renal disease. ***Administer:*** at night, on retiring. ***Evaluate:*** therapeutic effectiveness, compliance; adverse reactions such as CNS depression such as drowsiness, or occasionally the opposite reactions, such as restlessness, agitation and rage; respiratory function; suicidal tendencies; liver and renal function. ***Teach:*** to identify deviations from the therapeutic effect; to comply with the prescribed dose and not to carry out tasks which require concentration when drowsy; not to combine with other CNS depressants.

29
DRUGS USED IN NEUROLOGY

Rhondda Figgis Close

OBJECTIVES

At the conclusion of this chapter the reader should be able to:

1. define the terms "epilepsy", "migraine" and "Parkinsonism";
2. differentiate between the various types of each of these diseases;
3. list the drugs used in each of these diseases;
4. list the nursing implications associated with medication given in each of these diseases.

DEFINITIONS

Antiemetic — a drug capable of relieving or preventing nausea and vomiting.

Antiepileptics (*or anticonvulsants*) — drugs which work on the central nervous system to prevent epileptic seizures.

Catecholamine — a group of sympathomimetic drugs including adrenaline.

Epilepsy — a disorder of the central nervous system in which uncontrolled electrical discharge of brain cells results in transient episodes of unconsciousness or psychic dysfunction with or without convulsive movements.

Migraine — a paroxysmal intense pain in the head, commonly unilateral, and often, although not always, associated with nausea, vomiting and photophobia.

Paroxysmal — a sudden attack, a sudden reappearance of symptoms, or a sudden increase in the intensity of existing symptoms.

Psychotropic — pertaining to a drug having a special affinity for or effect on the psyche or mind.

Serotonin — a hormone released into the blood stream which imparts vasoconstrictor activity to the latter.

EPILEPSY

Epilepsy is a symptom rather than a disease, and it affects about one in every 100 people in the community. It is important that the nature of this condition be understood because there is so much misconception in relation to employment and social acceptance that the quality of life of epileptic patients can be severely impaired. Drug therapy is dependent upon the type of epilepsy so the various classifications will be looked at briefly.

Epilepsy may be classified as symptomatic or idiopathic.

SYMPTOMATIC EPILEPSY

Symptomatic (secondary) epilepsy may be due to *intracranial factors* such as infection (for example, meningitis, encephalitis, neurosyphilis, abscess, tuberculosis); trauma (for example, at birth, or head injury); vascular lesions; cerebal degeneration; tumours; or to *extracranial factors* such as anoxia; poisons (for example, alcohol, ethyl chloride, lead, cocaine); metabolic disturbances (for example, with uraemia, alkalosis, liver failure, hypoglycaemia); withdrawal of medications (hypnotics, opiates).

IDIOPATHIC EPILEPSY

Epilepsy is classified as idiopathic (primary) epilepsy when no cause (such as above) is present. It should be noted that all living brains have the capacity to produce a seizure if the stimulus is sufficient. Some individuals have spontaneous seizures without any provocative stimuli, others may be affected by such stimuli as a flickering light, excessive alcoholic intake, or severe fatigue, while still others may require electroconvulsive shock before seizure develops. The degree of stimulus needed to produce a seizure in a particular individual is the "***seizure threshold***" of that person.

There are several types of idopathic (or primary) epilepsy.

Tonic-clonic seizures

In this type of seizure, a patient, after varying periods of increasing tension (several minutes up to two days), simply loses consciousness and falls to the ground in a state of tonic rigidity. During this state the familiar "epileptic cry" is heard, air being forced out through the tightly abducted vocal cords. The rigidity of the muscles is followed by generalised jerking, which is then replaced by the limbs becoming flaccid. The patient may regain consciousness in about five to 15 minutes, may be confused for a further 15 minutes or so, and may then go into a deep sleep. These seizures are also known as major or grand mal seizures.

Simple absence seizures

These are only in children, who may have "little absences" of about 10 to 15 seconds where they stare straight ahead, sometimes blinking the eyelids or tilting the head backwards, and then return to their normal activity. These attacks may occur from five to 100 times per day. They are also known as true petit mal attacks.

Myoclonic seizure

This may occur as jerkiness of one limb or all limbs and is most obvious in the first hour after waking or in the hour before sleep. A child may appear to wilfully throw something across the table at breakfast or to drop articles. It may occur in patients having major epilepsy as well or be associated with various forms of symptomatic epilepsy.

Focal epilepsy (or Jacksonian epilepsy)

Hughlings Jackson first described seizures originating in the cortex in 1888. These seizures may remain localised and affect the appropriate part of the body. For example, a seizure in the motor cortex results in violent movements of a limb or part of a limb; in the sensory cortex, abnormal sensations appear in the other side of the body; and in the occipital region, impairment of vision such as brief flashes of light or confused visual hallucinations may occur. The seizures may also spread to adjacent areas producing a grand mal convulsion.

Temporal lobe epilepsy

This is a particular kind of focal seizure arising in the temporal lobe. It is the most common form of minor epilepsy seen in adults, accounting for one-third of all varieties of epilepsy. The following symptoms are usual: hallucinations referred to the senses of taste, smell, hearing and vision, visceral sensations, disorders of memory (*déjà vu*), dreamy states, automatic behaviour which may be violent.

Status epilepticus

This is a condition where seizures follow one another with no intervening periods of consciousness. Grand mal status epilepticus may persist for hours or days and can be fatal. This state may occur spontaneously or may be precipitated by a too-rapid withdrawal of anticonvulsants.

DRUGS USED IN EPILEPSY (ANTICONVULSANTS)

HYDANTOINS

Phenytoin, known also by the trade name *Epanutin,* is the best known and most used drug in this group.

The drug is thought to inhibit the spread of seizure discharge through the brain and to decrease intracellular sodium concentration.

It is the drug of first choice in grand mal and generally favoured for all forms of epilepsy except true petit mal (it may make this condition worse). It may be given in combination with other anticonvulsants.

Adverse Drug Reactions

Gum hypertrophy is a well-reported drug reaction — it is sometimes necessary to change to another anticonvulsant if this occurs. This may possibly be corrected by dental hygiene, or if not, dental surgery may be necessary.

Foetal hydantoin syndrome, which may lead to cleft palate, has been noted when the mother has taken phenytoin during pregnancy.

Dermatitis sometimes occurs, and this may be accompanied by fever and a blood disorder (eosinophilia). Unusual and excessive hair growth (hirsutism) has been reported, and acne is common.

When blood levels become too high so that phenytoin intoxication occurs, nystagmus (oscillating movements of the eyeballs), muscular incoordination and vertigo may be apparent. These effects usually may be removed by lowering the dose for two to three days after which the patient can usually go back to the previous dose.

Other less known drug reactions with chronic phenytoin usage include various blood disorders such as leucopenia, agranulocytosis and thrombocytopenia.

Drug Interactions

The metabolism of phenytoin may be affected significantly by the concomitant use of other drugs.

Barbiturates and ***carbamazepine*** may enhance the metabolism of phenytoin, resulting in lowered blood levels of phenytoin.

Coumarin anticoagulants, disulfiram, phenylbutazone and ***isoniazid*** may inhibit the metabolism of phenytoin, thus resulting in signs of phenytoin toxicity.

Tricyclic antidepressants in high doses may precipitate seizures so that the dose of phenytoin may have to be adjusted.

THE BARBITURATES

Members of this group are derived from barbituric acid and are closely related in structure. They include ***phenobarbitone*** and ***methyl phenobarbitone*** (*Prominal*), which is metabolised to phenobarbitone. Another in this group is ***primidone*** (*Mysoline*) which is metabolised to two other drugs, a compound known as PEMA and phenobarbitone; so it is in fact three anticonvulsants in one.

The barbiturates have generally come into some disrepute as sedatives, but as anticonvulsants they have a long and proven history of efficiency.

Barbiturates depress the CNS, that is, the cerebral cortex and the reticular formation. These drugs have been used for the treatment of major seizures of all kinds and are sometimes still used in paediatrics for febrile convulsions.

Adverse Drug Reactions

The barbiturates have a sedative effect and in some children produce irritability and aggravate any tendency to excessive movement associated with muscle spasm (hyperkinesia). Other well recognised side effects are incoordination of muscle action (ataxia) and rashes. They tend to produce tolerance and severe withdrawal effects. Other severe symptoms may develop from enhancement by alcohol and severe toxic effects may result from overdose. Because the drugs are inducers of liver enzymes, they cause increased metabolism and therefore decrease the effect of any other drugs which are metabolised by liver enzymes and given concomitantly.

THE SUCCINAMIDES

The succinamide drugs were developed for use in petit mal in the search for drugs with minimal side effects. This group includes ***ethosuximide*** (*Zarontin*).

The succinamides are used for the control of true petit mal.

Adverse Drug Reactions

These drugs may induce major seizures if there is a tendency to this condition, so it may be necessary to combine them with another drug effective against major epilepsy. Other side effects include anorexia, nausea and vomiting, and there have been rare reportings of bone-marrow depression, resulting in pancytopenia and leucopenia.

CARBAMAZEPINE

This drug is known also by the trade name of *Tegretol* and can be included in the miscellaneous group of drugs used in the treatment of epilepsy.

Carbamazepine may be given as drug of first choice in treatment of grand mal epilepsy or may be combined with other drugs for patients who have proved resistant to treatment. It is of particular use in the treatment of temporal lobe seizures, especially when associated with disturbed behaviour. Retarded children have been shown to benefit in some studies, both in the control of their epilepsy and behavioural disturbances. Carbamazepine has been successfully used in the treatment of tic douloureux and is drug of first choice in the treatment of trigeminal neuralgia.

Adverse Drug Reactions

Carbamazepine has produced side effects such as drowsiness, skin rashes and extremely rarely has produced aplastic anaemia (two or three cases).

SULTHIAME

Sulthiame is an anticonvulsant with a history of a high incidence of side effects. It has now been withdrawn voluntarily from the UK market.

Adverse Drug Reactions

These include nausea, vomiting, headache, difficulty in breathing, "tingling" of the skin, drowsiness and sometimes mental confusion. Some psychic side effects have been produced when given in conjunction with primidone in the treatment of temporal lobe seizures.

THE BENZODIAZEPINES

Drugs in this group are used in the treatment of various kinds of epilepsy. These drugs are diazepam (*Valium*), nitrazepam (*Mogadon*) and clonazepam (*Rivotril*).

Diazepam is an extremely useful drug in the treatment of status epilepticus when given intraventously, though it does not act as a potent anticonvulsant when given orally.

Nitrazepam is of more use in the treatment of myoclonic epilepsy occurring with grand mal.

Clonazepam is one of the newer benzodiazepines. It has been of use in a wide range of epilepsies in adults and children, including status epilepticus.

Adverse Drug Reactions

Drowsiness and sedation are side effects with all these drugs, and uncoordinated muscle movement (ataxia) may occur in high dosage. Ataxia may occur more frequently with clonazepam as well as fatigue, aggression and occasional instability in behaviour.

SODIUM VALPROATE (Epilim)

Sodium valproate is thought to maintain levels of a chemical in the brain called gamma amino butyric acid (GABA) by inhibiting the enzyme GABA transaminase which otherwise causes the breakdown of GABA.

It has been shown to be effective in the treatment of temporal lobe epilepsy, petit mal, grand mal, mixed epilepsy and myoclonic seizures. Children have performed better at school on this drug because it has a lesser sedative effect than other anticonvulsant drugs.

Adverse Drug Reactions

These were thought to be rare in the use of this drug, and reported adverse reactions included transitory indigestion, vomiting and drowsiness and an occasional tendency to cause bleeding. It had been reported to produce testicular damage in animals, although it is not known whether this occurs in man. Hair loss has also been reported.

There have been cases of hepatotoxicity, some of which have been fatal, with most reported deaths occurring in children. However, these cases are rare and so, as sodium valproate is such a useful drug, it continues to be used.

The following precautions are recommended however: avoidance in patients with altered liver function, regular monitoring of liver function and consideration of hepatotoxicity when a patient, especially a child, becomes unwell a few months after starting treatment with sodium valproate.

A report from France suggests a link between valproate being used in pregnancy and the incidence of spina bifida in the new-born child. The risk is thought to be between 1 in 50 and 1 in 100 births. This has not been confirmed by further research, but the facility for antenatal detection of spina bifida should be available.

It is important that medication is not stopped without medical advice, as this may precipitate an epileptic attack. Alternative drugs may be appropriate.

DRUGS USED IN STATUS EPILEPTICUS

Intravenous diazepam 10 mg may be given over five minutes. This may stop the seizure by the time the injection is completed. In children, doses of 1 mg every two to five minutes may be given up to a maximum of 10 mg in children more than five years of age, with about half of this dose being given to children under five years. The effect of the diazepam may be of short duration so it may be followed by intravenous phenytoin at the rate of 50 mg/min up to a loading dose of 500 mg to 1 gram for adults. Doses for children vary according to weight.

The rectal route may be used very effectively in status epilepticus in children. It can be administered as a rectal solution (diazepam 5 mg/2.5 ml and 10 mg/2.5 ml, *Stesolid*).

Clonazepam (1 to 4 mg IV) is sometimes given instead of diazepam. It has a longer effect than diazepam, but side effects such as respiratory depression and sedation may be more pronounced than with diazepam.

Paraldehyde has been used, but it is not favoured because of its toxicity and odour.

If these methods fail to control status epilepticus, short-acting barbiturate anaesthesia such as ***thiopentone sodium*** (*Intraval Sodium*) may be tried. In refractory cases, ***chlormethiazole*** (*Heminevrin*) has been used with success.

POST-TRAUMATIC EPILEPSY

Seizures may begin any time up to 24 months after trauma. This applies in about 10% of severe closed head injuries and 40% of penetrating head wounds. Patients with such injuries should receive prophylactic anticonvulsants (for example, phenytoin 100 mg three times daily) for up to three years to reduce the risk of seizures.

Anticonvulsants (for example, phenytoin 1 g/IV over 12 hours followed by 300 mg to 400 mg per day) may be given after skull fractures to protect against seizures. ***Osmotic diuretics*** (urea, mannitol, glycerol) given IV to reduce brain swelling should be reserved for preoperative use in patients with haematomas or for deteriorating patients. The benefit of corticosteroids used for this purpose is questionable.

NURSING IMPLICATIONS

The use of anticonvulsants is aimed at controlling seizures. Several types of anticonvulsants may be administered concurrently in an effort to obtain stability. It is essential that therapeutic blood levels be reached and maintained. This may take several days, and the length of time required will vary depending on the drug. Anticonvulsants should not be withdrawn suddenly. If a particular anticonvulsant is causing an adverse effect, a different drug should be considered.

When a patient is taking anticonvulsants, it is essential that the following points concerning drug education be made:

- Sudden discontinuation may induce seizures. In some cases status epilepticus may be induced.
- The dose should not be altered without consulting a medical officer.
- The concurrent use of alcohol is usually contraindicated, as alcohol is known to lower seizure threshold.
- Patients on anticonvulsant medication should be advised to wear or carry a medical identification tag.
- Maintain an adequate supply of medication at all times.
- Women taking anticonvulsants should discuss the risks associated with pregnancy with their physician prior to attempting conception.
- Inform the patient and relatives of known adverse and toxic effects and advise them to see a physician should these occur.
- If drowsiness occurs, patients should avoid activities which are potentially hazardous such as driving a motor vehicle or using machinery.
- Advise about driving and licensing requirements.
- Advise that the urine may change colour with the use of phenytoin.
- Regular blood screenings for therapeutic blood levels of anticonvulsants and haematological disorders should be carried out.
- Advise the patient to rise slowly from the recumbent position if taking barbiturates.
- Advise of the many potential drug interactions between the anticonvulsants and other medications that may be administered concurrently.

GENERAL

It is usually preferable to continue anticonvulsant medication during pregnancy since the risk to both mother and foetus of uncontrolled seizures may be more serious than that of the effects of the drug.

Most seizures are caused by non-compliance with medication regimes. It is therefore important that patients being treated for epilepsy take their medication as ordered and that they be given encouragement to do so. Reduction in the frequency of attacks will add immeasurably to their quality of life.

Many epileptics at one stage or another have experienced rejection, either socially or at the hands of a potential employer, or if the patient happens to be a child, at the hands of parents who cannot understand why their child has been afflicted in this way. There is still enormous misconception about epilepsy in the community, which on the whole regards it as a mental disorder.

Table 94
Drugs Used in Epilepsy

Generic Name	Trade Name	Specific Use	Drug Interactions	Adverse Effects
Phenytoin	*Epanutin*	All epilepsy except petit mal; first choice in grand mal	Barbiturates and carbamazepine enhance metabolism and hence lower phenytoin levels; coumarin anticoagulants, disulfiram, phenylbutazone, isoniazid inhibit phenytoin metabolism, hence, may cause phenytoin toxicity; tricyclic antidepressants may precipitate seizures	Gum hypertrophy; Foetal hydantoin syndrome — cleft palate; dermatitis, with fever and eosinophilia; hirsutism and acne; toxic effects — nystagmus, vertigo and muscular incoordination
Barbiturates				
Phenobarbitone		All major seizures, especially in paediatrics for febrile convulsions	Cause induction of metabolism of any other drugs metabolised in liver; actions enhanced by alcohol	Sedation; irritability in children; ataxia and rashes; tolerance; induction of liver enzymes
Methylphenobarbitone	*Prominal*			
Primidone	*Mysoline*			
Succinamides				
Ethosuximide	*Zarontin*	Petit mal		May induce major seizures, anorexia, nausea, vomiting
Carbamazepine	*Tegretol*	Grand mal, temporal lobe seizures	Enhances metabolism of warfarin phenytoin; phenobarbitone may stimulate metabolism of carbamazepine; d-propoxyphene inhibits metabolism	Drowsiness, skin rashes

Benzodiazepines				
Diazepam	*Valium*	Status epilepticus	Additive effects with alcohol; interaction with levodopa reported; metabolism enhanced by phenytoin	Drowsiness, sedation, ataxia with high dosage with all benzodiazepines; clonazepam: ataxia, fatigue aggression, behavioural instability
Nitrazepam	*Mogadon*	Myoclonic epilepsy		
Clonazepam	*Rivotril*	Wide range, including status epilepticus		
Sodium valproate	*Epilim*	Most types	May cause false positive in urine testing for glucose	Transitory indigestion; hair loss; severe liver damage; may cause spina bifida if used in pregnancy
Thipentone sodium	*Intraval sodium*	Status epilepticus	As with barbiturates	
Chlormethiazole	*Heminevrin*	Refractory status epilepticus		

PARKINSONISM

Parkinsonism is a neurological disorder which manifests itself as disturbances of posture, rigidity, tremor and hypokinesia (abnormally decreased muscular movement). It has been recognised as a disease entity for over 150 years, and it is a fairly common disorder. It has been said that it may affect as many as 1 in every 100 of the population over 50 years of age, although this figure has been disputed.

The disease symptoms are due to changes in the brain, that is, a reduction of dopamine receptors and cell loss in the substantia nigra. The two systems controlling movement become out of balance so that the dopaminergic system is defective and the cholinergic system is dominant. Drug treatment can therefore be utilised in restoring the dopaminergic system (L-dopa, amantadine) or depressing the cholinergic system (anticholinergic drugs, for example, benzhexol, orphenadrine hydrochloride).

DRUGS USED IN PARKINSONISM

LEVODOPA (Larodopa)

Levodopa has become drug of first choice in the treatment of Parkinsonism. Dopamine is not effective as it is poorly absorbed from the gut and does not pass the blood-brain barrier, whereas L-dopa, which is the immediate precursor to dopamine in the biochemical chain leading to noradrenaline, does. Levodopa is acted on by the enzyme decarboxylase to produce dopamine.

$$\text{Phenylalanine} \rightarrow \text{tyrosine} \rightarrow \text{dopa} \xrightarrow{\text{decarboxylase}} \text{dopamine} \rightarrow \text{noradrenaline}$$

Levodopa acts by replenishing dopamine in the corpus striatum, the beneficial response being related to the amount of dopamine present. L-dopa does not cure the disease. It acts as a replacement therapy as does insulin in diabetes.

L-dopa is generally more effective in the treatment of hypokinesia (abnormally decreased muscular movement) than in release of rigidity and tremor.

Adverse Drug Reactions

Anorexia, nausea, vomiting, postural hypotension, involuntary movements of face and lips or cardiac arrhythmias may result.

Drug Interactions

MAOIs decrease dopamine and noradrenaline degradation, resulting in increase of these amines and possibly leading to dangerous hypertension.

Reserpine *(Serpasil)* possibly depletes brain of dopamine and therefore antagonises levodopa.

Phenothiazines (for example, antihistamines such as promethazine) may block dopamine receptors and should not be given to people on L-dopa.

Pyridoxine reverses therapeutic effect of L-dopa, acting as a coenzyme in the decarboxylation of peripheral L-dopa to dopamine, hence leaving less L-dopa to penetrate the brain.

NURSING IMPLICATIONS

Assessment

This should begin with a review of the patient's history for the diagnosed cause of the Parkinsonian symptoms. Dopaminergic drugs should not be administered to patients whose Parkinsonian symptoms are secondary to the use of neuroleptic drugs. Also, confirmation of the order from the prescriber should be sought if the history shows evidence of psychoses of any kind, confusional states, postural hypotension, endocrine, cardiac, renal or hepatic impairment, diabetes or glaucoma. The patient's drug use should be reviewed, as the concurrent use of MAO inhibitors, tricyclic antidepressants, other sympathomimetic-type drugs, antipsychotic agents as well as pyridoxine are contraindicated because of the drug interactions which can occur.

Physical assessment will include the establishing of baseline observations of blood pressure (standing and lying), pulse rate, features of Parkinsonism (degree of joint movement, tremor, rigidity, ambulation, daily living activities and emotional state), and colour and temperature of extremities.

Administration

To avoid unpleasant gastrointestinal side effects, dopaminergic drugs are best given with food.

Evaluation

This will include the documentation of drug effectiveness, that is, both subjective and objective signs of improvement of Parkinsonian symptoms. Observe for adverse effects such as postural hypotension, cardiac arrhythmias, poor peripheral circulation and urinary retention. Observations for these will include monitoring blood pressure (lying and standing), pulse rate, colour and temperature of extremities and urinary output. Observation of the patient's mood and behaviour is essential for the prompt identification of any undesirable emotional effects of the drug.

Teaching

This should involve the patient and his family. They should be taught the indications of drug effectiveness and adverse effects and to report the latter to their physician. They should be advised that pyridoxine reduces the effectiveness of L-dopa and advised to avoid vitamin and food preparations and antinauseants which contain it. Over-the-counter cough and cold preparations containing sympathomimetic decongestants should be avoided. The patient and family need to be advised that the urine and perspiration may become darkened and that the full effects of the drug may not be experienced for several months. Such advice provides reassurance and enhanced compliance.

L-DOPA WITH DECARBOXYLASE INHIBITOR

These compounds have provided an advance in the treatment of Parkinsonism. Carbidopa is a decarboxylase inhibitor which does not pass the blood-brain barrier; by giving it with L-dopa, the peripheral breakdown of L-dopa to dopamine by the enzyme decarboxylase does not take place. This conversion does not occur until the drug reaches the brain where the carbidopa is excluded by the blood-brain barrier.

As L-dopa is not acted on until it reaches its target organ (the brain), a much smaller dose is needed (perhaps only 20% of that required if L-dopa was taken alone). This causes a corresponding drop in some side effects, such as nausea and vomiting. This particular combination of drugs appears on the market as *Sinemet*. *Madopar* is another L-dopa decarboxylase inhibitor combination. Pyridoxine does not appear to antagonise L-dopa in the presence of decarboxylase inhibitors.

AMANTADINE

Amantadine (*Symmetrel*) is an antiviral drug which was discovered to be of benefit when given to a Parkinsonian patient for influenza. It may act by increasing dopamine synthesis.

It is used where symptoms of dysarthria (impairment of articulation, or stammering), loss of manual dexterity and disorders of gait predominate.

Adverse Drug Reactions

These include skin pigmentation and hallucinations.

Drug Interactions and Precautions

Amantadine may potentiate the side effects (confusion and hallucinations) of high-dose anticholinergics; it is wise, therefore, to reduce the dose of the anticholinergic before giving amantadine. Epileptic patients might be adversely affected by amantadine which has produced adverse CNS effects.

ANTICHOLINERGICS

Anticholinergics may be used in the treatment of Parkinsonism. They include ***benzhexol*** (*Artane*), ***benztropine*** (*Cogentin*), ***orphenadrine*** (*Disipal*), and ***procyclidine*** (*Kemadrin*).

These drugs reduce cholinergic activity, thereby reducing the dominance of the cholinergic system present in Parkinsonism. They act by blocking acetylcholine in the CNS.

When symptoms are mild — rigidity and tremor with little or no gait disorder or akinesia — anticholinergics may be used.

Adverse Drug Reactions

These may occur from accumulation of the drug leading to a toxic state with confusion which may be attributed to the disease. Incipient glaucoma may be precipitated. Other side effects include dryness of mouth, urinary hesitancy or retention, nausea and drowsiness.

Another drug which has been tried for Parkinson's disease is ***bromocriptine*** (*Parlodel*). It is a derivative of ergot and has been found to have a direct stimulating effect on dopaminergic receptors. It has been used extensively in the US and Europe for its anti-Parkinson effects.

Bromocriptine 2.5 mg to 10 mg daily is equivalent approximately to levodopa 100 mg plus a decarboxylase inhibitor and probably is at its most effective when given with this combination. When the dosage exceeds 100 mg per day, distressing side effects such as nausea, vomiting and dyskinesia are common, but these may also occur at lower doses. Patients who show any evidence of loss of higher integrative function or dementia are more prone to have the side effects of mental clouding and confusion.

Bromocriptine is highly protein bound (90% to 96% to serum albumin). It is incompletely absorbed from the gastrointestinal tract, metabolised in the liver, and excreted mostly in the bile.

MIGRAINE

Migraine can be a disabling affliction which affects approximately 20% of the population, occurring on the average in twice as many women as men and causing the loss of a large number of working days in the year. Migraine is usually a sudden form of headache which is associated with nausea, vomiting and photophobia.

Migraine differs from other forms of headache, such as tension headaches which are not as severe or paroxysmal, but is a chronic dull pressing sensation which may go on day after day. Sufferers may have a combination of the two kinds of headache — dull continuous headache punctuated by episodes of the more severe migraine attacks.

The insidious progression of headaches of increasing severity together with other neurological symptoms should be investigated for the possibility of intracranial tumour.

Classical migraine is often preceded by visual disturbances such as blank flashing spots in the vision (fortification spectra), dysphasia, paraesthesia on one side of the body. Common migraine does not produce this form of symptoms. Migraine occurs mostly in adults, between puberty and 65 years. It does, however, occur in children, and in this group is often preceded by abdominal pain and vomiting.

Trigger factors are wide ranging and may be emotional (for example, stress, or relaxation after stress), physical (exertion, head injury), hormonal (premenstrual), or even foods (for example, cheese or red wine). Other factors are intrinsic body substances such as serotonin, bradykinin and histamine.

DRUGS USED IN MIGRAINE

Treatment of migraine attack may be divided into long-term management and prevention, and treatment of the acute attack.

LONG-TERM MANAGEMENT AND PREVENTION

Non-drug treatment may include such factors as avoidance of precipitatory factors (certain foods, situations and so on) and use of psychotherapy, physiotherapy and, in some cases, acupuncture.

Prophylactic drug treatment may be indicated if attacks occur more than once or twice each month. Drugs used are those which alter catecholamine action, anti-serotonin drugs and others.

Drugs which alter catecholamine action

Clonidine ((*Dixarit*) in small doses (25–50 mcg) sometimes used in long-term therapy for the prevention of migraine. It has been given a different trade name in the 25 mcg dosage from its counterpart used in hypertension (*Catapres*, 100 and 300 mcg tablets, 250 mcg sustained-release preparation) so as to avoid confusion. If a person taking *Catapres* for hypertension also has migraine, it is clearly useless to give *Dixarit* as well.

Adverse Drug Reactions

These include depression, drowsiness and dry mouth when taken in high doses.

Beta Adrenergic Blocking Drugs (β-blockers) are drugs which block the beta effects of adrenaline. It has been observed that some patients, previously migraine sufferers, no longer seemed to get migraine attacks when treated by these drugs for hypertension. They seem to have a place in treatment of migraine for some people. Propranolol (*Inderal*) has been shown to be useful as a migraine preventative.

Adverse Drug Reactions

These include cardiac failure, bronchoconstriction, hypoglycaemia.

Tricyclic antidepressant drugs (for example, amitriptyline) act by blocking noradrenaline re-uptake at nerve terminals, thus making more noradrenaline available for action in vessel walls and in the central nervous system. There have been some encouraging results with amitriptyline in the treatment of migraine at doses of 10 to 60mg given at night.

Adverse Drug Reaction

The main adverse reactions of amitriptyline are due to its anticholinergic actions, such as dry mouth, constipation, urinary retention, blurred vision. Other side effects include nausea, vomiting, hypertension, dizziness, sweating, tremor, excitement and skin reactions.

Monoamine oxidise inhibitors (MAOIs) act by preventing the breakdown of both noradrenaline and serotonin (5 hydroxytryptamine or 5HT) thus making more of both these neurotransmitters available. They have been shown in some studies to be useful in the prevention of migraine, but unfortunately there are a large number of potentially dangerous side effects associated with the use of these drugs, so they should probably only be tried after all other therapy has failed. An example of the group is phenelzine (*Nardil*)

Adverse Drug Reactions

Common reactions are postural hypotension and attacks of giddiness. Other effects include convulsions, jaundice, agitation, headache, tremors, dryness of mouth, blurred vision, skin rash, blood disorders and psychotic disturbances in susceptible persons. Severe reactions, sometimes fatal, may occur if these drugs are given simultaneously with some foods rich in tyramine, such as cheese (especially cheddar cheese), chianti wine, protein extracts such as Marmite. The reactions are characterised by prolonged rise in blood pressure, intracranial haemorrhage or acute cardiac failure.

Antiserotonin Drugs

Antiserotonin Antihistamines

Cyproheptadine (*Periactin*) This drug has been helpful to some people in the control of migraine attacks. It acts as a serotonin antagonist given in doses of 4 to 8mg three times daily.

Adverse Drug Reactions

It has appetite stimulating properties. This is possibly advantageous to some, but disadvantageous to others. Other side effects common to all antihistamines include drowsiness, inability to concentrate, lassitude, dizziness, hypertension, muscle weakness and incoordination. Other effects may be gastrointentinal and include nausea, vomiting, diarrhoea or constipation and colic.

Pizotifen malate (*Sanomigran*) is also an antiserotonin antihistamine and is structurally similar to cyproheptadine. It has mild anticholinergic properties. It is usually given in dose of 0.5mg once to three times daily for migraine prophylaxis.

Adverse Drug Reactions

These are similar to cyproheptadine.

Methysergide (*Deseril*) is an antiserotonin drug related to ergotamine and is effective in the prophylactic treatment of migraine. It has, however, an unpredictable side effect, which although rare is extremely serious that is, retroperitoneal fibrosis (obstructive renal disease), fibrosis of the heart, and pleura of the lung. Consequently, its use is no longer justified.

Miscellaneous Anti-migraine Drugs

Phenytoin (*Epanutin*) is generally not of any use except in migraine in children, where it can be extremely efficacious, and in treatment of a rare condition in adults where migraine has an aura of unilateral sensory symptoms or of aphasia.

Adverse Drug Reactions

See under phenytoin and anticonvulsants.

Anxiolytics (for example, the benzodiazepine drug *Valium*) can be useful for some people but generally do not appear to have much place as there is little evidence to show they are any better than placebos.

Adverse Drug Reactions

These drugs enhance the effects of CNS depressants, such as alcohol, and therefore may reduce a patient's ability to drive a car or use machinery safely.

Sex Hormones Although it has been noticed that migraine-prone patients do not have migraine attacks while pregnant, the results of the use of oestrogens have proved disappointing. The increased risk of a stroke is another deterrent to using this therapy.

Ergotamine tartrate will be discussed later in the text.

In the preventative use of all these drugs, it is necessary to try the drug for a few weeks. If no response is forthcoming, a larger dose is used before another drug is tried. Dosage must be tailored to the individual patient's needs.

THE ACUTE ATTACK OF MIGRAINE

The treatment of the acute attack of migraine may be divided into drug and non-drug treatment.

Non-Drug Treatment

A therapeutic atmosphere should be provided for the patient, who is encouraged to sleep. Most patients respond well if they can go to sleep.

Drug Treatment

Analgesics

Aspirin's action in the treatment of migraine is as an analgesic and possibly as an antiprostaglandin agent. It should be given in a dose of 900mg (three tablets) in the soluble form for better absorption.

Adverse Drug Reactions

The adverse effects of this drug are well known when given in high doses — intoxication causes sweating, nausea, vomiting, mental confusion, tinnitus, among others. However, in small doses, irritation of the gastric mucosa may occur with slight blood loss in 70% of patients. This is not usually of clinical significance.

Paracetamol should be given in a dose of 1g (two tablets) in the effervescent form.

It is important that both aspirin and paracetamol should be given in the soluble form as absorption is impaired during the acute attack of migraine because of gastric stasis.

Antiemetics

Metoclopramide (*Maxolon*) is the antiemetic of choice as it stimulates gastric motility and so counteracts gastric stasis encountered during an attack. It has central nervous effects, but little effect on a normal stomach. It has been found to be of benefit if a 10mg dose is given 10 minutes before the dose of aspirin or paracetamol in a migraine attack. The absorption of the analgesic then becomes almost normal.

Combined preparations include *Migravess* (metoclopramide 5 mg plus aspirin 325 mg) effervescent tablets and *Paramax* (metoclopramide 5 mg plus paracetamol 500 mg) tablets.

Toxic effects include diarrhoea or constipation. Extrapyramidal reactions and drowsiness and lassitude have been reported.

Other antiemetics include: thiethylperazine (*Torecan*) and prochlorperazine (*Stemetil*).

Tranquillisers Most patients respond to treatment of the acute attack if they can go to sleep. This is helped by use of a tranquilliser such as diazepam 5 to 10 mg (see previous description).

Ergotamine Tartrate 2 mg (*Lingraine*): Ergotamine is also presented in combination with an antihistamine and caffeine, as *Migril, Cafergot.*

Ergotamine is a powerful vasoconstrictor used in the treatment of migraine. There is diversity of thought on the maximum dosage which should be allowed in any one week, but it is thought to be 6 to 10mg.

Adverse Drug Reactions

Large doses of ergotamine, from 10 to 20 mg per week, can lead to ergotism or ergotamine toxicity. The toxic symptoms may be manifested by the three-day headache, which can be relieved only by more ergotamine. This withdrawal headache may take a few days to clear before ergotamine can be used again therapeutically. The combinations of ergotamine with caffeine mentioned before should be avoided at night as caffeine is a CNS stimulant. They may be helpful in daytime attacks, if, for example, the patient is at work.

NURSING IMPLICATIONS

The drugs used in migraine may be considered in terms of the management of the acute attack and long-term management and prevention. It is important to assess the headache profile, including family history, description of prodromontary signs, precipitating factors, duration, temporal profile and relieving factors.

Baseline vital signs such as BP, pulse rate and weight should be considered. A history of vascular, hepatic, renal or cardiac disease should form part of the assessment. Current pregnancy, infection or hypertension must be recorded.

The patient should be advised to avoid precipitating factors associated with the headache. In the acute attack, ergotamine is usually administered within two hours of the onset of the attack. In the long term, the drug should be administered with meals. It is important to evaluate the therapeutic effect. Record BP (lying and standing), and observe and report non-transient claudication, coldness of extremities, nausea, vomiting, anorexia, dysuria, backache, chest pain or depression.

Patient education includes advising the patient to rise slowly from the lying position to avoid postural hypotension. The patient should learn to recognise deviations from the therapeutic effect and seek medical advice if necessary.

Drugs administered for long-term management and prevention include those drugs which alter catecholamine action, for example, clonidine, beta adrenergic blockers, tricyclic antidepressants and monoamine oxidase inhibitors. Beta blockers may prolong insulin induced hypoglycaemia and if possible are probably best avoided in diabetic patients. The diet of patients taking monoamine oxidase inhibitors should be assessed and adequate instruction as to necessary dietary restrictions given (see Chapter 28). Pethidine and other narcotics should not be administered to patients receiving MAOI therapy. Antiserotonin drugs may also be used for long-term management, and patients should be advised as to adverse GIT and CNS effects of these including a possible increase in appetite.

Nursing implication for analgesics are listed in Chapter 16.

SELF-EVALUATION TEST

1. Define the term "epilepsy".
2. List extracranial factors which may lead to secondary epilepsy.
3. Describe types of primary epilepsy.
4. List drugs used in epilepsy.
5. State nursing implications of:
   (a) giving phenytoin by injection;
   (b) timing blood sampling for drug assays.
6. Define classical and common migraine.
7. Describe three classes of drugs used in long-term management of migraine.

8. List the drugs in each class.
9. State any nursing implications of drugs in this group.
10. List drugs used in an acute attack of migraine.
11. Why may it be of benefit to give metoclopramide 10 minutes before other medication in the acute migraine attack?
12. What effect does large doses of ergotamine have?
13. Describe Parkinsonism and the symptoms of this disease.
14. Describe how a decarboxylase inhibitor added to levodopa benefits the patient.
15. List other drugs used in Parkinsonism.
16. State any nursing implications associated with medication in Parkinsonian patients.

Table 95
Drugs Used in Neurology

Drug Group	Drug Name	Use	Action	Adverse Reactions	Nursing Implications
Anticonvulsant drugs					
Hydantoins	Phenytoin sodium	All types of epilepsy except petit mal	Alteration in CNS electrolyte concentrations and inhibition of spread of seizure discharge	Gum hypertrophy, foetal hydantoin syndrome, hirsutism, acne, nystagmus, vertigo, incoordination.	***Assess:*** baseline vital signs, BP, pulse rate, the presence of pregnancy or lactation, epilepsy profile and the number of seizures, current medications or alcohol use, previous drug reaction, history of head injury, alcohol abuse, allergic reaction, cardiac disease, hypertension or diabetes mellitus. ***Administer:*** orally with meals to prevent GIT irritation, may be given in suspension form; shake the bottle well before administration; parenteral: do not give IM; do not mix with other drugs; IV administration is usually given slowly at a dose not exceeding 50 mg/min; it is not advisable to administer phenytoin (*Epanutin*) with IV solutions other than normal saline; administered with an IV infusion, it may be given into a fast-running infusion of normal saline via a Y-injection site, or in a burette at a concentration of no greater than 1 mg/mL; should be administered carefully as sudden hypotension or cardiac arrhythmias may occur. ***Evaluate:*** BP, pulse rate, therapeutic effectiveness as observed by a reduction in the number of seizures; adverse effects involving the CNS such as drowsiness, ataxia or nystagmus; regular blood screenings for folic-acid depletion, megaloblastic anaemia, and hypoglycaemia; known diabetic patients may have to increase their insulin dose

					evaluation for side effects, signs of toxicity and therapeutic effect; to maintain adequate supply of medication and not to alter dose without consulting medical officer; to avoid the use of alcohol.
Barbiturates	Phenobarbitone Methylpheno-barbitone	All major seizures	Inhibition of spread of seizure discharge	Sedation, irritability, ataxia, rashes, tolerance, liver enzyme induction	***Assess:*** baseline vital signs BP, temperature, respirations, weight and sleep patterns, epilepsy profile, and the number of seizures, previous drug reactions and alcohol intake, presence of pregnancy or lactation. ***Administer:*** according to legal requirements; ensure compliance; orally or parenterally according to manufacturer's instruction; observe for hypotension and respiratory depression. ***Evaluate:*** therapeutic effectiveness observed by a reduction in the number of seizures; adverse effects especially CNS manifestations such as drowsiness to which tolerance usually develops, slurred speech, ataxia or vertigo.
	Carbamazepine	Grand mal, temporal lobe epilepsy	As for phenobarbitone	As for phenobarbitone	***Assess:*** epilepsy profile and the number of seizures, concurrent medication (should not be administered concurrently with barbiturates), previous drug reactions, presence of pregnancy or lactation, history of kidney, liver, cardiovascular disease, bone-marrow suppression. ***Administer:*** orally with food. ***Evaluate:*** therapeutic effectivenss as demonstrated by a reduction in seizure number of severity; adverse reactions such as haematological disorders; ensure regular blood screening; CNS depression resulting in drowsiness.

continued

Drug Group	Drug Name	Use	Action	Adverse Reactions	Nursing Implications
Benzodiazepines	Diazepam Nitrazepam Clonazepam	Status epilepticus, myoclonic epilepsy	CNS depression prevention of seizure discharge	Drowsiness, sedation, ataxia, behavioural instability, tolerance	***Assess:*** epileptic profile and the number of seizures, baseline with signs such as BP, respiration rate; alcohol intake, previous drug reactions; history of respiratory disease in small children. ***Administer:*** orally or parenterally. ***Evaluate:*** therapeutic effectiveness as demonstrated by a reduction in the number or severity of seizures; adverse reactions, especially CNS problems such as behavioural disorders in children; in adults, psychosis, neurological signs such as ataxia or drowsiness.
Succinamides	Ethosuximide	Petit mal	Prevention of seizure discharge	Anorexia, nausea, vomiting, induction of major seizures, bonemarrow depression	***Assess:*** epilepsy profile and number of seizures, previous drug reaction, history of kidney or liver disease or psychiatric disturbances. ***Administer:*** orally with meals to reduce GIT irration. ***Evaluate:*** therapeutic effectiveness as observed by a reduction in the number or severity of seizures; adverse effects such as gum hypertrophy or haematological problems; CNS depression, psychiatric disturbances and drowsiness.
Sodium valproate	Sodium valproate	Temporal lobe epilepsy, grand mal, mixed seizures, myoclonic seizures	Inhibition of GABA transaminase	Indigestion, vomiting, drowsiness, bleeding, alopecia	***Assess:*** epilepsy profile and number of seizures, concurrent medications, previous drug reactions, presence of pregnancy or lactation, history of diabetes mellitus or liver disease.

					Administer: orally with food; the capsule should be swallowed whole and not chewed as this has been known to induce mouth ulcers and throat irritation. ***Evaluate:*** therapeutic effectiveness as demonstrated by a reduction in the number and severity of the seizures; diabetics for false positive ketones on urinalysis; there may be an increased bleeding time when administered concurrently with aspirin; liver function tests.
Treatment of migraine Clonidine — see Chapter 7 Beta-adrenergic blockers — see Chapter 7 Tricyclic antidepressants — see Chapter 28 Monoamine oxidase inhibitors — see Chapter 28 Analgesics — see Chapter 16					
Anti-serotonin drugs	Pizotifen malate Cyproheptadine	Long-term management and prevention of migraine	Antiserotonin	Appetite stimulant; may cause drowsiness, lack of concentration, lassitude, dizziness, hypotension, weakness, incoordination, nausea, vomiting, diarrhoea, colic, constipation.	***Assess:*** migraine profile, baseline vital signs,BP (lying and standing) pulse rate and weight, present medications, previous drug reactions, history of peripheral vascular disease, cardiac disease or hypertension. ***Administer:*** with drug holiday, e.g. one month off in every 4 to 6 months; monitor regime carefully. ***Evaluate:*** therapeutic effectiveness, BP (lying and standing) and adverse effects. ***Teach:*** to recognise adverse effects and to seek medical advice if any occur; to rise slowly from the lying position.

continued

Drug Group	Drug Name	Use	Action	Adverse Reactions	Nursing Implications
Treatment of Parkinsonism					
Dopaminergic drugs	Levodopa	Parkinsonism	Replenishes dopamine in corpus striatum	Anorexia, nausea, vomiting, postural hypotension, involuntary movement of face & lips, cardiac arrhythmias	***Assess:*** for history of Parkinsonism secondary to the use of neuroleptic drugs, dementia, memory loss, confusion, psychoses, postural hypotenstion, endocrine, renal, cardiac, hepatic impairment, diabetes, glaucoma; concurrent use of other drugs which can interact with levodopa; establish baseline blood pressure (lying and standing), colour and temperature of extremities, urinary output; document baseline observations of Parkinsonism symptoms and emotional state. ***Administer:*** with food. ***Evaluate:*** for therapeutic effect; sympathomimetic effect, i.e. blood pressure, pulse rate, colour and temperature of extremities, urinary output; psychological behaviour. ***Teach:*** to change position slowly to avoid postural hypotension; to avoid pyridoxine, e.g. vitamin supplements, and fortified cereals; that urine and perspiration may darken; drug efficacy may not occur for several months.
	Levodopa plus decarboxylase inhibitor	Parkinsonism	Replenishes dopamine in corpus striatum	As for levodopa, but less nausea and vomiting	As for levodopa, except that pyridoxine does not reduce effect

Anticholinergic drugs	Benzhexol Orphenadrine hydrochloride Benztropine Orphenadrine Procyclidine	Parkinsonism	Reduce dominance of cholinergic system	Confusion, glaucoma, see Chapter 5	See Chapter 5

30
DRUGS USED IN ANAESTHESIA

Bruce S. Clifton

OBJECTIVES

At the conclusion of this chapter, the student should be able to:

1. name the groups of drugs commonly used by the anaesthetist;
2. understand the reasons for their administration;
3. describe the pharmacology of the drugs used in anaesthesia and their undesirable side effects;
4. as a result of 1, 2 and 3 above, assist the anaesthetist with the anaesthetic and with preoperative and postoperative care;
5. most importantly, give factual and helpful information to patients who require anaesthesia and/or pain relief.

PREREQUISITE KNOWLEDGE

1. The structure and function of the nervous system, central and peripheral.
2. The structure and function of the autonomic nervous system, sympathetic and parasympathetic - See Chapter 5.
3. The mechanism of neuromuscular transmission.
4. Central nervous system (CNS) depressant drugs, sedatives and hypnotics, tranquillisers, narcotics and general anaesthetics. See Chapters 16 and 28.
5. Oxygen and its administration.

DEFINITIONS

Premedication — a drug or drugs ordered by the anaesthetist for administration in the ward before the patient leaves for the operating theatre.
Analgesic — a drug used to lessen pain without producing unconsciousness.
Neuroleptanalgesia — a deep trance-like state with a diminished pain.
General anaesthetic — a drug used to produce and/or maintain a state of unconsciousness.

Local anaesthetic — a drug used to produce an area of loss of sensation in the body without loss of consciousness.
Muscle relaxant — a drug used to paralyse the muscles of the body.
Antiemetic — a drug that depresses the CNS vomiting centre.
Antisialogogue — a drug that inhibits the secretion of saliva.

OXYGEN

Oxygen is by far the most important drug used in anaesthesia. Preoperatively, oxygen therapy may be required for patients with coma, shock or respiratory failure. During anaesthesia, there is always some depression of the respiratory and cardiovascular system and, for this reason, it is usual to administer at least 33% oxygen to anaesthetised patients. Postoperatively in the recovery room, the residual effects of general anaesthetics and relaxants cause hypoventilation; also, shivering increases the requirements for oxygen. For these reasons, most patients receive oxygen therapy in the recovery room.

In the modern operating suite, oxygen is piped to the anaesthetic rooms, operating theatres and recovery room. Mobile oxygen-therapy equipment is required to transport certain patients to and from theatres. The operating suite and each anaesthetic machine are supplied with oxygen cylinders in case there is a failure of the piped supply. Each anaesthetic machine has an oxygen flowmeter (usually of the rotameter type) colour-coded with a white knob and situated next to the nitrous oxide flowmeter, which is colour-coded blue. Connecting tubes from wall (or pendant) oxygen points to the anaesthetic machine are colour-coded black and white. In some operating suites, nitrous oxide is supplied via a pipeline. These connecting tubes are coloured blue, and the points are not the same size as the oxygen points.

PREMEDICANT DRUGS

Most patients about to have an operation are apprehensive concerning the possibilities of dying under the anaesthetic, the successful outcome of the surgery, and the effects of the hospitalisation on their family life and job. These are all normal fears. A reasonable explanation of the operation and the anaesthetic should always be given to the patient. This explanation, together with a considerate and sympathetic approach by all members of the hospital staff, is often sufficient to allay preoperative anxiety. However, many patients require the administration of a "calming" drug in the ward, so that they may arrive in the operating suite in a drowsy but cooperative mood.

The three groups of drugs used for their "calming" effect are:

(a) **the sedatives and hypnotics**
(b) **the tranquillisers**
(c) **the narcotics** (see Table 96).

Table 96
Drugs Used for Premedication

Main Action	Drugs	Examples	Trade Names
Sedative	Barbiturates	Pentobarbitone	*Nembutal*
Hypnotic		Amylobarbitone	*Amytal*
	Benzodiazepines	Diazepam	*Valium*
		Nitrazepam	*Mogadon*
		Lorazepam	*Ativan*
		Temazepam	*Normison*
Tranquilliser	Phenothiazines	Promethazine	*Phenergan*
Neuroleptic		Trimeprazine	*Vallergan*
	Butyrophenones	Haloperidol	*Serenace*
		Droperidol	*Droleptan*
Narcotic	From opium	Papaveretum	*Omnopon*
Analgesic		Morphine	
	Synthetic	Pethidine	
		Pentazocine	*Fortral*
Antisialogogue	Anticholinergics	Atropine	
Prevents bradycardia		Hyoscine	

Note: Barbiturates are not so popular since the introduction of the benzodiazepines.

All of these drugs are CNS depressants, so that excessive dosage will lead to stupor, unconsciousness, respiratory depression and hypotension. All cross the placenta and depress the respiratory centre of the foetus. For the latter reasons, these CNS depressants must be used with great caution, if at all, during labour.

The choice of the particular "calming" drug for premedication depends mainly on the personal preference of the anaesthetist. The sedatives and hypnotics are not very effective when the patient is in pain. The tranquillisers have mild sedative and analgesic actions together with antiemetic and anticholinergic side effects. The narcotics are powerful analgesics, and they produce marked euphoria (a feeling of well-being and inner peace). Their undesirable side effects are nausea and/or vomiting, respiratory depression and addiction. Addiction is a problem only with prolonged administration.

The anticholinergic drugs, atropine or hyoscine, are used for premedication to decrease salivation and bronchial secretions and/or to prevent bradycardia. Before an ether anaesthetic, atropine premedication was essential to avoid profuse salivation and bronchorrhoea, which could lead to serious airway obstruction. Ether is rarely used now. Modern intravenous and inhalational anaesthetics produce much less irritation of the respiratory passages. Except in children, vagal bradycardia due to a drug or due to reflexes on intubation or during surgery is uncommon. For these reasons, anticholinergic premedication is not always given routinely. Excessive dosage, particularly in children, leads to tachycardia, restlessness, flushing, absence of sweating, pyrexia and rarely convulsions.

Narcotic and/or anticholinergic premedication is usually administered intramuscularly about one hour before operation. Sedatives and tranquillisers are usually administered orally about two hours before operation or, less commonly, intramuscularly one hour before operation. Oral premedication may be in the form of a tablet, a syrup or an elixir. Dosage is varied according to the age, the size and the general health of the patient (see Table 97).

Table 97
Dosages of Premedicant Drugs

Drug	Average Adult (Healthy)	Small Adult (Sick)	Infant or Child
Pentobarbitone	200 mg orally	100 mg orally	—
Diazepam	15 mg orally	7 mg orally	0.2 mg/kg orally
Morphine	15 mg IM	7.5 mg IM	—
Pethidine	100 mg IM	50 mg IM	—
Atropine	0.6 mg IM	0.3 mg IM	—
Trimeprazine	—	—	2–4 mg/kg

Note: Dosage of premedicant drugs is varied with age, size and general health of the patient.

With careful dosage, premedication seldom causes unconsciousness or respiratory depression. If these rare complications do occur, oxygen therapy and/or artificial respiration must be given immediately. Once the patient has been oxygenated, the effects of a narcotic analgesic may be reversed by naloxone (*Narcan*), a narcotic antagonist (see also Chapters 4 and 16). Naloxone does not reverse the effects of sedatives, hypnotics or tranquillisers.

GENERAL ANAESTHETIC AGENTS

General anaesthesia is a reversible and controlled state of unconsciousness used to provide adequate conditions for surgery and is produced by the administration of one or more of a group of drugs called the general anaesthetics. These drugs act on the brain but, despite much research and many theories, their exact mechanism of action remains unknown.

A useful and frequent classification of the general anaesthetics depends on their route of administration, that is, intravenous or inhalational (see Tables 98 and 99). Intravenous anaesthetics are injected from a syringe as a bolus into a vein or into a rapidly running infusion. Less commonly, they may be given as a slow infusion. Inhalational anaesthetics are administered from an anaesthetic machine, which is equipped with a face mask, flowmeters, vapourisers, breathing tubes and reservoir bag.

During the unconscious state of general anaesthesia, the patient is completely free of pain and immobile except for breathing; also, there is a degree of muscle relaxation that varies with the depth of anaesthesia.

From 1846 to 1932, the early days of anaesthesia, muscle relaxation for abdominal surgery was obtained by the inhalation of high concentrations of ether or choloroform. These deep planes of anaesthesia had undesirable effects on the patient: marked depression of respiration and circulation, depression of hepatic and renal function, prolonged recovery time, and prolonged nausea and vomiting. Fortunately, in 1932, the muscle relaxants (neuromuscular blocking agents) were introduced into clinical practice, and deep general anaesthesia for muscle relaxation was no longer required.

The three clinical and chronological phases of general anaesthesia are:

(a) **induction**
(b) **maintenance**
(c) **recovery.**

Induction is the commencement of anaesthesia when the patient is rendered unconscious, maintenance is the period of unconsciousness during the operation and recovery is the return of consciousness at the completion of the operation. Anaesthesia is usually induced by an intravenous anaesthetic or less commonly by an inhalational anaesthetic. It is maintained usually by the continuous administration of inhalational anaesthetics from the anaesthetic machine or less commonly by the steady infusion of an intravenous anaesthetic. Recovery, of course, takes place when the administration of the anaesthetic ceases.

If the induction of anaesthesia is slow, the patient may pass through a stage of excitement. This may consist of coughing, breath holding, vomiting, struggling, rigidity of the limbs, trismus (clenching the jaws), salivation, sweating and even urination. The excitement stage occurs just after the loss of consciousnessness, and therefore it is not remembered by the patient. It may occur without apparent external stimulation but, more commonly, it is precipitated by loud noises, movement of the patient, insertion of a pharyngeal airway or premature surgical stimulation. The excitement stage occurs frequently during an inhalational induction, which is slow:

(a) because the anaesthetic agent takes some time to pass from the anaesthetic machine into the lungs and then into the blood stream;
(b) because this depends on the rate and depth of the patient's breathing which are not under the control of the anaesthetist.

On the other hand, intravenous induction is rapid because the anaesthetic is injected directly into the blood stream and the rate of injection is controlled by the anaesthetist. This, together with the patient's preference for a needle rather than the mask, accounts for the popularity of intravenous induction. Children, however, may prefer the mask.

All general anaesthetics, intravenous and inhalational, produce some depression of the respiratory and cardiovascular systems. The severity of the depression is directly proportional to anaesthetic dosage and depth, that is, the higher the dosage, the deeper the anaesthesia and the greater the depression. Certain patients are particularly susceptible to these depressant effects — infants, the elderly, the very ill or those with heart disease, lung disease, respiratory obstruction or hypovolaemia (shock).

Therefore, the anaesthetist assesses the age, the size and the general condition of the patient before anaesthesia and carefully controls both the dose and rate of injection of intravenous anaesthetics and the concentration setting for the inhalational anaesthetics on the anaesthetic machine.

It is important to monitor the response of the patient during anaesthesia — rate and depth of breathing, colour of the skin, pulse, blood pressure and electrocardiography. Severe depression of respiration will lead to respiratory acidosis, hypoxia with cyanosis and possibly apnoea (no respiration). Severe cardiovascular depression will lead to arterial hypotension, bradycardia and cardiac arrest. In high dosage, some inhalational anaesthetics increase cardiac irritability, and this leads to ventricular ectopic beats, particularly when the patient has respiratory acidosis or when the surgeon injects adrenaline. All of the halogenated hydrocarbons have this effect.

All general anaesthetics relax the pregnant uterus. They cross the placenta rapidly and depress the respiration of the foetus or neonate. These undesirable effects become more marked as the depth of anaesthesia increases. To avoid uterine haemorrhage and foetal or neonatal depression, "light" anaesthesia must be used in pregnancy.

Table 98
Some Intravenous Anaesthetic Drugs

Chemical Grouping	Intravenous Anaesthetic	Trade Names
Barbiturates	Thiopentone	*Intraval*
	Methohexitone	*Brietal*
Benzodiazepines	Diazepam	*Valium*
	Midazolam	*Hypnovel*
Narcotics	Morphine	
	Fentanyl	*Sublimaze*
Imidazole	Etomidate	*Hypnomidate*
	Ketamine	*Ketalar*

Note: Intravenous anaesthetics are presented in ampoules or vials, already in solution or as a powder that has to be dissolved just before use.

During injection, intravenous anaesthetics pass rapidly to the brain because the latter has a relatively high perfusion (blood flow). The effect of a bolus (single dose) is short, and the patient recovers quickly (five to 10 minutes) because the anaesthetic is redistributed from the brain to other, less well-perfused organs. However, after repeated doses of an intravenous anaesthetic, recovery becomes increasingly prolonged because it depends on biotransformation (metabolic breakdown) in the liver.

All the metabolites are non-toxic and, except for diazepam, non-active. One of the metabolites of diazepam is a CNS depressant, and this accounts for its prolonged duration of action.

At one time it was thought that all the inhalational anaesthetics were excreted unchanged via the respiratory tract. It is now known that some biotransformation occurs in the liver and that this varies from 0.2% with isoflurane to 45% with methoxyflurane. Fortunately, with one exception, the metabolites have not been shown to be toxic. The exception is methoxyflurane which is metabolised to inorganic fluoride, a potential nephrotoxin. Great care is taken to limit the concentration and the duration of administration of the anaesthetic.

Trace amounts of inhalational anaesthetics enter the atmosphere of the operating theatre from the anaesthetic machine and from the patient. As a result of some epidemiological surveys, it has been alleged that waste anaesthetic gases and vapours have adverse effects on operating theatre personnel, causing an increased incidence of spontaneous abortion, congenital abnormalities, hepatic and renal diseases, and cancer as well as changes in mood and intellectual function. Although these allegations are unproven and although other factors in the operating theatre could be involved, various scavenging devices are available to collect and remove waste anaesthetics from the anaesthetic machine before they "pollute" the atmosphere.

INTRAVENOUS ANAESTHETICS

Some of the desirable properties for an "ideal" intravenous anaesthetic are:

(a) **water soluble and stable in solution;**
(b) **non-irritating to tissues and not painful during IV injection;**
(c) **no psychic or muscular excitation during induction;**
(d) **predictable actions on respiration and circulation;**
(e) **rapidly destroyed in the body, metabolites inactive and non-toxic;**
(f) **rapid recovery without delirium or restlessness;**
(g) **low incidence of histamine release and allergy;**
(h) **low incidence of post-anaesthetic nausea and vomiting.**

Unfortunately, the "ideal" IV anaesthetic has not been discovered. Those listed in Table 98 all have problems for the patient and hence for the anaesthetist. Although thiopentone (*Intraval*) was introduced many years ago (1936), it remains the most popular IV induction agent, being used in more than 90% of patients.

Thiopentone is an ultra-short acting barbiturate. It is a yellow powder, rapidly soluble in water. While it is sealed in its ampoule in an atmosphere of nitrogen, the drug is stable for years, but once mixed with water, it becomes unstable due to hydrolysis. For this reason, thiopentone is always dissolved in sterile water for injection just before use. A 2.5% solution (25 mg/mL), the standard strength used in most countries, is injected intravenously by the anaesthetist. If the needle is accidentally inserted outside the vein, the thiopentone may damage the local tissues. Accidental intra-arterial injection, a very rare complication, causes extreme pain in the hand and may lead to thrombosis and gangrene. Thiopentone anaesthesia commences within one minute and lasts five to 10 minutes, depending on the dose, the patient's general condition and the degree of surgical stimulation. This short duration of action is due to redistribution from brain to muscle and other organs. The drug undergoes biotransformation in the liver, and the metabolites are excreted by the kidneys over 24 hours. Patients recovering from thiopentone have a "hangover"; they are sleepy but rousable. This is an advantage for the hospitalised patient but a disadvantage for "day only" patients, who should be instructed not to drive home and to arrange for a relative or friend to act as an escort. Thiopentone does not stimulate during induction, it has predictable depressant actions on respiration and circulation, allergic reactions are rare, and there is a low incidence of delirium or nausea and vomiting during recovery.

INHALATIONAL ANAESTHETICS

Some of the desirable properties for an "ideal" inhalational anaesthetic are:

(a) **non-flammable, stable chemically, non-toxic;**
(b) **pleasant to inhale, not irritant to the respiratory tract;**
(c) **high potency (effective in low concentrations);**
(d) **predictable and minimal cardiac effects;**
(e) **rapid action, quick recovery,**
(f) **low incidence of post-anaesthetic nausea and vomiting.**

Unfortunately, the "ideal" inhalational anaesthetic has not been discovered. Those listed in Tables 99 and 100 all have problems for the patient and hence for the anaesthetist. In the UK nitrous oxide, halothane and enflurane are the most frequently used.

Nitrous oxide is a colourless gas with a slightly sweetish odour. It is neither flammable nor explosive, but it will support combustion. It is compressed to a liquid by the manufacturers and supplied in bue cylinders of various sizes. The smaller cylinders are pin-indexed for coupling to the anaesthetic machine. The larger cylinders are stored outside the operating suite as a bulk supply, and the nitrous oxide is piped to the suite.

Normally, we breathe air which contains approximately 79% nitrogen and 21% oxygen. Because anaesthesia produces respiratory and cardiovascular depression, the inspired concentration of oxygen is increased to at least 33% in all patients and to 50% in poor-risk patients. This limits the concentration of nitrous oxide to 67% or 50%, respectively. At these levels, nitrous oxide produces analgesia but not anaesthesia. Therefore, the mixture of nitrous oxide and oxygen is supplemented with small percentages (0.25 to 1.0%) of halothane or enflurane or with intravenous anaesthetics.

Table 99
Some Inhalational Anaesthetics

Classification	Inhalational Anaesthetics	Trade Name
Anaesthetic gases	Nitrous oxide	
	Cyclopropane	
Anaesthetic ethers (liquids)	Diethyl ether*	*Ether*
	Methoxyflurane	*Penthrane*
	Enflurane	*Ethrane*
	Isoflurane	*Forane*
Halogenated hydrocarbons (liquids)	Chloroform**	
	Trichlorethylene	*Trilene*
	Halothane	*Fluothane*

* Largely superseded by other agents in this country.
**No longer used; toxic to liver and heart.
Note: The gases are supplied in cylinders. The liquids are supplied in brown bottles, usually of 125 to 250 mL capacity.

Entonox is a mixture of 50% oxygen and 50% nitrous oxide compressed in cylinders of various sizes. These cylinders have a blue body and white-and-blue shoulder quadrants. *Entonox* may be used to produce analgesia for short-period procedures in the ward or the emergency department.

Halothane is a colourless liquid with a sweet, non-irritating odour. It decomposes on exposure to light and is supplied in amber glass bottles. Halothane is non-flammable and non-explosive. It is administered by passing oxygen or a nitrous oxide/oxygen mixture through a vapouriser (metal container) attached to the anaesthetic machine. This *Fluotec* vapouriser is calibrated from 0% to 5%. As with all the inhalational anaesthetics, the anaesthetic potency of halothane is expressed in terms of MAC, which is the minimum alveolar concentration at which 50% of patients do not move on surgical stimulation. Halothane is a potent anaesthetic with a MAC of 0.75%, and 1% (1.3 times MAC) is sufficient to prevent movement in most patients.

Induction with halothane is not nearly as rapid as with thiopentone but still fast enough for halothane to be used for induction if required. Once anaesthesia is induced, maintenance of a stable anaesthetic level is easily achieved. Halothane produces a fall in arterial pressure due to peripheral vasodilatation and cardiac depression, and this property may be used to reduce operative bleeding (the technique of induced hypotension). Halothane may, rarely, cause liver damage ("halothane hepatitis"). The incidence of this complication is reported to vary from 1 in 10,000 to 1 in 100,000 administered anaesthetics and the cause is unknown. Like all the halogenated anaesthetics, halothane increases cardiac irritability and, to avoid serious ventricular arrhythmias, it should not be used when adrenaline is to be injected as a vasoconstrictor.

Enflurane is a non-flammable, volatile liquid administered from a calibrated vapouriser called an *Enfluratec*. It is not as potent as halothane and has a MAC of 1.68%. The effects of enflurane on the heart are similar to those of halothane.

Table 100
Inhalational Anaesthetics

Anaesthetic (date)*	**MAC****	**F*****	**Comments**
Nitrous oxide (1844)		NF	Not potent enough to produce anaesthesia; used for analgesia and to supplement other anaesthetics
Diethyl ether (1842)	1.92%	2 to 82%	Used in Third-World countries; no diathermy
Chloroform (1847)	0.5%	2 to 60%	No longer used; toxic to liver and heart
Trichlorethylene (1934)	0.2%	10 to 65%	Rarely used; moderate cardiac effects; reacts with sodalime to give a toxic product
Cyclopropane (1933)	9.2%	2 to 60%	Rarely used; moderate cardiac effects, no diathermy
Halothane (1956)	0.75%	NF	Frequently used; moderate cardiac effects; liver damage rare
Methoxyflurane (1960)	0.16%	5 to 28%	Less frequently used; slow recovery; nephrotoxic in high dosage
Enflurane (1968)	1.68%	NF	Frequently used; mild cardiac effects
Isoflurane (1980)	1.15%	NF	Mild cardiac effects

* — date of introduction into anaesthetic practice.
** — MAC: minimum alveolar concentration; see text for explanation.
*** — F: flammability in oxygen (% vol/vol).
NF — not flammable.

MUSCLE RELAXANTS

Although deep general anaesthesia produces moderate relaxation of the muscles, the general-anaesthetic drugs are not called muscle relaxants. The muscle relaxants or neuromuscular blocking agents are a special group of drugs which block neuromuscular transmission at the endplates in skeletal (striated) muscle. This leads to complete paralysis and respiratory arrest (apnoea). The relaxants have no effect on the brain, they do not produce unconsciousness, and fortunately, they do not paralyse the plain (unstriated) muscle of the heart, the uterus or the bowel; those in clinical use do not cross the placenta. Pharmacologically the muscle relaxants are classified into two groups: depolarising and non-depolarising.

Suxamethonium (*Anectine* or *Scoline*) is the only depolarising muscle relaxant in frequent use. About 20 to 30 seconds after IV injection, suxamethonium depolarises the muscle endplates as does acetylcholine, the physiological transmitter. During the process of depolarisation, there is a five to 10-second period of widespread muscular twitching (fasciculations), and after this the patient becomes completely paralysed. Suxamethonium has a short duration of action (3 to 5 minutes) because it is destroyed rapidly by pseudocholinesterase, an enzyme that is formed in the liver and circulates in the plasma; however, the period of relaxation may be extended by giving repeated injections. Suxamethonium is used to produce total but brief relaxation for instrumentation procedures, such as endotracheal intubation or oesophagoscopy. It is always used for intubation when the patient has a full stomach and/or is likely to regurgitate, because it is so rapid in action and because the relaxation is complete.

There are certain problems associated with the use of suxamethonium: "after" pains, prolonged action, bradycardia and hyperkalaemia. Some patients complain of muscle pains for 24 to 36 hours after suxamethonium. These unexplained pains occur more commonly in ambulant patients, for example "day only" patients. They may be severe, and they affect particularly the muscles around the shoulders and the costal margins. Usually, there is sharp pain on inspiration. Symptomatic relief may be obtained with aspirin or paracetamol.

Rarely, suxamethonium may have an unexpectedly prolonged effect. This problem occurs when the patient has a congenitally abnormal or reduced level of the enzyme pseudocholinesterase. As there is no pharmacological antidote for suxamethonium, the patient must have artificial respiration until the paralysis wears off.

Bradycardia occurs mainly in children, particularly with repeated doses, and it is prevented by atropine. Suxamethonium releases potassium from the muscles, and in normal patients this results in a slight rise of the serum potassium level. In patients with pre-existing hyperkalaemia and/or extensive tissue damage (for example, trauma, burns), the drug may cause a greater and potentially dangerous rise in serum potassium.

Suxamethonium is supplied in 2 mL ampoules, 50 mg/mL. The dosage for intubation is usually 20–100 mg intravenously. It is an unstable drug, and should be stored in a refrigerator.

Tubocurarine (*Tubarine*), ***pancuronium*** (*Pavulon*), and ***alcuronium*** (*Alloferin*) are the most frequently used non-depolarising relaxants. They compete with acetylcholine for access to receptor sites on the muscle endplates. Sometimes these are referred to as competitive blocking agents.

Neostigmine (*Prostigmin*), an inhibitor of cholinesterase, is an antidote for the non-depolarising relaxants. It allows the accumulation of acetylcholine at the endplate, and hence the relaxant is displaced from the receptor sites. Therefore, at the end of the anaesthetic, a large dose of neostigmine is injected IV to reverse the paralysis. A large dose of atropine (0.6–1.2 mg) must be injected IV beforehand or with the neostigmine, otherwise the latter will cause dangerous bradycardia or perhaps cardiac arrest.

Tubocurarine, pancuronium and alcuronium are injected IV, and the dosage is varied with the age, the size and the general health of the patient. Significant paralysis occurs in two to five minutes, at which time the patient can be intubated. Their duration of action is about 25 to 35 minutes, and further doses are given to maintain relaxation until the operation is completed. During the period of paralysis, the patient must receive intermittent positive pressure ventilation (IPPV) via a cuffed endotracheal tube using the anaesthetic machine and hand ventilation or a mechanical respirator. A small, battery-powered, nerve stimulator may be used to monitor the degree of paralysis and its reversal at the end of the operation.

There are certain problems associated with the use of these long-acting non-depolarisers:

(a) **awareness**
(b) **incomplete reversal**
(c) **cardiovascular effects.**

As mentioned earlier, the great value of the muscle relaxants lies with the avoidance of the undesirable effects of deep anaesthesia. However, unless sufficient anaesthesia is maintained, it is possible for a paralysed patient on IPPV to be completely conscious, in pain and incapable of movement. This rare complication is called awareness.

Occasionally, despite the injection of 5 mg neostigmine, the reversal of paralysis may not be immediate or complete. In this circumstance, the endotracheal tube is not removed, and the patient is ventilated in the recovery room until the paralysis wears off. Extra neostigmine is not given because it may produce neuromuscular block.

Non-depolarising relaxants may have slight effects on the cardiovascular system, for example, hypotension with tubocurarine and tachycardia and/or hypertension with pancuronium.

Tubocurarine (10 mg/mL), pancuronium (2 mg/mL) and alcuronium (5 mg/mL) are supplied in 2 mL ampoules. Dosages vary. In adults, tubocurarine's initial dose is 10–15 mg, then 5 mg as required up to a maximum of 40 mg; pancuronium 50–100 mcg/kg body weight, then 10–20 mcg/kg as required; and alcuronium 200–250 mcg/kg then incremental doses of one sixth to one quarter of the initial dose as required. Allergic reactions occur, but they are uncommon. These relaxants are eliminated from the body by the kidney and liver, so that prolonged paralysis may occur when these two organs are functioning poorly.

LOCAL ANAESTHETICS

Local anaesthetics are drugs that act locally on nerves, producing a reversible block of nerve conduction. Despite several theories, their exact mechanism of action is unknown. Depending on the percentage concentration (strength) of the local anaesthetic used, the conduction block may affect all the different fibres in the nerve — motor, sensory and sympathetic (autonomic). Therefore, in the area supplied by the nerve, there may be paralysis of muscles, anaesthesia (loss of pain, touch and temperature sensations) and vasodilatation. Of course, if the particular nerve does not contain motor fibres, the block will not lead to muscle paralysis. The greater the diameter of the nerve fibre, the higher the concentration of local anaesthetic required to produce conduction block. The motor fibres are larger than the sensory and autonomic fibres and, by selecting the appropriate anaesthetic concentration, it is possible to produce local anaesthesia without significant paralysis. This may be helpful for analgesia in the labour ward. Another factor influencing the local anaesthetic concentration for block is the size of the nerve itself — the larger the nerve, the higher the required concentration.

The techniques of local anaesthesia are classified according to the method of administration or the site of injection:

(a) **topical**
(b) **infiltration**
(c) **nerve or plexus block**
(d) **epidural (extradural) block**
(e) **subarachnoid block**
(f) **intravenous regional.**

With topical anaesthesia, the local anaesthetic is applied directly to the mucous membranes of the nose, the eye, the throat, the trachea, the urethra or the conjunctiva. Relatively high concentrations are needed to permit penetration of the mucous membrane. Solutions, aerosols, drops, ointments and jellies are supplied for this purpose. Topical anaesthesia is suitable only for minor, superficial operations or endoscopies. Local anaesthetics, even in high concentrations, do not penetrate or anaesthetise normal skin because its cornified layer is impervious.

With infiltration anaesthesia, the anaesthetic solution is injected into and around the site of the operation. Here, the nerve branches are quite small, and for this reason, lower anaesthetic concentrations produce satisfactory anaesthesia. Infiltration anaesthesia is suitable for minor, superficial procedures such as biopsy or excision of skin lesions and vascular cannulations.

With nerve or plexus block, the anaesthetic solution is injected around a nerve or plexus of nerves. Higher concentrations are required for this technique. Anaesthesia is produced in the area of distribution of the nerve or plexus; that is, a brachial-plexus block will anaesthetise the upper limb.

With epidural block, the anaesthetic solution is injected deeply into the epidural (extradural) space, usually in the lumbar area. Higher concentrations are required to effectively block the large nerves as they leave the spinal cord. A lumbar epidural produces anaesthesia of the lower half of the body and it relieves the pains of labour. A fine, plastic catheter may be left in the epidural space and repeated injections ("top ups") via this catheter provide prolonged pain relief.

With subarachnoid block, the anaesthetic solution is injected into the subarachnoid space. This space contains cerebrospinal fluid, and a fine, lumbar puncture needle is used for the injection. The large nerves leaving the spinal cord are blocked, and anaesthesia is produced in the lower half of the body.

With the intravenous regional technique, an arterial tourniquet is applied to a limb, and then the anaesthetic solution is injected intravenously into that limb. The solution diffuses from the veins into the tissues and blocks the nerves. Anaesthesia is maintained as long as the tourniquet remains inflated. This technique is suitable only for limb surgery. Accidental deflation of the tourniquet soon after the IV injection of the local anaesthetic leads to severe and perhaps fatal systemic toxicity.

From the site of administration, local anaesthetics are absorbed into the blood stream and metabolised by the liver. The shorter-acting, ester type are also destroyed in the blood stream by cholinesterase. Local anaesthetics are toxic drugs, and great care must be taken to avoid overdosage or accidental intravascular injection, both of which result in high anaesthetic blood levels. Systemic toxicity affects the central nervous and cardiovascular systems. Stimulation of the brain (with restlessness, tremors, twitchings and convulsions) is followed by depression with drowsiness, respiratory failure and coma. The depression of the cardiovascular system leads to hypotension, bradycardia and perhaps cardiac arrest. Management of these toxic effects consists of oxygen therapy, anticonvulsants (relaxants or diazepam), artificial respiration, vasopressors and perhaps cardiopulmonary resuscitation (CPR). There are no antidotes for local anaesthetic toxicity. Allergic reactions have been reported, but they are uncommon.

The rate of absorption from the site of administration may be reduced by adding a vasoconstrictor drug to the local anaesthetic. As a result, more anaesthetic may be injected without the danger of systemic toxicity, and the duration of anaesthesia is prolonged. The catecholamine, ***adrenaline***, and the peptide, ***felypressin*** (*Octapressin*), are the vasoconstrictor drugs most frequently used for this purpose. Excessive dosage of the vasoconstrictors may lead to a hypertensive crisis, and with adrenaline, dangerous beta-adrenergic effects on the heart, such as gross tachycardia, multiple ventricular ectopic beats and even ventricular fibrillation. Therefore, great care must be taken to use a low concentration of vasoconstrictor and not to exceed the maximum recommended dosage. Vasoconstrictor drugs must not be injected in fingers or toes or around the base of the penis because the vascular spasm may lead to ischaemia and perhaps gangrene.

Some of the frequently used local anaesthetics are listed in Table 101.

Table 101
Local Anaesthetics

Chemical Group	Local Anaesthetics*	Trade Names*	% Concentration Required** Topical	Infiltration	Plexus, Epidural	Spinal	Max Dose with Adrenaline*** (mg/kg)	Onset, Duration
Esters	Cocaine	—	Too toxic for injections; 4% to 20% still used for topical anaesthesia; has vasoconstrictor action on its own.					
	Procaine		—	0.25–1	1–2	5	10	Slow onset, short acting (30 to 45 min)
Amides	Lignocaine	*Xylocaine*	2–10	0.25–0.5	1.5–2	5	7	Rapid onset, medium acting (1 to 2 h)
	Mepivacaine	*Carbocaine*	—	1	1.5–2	—	7	Slow onset, medium acting (1.5 to 3 h)
	Prilocaine	*Citanest*	—	0.5–1	2–3	—	10	Slow onset, medium acting (1 to 2 h)
	Bupivacaine	*Marcain*	—	0.25–0.5	0.25–0.5	—	2	Slow onset, long acting (4 to 8 h)
	Cinchocaine	*Nupercaine*	Very toxic; used only for spinal blocks as 0.5% solution; 6% dextrose already added to make heavier than CSF (hyperbaric)					

** % concentration is expressed as grams of the drug per 100 mL of solution.
*** Maximum dosage should be reduced by a half if vasoconstrictor not added.

For topical anaesthesia, ointments, jellies, pressure-packs and solutions are supplied. The topical solutions are often coloured artificially to indicate that they are not meant for injection. Local anaesthetics for injection are supplied in ampoules or vials with or without vasoconstrictor. All of these preparations have an expiry date. A partially used ampoule or vial should be discarded to avoid contamination and decomposition.

The local anaesthetic, lignocaine, is used as a cardiac antiarrhythmic for the control of ventricular ectopic beats. For this purpose and to facilitate its administration by continuous infusion, lignocaine is supplied in solution of 20 mg/mL and 200 mg/mL as *Xylocard.*

POSTOPERATIVE ANALGESICS

The analgesic drugs have been considered in some detail in Chapter 16. They are frequently used postoperatively. After minor surgery and particularly after "day-stay" surgery, the mild analgesics are prescribed for oral administration — aspirin, paracetamol, codeine and dextropropoxyphene. After more extensive surgery, pentazocine or narcotics are usually prescribed for intramuscular injection every four hours, for example, morphine, pethidine or papaveretum. The age, the size and the general condition of the patient are considered when choosing the appropriate dosage (see section on premedicant drugs and Table 97 in this chapter). Other and more complicated techniques for postoperative analgesia are under investigation in various parts of the world:

(a) continuous intravenous infusion of narcotics using mechanically driven syringes;
(b) self-administration of narcotics by the patient;
(c) continuous regional infusion or intermittent injection of local anaesthetics;
(d) epidural morphine;
(e) transcutaneous electrical nerve stimulation (TENS).

NURSING IMPLICATIONS

The patient receiving an anaesthetic agent must be considered in terms of preoperative, intraoperative and postoperative care. Several groups of nursing staff may be involved so that accurate and consistent recording of information is essential.

Preoperative assessment

This is the most important aspect of the preoperative period. A nursing history should include the following information.

- Known or suspected allergies.
- Past and present illness.

- Past surgical procedures.
- Present drug regime. Several factors are important. Patients on steroids have a decreased ability to handle the stress of surgery. There may be an increased risk of wound infection and delayed wound healing. Prolonged phenothiazine treatment may hinder postanaesthetic recovery.
- An assessment of vital signs will establish a baseline from which intraoperative and postoperative status can be evaluated.
- Information concerning smoking patterns will assist in planning pulmonary care. Psychological attitudes to surgery must be evaluated.
- Assess the patient's understanding of anaesthesia and surgery.
- Assess pulmonary function.
- Urinalysis.
- Weight.

Management

It may be necessary to initiate pulmonary care several days before surgery. The patient's premedications are usually ordered to be given at a specific time. In some cases they may be ordered "on call". They must be administered at the correct time and via the correct route, which is usually intramuscular. Drugs must not be mixed in syringes unless specific instructions to that effect are given by a medical officer or advice sought from the pharmacist. A patient should remain in bed after a premedication has been given, as hypotension may precipitate an injury if he or she is mobile.

Evaluation

Evaluate the effects of premedication which includes settling and drowsiness. These should be noticeable approximately 20 minutes after injection. Note any unwanted effects and report these to the appropriate staff. These effects should be fully documented.

Intraoperative assessment

Documentation of the preoperative vital signs and status should be available for evaluation. Ensure that the anaesthetist is aware of any abnormalities. The nurse receiving the patient should also assess the patient herself.

Excitability is associated with stage II anaesthesia so that a quiet environment is essential during this stage. Correct positioning of the patient and padding will reduce the incidence of pressure areas. These may occur as a complication of hypotension and immobility induced by anaesthesia.

As profound hypotension may occur during general anaesthesia, the patient should be handled gently and carefully while re-positioning. Ongoing evaluation of the patient's vital signs and status is usually maintained by the anaesthetist. If a local anaesthetic is used, the nurse may be asked to assist with observation and management.

Local anaesthetics

In patients who are anxious or fearful, vaso-vagal syncope may occur in reaction to the insertion of the needle and relief on its withdrawal. If this occurs, the patient should be placed flat immediately. Shock and convulsions can occur if the local anaesthetic is injected via the general circulation.

Postoperative assessment

In the recovery room, this includes the noting of the type of anaesthetic and any adjustments administered by the anaesthetist. Vital signs should be assessed and comparisons made with preoperative and intraoperative status. Recovery from anaesthesia proceeds in stages with return of function occurring in an orderly way. The following assessments should be made: cardiopulmonary, laryngeal or cough reflex, corneal reflex, swallowing (pharyngeal or gag) reflex, motor activity, vomiting, and mental state and consciousness. Improvements in these signs indicate recovery from a deep level of anaesthesia to consciousness. On transfer to the ward, monitoring of vital signs should continue. Observe the patient for the common complications of general anaesthesia, which include: hypotension, nausea or vomiting due to excitation of the vomiting centre, hypoventilation, oliguria, intestinal distension, nerve injury, thrombophlebitis due to venous stasis, and muscle pains or weakness.

Management

Of the above complications, most common are pulmonary and are related to bronchospasm. Protection of the restless, excitable patient by the use of rails may be necessary. This is particularly relevant to the asthmatic patient.

Patients taking steroids preoperatively must remain on them following surgery.

The patient who experiences pain when the anaesthetic is "wearing off" presents a particular management problem. How much analgesic drug the patient should receive at this time may require careful consultation with a medical officer. Parameters which may be used in the evaluation of analgesia and pain include: blood pressure, pulse rate, anaesthetic agent, length of anaesthesia and level of consciousness. Care should be taken when administering narcotic analgesics to patients with a history of myocardial infarction. The choice and dose of analgesic given will be determined by the extent to which the above parameters are affected. Once the anaesthetic effect has completely worn off, then decisions about analgesia are more straight-forward.

In some cases where parasympatholytic drugs have been used, the occurrence of a dry mouth will necessitate adequate oral hygiene. Some patients may feel cold and shivery with the use of particular anaesthesics. Keep the patient warm and dry without overheating. As anticholinergic drugs prevent sweating, overheating or the presence of a fever (combined with reduced fluid loss) may result in seizures, especially in children.

Observation of bladder distension and voiding is necessary as the anaesthetic or other drugs may inhibit the voiding reflex. Preoperative fasting and intraoperative fluid loss may contribute to decreased urine production. Methods used to intervene in this situation will depend on patient status and stability, the type of operation, degree of pain and the degree to which the patient can be mobilised. Catheterisation may be an option.

Local anaesthetic reactions tend to be related to three main factors: toxic overdose, entry of the drug into the general circulation, and hypersensitivity reactions. These are manifested by changes in the normal functioning of the following systems:

(a) central nervous system; mainly stimulation followed by depression resulting in unconsciousness and death;
(b) cardiovascular system; these changes are mainly bradycardia and hypotension terminating in cardiac arrest; cardiac arrhythmias may occur when adrenaline is combined with cyclopropane or halothane;
(c) hypersensitivity reactions are uncommon and are usually only mild rashes; occasionally anaphylaxis may occur.

Any patient discharged from hospital within 24 hours of an anaesthetic should not drive a motor vehicle or carry out any activities needing full alertness until they have had a full night's sleep.

SELF-EVALUATION TEST

1. Which of the following drugs may be used for premedication?
   (a) alcuronium
   (b) atropine
   (c) pentazocine
   (d) cimetidine
   (e) morphine
   (f) methohexitone
2. Which of the following drugs are used as general anaesthetics?
   (a) thiopentone
   (b) naloxone
   (c) felypressin
   (d) nitrogen
   (e) enflurane
3. Which of the following drugs are likely to cause hypotension?
   (a) adrenaline
   (b) halothane
   (c) atropine
   (d) neostigmine
   (e) alfathesin
   (f) nitrous oxide
4. Which of the following drugs are used as muscle relaxants?
   (a) suxamethonium
   (b) pancuronium
   (c) neostigmine
   (d) procaine
   (e) tubocurarine
   (f) droperidol

5. Which of the following drugs are used as local anaesthetics?
   (a) hyoscine
   (b) felypressin
   (c) thiopentone
   (d) bupivacaine
   (e) lignocaine
   (f) *Xylocard*
6. Which of the following is true about nitrous oxide?
   (a) it can be used when the surgeon uses diathermy;
   (b) it is a potent general anaesthetic;
   (c) it is supplied in blue cylinders;
   (d) it reacts chemically with sodalime;
   (e) it usually produces unconsciousness at 50% concentration;
   (f) it sensitises the heart to adrenaline.
7. Thiopentone has which of the following properties:
   (a) it is a yellow powder;
   (b) it is freely soluble in water;
   (c) it is destroyed by the liver;
   (d) it is locally irritating to tissues;
   (e) it frequently causes allergic reactions;
   (f) it frequently causes hypotension.
8. Suxamethonium has which of the following properties:
   (a) it is stable in solution;
   (b) it is a depolarising relaxant;
   (c) it may produce fasciculations;
   (d) it is a long-acting relaxant;
   (e) it causes "after pains";
   (f) it is reversed by neostigmine.
9. Lignocaine has which of the following properties:
   (a) it is a long-acting local anaesthetic;
   (b) it may be used for topical anaesthesia;
   (c) it may lead to CNS stimulation;
   (d) it may lead to CNS depression;
   (e) it is always mixed with adrenaline;
   (f) it may be infused intravenously.
10. Halothane has which of the following properties:
   (a) it is a volatile liquid;
   (b) it is an inhalational anaesthetic;
   (c) it is potent;
   (d) it may cause respiratory depression;
   (e) it is flammable;
   (f) it is administered from an *Enfluratec* vapouriser.

Table 102
Drugs Used in Anaesthesia

Drug Group	Drug Name	Use	Action	Adverse Reactions	Nursing Implications
Inhalational anaesthetics	Nitrous oxide	General anaesthetic	CNS depressant	Nausea, vomiting, excitability	***Assess:*** respiration rate, BP, pulse rate, ECG if required, mental state, patient safety. ***Evaluate:*** for adverse effects.
	Halothane	General anaesthetic	CNS depressant	Nausea, vomiting, cardiac arrhythmias, hypoventilation, hypotension, liver damage	***Assess:*** BP, respiration rate, pulse rate, ECG if required. ***Evaluate:*** for adverse effects, safe emergence from anaesthesia.
	Enflurane	General anaesthetic	CNS depressant	Nausea, vomiting, cardiac arrhythmias, hypoventilation, hypotension	***Assess:*** as for halothane, history of convulsions. ***Evaluate:*** pulse rate, convulsions, safe emergence from anaesthesia.
Intravenous anaesthetics	Thiopentone	General anaesthetic, induction agent	CNS depressant	Severe local tissue damage if extravasation occurs, hangover, depression of respiration and circulation, low incidence of delirium, nausea and vomiting on recovery	***Assess:*** baseline vital signs such as BP, pulse rate, respiration rate and pattern, temperature and sleep patterns; previous drug reactions or dependency on barbiturates; presence of pregnancy or lactation; history of chronic respiratory conditions, hypotension, liver or thyroid disease. ***Administer:*** carefully and according to legal regulations; slow IV, monitoring flow rate; avoid tissue extravasation. ***Evaluate:*** respiratory status and temperature, BP, pulse rate, adverse effects of delirium, nausea or vomiting; emergence from anaesthetic, consciousness state and hang-over effect, allergic reactions. ***Teach:*** do not allow patient to drive home if "day only" patient

Muscle relaxants	Suxamethonium	Muscle relaxation during surgery	Depolarising muscle relaxant	"After pains", bradycardia, hyperkalaemia, rarely prolonged effect	***Assess:*** BP, pulse rate, respiration rate, history of kidney disease, asthma, muscle disease or myasthenia gravis; electrolyte status, especially serum potassium and blood pH; present history of extensive tissue damage. ***Evaluate:*** emergence from effect of the neuromuscular blockers, e.g. limb, diaphragm and intercostal muscle movement, dysarthria or diplopia; muscle pain especially on inspiration; respiratory function, bradycardia and serum potassium levels.
	Tubocurarine Pancuronium Alcuronium	Muscle relaxation during surgery	Non-depolarising muscle relaxant	Awareness, incomplete reversal, hypotension, tachycardia, allergic reactions	***Assess:*** BP, pulse rate, respiration rate, consciousness, history of respiratory, kidney, liver or muscle disease, or myasthenia gravis, or cardiac disease. ***Evaluate:*** level of consciousness; reversal of paralysis as above; cardiovascular status, hypotension with tubocurarine, hypertension and tachycardia with pancuronium, pain level.
Local anaesthetics	Cocaine Cinchocaine Procaine Lignocaine Mepivacaine Prilocaine Bupivacaine	Topical or infiltration anaesthesia nerve or plexus block, epidural block, subarachnoid block, intravenous regional anaesthetic	Produce a reverse block of nerve conduction	Effects of overdose. CNS stimulation (convulsions) respiratory failure, coma, cardiovascular depression, allergic reaction	***Assess:*** liver function, BP, pulse rate, respiration rate, consciousness, history of cardiovascular or liver disease, or hypersensitivity. ***Evaluate:*** for adverse effects — restlessness, convulsions, respiratory depression, hypotension, bradycardia, allergic reactions

SECTION 9

31

DRUGS USED IN TREATMENT OF DISORDERS OF THE ALIMENTARY SYSTEM

Michael Wyer and Robyn Ronai

OBJECTIVES

At the end of this chapter the student should be able to:

1. define drug groups used to treat abnormal conditions of the mouth and pharynx, oesophagus, stomach and duodenum, liver and intestinal tract;
2. understand and describe simple mechanisms of action of drugs used to treat the various conditions;
3. identify by name and classify drugs commonly used to treat various conditions of the alimentary tract;
4. list the common and dangerous side effects of these drugs;
5. describe the important aspects of drug usage which will maximise drug effects through correct administration and patient care.

PREREQUISITE KNOWLEDGE

Students should review the physiology of the alimentary tract with particular reference to secretions, the digestive process, gastric function, hepatic function, intestinal function, and nausea and vomiting.

DEFINITIONS

Antacid — drug which partially neutralises gastric acid.
Anticholinergic — drug which reduces gastric-acid secretion and gastrointestinal motility.
Antiflatulent — drug used to relieve gaseous distension of the stomach (also known as carminative).
Antispasmodic — drug which relaxes muscle spasm and reduces hypermotility of the gastrointestinal tract.
Laxative — drug used to promote defecation or evacuation of bowel contents.
Anthelmintic — drug used to treat parasitic worm (helminth) infestation.
Antiemetic — drug used to relieve nausea and vomiting.

PEPTIC ULCERS

Peptic ulcers usually occur in the stomach (gastric ulcer) or in the duodenum (duodenal ulcer). They result from damage to the mucosa in the gastrointestinal tract. Whatever the cause of the ulcer, any ulcer is aggravated by the acid secretions hydrochloric acid and pepsin. The effects of these acids on the ulcer cause pain and possibly vomiting. Treatment, therefore, is directed towards abolishing the effects of acid on the ulcer. This in turn should be associated with relief of symptoms (pain and vomiting), the promotion of healing and the prevention of relapse.

Treatments have included hospital admission and bed-rest; cessation of smoking; cessation of analgesic drugs; drug therapy; appropriate diet and eating habits; and bed-rest.

Historically, antacids and anticholinergic drugs have been used in the treatment of peptic ulcers, and they still are. However, major therapeutic advances have been made in the treatment of peptic ulcers in recent years. For many years carbenoxolone has been used, but side effects limit its use, and modern drugs are more commonly used. The modern drugs which have made a marked advance in the treatment of ulcers are tripotassium dicitrato bismuthate (*De-Nol*) and cimetidine (*Tagamet*).

ANTACIDS

The pH of the stomach is acid, and acid secretion increases following food intake. Ulcer pain is most severe at this time. Antacids to a large degree neutralise the acid secretions. At standard doses (10 to 15mL of most liquids), antacids will only ease the pain, but with frequent high doses a positive healing effect on the ulcer can be obtained. Such dosages are usually in the range of 20 to 40 mL and may be given as frequently as every hour during waking hours.

Antacids are used in the treatment of gastric ulcers, duodenal ulcers, dyspepsia and oesophagitis.

Antacid agents include ***aluminium hydroxide, magnesium hydroxide, magnesium carbonate, magnesium trisilicate and calcium carbonate.*** These agents form the basis of most of the many commercial preparations. Aluminium hydroxide is often used alone as a mixture or tablets. Aluminium hydroxide and magnesium hydroxide mixture is a common combination used to balance the opposing side effects of constipation and diarrhoea which may be seen with these two drugs (see Adverse Drug Reactions below.) Common trade preparations containing these two drugs include *Aludrox, †Antasil, Mucogel* and *Mucaine* (which also contains a local anaesthetic). Aluminium hydroxide and magnesium carbonate are combined in *†Dijex* preparations.

†Antasil, Asilone and *†Polycrol Forte* contain the antiflatulent dimethicone which aids the expulsion of gastric gas associated with flatulence or a "bloated" feeling.

Antacids should be given immediately after meals and at bedtime. Additional doses may be taken in between to relieve pain. The dosage is

5 to 40 mL for most liquids, or 1 or 2 tablets which should be sucked or chewed for prompt relief.

Adverse Drug Reactions

Aluminium salts may cause constipation; magnesium salts may cause diarrhoea; aluminium hydroxide on prolonged use may cause phosphate depletion; calcium carbonate may cause constipation and renal stones with renal failure; sodium bicarbonate has been used, but the danger of systemic alkalosis and fluid retention from this soluble salt restricts its use.

Antacids may interfere with the absorption of antibiotics, particularly tetracycline. They are contraindicated in cases of renal insufficiency.

NURSING IMPLICATIONS

Assessment

Before the administration of antacids, the patient's history should be assessed for the presence of renal insufficiency, oedema or hypertension where substances which contain calcium carbonate or sodium bicarbonate are to be used. Check current drug profile for use of salicylates or tetracyclines. Antacids can lower the plasma salicylate level, and they prevent the absorption of tetracyclines.

Administration

Shake mixtures well before pouring the dose. Patients should be instructed to chew or suck tablets because if they are swallowed whole, there is a risk of intestinal obstruction. Antacids are usually given after meals and at bedtime or more frequently if required.

Evaluation

Assess for relief of discomfort. If diarrhoea or constipation occur, request a change to another type of antacid.

Patient teaching

Patients and the general public should be warned against the over-use of sodium bicarbonate due to the risk of alkalosis and sodium retention. Sodium bicarbonate can cause severe gastric distension due to the formation of carbon-dioxide gas in the stomach which could lead to perforation in ulcer patients. These patients should be warned not to take aspirin and that some over-the-counter preparations for "upset stomach" do contain aspirin.

ANTICHOLINERGICS

The commonly used anticholinergics are listed in Table 103.

Anticholinergic drugs decrease gastric-acid secretion by inhibiting vagal nerve activity. This action causes reduced gastrointestinal motility which gives them an antispasmodic effect. They are used in the treatment of gastric ulcer, duodenal ulcer, and spastic colon (colitis).

When used alone or with antacids, the dosage is usually increased until limited by side effects. Since the introduction of cimetidine, anticholinergic drugs are mainly used as a supplementary drug at lower dose levels. They are usually given 30 to 60 minutes before meals and at bedtime.

Table 103
Commonly Used Anticholinergics

Generic Name	Trade Name	Tablet Strength
Belladonna compounds	Various	Various
Glycopyrronium bromide	*Robinul*	1 mg
Hyoscine butylbromide	*Buscopan*	10 mg
Dicyclomine hydrochloride	*Merbentyl*	10 mg
Penthienate methobromide	*Monodral*	5 mg
Propantheline bromide	*Pro-Banthine*	15 mg

Adverse Drug Reactions

These include dry mouth, blurred vision, dilated pupils, tachycardia, constipation, difficulty in passing urine, dizziness, mental confusion and impotence.

Reduced gastric motility may delay passage of drugs through the stomach, causing altered absorption rates. Anticholinergics are contraindicted in glaucoma, enlarged prostate, oesophageal reflux and oesophagitis.

NURSING IMPLICATIONS

Assessment

Anticholinergic drugs are used in a wide variety of situations, not just gastrointestinal conditions. The nursing implications for anticholinergic drugs (including drugs with atropine-like properties) will be similar, no matter what condition they are used for.

Prior to administration of an anticholinergic drug, the nurse should assess the patient's history for evidence of glaucoma, hypertension, coronary artery disease, enlarged prostate or urinary hesitancy, oesophageal reflux or hiatus hernia. Current drug profile should be assessed for use of other atropine-like drugs such as antihistamines or tricyclic antidepressants.

Administration

The nurse should evaluate the patient for signs of the desired response to the drug and observe for adverse effects. Initially the patient may experience a dry mouth. This can be alleviated by giving extra fluids or sweets to suck. Be alert for reports from the patient of urinary hesitancy or retention. Reports of visual disturbances such as seeing haloes around lights could be a symptom of glaucoma. Restlessness or confusion are signs of toxicity and may indicate the need to reduce the dose. Observe bowel function as constipation may occur.

Teaching

Reassure the patient that the side effects of dry mouth and blurred vision may occur initially, but should pass as his body adjusts to the dose. He should also be advised that if blurred vision and drowsiness occur, driving a car or operating machinery would be dangerous.

CARBENOXOLONE

Carbenoxolone is marketed as *Biogastrone* (tablets 50 mg), *Duogastrone* (capsules 50 mg) and *Pyrogastrone* (carbenoxolone plus antacids).

Carbenoxolone is a liquorice derivative whose mode of action in promoting healing of ulcers is unclear. Possible actions are an anti-inflammatory effect, and a local effect, stimulating mucin production and enzyme processes involved in cellular regeneration.

Biogastrone is used for gastric ulcers, and *Duogastrone* for duodenal ulcers.

Gastric ulcer patients should take carbenoxolone after a meal or, if heartburn occurs, with milk. Duodenal ulcer patients should take carbenoxolone 15 to 30 minutes before a meal.

Adverse Drug Reactions

These include fluid retention and oedema, hypertension, hypokalaemia and heartburn; headache and nausea are rare. These effects have restricted the use of this drug in elderly patients and in hypertensive patients who are often prone to ulcers.

Carbenoxolone is contraindicated when a patient is taking spironolactone (*Aldactone*) and in patients with cardiac and/or renal disease.

NURSING IMPLICATIONS

Watch for signs of oedema, increased blood pressure, and signs of hypokalaemia such as weakness and muscle cramps.

CIMETIDINE AND RANITIDINE

Cimetidine is marketed as *Tagamet* (tablets 200 mg, 400 mg and 800 mg, ampoules 200 mg/2 mL). ***Ranitidine*** is marketed as *Zantac* (tablets 150 mg, ampoules 50 mg/2 mL).

Cimetidine and ranitidine are histamine-2 (H_2) receptor antagonists. Histamine is a physiological substance found in many parts of the body. Apart from its better-known vascular effects as in allergies (histamine-1 receptors), it also causes increased gastric-acid secretion. This effect occurs through histamine-2 receptors in the stomach. Cimetidine and ranitidine block this action of histamine on the H_2 receptors and inhibit basal and nocturnal gastric-acid secretion. The drug is used in cases of gastric ulcer, duodenal ulcer and Zollinger-Ellison syndrome.

Dosage for treatment is as follows: cimetidine — 400 mg in the morning and 400 mg at night; ranitidine — one tablet (150 mg) twice daily. The course is usually four to six weeks and may be repeated. Patients with frequent relapse or hypersecretory problems may require long-term treatment on a full dose or just a maintenance dose. The maintenance dose for cimetidine is 400 mg at night, and for ranitidine, it is 150 mg at night.

Cimetidine tablets should be taken with meals. Injections are used in emergencies for stress ulcers associated with hospitalisation. Concurrent administration of antacids for pain relief after meals may be necessary.

Ranitidine tablets do not need to be taken with meals. Injections are used as for cimetidine. As for cimetidine, concurrent administrations of antacids for pain relief after meals may be necessary.

Adverse Drug Reactions to Cimetidine

Side effects are not common but include headache, diarrhoea, dizziness, muscular pain, rash, increased serum creatinine and mild gynaecomastia.

Adverse Drug Reactions to Ranitidine

Rash, pruritus, diarrhoea or flatulence, and tiredness or lethargy are among the side effects.

NURSING IMPLICATIONS

Blood pressure and pulse rate should be monitored during IV administration of cimetidine and ranitidine, since hypotension and tachycardia or bradycardia may occur.

Give IV injections slowly.

TRIPOTASSIUM DICITRATO BISMUTHATE (TDB)

TDB appears under the trade name of *De-Nol*. In an acid medium, TDB combines with proteins at the site of the ulcer to form a protective layer. In addition, acid precipitates bismuth oxide which has an affinity for granulation tissue in the ulcer base, that is, TDB protects the ulcer from acid. It is used in cases of gastric ulcer and duodenal ulcer.

Exact adherence to the dosage schedule is important. No liquids should be given for half an hour after a dose. Antacids and milk should be avoided during treatment as they prevent effective binding of the bismuth compound at the ulcer site.

Adverse Drug Reactions

These are few, but include blackening of stools. TDB is contraindicated in severe renal insufficiency.

NURSING IMPLICATIONS

Patient education is important as compliance is necessary if treatment is to be effective. Teach the patient the correct dosage regime and to avoid antacids and milk during treatment. Explain to the patient that stools will probably be darker than normal.

SUCRALFATE

Sucralfate is marketed as *Antepsin* (tablets 1 g). Sucralfate is a new agent which has three actions. First, it combines with protein at the ulcer site and hence forms a protective barrier. Second, it blocks the back diffusion of gastric acid across the barrier, and third, it inhibits the action of pepsin and bile.

Sucralfate is recommended only for use in acute ulcerous conditions (up to 8 weeks).

The dosage for treatment is 1 g three times a day, one hour before meals and 1 g at bedtime.

Adverse Drug Reactions

These have been reported only in a small percentage of patients, the main adverse effect being constipation (2% to 3%). Other adverse effects include: headache, urticaria, nausea, diarrhoea, gastric discomfort, indigestion, dry mouth, skin rash, pruritus, back pain, dizziness, sleepiness and vertigo.

NURSING IMPLICATIONS

Antacids may be given concurrently to relieve pain, but they should not be given within half an hour before or after sucralfate intake.

Care should be taken in patients with impaired renal function as each 1 g dose of sucralfate contains 190 mg of aluminium.

The drug should be given on an empty stomach. Watch for constipation. Avoid the concurrent administration of antacids and H_2 blockers as the antacid can reduce the uptake of the H_2 blocker.

ANTIFLATULENTS

Drugs used as antiflatulents include ***peppermint water, dill water*** (*Gripe Water*), ***pipenzolate*** (*Piptal*) and ***dicyclomine*** (*Merbentyl*).

These drugs alter the surface activity of gas in the gastrointestinal tract. This assists in removal of the gas by belching or passage through the intestine. Dicyclomine and pipenzolate have an antispasmodic effect.

The antiflatulents are used for flatulence and infant colic.

Adverse Drug Reactions

There is little likelihood of side effects at standard doses. *Piptal* may, however, have some anticholinergic effects.

ANTISPASMODICS

Drugs with predominantly antispasmodic action include ***mebeverine*** (*Colofac*), ***hyoscine-N-butylbromide*** (*Buscopan*), ***dicyclomine*** (*Merbentyl*), and ***mepenzolate bromide*** (*Cantil*).

Antispasmodic drugs relax the smooth muscle of the gastrointestinal, biliary and renal tracts. They are used for gastrointestinal spasm, irritable colon syndrome, biliary colic and renal colic.

Adverse Drug Reactions

At higher dosage levels, anticholinergic side effects may occur.

NURSING IMPLICATIONS

Because anticholinergic (atropine-like) side effects may occur with some of the antispasmodics, the nurse needs to evaluate her patient's response and reaction to the drug accordingly (see nursing implications under the heading of anticholinergic drugs).

Note that mebeverine (*Colofac)* exerts its main action specifically on the colon and is claimed to be wholly free of atropine-like side effects at therapeutic doses.

LAXATIVES

Laxatives are used for treating constipation and for preoperative bowel emptying. There are a number of different types of laxatives with differing actions.

SALINE LAXATIVES

Saline laxatives include ***magnesium sulphate*** (*Epsom Salts*), ***sodium phosphates*** (*Fletchers' Phosphate Enema*) and ***sodium citrate*** (a component of *Microlax*). These substances are not well absorbed, and after oral or rectal administration they remain in the bowel where they attract water which softens the faeces and increases the bulk of the bowel content. This promotes peristalsis and bowel evacuation. Taken orally, drug effects occur in three to six hours.

STIMULANT LAXATIVES

Stimulant laxatives include vegetable extracts such as ***senna*** (*Senokot*) and ***castor oil***, and synthetic drugs such as ***bisacodyl*** (*Dulcolax*), ***danthron*** (a component of *co-danthramer*), ***phenolphthalein*** and *Alophen†*.

The stimulant laxatives act by stimulating peristalsis by irritation of the intestinal mucosa or smooth muscle. With the exception of castor oil, they act on the colon or large intestine and take approximately six hours to act. Night-time dosage is therefore common. Castor oil acts within three hours.

BULK LAXATIVES

Bulk laxatives include ***methylcellulose*** (*†Cologel*), vegetable mucilaginous extracts such as ***ispaghula*** (*Isogel, Fybogel*) and ***sterculia*** (*Normacol*), and ***unprocessed bran.***

The bulk laxatives are indigestible. In the bowel they absorb water and swell, thus increasing the bulk of the bowel content. This causes reflex peristaltic contraction. They also become mucilaginous and lubricate the intestinal wall. These drugs are usually in granule form.

Bulk laxatives should be taken with copious amounts of water. They are sometimes given for diarrhoea not responding to other drugs, in which case the drug's action is to absorb excess water in the faeces, so minimal water should be taken in this instance.

LUBRICANT LAXATIVES

Lubricant laxatives include ***glycerin*** (as a suppository), ***liquid paraffin*** and ***liquid paraffin emulsion.***

These drugs work by lubrication of the intestinal wall and softening of faeces which allows defecation without straining.

Adverse Drug Reactions

1. May interfere with the absorption of fat-soluble vitamins and some drugs, for example, phenindione, the anticoagulant.
2. Regular ingestion during pregnancy may reduce absorption of vitamin K and produce hypoprothrombinaemia.
3. Anal leakage of oil may occur.
4. Lipid pneumonia may occur if the oil gains access to the lungs.
5. Habituation.

SURFACE ACTIVE LAXATIVES

Surface-active agents include ***dioctyl sodium sulphosuccinate*** (*Dioctyl*) and ***sodium lauryl sulphoacetate*** (a component of *Microlax*). These drugs have a detergent-like effect facilitating penetration of the faecal mass by water and fats and thus softening the faeces.

Adverse Drug Reactions Recommended dosages are well tolerated, but large doses may cause anorexia, vomiting and diarrhoea.

LACTULOSE

Lactulose (*†Duphalac*) is a disaccharide which is not broken down in the gut or upper intestine, but in the colon is broken down into low-molecular-weight organic acids. These cause mild irritation and promote peristalsis.

Lactulose also provides nutrient for saccharolytic bacterial growth in the colon. This maintains a balance with colonic proteolytic bacteria which is necessary for normal bowel function.

NURSING IMPLICATIONS

Assessment

Before the administration of a laxative, the nurse should ensure the patient is not suffering from intestinal obstruction or perforated bowel, the signs and symptoms of which include nausea, vomiting, abdominal pain and distension. All laxatives are contraindicated in these situations. Patients who are receiving anticoagulant therapy and those who are debilitated should not be given lubricant laxatives as decreased vitamin absorption can occur with these. Saline-type laxatives should be avoided when the patient's sodium intake is restricted, or where there is an existing or potential risk of fluid and electrolyte imbalance.

Administration

This should occur so that the drug's onset and peak of action occurs at a convenient time and not during the night. Ensure that bulk laxatives are given with a large glass of water. They require a high fluid intake to be effective.

Evaluation

Check for the relief of constipation and record appropriately. If the patient remains constipated after the administration of bulk laxatives, check on fluid intake and assess further for signs of intestinal obstruction such as pain and distension. Observe the patient for signs of dehydration and electrolyte imbalance, especially where saline laxatives have been used or if the patient is very ill or debilitated.

Patient teaching

The nurse has an important role as an educator to both patients and the general public regarding how to maintain normal bowel function. Some people have "bowel phobia" and become habitual laxative users, which can then lead to the "lazy bowel" syndrome. A high fibre diet, plenty of fluids and regular exercise all contribute to maintaining normal bowel function. Nurses should be continually alert to prevent the development of constipation in their patients. Prevention or treatment must be carried out in order to avoid the problem of severe faecal impaction.

ANTIDIARRHOEAL DRUGS

Diarrhoea is a symptom of abnormal bowel function which exhibits as frequent passing of faeces, usually watery in nature. The watery stools can result in excess fluid loss with dehydration and electrolyte loss. Diarrhoea may be accompanied by colonic spasm and pain.

Diarrhoea has many causes such as antibiotic use, lactose intolerance, bacterial infection and *Giardia lamblia*. Specific drugs may be necessary to treat the cause.

Drugs used to treat the symptom of diarrhoea fall into two main categories: absorbents which reduce the amount of free water in the bowel, and antimotility drugs which relieve colonic spasms and may relieve pain. Adjuvant therapy may be necessary in the form of fluid replacement, electrolyte replacement and dextrose (glucose) administration.

Administration may be by the intravenous route in severe cases, but generally the oral route is satisfactory. One preparation for oral use is *Dioralyte*, which contains potassium, sodium and chloride ions as well as some dextrose.

ABSORBENTS

Absorbent drugs include ***kaolin*** and ***aluminium hydroxide***. They are used alone or in combination in many commercial preparations, for example, *Kaolin Mixture, Kaopectate, KLN*.

ANTIMOTILITY DRUGS

Antimotility drugs include ***codeine phosphate***, ***diphenoxylate*** (*Lomotil*), and ***loperamide*** (*Imodium*).

These drugs have a suppressant effect on intestinal motility, thus reducing peristaltic action. Codeine phosphate is a narcotic analgesic and relieves pain associated with diarrhoea. Diphenoxylate is related to pethidine and has an opiate activity, but is non-addictive. Loperamide is similar to diphenoxylate but does not have opiate activity.

Adverse Drug Reactions

1. Overdosage may cause nausea, vomiting, constipation and respiratory depression.
2. Addiction may occur with codeine phosphate.
3. *Lomotil* also contains atropine as a guard against excessive dosage. Anticholinergic effects such as dry mouth and tachycardia may therefore occur.

NURSING IMPLICATIONS

Assessment

If the patient has diarrhoea, the nurse should first establish the cause if known, as then it may be treated with specific therapy. Assess the patient's fluid and electrolyte status, and document the number, frequency and consistency of all bowel actions. It may be inadvisable to administer opiate derivates to patients with compromised respiratory function.

Administration

Absorbents may be given frequently, such as after each bowel action. Antimotility drugs have a structured dosage schedule, and excessive dosage of these must be avoided.

Evaluation
Observe for reduction in number of stools and consistency. Record stool chart and fluid-balance chart in severe cases. Observe for atropine-like side effects with antimotility drugs such as diphenoxylate.

Patient teaching
Where the patient is taking the drug at home, he should be instructed on the correct dosage regime, and if taking opium derivatives and antimotility drugs, he should be advised against excessive dosage.

DRUGS FOR SPECIFIC DIARRHOEA-CAUSING SITUATIONS

Lactobacillus (from yoghurt). This is used to re-establish or maintain lactobacillus content of intestinal flora in conditions such as prolonged antibiotic taking and monilial infections.

Tinidazole (*Fasigyn*) and ***metronidazole*** (*Flagyl*). These drugs are used in giardiasis and amoebic dysentery. Metronidazole, in particular, is being used before and after bowel surgery for prophylaxis and therapy against anaerobic infections.

Neomycin sulphate This has been used for bacillary dysentery but is not now recommended. It has been used for preoperative bowel sterilisation.

Natamycin (*Pimafucin*) and ***nystatin*** (*Nystan*). These drugs may be used orally to treat intestinal monilial infection which may be caused by large doses and/or prolonged therapy with antibiotics.

ANTIEMETICS

Antiemetics are used for the control of nausea and vomiting. Antiemetics do not treat the underlying cause of the nausea and vomiting; they merely alleviate the symptoms and hence are considered palliative treatment.

Nausea and vomiting can be prevented or treated by drugs acting on central or peripheral receptor sites, or both.

Adverse Drug Reactions

Phenothiazines — adverse reactions to and nursing implications of the phenothiazines are discussed in Chapters 28 and 30 of this book.
Antihistamines — sedation, dizziness, anticholinergic side effects (for example, dry mouth, gastrointestinal disturbances), hallucinations, potentiation of effects of CNS depressants such as alcohol.
Anticholinergics — dry mouth, blurred vision, urinary retention, constipation.
Metoclopramide — dystonia, drowsiness.

Table 104
Commonly Used Antiemetics

Drug Class	Site of Action	Generic Name	Trade Name	Tablet	Ampoule	Suppository
Phenothiazines	Act on chemoreceptor trigger zone	Prochlorperazine	*Stemetil*	5 mg, 25 mg	12.5 mg	5 mg, 25 mg
		Perphenazine	*Fentazin*	2 mg, 4 mg, 8 mg	5 mg	
		Thiethylperazine	*Torecan*	10 mg	6.5 mg	6.5 mg
		Chlorpromazine	*Largactil*	10 mg, 25 mg 50 mg, 100 mg	25 mg, 50 mg	
Antihistamines	Act mainly on CNS vomiting centre (effective in motion sickness)	Dimenhydrinate	*Dramamine*	50 mg		
		Cyclizine	*Valoid*	50 mg	50 mg	
		Meclozine	*Ancoloxin*	25 mg		
		Promethazine	*Phenergan*	10 mg, 25 mg	25 mg, 50 mg	
Anticholinergics	Act on CNS vomiting centre; central cholinergic pathways (effective in motion sickness)	Hyoscine	*Merbentyl*	300, 600 mcg		
		Dicyclomine		10 mg		
Metoclopramide	Peripheral action, enhances motility and increases the rate of gastric emptying	Metoclopramide	*Maxolon*	10 mg	10 mg	
Vitamin B_6	Unknown	Pyridoxine	*Paxadon*	25 mg		
			Benadon	100 mg		

NURSING IMPLICATIONS

Assessment

Before the administration of an antiemetic, the patient's history should be assessed in relation to the type of drug to be used (see Table 104).

Administration

Metoclopramide should always be given 15 to 30 minutes before meals. Avoid spilling injectable phenothiazines on the skin.

Evaluation

Response to the drug should be monitored, and observations should be carried out for possible adverse effects. Watch for dystonic reactions, and report them if they occur. For example, oculogyric crisis has been known to occur after a single dose of a phenothiazine. Watch for anticholinergic side effects, and offer appropriate explanation to the patient should they occur.

Patient teaching

Advise patients that drowsiness, blurred vision and dry mouth may occur. Suggest the use of sunscreens to patients taking high doses of phenothiazines, especially chlorpromazine. Warn the patient that increased sedation and hypotension may occur when other CNS depressant drugs (such as alcohol, sedatives, narcotic analgesics) are used concurrently with antihistamines or phenothiazines, and therefore driving a car or operating machinery could be dangerous.

DIGESTIVE SUPPLEMENTS

In conditions where natural secretions used in the digestive process are absent or reduced, replacement or supplementary therapy will be necessary.

GASTRIC SUBACIDITY OR ACHLORHYDRIA

This condition can be helped by the administration of ***betaine hydrochloride/pepsin*** (*Acidol-Pepsin*) or ***glutamic acid hydrochloride*** (*Muripsin*).

PANCREATIC DISEASE

Pancreatitis is a nonbacterial inflammatory condition of the pancreas and may be caused by many different aetiological factors, for example, alcohol or gallstones. Acute pancreatitis has associated pain, shock and electrolyte imbalance. Pethidine is the drug of choice for treatment of the pain. Morphine and its derivatives are contraindicated because of their constricting action on the sphincter of Oddi.

The treatment of pancreatitis (and associated pancreatogenic shock) may include ***aprotinin*** (*Trasylol*).

Aprotinin is a proteinase inhibitor. Excessive amounts of proteinases such as trypsin, chymotrypsin, plasmin and leukocytal or tissue proteases have been found in an active form in many pathophysiological processes. The perpetuation of certain aspects of shock and inflammation have been associated with protein metabolism. Aprotinin has therefore been used in haemorrhagic shock and hyperfibrinolytic haemorrhage.

Dosage recommendation is high, with 500 000 KI units being injected slowly initially (maximum rate 5 mL/minute). Thereafter, 200 000 KI units are administered every four hours by slow intravenous injection or by continuous intravenous infusion.

Adverse Drug Reactions

Aprotinin may occasionally cause gastrointestinal upset, muscle pain or an allergic reaction with urticaria and bronchospasm. Blood pressure changes have been reported. In chronic pancreatitis, pancreatic steatorrhoea may be present and pancreatic replacement therapy necessary. Supplements used for this purpose reduce the diarrhoea and improve fat absorption. Pancreatin, the main substance used, is contained in *Cotazym, Creon, Nutrizym, Pancrex* and *Pancrex-V*.

These preparations are used in other conditions such as cystic fibrosis and after gastrectomy or cholecystectomy, where fat malabsorption is an associated problem.

ANTHELMINTICS

Anthelmintics are used to treat parasitic worm (helminth) infestation in humans due to roundworm, threadworm (pinworm), hookworm, whipworm and tapeworm. Roundworm and threadworm infestations are a common occurrence, particularly in childhood. Treatment is easy and generally uncomplicated.

Drugs include ***mebendazole*** (*Vermox*), ***niclosamide*** (*Yomesan*), ***piperazine*** (*Antepar, Pripsen*), ***pyrantel*** (*Combantrin*) and ***thiabendazole*** (*Mintezol*).

Piperazine and pyrantel are thought to cause paralysis of the worms which are then excreted in the faeces. In some cases the use of a purgative agent as well may be necessary. The action of the other drugs on the worms is uncertain, but metabolic interference is most likely.

Mebendazole is a broad spectrum drug and is effective against all the above worms. The dose will vary for some of the different worm types being treated. Thiabendazole is similar. Piperazine and pyrantel are used for threadworms and roundworms. Niclosamide may be used to treat tapeworm infestation. For roundworms and threadworms, the dose is usually given as a single dose and repeated in one to two weeks.

Adverse Drug Reactions

Mebendazole — mild diarrhoea and abdominal pain.
Piperazine — nausea and vomiting occasionally; urticaria; overdose may cause neurotoxicity with vertigo, spasm and loss of reflexes.
Niclosamide — mild colic and diarrhoea.

Thiabendazole — common reactions include anorexia, nausea, vomiting, epigastric distress, vertigo; less common reactions include skin rash and pruritus, diarrhoea, headache, fatigue, bradycardia and hypotension.
Pyrantel — anorexia, nausea and diarrhoea occur infrequently.

NURSING IMPLICATIONS

As the mouth is the main route of entry for worms in humans, hygiene is important. Ensure patient understands that the follow-up dose is necessary. If bowel actions are uncertain, give a laxative to ensure quick evacuation of worms after dose of the anthelmintic.

MISCELLANEOUS DRUGS

GAVISCON

Gaviscon is a combination of ***alginates*** and ***antacids***. Alginates gel on contact with water. The antacids neutralise excess gastric acid. The gel floats on top of gastric contents and protects the oesophagus from acid irritation if gastric reflux occurs. *Gaviscon* is used for gastric reflux, reflux oesophagitis and hiatus hernia.

Adverse Drug Reactions

No major side effects are known. However, the gel nature and high sugar content of *Gaviscon* has been thought to be associated with increased incidence of dental decay after prolonged use of the medication, if adequate rinsing of the mouth with water does not take place after each dose. The high sugar content may restrict use in diabetics.

SULPHASALAZINE

Sulphasalazine (*Salazopyrin*) is used in the treatment of ulcerative colitis.

Sulphasalazine is poorly absorbed from the gastrointestinal tract and in the intestine is broken down into sulphonamide compounds and a salicylate. The exact mode of action of these compounds in ulcerative colitis is not clear, but the salicylate effect is most likely anti-inflammatory.

Adverse Drug Reactions

1. Nausea, vomiting and anorexia are common.
2. Skin rash, Stevens-Johnson syndrome.
3. Giddiness and intense headache.
4. Blood dyscrasias — haemolytic anaemia, agranulocytosis.
5. Drug fever.
6. Cyanosis.
7. Neurotoxicity — peripheral neuritis, mental depression.

Most side effects are dose related and subside on drug withdrawal. The drug may then be reintroduced at a lower dose.

TREATMENT OF THE MOUTH AND THROAT

While there are many pharmaceutical preparations used for conditions of the mouth, most mouth conditions are not serious. They are often not primary in nature but secondary to an underlying systemic disease or reflect a poor nutritional status. Conditions most commonly seen are mouth ulcers, inflammation, damage to the mucous membrane, infections or drying of mucus and saliva. Local application of medicaments is usual.

MOUTHWASHES AND GARGLES

These are liquid preparations used to rinse or bathe the mouth and pharynx which have an antiseptic and often astringent and deodorant effect. They are often alkaline in nature and dissolve dry mucus and saliva which provides a medium for bacterial growth.

Usually, the preparations are not swallowed after rinsing of the mouth or gargling, but this will vary with the preparation used.

Some of the commonly used preparations are as follows.

Thymol glycerin compound

Thymol, the main component, is a mild phenolic antiseptic. The preparation should be diluted one part with three parts of water before use. It is widely used for general oral hygiene and prophylactically against infections.

Hexetidine *(Oraldene)* and ***Cetylpyridinium chloride solution*** *(Merocet)* are antiseptic deodorant preparations. ***Chlorhexidine*** mouthwashes *(Corsodyl, Eludril)* perform a similar function. ***Benzydamine*** *(Difflam Oral Rinse)* has an analgesic action useful in ulcerated mouths.

Sodium bicarbonate 5% solution is an alkaline mouthwash used to dissolve dried mucus.

Perborate compounds *(Bocasan)*

Bocasan powders are dissolved in water and used as a mouthwash for oral hygiene in conditions such as mouth infections, gingivitis and bleeding gums. Perborate liberates oxygen and so is mildly antiseptic.

MOUTH PAINTS

Mouth paints are thickened or concentrated liquid preparations for local application in the mouth. They may be antiseptic, anaesthetic, astringent and/or cleansing.

Glycerin alone or flavoured, when painted in the mouth is hygroscopic and stimulates flow of saliva. This has a cleansing effect in the mouth. If glycerin is required to moisten the mouth, it must be used in a diluted form of less than 40% concentration so that moisture is drawn from the diluent to the tissues. If the solution is stronger it absorbs moisture and leads to dehydration.

LOCAL PROTECTANTS

Local protectants for use in the mouth usually come in the form of gel-based compound containing antiseptics and/or anti-inflammatory drugs such as *Bonjela, Bioral Gel, Adcortyl in Orabase* and *Orahesive.*

LOCAL ANAESTHETICS

Pain associated with mouth abrasions can be relieved by the use of anaesthetic preparations, which also may be used to allow minor surgical procedures to be carried out. These include ***benzocaine*** (*AAA Throat Spray*) and ***lignocaine*** (*Xylocaine Spray*).

ANTIFUNGAL DROPS

Thrush, a common mouth infection in adults and children, may be associated with bad hygiene or antibiotic therapy. Thrush is caused by the fungal organism *Candida albicans* and is also known as moniliasis. It is treated by the local application of antifungal drops such as ***amphotericin*** (*Fungilin*), ***natamycin*** (*Pimafucin*), or ***nystatin*** (*Nystan*).

NURSING IMPLICATIONS

Preparations containing antifungal agents

As the antifungal preparations are suspensions of insoluble powders, remember to shake the bottle well immediately before administering the dose. Ensure that when the suspension is applied to the lesion, it is retained in the mouth for some time before swallowing, to ensure maximum local effect. The patient should avoid rinsing the mouth, eating or drinking for some time after administration.

Preparations containing local anaesthetics

Observe the local adverse effects. Instruct the patient to avoid hot liquids and hot or abrasive food until local anaesthetic effect wears off.

Assess the patient for hypersensitivity to the active ingredient. Administer the preparation as prescribed. Shake the bottle well if the preparation is a powder suspension. Evaluate the patient for effectiveness of preparation and for any adverse reactions. Teach the patient to retain the substance in the mouth for a while before swallowing.

DRUGS AND LIVER FAILURE

Liver disease can be classified into:

(a) acute liver failure caused by, for example, viral hepatitis;
(b) chronic liver failure caused by, for example, chronic hepatitis and cirrhosis.

Treatment usually combines bed rest, diet and medication.

Phenothiazines are used to treat nausea and vomiting, but these symptoms are usually self-limiting and will improve in a few days.

Fat-soluble vitamins (A,D,E,K) may need to be supplemented since fat absorption is impaired in viral hepatitis. These can be given orally as water-soluble preparations.

Corticosteroids have been used to decrease the inflammation in acute viral hepatitis, but these now seem to be contraindicated due to their immunosuppressive action. However, in prolonged cholestasis due to viral hepatitis, prednisolone 10 mg three times a day produces a dramatic fall in serum bilirubin and may shorten the illness.

Normal Immunoglobulin (Human) is a preparation containing 16% gamma globulins from normal human plasma. Normal Immunoglobulin (Human) can be given as a prophylaxis against Hepatitis A. It is not so effective against Hepatitis B. Also, it can be given after exposure to Hepatitis A to minimise the course of the disease. It is not effective for the treatment of active clinical disease nor if given more than six weeks after exposure.

Dosage

The recommended dose is 0.02 to 0.2 mL/kg body weight. Usually 2 mL is given IM as the adult "contact" dose. This dose should provide protection for three to four weeks. The duration of protection is increased to four to six months if this dose is doubled. Hence, for prophylaxis in adult overseas travellers, a 5 mL dose is used.

Adverse Drug Reactions

Severe allergic reactions may occur. For this reason, the IM route is normally used and not the IV route. There is a special 6% preparation available for IV use in cases where high doses of immunoglobulin are required.

Tenderness and stiffness may occur at the site of injection and may persist for several hours. Rarely, mild pyrexia, urticaria and malaise have been reported.

Hepatitis B vaccine (*H-B-VAX*) is a non-infectious subunit viral vaccine which provides immunisation against infection caused by Hepatitis B virus. It is ineffective if the patient already has Hepatitis B infection and so should only be used prophylactically.

It is indicated in people who are in constant contact with infected individuals, or else those people who handle the secretions (saliva, urine, tears, semen, vaginal secretions, bile, breast milk) of infected individuals. These may include health-care workers, renal dialysis patients, parenteral-drug abusers, promiscuous homosexuals, and travellers to and from endemic areas.

Dosage

It should be given only intramuscularly, and the dosage regimen consists of three doses: first dose — at elected date; second dose — one month later; third dose — six months after first dose. The vaccine should be refrigerated but not frozen.

Adverse Drug Reactions

In 25% of patients, adverse drug reactions include some local or systemic complaint such as local soreness, erythema, low-grade fever, malaise, fatigue, headache, nausea or arthralgia.

CHRONIC LIVER FAILURE

In chronic active hepatitis, ***corticosteroids*** and ***azathioprine*** can significantly alter the course and prognosis of the disease.

Dosage

Therapy starts with ***prednisolone*** 20 mg three times a day. This dose is decreased following improvement in conditions, either clinically or biochemically. Maintenance dose is 10 to 15 mg daily.

Azathioprine is used when corticosteroids are contraindicated, for example, in diabetes mellitus or when prednisolone alone is not adequate. Dosage starts at 25 to 50 mg daily with a gradual increase to approximately 100 mg per day, provided there are no adverse effects.

Adverse Drug Reactions

There is a possibility of an increase in jaundice and development of hepatic coma. Adverse drug reactions of corticosteroids and nursing implications are discussed in Chapter 11.

Vitamin K_1 (phytomenadione) should be given daily (10 mg) if there is a prolonged prothrombin time.

CHRONIC PERSISTENT HEPATITIS

This disease usually resolves spontaneously. Corticosteroids or azathioprine have no place in the therapy. Diet does not need to be restricted.

CIRRHOSIS

Cirrhosis cannot be reversed, nor can the progression of the disease be arrested. Therapy can only alleviate the symptoms and hence improve the general health of the patient. The main aims of treatment are to control the sequelae of cirrhosis, namely, chronic cholestasis, ascites, oedema, bleeding oesophageal varices, hepatic encephalopathy and malnutrition.

NUTRITION

It is imperative that patients with alcoholic cirrhosis avoid alcohol intake. This may in itself produce an improvement in condition. They should be given a high-protein, nutritious diet which usually negates the need for supplementary vitamins. If however there is evidence of hypoprothrombinaemia, Vitamin K_1 (phytomenadione) should be given (10 mg) daily.

CHRONIC CHOLESTASIS

Prednisolone seems to be effective in lowering serum bilirubin levels although the mechanism is unclear. Prednisolone can be given for refractory cases but only for a short course, for example, 20 to 40 mg daily for 10 to 14 days.

The main symptom of cholestasis requiring treatment is pruritus, probably due to bile acids. Anion binding resins such as ***cholestyramine*** (*Questran*), 4 to 16 g per day, bind the bile acids in the intestine and increase their excretion in the stool. The powder is mixed in fruit juice before being taken. Since it can bind other drugs in the gut and decrease their absorption, it is important that other drugs be given one hour before or three hours after the cholestyramine. Following the therapy, pruritus will usually disappear within a week.

Malabsorption of fat-soluble vitamins and calcium and steatorrhoea can be associated with cholestasis. Decreasing fat intake will alleviate the steatorrhoea. Vitamins A, D and K should be given by injection or water-soluble analogues of them should be taken orally. Calcium supplements also need to be given.

OEDEMA AND ASCITES

Dietary sodium needs to be restricted to 1 to 2 g per day, even if hyponatraemia is present. The hyponatraemia is dilutional and paradoxically is treated by fluid and sodium restriction. Fluid intake should be approximately 1.5 litres daily, irrespective of whether diuretics are being administered concurrently. In ascites the aim is to produce a slow and gradual diuresis of approximately 0.5 kg weight per day.

In cirrhosis there is nearly always secondary hyperaldosteronism present. ***Spironolactone*** is the diuretic of choice because of its aldosterone antagonistic effect. It is potassium sparing which is important since hypokalaemia may precipitate encephalopathy. Dosage used is 50 to 200 mg daily.

Adverse Drug Reactions

Adverse drugs reactions include gynaecomastia (disappears on withdrawal), breast soreness, amenorrhoea, decreased libido and impotence. If the above measures do not produce a diuresis, frusemide (*Lasix*) may be added (80 to 160 mg daily). Serum electrolyte levels need to be checked regularly.

Salt-poor human albumin (25 g IV over three hours) produces a diuresis when ascites is associated with severe hypoalbuminaemia. However it often is not effective.

BLEEDING OESOPHAGEAL VARICES

Vasopressin (20 U IV in 150 mL 5% dextrose over 15 minutes) will decrease portal pressure causing stasis of the blood. This therapy can be given again in three to four hours; however, effectiveness decreases on repeated dosage.

Adverse Drug Reactions

Abdominal colic, nausea and coronary artery constriction are some of the important adverse drug reactions.

HEPATIC ENCEPHALOPATHY

Treatment is aimed at reducing blood ammonia concentration. Firstly, all dietary protein must be stopped. The diet should be high in carbohydrate and calories. Bowel flora needs to be reduced since intestinal bacteria produce ammonia. ***Oral neomycin*** (0.5 to 1 g every six hours) is given with ***lactulose*** (orally 10 to 45 mL three times a day) to produce two to three soft-formed bowel movements per day. Lactulose works by increasing catharsis, acidifying the colonic contents and hence decreasing reabsorption of ammonia.

Hepatic encephalopathy can be precipitated by many factors including excessive diuretic therapy and subsequent hypokalaemia, high doses of potent analgesics, sedatives and hypnotics (due to increased sensitivity to CNS depression), and oral ammonium compounds. Examples of oral ammonium compounds include *ammonia and ipecacuanha mixture* and *ammonium chloride mixture.*

USE OF DRUGS IN LIVER DISEASE

Because the liver is the major organ of drug metabolism, it follows that in liver disease the pharmacology and pharmacokinetics of many drugs will be altered. When drugs are used in patients with liver disease, it is important to know how these drugs are eliminated from the body and whether they need to undergo hepatic biotransformation.

There are a number of classes of drugs which can cause problems in patients with liver disease, either because of altered response to these drugs or because they are directly hepatotoxic. Because of this, it is important to evaluate the benefits against the risks to the patients of using the drugs. As a general rule it is better to choose drugs which are eliminated renally, have no potential hepatotoxicity and have no sedative effect on the central nervous system.

The normal response to the following classes of drugs may be affected if used in liver disease: benzodiazepines, barbiturates, narcotics and analgesics, corticosteroids (particularly prednisone), some antibiotics, oral anticoagulants, anticonvulsants and lignocaine.

SELF-EVALUATION TEST

1. What steps would you take to aid patient acceptance of taking *De-Nol*?
2. Antacids act by:
   (a) reducing acid secretion;
   (b) neutralising acid secretions;
   (c) forming a protective coating on the ulcer;
   (d) forming a gel with stomach contents.
3. Which side effect is not associated with anticholinergic drugs?
   (a) tachycardia
   (b) bradycardia
   (c) constipation
   (d) urine retention.
4. Cimetidine is indicated for:
   (a) stress hyperacidity
   (b) gastric ulcer
   (c) duodenal ulcer
   (d) all of the above.
5. Saline laxatives depend for their action on:
   (a) fluid retention in the bowel;
   (b) irritation of bowel wall;
   (c) lubrication of bowel wall;
   (d) growth of bowel bacteria.
6. Diphenoxylate is used to treat diarrhoea because it:
   (a) has an analgesic effect on gripe pain;
   (b) absorbs excess fluid in the bowel;
   (c) has an astringent effect on the bowel;
   (d) reduces bowel motility.
7. Anthelmintic drugs are used to treat:
   (a) gastric flatulence in infants;
   (b) constipation in all age groups;
   (c) parasitic worm infestation in humans;
   (d) monilial diarrhoea during antibiotic therapy.
8. Nystatin (oral drops) used in the treatment of thrush:
   (a) has a systemic effect after absorption;
   (b) is better absorbed if given after food;
   (c) has a local effect after topical application;
   (d) is less effective if given after food.

Table 105
Drugs Used in the Alimentary System

Drug Group	Drug Name	Use	Action	Adverse Reactions	Nursing Implications
Antacids	Aluminium hydroxide Magnesium hydroxide Magnesium carbonate Magnesium trisilicate Calcium carbonate	Gastric and duodenal ulcers	Neutralisation of acid secretion, ease ulcer pain, ulcer healing effect in high doses	Aluminium salts: constipation; magnesium salts: diarrhoea; long-term therapy with antacids causes phosphate depletion; calcium carbonate: constipation, renal stones and failure; antacids interfere with absorption of other drugs	***Assess:*** presence of renal insufficiency, diarrhoea or constipation, presence of oedema or hypertension, concurrent use of other drugs such as tetracyclines. ***Administer:*** as ordered, usually after meals and at bedtime, and more frequently if required. ***Evaluate:*** effectiveness of preparation, presence of diarrhoea or constipation. ***Teach:*** current dosage regime; warn against over-medication with sodium bicarbonate and that some preparations advertised for "upset stomachs" contain aspirin.
Anticholinergics	Atropine Belladonna compounds Glycopyrronium Bromide Hyoscine Penthienate Propantheline	Peptic ulcers, reduce GIT motility	Inhibition of vagal nerve activity, which reduces acid secretion	Dry mouth, blurred vision, dilated pupils, tachycardia, constipation, urinary hesitancy, dizziness, mental confusion, impotence, see Chapter 5	***Assess:*** for signs of glaucoma, enlarged prostate, oesophageal reflux, hiatus hernia; ascertain whether currently taking other atropine-like drugs such as tricyclic antidepressants or antihistamines. ***Administer:*** as prescribed — usually up to one hour before meals and at bedtimes. ***Evaluate:*** response to drug, bowel function, urinary output, visual function, mental state, pulse rate. ***Teach:*** advise patient that blurring of vision and drowsiness may occur and therefore driving a car or operating machinery may be dangerous.

continued

Drug Group	Drug Name	Use	Action	Adverse Reactions	Nursing Implications
Liquorice derivatives	Carbenoxolone	Promotion of ulcer healing	Anti-inflammatory, stimulates mucin production	Fluid retention, oedema, hypertension, hypokalaemia, heartburn, headache, nausea	***Assess:*** for presence of hypertension, or tendency to oedema, concomitant use of other drugs (e.g. spironolactone, anticholinergics). ***Administer:*** gastric ulcer — as prescribed after meals and with milk if heartburn occurs; duodenal ulcer — give 15 to 30 minutes before meals. ***Evaluate:*** for signs of oedema, elevated blood pressure, signs of hypokalaemia (weakness, muscle cramps). ***Teach:*** correct administration procedure and to report development of oedema.
H_2 receptor antagonists	Cimetidine Ranitidine	Promotion of ulcer healing, Zollinger-Ellison syndrome	Block action of histamine on H_2 receptors, thereby diminishing acid secretion	Cimetidine: headache, diarrhoea, dizziness, muscle pain, rash, raised serum creatinine, gynaecomastia; ranitidine: rash, pruritus, diarrhoea, flatulence, tiredness, lethargy	***Assess:*** renal function; if lactating. ***Administer:*** tablets — as ordered; IV injection: cimetidine — 200 mg diluted to 20 mL with normal saline; continuous infusion rate should not exceed 75 mg/h during 24 h; ranitidine (more potent than cimetidine) — 50 mg diluted to 20 mL normal saline by slow IV injection; intermittent IV infusion — 25 mg for 2 h at 6 to 8 h intervals. ***Evaluate:*** pulse rate and blood pressure during IV administration. ***Teach:*** correct dosage regime and to report any adverse reactions which may occur.

Bismuth compounds	Tripotassium dicitrato bismuthate (TDB)	Gastric and duodenal ulcer	Combines with proteins at ulcer site to form a protective layer	Blackening of stools	***Assess:*** for presence or history of renal insufficiency. ***Administer:*** 5 mL plus 15 mL of water four times a day half an hour before meals and two hours after last meal. ***Evaluate:*** patient's tolerance to odour of drug, effectiveness of therapy and incidence of blackened stools. ***Teach:*** specific dosage regime, to avoid antacids and milk during treatment.
Miscellaneous	Sucralfate	Gastric and duodenal ulcer	Combines with protein at ulcer site to form protective layer, blocks back-diffusion of gastric acid, inhibits action of pepsin and bile	Constipation, headache, urticaria, nausea, diarrhoea, gastric discomfort, indigestion, dry mouth, rash, pruritus, back pain, dizziness, vertigo, sedation	***Assess:*** for signs of renal insufficiency. ***Administer:*** 1 g three times a day, one hour before meals and 1 g at bedtime; antacids may be given only within half an hour before or after sucralfate intake. ***Evaluate:*** bowel function and side effects. ***Teach:*** correct administration procedure and that drug must be taken on an empty stomach; advise that constipation may occur and to report to doctor if this becomes a problem

continued

Drug Group	Drug Name	Use	Action	Adverse Reactions	Nursing Implications
Saline laxatives	Magnesium sulphate Sodium sulphate Sodium phosphate Potassium phosphate Sodium citrate	Constipation, preoperative bowel evacuation	Attract water, soften faeces, increase bulk	Diarrhoea, electrolyte imbalance	***Assess:*** for presence of nausea, vomiting, abdominal pain, possibility of intestinal obstruction or perforated bowel as all laxatives are contraindicated in these situations; assess hydration and electrolyte status; sodium restriction (saline laxatives), anticoagulant therapy (lubricant laxatives). ***Administer:*** so that the drug's onset and peak of action occurs at a convenient time and not during the night; give bulk laxatives with a large glass of water; avoid giving bisacodyl tablets with mild or antacids as this could cause premature dissolution of enteric coating, leading to nausea and vomiting. ***Evaluate:*** for required effect of drug and record appropriately; for signs of intestinal obstruction (bulk laxatives); for signs of electrolyte imbalance (especially saline laxatives). ***Teach:*** about normal bowel function and how to prevent constipation with correct diet, fluids and exercise; that the continual use of drugs to relieve constipation can lead to the ''lazy bowel syndrome''; advise approximate time the

					laxative effect of the drug will occur; advise to seek medical advice if constipation remains a problem or if the laxative is not effective
Stimulant laxatives	Senna Cascara Castor oil Bisacodyl Danthron	Constipation	Irritation of intestinal mucosa and stimulation of peristalsis	Nausea, diarrhoea, cramping, habituation	
Bulk laxatives	Methylcellulose Ispaghula Sterculia Bran	Constipation	Absorb water and swell causing reflex peristalsis	Diarrhoea, cramping, habituation	
Lubricant laxatives	Glycerin Liquid paraffin	Constipation	Lubricate intestinal wall and soften faeces	Cramps, diarrhoea, interfere with absorption of fat soluble vitamins and other drugs, anal leakage of oil, lipid pneumonia, habituation	
Surface-active laxatives	Dioctyl sodium sulphosuccinate	Constipation	Detergent-like effect on faecal mass allowing penetration of water and fats, thus softening faeces	Anorexia, vomiting, habituation	
Miscellaneous	Lactulose	Constipation	Lactulose is broken down in colon into organic acids which cause mild irritation and promote peristalsis	Cramps, diarrhoea, nausea, vomiting	

continued

Drug Group	Drug Name	Use	Action	Adverse Reactions	Nursing Implications
Absorbents	Kaolin Aluminium hydroxide Ceratonia	Diarrhoea	Absorb toxins	Constipation	***Assess:*** possible cause of diarrhoea. ***Administer:*** absorbents — frequently as required and after each bowel action until diarrhoea ceases; antimotility drugs — as per ordered dosage schedule. ***Evaluate:*** response to drug; record stool chart; observe for atropine-like side effects with diphenoxylate. ***Teach:*** correct dosage regime and advise patients taking opium derivatives and antimotility drugs such as diphenoxylate to avoid excessive dosage.
Antimotility drugs	Codeine phosphate Diphenoxylate Loperamide	Diarrhoea	Suppression of intestinal motility	Overdose: nausea, vomiting, constipation, respiratory depression; codeine phosphate is habituating	
Phenothiazines	Prochlorperazine Perphenazine Thiethylperazine Chlorpromazine	Nausea, vomiting	Acts on chemoreceptor trigger zone	Extrapyramidal effects, sedation; see Chapter 28	***Assess:*** for known hypersensitivity to drug, liver function, blood pressure, concurrent use of other CNS depressants, including alcohol and over-the-counter cough and cold remedies and antacids (the latter interfere with the absorption of phenothiazines). ***Administer:*** as ordered; avoid spilling injectable solutions on

					skin. ***Evaluate:*** for signs of extrapyramidal side effects and hypotension (especially after injected doses), signs of skin irritation at injection sites, and body temperature. ***Teach:*** advise use of sunscreening agent if necessary and to avoid concurrent use of other CNS depressants and that the sedating effect of the drug could make driving a car or operating machinery dangerous
Antihistamines	Dimenhydrinate Cyclizine Meclosine Promethazine	Nausea, vomiting	Acts on CNS vomiting centre	Sedation, dizziness, anticholinergic effects; see Chapter 20	Note that some antihistamines belong in the phenothiazine group. ***Assess:*** for known hypersensitivity, blood pressure, concurrent use of other anticholinergic-like drugs and CNS depressants. ***Administer:*** as ordered. ***Evaluate:*** for drowsiness, anticholinergic side effects, hypotension (the latter especially after IV injection). ***Teach:*** warn that drowsiness and dry mouth may occur; advise of potential dangers when driving and operating machinery and the potentiating of sedative effect by other drugs.
Anticholinergics	Hyoscine Dicyclomine	Nausea, vomiting	Acts on CNS vomiting centre and central cholinergic pathways	Dry mouth, blurred vision, urinary retention, constipation; see Chapter 5	As for anticholinergic drugs — see this chapter

Drug Group	Drug Name	Use	Action	Adverse Reactions	Nursing Implications
Miscellanous	Metoclopramide	Nausea, vomiting	Enhances GIT motility and gastric emptying	Dystonia, drowsiness	***Assess:*** for concurrent use of other atropine-like drugs or phenothiazines. ***Administer:*** 10 mg eight hourly, oral IM or IV as ordered, usually 15 to 30 minutes before meals. ***Evaluate:*** for signs of extrapyramidal side effects, drowsiness. ***Teach:*** to take 15 to 30 minutes before meals.
Anthelmintics	Mebendazole	Roundworm, threadworm, hookworm, whipworm	Inhibition of metabolism in parasite	Mild diarrhoea, abdominal pain	***Assess:*** ability of patient to understand hygiene principles to prevent re-infection; presence of constipation; age and weight of patient. ***Administer:*** as per recommended dosage regimen for drug prescribed; therapeutic dose is usually calculated according to body weight; give laxative if indicated. ***Evaluate:*** record if and when bowel action occurs; note presence of helminths; observe for side effects of drug. ***Teach:*** principles of hygiene to prevent re-infection; correct dosage and date to take follow-up dose.
	Niclosamide	Tapeworm	Causes disintegration of parasite	Colic, diarrhoea	
	Piperazine	Threadworm, roundworm	Paralysis of worms	Nausea, vomiting, urticaria	

	Pyrantel	Threadworm, roundworm	Paralysis of worms	Nausea, vomiting, urticaria	
	Thiabendazole	Roundworm, threadworm, hookworm, whipworm	Inhibition of metabolism in parasite	Anorexia, nausea, vomiting, epigastric distress, vertigo, rash, pruritus, diarrhoea, headache, fatigue, hypotension, bradycardia	
Alginate and antacid	Gaviscon	Gastric reflux suppression	Neutralises excess acid and protects oesophagus from acid irritation if reflux occurs	No major adverse effects; high sugar content may cause dental decay	***Assess:*** for presence of diabetes mellitus. ***Administer:*** as prescribed. ***Evaluate:*** for relief of symptoms. ***Teach:*** to rinse mouth well after each dose to avoid risk of dental decay.
Sulphonamides	Sulphasalazine	Ulcerative colitis	Sulphasalazine breaks down in gut to sulphonamide and salicylate; action is probably anti-inflammatory	Nausea, vomiting, anorexia, rash, Stevens-Johnson syndrome, giddiness, headache, blood dyscrasias, drug fever, cyanosis, neurotoxicity	***Assess:*** for previous hypersensitivity to sulphonamides and salicylates, pregnancy, lactation. ***Administer:*** with food or following meals, as prescribed at equal intervals. ***Evaluate:*** for drug effectiveness, adverse effects, renal function (proteinuria, haematuria, adequate urinary output). ***Teach:*** correct method or administration; that urine colour might turn orange, importance of adequate fluid intake and to recognize indications of adverse effects.

32
ENTERAL FEEDING

Nita Whipp and Joy B. Hobbes

OBJECTIVES

At the conclusion of this chapter, the student should be able to discuss:

1. how to recognise the malnourished patient;
2. the role of enteral feeding in nutrition;
3. when to introduce enteral feeding as a nutritional support;
4. how to reduce the incidence of side effects due to enteral feeding;
5. some of the products available in Great Britain for tube feeding;
6. the relationship between "normal feeding", enteral feeding and parenteral feeding.

PREREQUISITE KNOWLEDGE

1. Principles of nutrition as they apply to health and disease states.
2. Physiology of the gastrointestinal tract.
3. Physical properties of solutions, for example, osmosis, isotonicity, molarity, molality.
4. Parenteral feeding.
5. Basic theory of drug absorption.

DEFINITIONS

Aspiration — the act of withdrawal by suction of fluids or gas from any of the cavities of the body.
Catabolism — the breaking-down of tissues so that the constituents of living matter are reduced to waste material and are eliminated from the body (applies to catabolic diseases which cause wasting).
Enteral — by the intestinal route.
Enteral feeding — nutritional support via the gastrointestinal tract.
Gastrostomy — the establishment by abdominal operation of a communication between the interior of the stomach and the skin surface for tube feeding in patients who are unable to swallow.
Hypoproteinaemia — a condition in which there is an abnormally

reduced quantity of protein in the plasma, such as occurs in nephrosis, hepatic dysfunction or as the result of too little protein in the diet.
Hypovolaemia — a condition in which the blood volume in the body is diminished.
Jejunostomy — the establishment of an opening into the jejunum through the wall of the abdomen.
Parenteral — introduced intravenously or by any route other than by way of the digestive tract.

Enteral feeding refers to nutritional support by feeding via the gastrointestinal tract. It may be supplementary to normal eating, or the total nutritional needs of the patient may be provided by a special feeding. The feeding may be taken orally or administered by tube. If the gastrointestinal tract is functional, enteral feeding is the easiest, cheapest and safest way of administering nutritional support.

If it is necessary to substitute feeding by nasogastric tube or parenteral feeding for normal meals, it is important to understand the psychological deprivation experienced by the patient. The importance of the regime should be fully explained to the patient whenever this is possible, and the patient should be encouraged to take an interest in the treatment and the monitoring of results.

All patients need the understanding and support of the health-care team with respect to their nutrition. A team effort involving the doctor, nurses, dietitian, pharmacist and biochemist is essential to achieve a satisfactory outcome. The nurse has a vital role in offering psychological support to the patient.

REQUIREMENTS FOR NUTRIENTS

The nutrient requirements of healthy individuals vary over a wide range, and the requirements of any one individual vary over time under different conditions. Tables of dietary allowances take this variation into account, and the levels suggested are believed to meet the needs of "practically all healthy persons". It is recognised that a small number of healthy people may have needs in excess of the standard. For this reason, dietary allowances are meant to be used as a guide for the feeding of groups of healthy people. When they are used as a guide for individuals, it is important to realise their limitations.

The ***DHSS report by the Committee on Medical Aspects of Food Policy*** has established a guide which is set out in Table 106: Recommended Daily Amounts of Food Energy and some Nutrients for Population Groups in the UK, and in Table 107: Recommended Daily Amounts of Food Energy and Protein for Infants (1979). If the nutrients listed in the Allowances are checked against the nutrients contained in various enteral and parenteral feedings, it will be found that allowances are not suggested for many of the nutrients present in the feedings. The Committee explains the reason for this as follows:

If the nutrients specified in daily allowances are provided by a mixed diet, it is unlikely that such a diet would be deficient in the other essential nutrients such as manganese, magnesium and copper. Some of these nutrients are referred to as trace elements or microtrace elements because they occur in our food and in our body in minute quantities. However, they are essential for normal body function.

It is when we consume a diet made up of a narrow range of foods that we are at risk of developing nutritional deficiences. Some of the early attempts at enteral and parenteral feeding encountered problems relating to deficiencies of these trace elements, and great care is now devoted to formulation and the monitoring of the patient's nutrient levels.

NUTRITIONAL NEEDS OF PATIENTS

In recent years there have been a number of reports of iatrogenic (treatment-induced) malnutrition or "hospital" malnutrition, that is, malnutrition which has developed while the patient was undergoing hospital treatment. The nurse has a vital role in the early identification of such malnutrition.

Disease alters nutritional needs and it may alter the ability of patients to digest, absorb or metabolise nutrients, or it may alter the mechanisms of excretion. Each patient should be monitored to provide appropriate nutritional assessment and to draw attention to the need for nutritional support as soon as possible. Symptoms associated with malnutrition are:

loss of weight
reduced muscle mass
hypoproteinaemia
oedema
increased susceptibility to infection
poor wound healing
apathy.

Some patients are particularly at risk of developing malnutrition. For example the unconscious patient, patients with swallowing disorders or malabsorption, patients suffering severe shock or trauma, patients suffering from psychological disorders such as anorexia nervosa and severe depression or patients suffering from severe anorexia which may result from disease or from therapy. Also patients suffering from cancer and some post-operative patients. In these cases nutritional support should be given routinely and early.

The routine recording of height and weight on admission and the regular monitoring of weight are essential. Diminution in muscle mass, apathy and depression are indicators which should be heeded as symptoms often associated with malnutrition. Food intake should be monitored and patients who are consistently unable to consume an adequate diet should be given individual attention. Supplementary oral feeding introduced at this stage may give sufficient support.

Correct nourishment of the surgical patient is advantageous because postoperative recovery is enhanced, postoperative morbidity is reduced, wound healing is accelerated, and the patient is discharged from hospital earlier as a result.

Age range[a] years	Occupational category	Energy[b] MJ	Energy[b] Kcal	Protein[d] g	Thiamin mg	Riboflavin mg[1]	Nicotinic acid equivalents mg[f]	Total folate[g] µg	Ascorbic acid mg	Vitamin A retinol equivalents µg[h]	Vitamin D[i] cholecalciferol µg	Calcium mg	Iron mg
Boys													
under 1		(c)	(c)	(e)	0.3	0.4	5	50	20	450	7.5	600	6
1		5.0	1200	30	0.5	0.6	7	100	20	300	10	600	7
2		5.75	1400	35	0.6	0.7	8	100	20	300	10	600	7
3–4		6.5	1560	39	0.6	0.8	9	100	20	300	10	600	8
5–6		7.25	1740	43	0.7	0.9	10	200	20	300	(i)	600	10
7–8		8.25	1980	49	0.8	1.0	11	200	20	400	(i)	600	10
9–11		9.5	2280	57	0.9	1.2	14	200	25	575	(i)	700	12
12–14		11.0	2640	66	1.1	1.4	16	300	25	725	(i)	700	12
15–17		12.0	2880	72	1.2	1.7	19	300	30	750	(i)	600	12
Girls													
under 1		(c)	(c)	(e)	0.3	0.4	5	50	20	450	7.5	600	6
1		4.5	1100	27	0.4	0.6	7	100	20	300	10	600	7
2		5.5	1300	32	0.5	0.7	8	100	20	300	10	600	7
3–4		6.25	1500	37	0.6	0.8	9	100	20	300	10	600	8
5–6		7.0	1680	42	0.7	0.9	10	200	20	300	(i)	600	10
7–8		8.0	1900	47	0.8	1.0	11	200	20	400	(i)	600	10
9–11		8.5	2050	51	0.8	1.2	14	300	25	575	(i)	700	12[k]
12–14		9.0	2150	53	0.9	1.4	16	300	25	725	(i)	700	12[k]
15–17		9.0	2150	53	0.9	1.7	19	300	30	750	(i)	600	12[k]
Men													
18–34	Sedentary	10.5	2510	63	1.0	1.6	18	300	30	750	(i)	500	10
	Moderately active	12.0	2900	72	1.2	1.6	18	300	30	750	(i)	500	10
	Very active	14.0	3350	84	1.3	1.6	18	300	30	750	(i)	500	10
34–64	Sedentary	10.0	2400	60	1.0	1.6	18	300	30	750	(i)	500	10
	Moderately active	11.5	2750	69	1.1	1.6	18	300	30	750	(i)	500	10
	Very active	14.0	3350	84	1.3	1.6	18	300	30	750	(i)	500	10
65–74 }	Assuming a	10.0	2400	60	1.0	1.6	18	300	30	750	(i)	500	10
75+ }	sedentary life	9.0	2150	54	0.9	1.6	18	300	30	750	(i)	500	10
Women													
18–54	Most occupations	9.0	2150	54	0.9	1.3	15	300	30	750	(i)	500	12[k]
	Very active	10.5	2500	62	1.0	1.3	15	300	30	750		500	12[k]
55–74 }	Assuming a	8.0	1900	47	0.8	1.3	15	300	30	750	(i)	500	10
75+ }	sedentary life	7.0	1680	42	0.7	1.3	15	300	30	750	(i)	500	10
Pregnancy		10.0	2400	60	1.0	1.6	18	500	60	750	10	1200[j]	13
Lactation		11.5	2750	69	1.1	1.8	21	400	60	1200	10	1200	15

(a) Since the recommendations are average amounts, the figures for each age range represent the amounts recommended at the middle of the range. Within each age range, younger children will need less, and older children more, than the amount recommended.
(b) Megajoules (10^6 joules). Calculated from the relation 1 kilocalorie = 4.184 kilojoules, that is to say, 1 megajoule = 240 kilocalories.
(c) See Table 107.
(d) Recommended amounts have been calculated as 10% of the recommendations for energy.
(e) See Table 107.
(f) 1 nicotinic acid equivalent = 1 mg available nicotinic acid or 60 mg tryptophan.
(g) No information is available about requirements of children for folate. Graded amounts are recommended between the figure shown for infants under 1 year, which is based upon the average folate content of mature human milk, and the 300 mg daily which is suggested for adults.
(h) 1 retinol equivalent = 1 µg retinol or 6 µg β-carotene or 12 µg other biologically active carotenoids.
(i) No dietary sources may be necessary for children and adults who are sufficiently exposed to sunlight, but during the winter children and adolescents should receive 10 µg (400 i.u.) daily by supplementation. Adults with inadequate exposure to sunlight, for example those who are housebound, may also need a supplement of 10 µg daily.
(j) For the third trimester only.
(k) This intake may not be sufficient for 10% of girls and women with large menstrual losses

Table 107
Recommended Daily Amounts (RDA) for Food Energy and Protein for Infants

Age range (months)	Body weight (kg)		RDA food energy (mean)				RDA protein (g)	
	Boys	Girls	MJ Boys	MJ Girls	kcal Boys	kcal Girls	Boys	Girls
0–3	4.6	4.4	2.2	2.1	530	500	13	12.5
3–6	7.1	6.6	3.0	2.8	720	670	18	17
6–9	8.8	8.2	3.7	3.4	880	810	22	20
9–12	9.8	9.0	4.1	3.8	980	910	24.5	23

More sophisticated physical measurements such as skinfold thickness and mid-arm circumference may be used, and biochemical and haematological tests such as prothombin time, levels of vitamins in body tissues, serum albumin, serum calcium and phosphorus, haemoglobin levels and red-cell counts may be used, but attention to weight and food intake are more likely to provide an early warning.

NUTRITIONAL SUPPORT

The decision to introduce enteral or parenteral feeding will depend upon gastrointestinal function, the degree of malnutrition and the patient's willingness to take food. If gastrointestinal function is efficient and malnutrition not extreme, enteral feeding is indicated and is the preferred method. If there is gastrointestinal failure, severe acute pancreatitis or vomiting or extreme malnutrition, parenteral feeding is indicated. ***Parenteral feeding*** may gradually be replaced by enteral feeding which in turn is replaced by normal feeding.

Enteral feeding is easier to administer, cheaper, less likely to introduce infection, more readily available and more flexible than parenteral feeding. It is relatively easy to regulate the amount of feeding administered by a given time. If the patient is able to eat normal foods, he or she should be encouraged to do so, and detailed attention should be given to planning the meals and to the food intake. The food consumed should be monitored, and the intake of nutrients calculated and compared with estimated requirements. This should be done by the dietitian. Enteral feeding may be administered orally or by tube.

Even though complications following enteral therapy are few, there are several dangers which should be noted.

1. ***Dehydration*** due to administration of hyperosmolar feeds.
2. ***Accidental intravenous administration*** of a tube feed due to hooking up the tube-feed containers to an IV giving set.
3. ***Microbial contamination*** of the feed during preparation and setting up in the ward. Correct storage conditions must be maintained at ward level to minimise bacterial contamination.
4. ***Tissue perforation*** in children.

Table 108
Alternative Methods of Enteral Feeding

1. Oral feeding
   - total nutritional requirements supplied by liquid feedings
   - sip feeding supplementary to normal food
   - other supplementary feedings
2. Tube feeding
   - nasogastric
   - gastrostomy
   - jejunostomy

If the feeding is taken by mouth, special attention must be given to flavour, consistency, the frequency of administration and amount given, as well as to the nutrients. It is important to watch for signs of "taste fatigue" which refers to the change in attitude to a flavour after a period of time. It may be necessary to vary flavours in order to encourage patients to continue with the treatment.

The sip feeding is taken in small quantities by the patient every 10 to 15 minutes over a prolonged period. This avoids gastric overload and is a simple method of administering a supplementary feeding. This method also reduces the likelihood of diarrhoea. Gastrostomy and jejunostomy feedings make up only a small percentage of enteral feedings. Gastrostomy may be used for patients with severe oesophageal obstruction. Jejunostomy is indicated in the presence of pyloric obstruction, upper gastrointestinal enterocutaneous fistulae and postoperatively when surgery involves the stomach and pylorus.

ENTERAL FEEDING

The factors to be considered with nasogastric feeding are:

method of administration
nutritional adequacy and content of feeding
water and electrolyte balance
osmolar load
possible complications
selecting the feeding.

Method of Administration

The thin, fine bore plastic tube with an internal diameter of 1 mm is the preferred method for nasogastric feeding. The feeding is best administered by slow, continuous drip. If necessary, the fine-bore tube can be left *in situ* for several weeks. It is important to select a feeding of a suitable consistency to flow through the tube. Previously the thick bore Ryle's tube or the double lumen tube were used. These were uncomfortable for the patient, and they were frequently associated with nasopharyngeal ulceration and gastro-oesophageal reflux and sometimes stricture. The feeding was usually administered by the bolus method when a given amount of feeding was syringed into the tube at set intervals.

Nutritional Adequacy

It would be expected that the average requirement of patients on enteral feeding would exceed the daily allowances suggested for healthy individuals (Tables 106 and 107).

Table 109 shows the range of protein and energy requirements for different patients. In addition, there is a need for vitamins, minerals, essential fatty acids, electrolytes and water.

The form in which nutrients are included in the feeding, (for example, protein such as casein or as dipeptides, tripeptides or amino acids) will depend upon the needs of patients.

Table 109
Guide to Protein and Energy Requirements

Patient	Protein (g)	Energy kJ	Calories
Medical patient (uncomplicated)	45-75	6300-8400	1500-2000
Surgical patient (uncomplicated)	75-125	8400-14 700	2000-3500
Hypercatabolic state (e.g. major burns)	125-300	14 700-21 000	3500-5000

Elemental diets are sometimes used for enteral feeding. In these feedings the nutrients occur in simple forms which can be absorbed without further digestion. In these diets, protein was supplied as amino acids, carbohydrate as glucose and fats as fatty acids. However, it is now realised that there is some advantage in supplying protein as dipeptides or tripeptides (two or three amino acids linked together), the carbohydrate as polymers of glucose and the fat as medium-chain triglycerides (MCT) which are relatively water soluble and can pass into the portal tract.

Elemental feedings are expensive because of the processing involved.

Water and Electrolytes

Many patients are hypovolaemic when enteral feeding begins, and they require sufficient fluid to restore normal blood volume. Potassium is concentrated in the intracellular fluids, and as tissues are restored, potassium needs increase. As protein requirements increase, potassium requirements increase. Sodium is concentrated in the intercellular fluids. H.A. Lee's suggested requirements are listed in Table 110.

Table 110
Water and Electrolyte Requirements

	per kg body weight
Water (mL)	30-45
Sodium (mmol)	0.9-1.2
Potassium (mmol)	0.7-0.9

(*After H. A. Lee*)

It is important that sufficient water be given to control the osmolarity of the feeding and to facilitate renal function. The more protein administered, the more water will be required. Pyrexia increases water losses, and each 1° elevation in body temperature increases daily water requirements by 500 to 750 mL.

Osmolar Load

The terms ***osmolarity*** and ***osmolality*** refer to the number of osmotically active particles in a given amount of solution. Osmolarity is the number of osmotically active particles in 1 litre of solution. Osmolality is the number of osmotically active particles in 1 kg of solution.

The contents of the gut are rendered isotonic (the same osmolality) with the body fluids in the duodenum, and they remain isotonic during the various stages of digestion and absorption. An osmolality of 300 mOsm/kg is isotonic. If the gut contents have a higher osmolarity than the body fluids, water and electrolytes will be transferred across the mucosa of the gut until a balance is achieved. If nutrients such as glucose are unabsorbed and remain in the gut, water is absorbed into the colon and diarrhoea results.

The osmolarity of a feeding is important because it affects the amount of fluid drawn from the tissue into the gut and therefore the transit time of food through the gut and the absorption of nutrients. If large amounts of water are drawn into the gut and diarrhoea results, the food passes through the gastrointestinal tract more rapidly, and there is insufficient time to absorb nutrients. Water and electrolytes as well as other nutrients will be depleted.

It is important to choose a feeding of low osmolality. Problems with diarrhoea and absorption are lessened if an isotonic mixture is introduced and administered using a slow continuous drip and small hourly volume. The volume of feed per hour is increased slowly. Dilute mixtures should be avoided as they do not provide sufficient nutrients.

Feeding carbohydrate as polymers of glucose and protein as dipeptides and tripeptides (rather than feeding glucose or sucrose and amino acids) reduces osmolarity by reducing the number of particles.

Lactose (sugar of milk) intolerance may also cause diarrhoea in patients with lactase deficiency. This is discussed later in the text.

Possible Complications

Nasopharyngeal ulceration and gastric erosion may occur, particularly if inflexible, wide bore tubes are used. In the severely debilitated, elderly or comatosed patient, aspiration may occur. However, diarrhoea is the most common complication, and it can be largely avoided by attention to the components of the feeding and its administration.

Diarrhoea can be caused by administration of bolus feeds, concurrent administration of antibiotics, lactase deficiency, or rapid gastric-emptying time after surgery or from drugs such as metoclopramide.

It should be remembered that digestion and absorption are impaired in malnourished patients. Deficiencies of enzymes in the gastric mucosa are common. For example, lactose (sugar of milk) intolerance is common because of the deficiency of the enzyme lactase. Milk-based foods and feedings are unsuitable for lactase deficient patients.

Selecting the Feeding

Feedings should be selected with close attention to the individual needs of the patient. If the need for nutritional support is recognised early, it may be possible to nourish the patient with small normal meals and milk-based nutritional supplements, taken orally between meals. It is always desirable to maintain the patient's normal meals if possible.

There are a number of commercial feeds available which have been prepared with special attention to nutritional needs, electrolytes and consistency. Details of these are given in Tables 111, 112, 113, 114, 115 and 116.

Table 111 shows a comparison of *Clinifeed ISO, Clinifeed Favour, Clinifeed 400, Ensure, Ensure Powder, Enteral 400, Fortison Standard, Isocal* and *Nutrauxil.* Table 112 shows feeds available when there is an increase in metabolic requirements.

Tables 113 and 114 give details of MCT based feeds and peptide based feeds.

Table 115 gives details of *Elemental 028, Flexical, Vivonex High Nitrogen* and *Vivonex Standard,* which are elemental feeds. They supply nutrients in a readily absorbable form and are useful for nourishing patients with gastrointestinal problems (for example, lack of enzymes due to surgery), so avoiding the use of the more expensive method of total parenteral nutrition.

Table 116 gives details of miscellaneous feeds.

Feedings are available in powdered and liquid form. Particular attention should be given to the conditions under which feedings are prepared and stored to avoid bacterial contamination. Feedings should be stored under refrigeration but brought to room temperature before they are administered.

Monitoring

The aim of the treatment should always be to restore the nutritional status of the patient and to return the patient to normal eating as speedily as possible. The following measures are useful in monitoring the efficacy of treatment, as noted by H.A. Lee:

daily weight
urine volume
stool frequency, consistency and volume
serum and urine osmolarities
blood glucose
haemoglobin and packed cell volume
serum electrolytes and blood urea
serum albumin.

Table 111
"Normal" metabolic requirements

Parameters	Clinifeed ISO	Clinifeed Favour	Clinifeed 400	Ensure	Ensure Powder	Enteral 400	Fortison Standard	Isocal	Nutrauxil
Protein source	Milk/whey	Casein/soya	Milk/whey	Casein/soya protein isolate	Casein/soya protein isolate	Whey	Casein	Soy/casein	Casein/soya
Protein formulation	Whole	Whole	Whole	Whole	Whole	Whole	Whole	Whole	Whole
Gluten free	√	√	√	√	√	√	√	√	√
Fat source	Veg. oil, butter fat	Maize oil, MCT, soya oil	Egg yolk, maize oil, soya oil	Corn oil	Corn oil	Arachis oil MCT oil	Corn, palm and coconut oils	Soy oil MCT oil	Sunflower oil
Fat formulation	NS	NS	NS	NS	NS	25% MCT	NS	20% MCT	13% MCT
Carbohydrate formulation	80% Malto-dextrin 14% Lactose	80% Malto-dextrin 15% Glucose	70% Malto-dextrin 17% Lactose	Corn starch Sucrose	Corn starch Sucrose	Maltodextrin	Maltodextrin	Glucose syrup Solids	Oligo-, poly-saccharides
Lactose free	X	√	X	√	√	Low	Trace	√	√
Pack	Can	Can	Can	Can and bottle (large can)	Can	Box	Bottle	Can	Bottle
Pack size	375 mL	375 mL	375 mL	237 mL (946 mL)	400 g	86 g	500 mL	250 mL	500 mL
'2000 cals.' Packs needed	5 cans	5 cans	5 cans	8 cans 8 bottles (2 cans)	1 can	5 boxes	4 bottles	8 cans	4 bottles
Protein g	52 (11%)	70 (14%)	75 (15%)	70 (14%)	70 (14%)	57 (11%)	80 (16%)	64 (13%)	76 (15%)
Fat g	77 (37%)	62 (30%)	67 (30%)	70 (32%)	70 (32%)	78 (35%)	80 (36%)	84 (37%)	68 (30%)
CHO g	245 (52%)	262 (56%)	275 (55%)	275 (55%)	275 (55%)	287 (57%)	240 (48%)	252 (50%)	276 (55%)
Sodium mmol	28	57	36	70	70	53	70	44	66
Potassium mmol	72	53	62	76	76	60	76	64	64
Calories	1875	1875	2000	2000	2000	2000	2000	2020	2000
Final volume	1875 mL	1875 mL	2000 mL	1900 mL	1900 mL	2000 mL	2000 mL	2000 mL	2000 mL
Osmolarity (mOsm/L)	270	335	255 (undil. 346)	380	380	330	260	NS	NS
Osmolality (mOsm/kg)	NS	NS	NS	NS	NS	NS	300	300	350
'ACBS' listed	√	√	√	√	√	√	√	√	√
Flavours	Vanilla	Neutral	Vanilla	237 mL can in Vanilla, Coffee, Egg Nog. Bottle and large can in Vanilla	Vanilla	Enteral Flavour: Chicken & Herb, Savoury Tomato, Orange & Nougat, Butterscotch, all at extra cost.	Vanilla	Unflavoured	Vanilla

Table 112
Increased Metabolic Requirements

Parameters	Ensure Plus	Fortison Energy Plus	Clinifeed Protein Rich	Stressnutril	Twocal HN
Protein source	Casein/soya protein isolate	Casein	Milk/whey/ casein	See formulation	Casein/soya protein isolate
Protein formulation	Whole	Whole	Whole	Oligopeptides Amino acids	Whole
Gluten free	√	√	√	NS	√
Fat source	Corn oil	Corn, palm and coconut oils	Soya oil	NS	Corn oil, coconut oil
Fat formulation	NS	NS	NS	78% MCT	NS
Carbohydrate formulation	Corn starch Sucrose	Maltodextrin	56% Maltodextrin 28% Sucrose	Poly- and disaccharides	Corn syrup Sucrose
Lactose free	√	Trace	X	NS	√
Pack	Can	Bottle	Can	Packet	Can
Pack size	237 mL	500 mL	375 mL	91 g	237 mL
'2000 cals.' packs needed	6 cans	3 bottles	4 cans	5 packets	4 cans
Protein g	78 (15%)	75 (13%)	120 (24%)	80 (16%)	80 (17%)
Fat g	76 (32%)	98 (39%)	44 (20%)	NS (34%)	86 (40%)
CHO g	284 (53%)	269 (48%)	280 (56%)	NS (50%)	206 (43%)
Sodium mmol	70	53	51	90	44
Potassium mmol	85	57	86	65	56
Calories	2130	2250	2000	2000	1900
Final volume	1400 mL	1500 mL	2000 mL	2000 mL	950 mL
Osmolarity (mOsm/L)	460	320	399 (undil. 562)	'Hyperosmolar'	NS
Osmolality (mOsm/kg)	NS	410	NS	NS	NS
'ACBS' Listed	√	√	√	√	X
Flavours	Vanilla	Vanilla	Vanilla	'Flavouring added' — NS	Vanilla

Table 113
MCT Based Feeds

Parameters	Hipernutril MCT	MCT Enteral 400	Osmolite	Salvimulsin MCT	Triosorbon
Protein source	Casein/ lactalbumin	Whey	Casein/soya protein isolates	Casein/ lactalbumin	Whey/casein
Protein formulation	Whole	Whole	Whole	Whole	Whole
Gluten free	√	√	√	√	√
Fat source	NS	MCT Monoglycerides	MCT, corn oil, soya oil	50% soya bean oil, 50% MCT	MCT Sunflower oil
Fat formulation	75% MCT	NS	50% MCT	50% MCT	80% MCT
Carbohydrate formulation	Di- and poly-saccharides	NS	Glucose polymers	Maltodextrin	Oligo- and polysaccharides
Lactose free	√	Trace	√	Trace	Trace
Pack	Packet	Box	Can	Bottle	Foil sachet
Pack size	90 g	86 g	237 mL (946 mL)	500 mL	85 g
'2000 cals.' Packs needed	5 packets	5 boxes	8 cans (2 cans)	4 bottles	5 sachets
Protein g	96 (20%)	57 (11%)	70 (14%)	96 (19%)	81 (16%)
Fat g	NS (30%)	NS	73 (31%)	60 (27%)	81 (36%)
CHO g	NS (50%)	NS	274 (55%)	270 (54%)	238 (48%)
Sodium mmol	89	NS	45	80	85
Potassium mmol	89	NS	49	60	85
Calories	2000	2000	2000	2000	2000
Final volume	2000 mL	2000 mL	1900 mL	2000 mL	2000 mL
Osmolarity mOsm/L	350	NS	250	300	215
Osmolality mOsm/kg	NS	NS	NS	NS	NS
'ACBS' listed	X	√	X	X	√
Flavours	'Flavouring added' — NS	NS	Unflavoured	Neutral Chocolate Nut vanilla	Neutral

Table 114
Peptide Based Feeds

Parameters	Nutranel	Pepdite 2+	MCT Pepdite 2+	Peptisorbon	Salvipeptid
Protein source	Hydrolysate of whey	Hydrolysed meat & soya protein	Hydrolysed meat & soya protein	Hydrolysate of lactalbumin	Hydrolysed lactalbumin
Protein formulation	80-85% peptides 15-20% amino acids	Peptides	Peptides	80% oligopeptides 20% amino acids	65% oligopeptides 25% amino acids 10% polypeptides
Gluten free	√	√	√	√	√
Fat source	Corn Oil MCT Oil	Coconut, Animal fat. Groundnut oil	Coconut oil Linoleic acid	MCT Sunflower oil	Soya bean oil
Fat formulation	50% MCT	35% MCT	83% MCT	60% MCT	NS
Carbohydrate formulation	Maltodextrin	Maltodextrin	Maltodextrin	Maltodextrin	Maltodextrin
Lactose free	Low	√	√	√	Low
Pack	Tin	Sachet	Sachet	Foil sachet	Sachet
Pack size	101 g	100 g	100 g	83.3 g	128.5 g
'2000 cals.' Packs needed	5 tins	4 sachets	4 sachets	6 sachets	4 sachets
Protein g	80 (16%)	56 (12%)	56 (12%)	81 (18%)	67 (13%)
Fat g	20 (9%)	72 (35%)	75 (37%)	26 (12%)	24 (11%)
CHO g	372 (75%)	252 (53%)	250 (51%)	350 (70%)	380 (76%)
Sodium mmol	40	37	54	120	120
Potassium mmol	72	52	52	60	60
Calories	2000	1800	1840	2000	2000
Final volume	2000 mL	2000 mL	2000 mL	2000 mL	2000 mL
Osmolarity mOsm/L	410	NS	NS	400	450
Osmolality mOsm/kg	480	288	360	NS	NS
'ACBS' listed	√	√	√	X	X
Flavours	Neutral	Neutral 10 g vanilla and strawberry flavour sachets	Neutral 10 g vanilla and strawberry flavour sachets	Neutral	Peppermint

Table 115
Elemental Feeds

Parameters	Elemental 028	Flexical	Vivonex High Nitrogen	Vivonex Standard
Protein source	Amino acids	Hydrolysed casein	Amino acids	Amino acids
Protein formulation	Amino acids	Peptides Amino acids	Amino acids	Amino acids
Gluten free	√	√	√	√
Fat source	Arachis oil	Soy oil MCT	Purified sunflower oil	Purified sunflower oil
Fat formulation	NS	NS	80% as triglyceride of linoleic acid	80% as triglyceride of linoleic acid
Carbohydrate formulation	Maltodextrin	Glucose solids tapioca starch	Glucose solids	Glucose solids
Lactose free	√	√	√	√
Pack	Box	Can	Sachet	Sachet
Pack size	100 g	454 g	80 g	80 g
'2000 cals.' Packs needed	5 boxes	1 can	7 sachets	7 sachets
Protein g	50 (10%)	45 (9%)	88 (18%)	36 (8%)
Fat g	33 (15%)	68 (30%)	2 (1%)	3 (1.5%)
CHO g	389 (78%)	304 (61%)	570 (81%)	483 (90.5%)
Sodium mmol	54	30	70	78
Potassium mmol	60	64	37	63
Calories	2000	2006	2100	2100
Final volume	2000 mL	2000 mL	2100 mL	2100 mL
Osmolarity mOsm/L	600	NS	800	550
Osmolarity mOsm/kg	720* and 450**	550	NS	NS
'ACBS' listed	√	√	√	√
Flavours	*Orange and **unflavoured 10 g flavour sachets — vanilla and strawberry	Unflavoured	Unflavoured Flavour sachets — orange, tomato, strawberry, beef broth	Unflavoured Flavour sachets — orange, tomato, strawberry, beef broth

Table 116
Miscellaneous

Parameters	Enrich	Fortison Low Sodium	Fortison Soya	Hepatonutril	Nefronutril Plus
Protein source	Casein/soy protein isolate	Casein	Soy protein isolate	See formulation	See formulation
Protein formulation	Whole	Whole	Whole	Oligopeptides Amino acids	Oligopeptides 80% amino acids
Gluten free	√	√	√	NS	NS
Fat source	Corn oil	Corn, palm and coconut oils	Corn, palm and coconut oils	NS	NS
Fat formulation	NS	NS	NS	75% MCT	75% MCT
Carbohydrate formulation	Corn syrup, sucrose, soya polysaccharides	Maltodextrin	Maltodextrin	Poly-, di-, and monosaccharides	Di- and polysaccharides
Lactose free	√	Trace	√	NS	NS
Pack	Can	Bottle	Bottle	Packet	Packet
Pack size	237 mL	500 mL	500 mL	98 g	91 g
'2000 cals.' Packs needed	8 cans	4 bottles	4 bottles	5 packets	5 packets
Protein g	75 (14%)	80 (16%)	80 (16%)	60 (12%)	50 (10%)
Fat g	70 (31%)	80 (36%)	80 (36%)	NS (15%)	NS (17%)
CHO g	306 (55%)	240 (48%)	240 (48%)	NS (72%)	NS (74%)
Sodium mmol	70	22	70	19	'Low electrolyte'
Potassium mmol	76	76	76	38	'Low electrolyte'
Calories	2080	2000	2000	2000	1900
Final volume	1900 mL	2000 mL	2000 mL	2000 mL	2000 mL
Osmolarity mOsm/L	NS	220	260	799	590
Osmolality mOsm/kg	NS	260	300	NS	NS
'ACBS' listed	X	√	√	X	X
Flavours	Vanilla	Vanilla	Vanilla	NS	'Flavouring added' — NS

NURSING IMPLICATIONS

Assessment

Before the patient commences an enteral feeding programme, the nurse should establish baseline documentation of height and weight, current nutritional state and fluid and electrolyte status. Before preparing to administer the feeding, the nurse should check the type and amount of feeding to be given, and the rate and frequency of administration.

Administration

This is usually done by a slow continuous drip, using a fine-bore intragastric tube. When preparing and setting up, avoid contamination of the feed, and avoid accidentally connecting the feed to an IV line. Check that the feed is administered via the correct enteral administration set and that the container is not left suspended for long periods as bacterial contamination of the line could occur.

Evaluation

Keep a careful record of fluid intake and output. Monitor weight three times weekly. Check the rate of administration during feeding. Observe for signs of delayed gastric emptying such as nausea, vomiting, regurgitation, distension. Monitor carefully for signs of hyperglycaemia, glucosuria, dehydration and diarrhoea, and report if these occur.

Teaching

Explain the feeding regime to the patient, and where possible, encourage the patient to take an active interest in the treatment and progress.

SELF-EVALUATION TEST

1. Explain the reason for emphasis on the osmolality of enteral feedings.
2. What are three indications for enteral feeding which would be routinely recorded by the nursing staff?
3. What are the advantages of commercial feedings?
4. How would you define an elemental feed?
5. What are three causes of diarrhoea in patients receiving enteral feeding?
6. Explain the difference between bolus feeding and continuous drip feeding.

(Tables 111-116 are adapted from tables produced by the British Dietetic Association and circulated with its product information booklet ADviser. Reproduced in this publication by kind permission of Blackpool, Wyre and Fylde Health Authority and the British Dietetic Association.)

33
A NURSE'S GUIDE TO PARENTERAL NUTRITION

Melvyn R. Davis

OBJECTIVES

This chapter is intended to provide a basic orientation to the principles of nutritional support and particularly to foster an understanding of parenteral nutrition (PN). It does not seek to provide detailed descriptions of nursing procedures involved in the care of patients receiving PN; monographs referred to in the text adequately satisfy this need. By presenting a sample parenteral-nutrition protocol as an appendix, it provides the student with the opportunity to observe the practical application of much of the theory discussed here.

At the end of this chapter the reader should be able to:

1. identify nutritional requirements for patients receiving parenteral nutrition;
2. assess the value of energy sources in kiloJoules;
3. list which trace elements may become deficient after several weeks of total parenteral nutrition;
4. describe the use of amino acids in parenteral nutrition;
5. list the nursing implications of the use of parenteral nutrition.

PREREQUISITE KNOWLEDGE

1. Comprehension of human physiology.
2. Knowledge of biochemical principles.
3. An appreciation of the factors involved in sepsis.
4. The means of avoiding sepsis.

DEFINITIONS

Parenteral nutrition — the administration of all or a portion of a patient's nutritional requirements by the venous route.

Total parenteral nutrition (TPN) — the administration of all nutrients by the venous route.
Hyperalimentation, parenteral hyperalimentation — formerly used to described the technique now referred to as TPN. The term "hyperalimentation" is infrequently used today to describe the administration of nutrients considerably in excess of the normal oral intake.
Assisted, partial or supplementary parenteral nutrition — the use of intravenous feeding to supplement a patient's oral food intake.
Peripheral parenteral nutrition — the administration of nutrients through a peripheral vein, a practice popular in countries where fat emulsions can be cheaply employed as a source of energy. The solutions used must approach iso-osmolarity to prevent venous irritation or destruction.
Enteral nutrition — an alternative to parenteral nutrition for patients whose alimentary tract is intact and who can be fed by nutrient solutions introduced by drinking, sipping or by a nasogastric tube.
Osmolarity — a term used to describe the strength of solutions. It describes the number of particles present in solution which determines *osmotic pressure.* The unit of osmotic pressure is the *osmole* and the values are expressed in *milliosmoles* (mOsm) per litre: Blood plasma has an osmolarity of 282 mOsm/L.
Isosmolar — a solution having an osmolarity equal to or approaching that of blood plasma, for example, sodium chloride 0.9% in water.
Hyperosmolar — a solution having an osmolarity greater than that of blood plasma, for example, 20% dextrose injection.
Isotonic and hypertonic — for the purpose of this discussion, isotonic and hypertonic solutions may be regarded, respectively, as isosmolar and hyperosmolar solutions (see above).
Anabolic — a state in which the patient is in positive nitrogen balance and protein synthesis is taking place. This is a desirable situation in PN.
Catabolic — the patient is in negative nitrogen balance and his muscle mass is being consumed to manufacture glucose in a process called gluconeogenesis.
Hypercatabolic — a state of profound catabolism.

Parenteral nutrition may be employed to metabolically support patients who cannot eat, who cannot eat enough, who should not eat, who will not eat and those whose nutritional needs are greater than can be provided by a normal diet.

The technique of administering total nutritional requirements of an individual through a catheter introduced into the superior vena cava was first described by Doctors Stanley Dudrick and Douglas Wilmore at the University of Pennsylvania in 1968. These workers used the term "parenteral hyperalimentation" to describe their method, which differed markedly from some of the earlier European techniques of intravenous feeding.

Dudrick and Wilmore's hyperalimentation consisted of administering a precisely formulated solution of hypertonic glucose, protein hydrolysate, vitamins and minerals in such a manner that the totality of the patient's nutritional needs were satisfied even though oral intake had ceased. They were successful in developing a life-saving technique which, in the space of sixteen years, has become widely employed throughout the western world. With the increasing use of parenteral nutrition in the home (HPN), this method of supporting patients who would otherwise starve is becoming commonplace.

THE BODY'S RESPONSE TO STARVATION

The human body, even in a state of little or no activity, constantly expends energy in order to maintain essential life processes, for example, brain function, cardiac activity, respiration and so on. It uses ingested food or nutrients from a normal diet to provide this energy. In the starving state, these processes continue and the body's demands for energy to maintain them also continues. In this case, the only energy sources are the body's own stores of glycogen (normally depleted in about 24 to 48 hours), its fat (adipose tissue) and muscle mass (protein).

BRIEF STARVATION (0-72 HOURS)

Within about forty-eight hours of a patient's inability to maintain adequate nutritional intake, he enters a period of brief starvation. The two major components of diet, an energy source (carbohydrate) and protein are no longer available, so the body begins to adjust to the deficiency of carbohydrate intake by increased gluconeogenesis. This is a process in which protein obtained from the breakdown of skeletal muscle are converted in the liver to glucose; the brain becomes the principal recipient of this glucose.

Protein loss is accompanied by rapid urinary nitrogen loss, and it is not uncommon for the body to lose up to 15 to 20 g of nitrogen in the urine over a 24 hour period of starvation. Since there is 1 g of nitrogen in every 6.25 g of protein, something in the order of 100 g (6.25 x 17) of protein will therefore have been lost from skeletal muscle during this period. Had 100 g of carbohydrate (glucose, for example) been provided as an energy source over the 24 hours, loss of nitrogen could have been reduced to between 2 to 5 g. The ability of carbohydrate to "spare" (reduce the loss of) protein during starvation is extremely important and is one of the principles upon which parenteral nutrition is based.

During the gluconeogenic process, a small amount of the body's fat mass will be broken down into its constituent parts, glycerol and free fatty acids. These components are transported to the liver where they will be converted into ketone bodies for use as an additional fuel source. Thus during a brief period of starvation, the major energy source comes from the breakdown of protein while only a small percentage of the needed energy is obtained from the degradation of body fat.

PROLONGED STARVATION (GREATER THAN 72 HOURS)

As the duration of starvation continues, the muscle mass is further degraded to liberate its constituent amino acids which will be converted by the liver into glucose as a source of energy. However the labile fat mass of the body's adipose tissue now becomes the major source of fuel. Ketones become the most significant substrate for the brain's activity. Serum ketones become elevated as an indication of the conversion from protein-based metabolism to fat as a source of energy. Loss of urinary nitrogen is substantially reduced to approximately 10 to 12 g every twenty-four hours as the body strives to conserve its protein. If intervention to arrest or reverse this process does not occur, death will ultimately ensue.

BASIC NUTRITIONAL REQUIREMENTS

The body functions and heals optimally when supplied with the correct type and amount of nutrients. It is not enough only to meet some of the body's nutritional needs; it demands an adequate and balanced supply of all of its requirements—the seven basic nutrients.

Seven substances or groups of substances are essential for maintenance of a normal physiological state, and these occur in the regular diet. Other substances are of less importance but may have to be considered in the long term (see Table 117).

Table 117
Basic Nutritional Requirements

Item	Examples
Carbohydrate	Potatoes, sugar (sucrose)
Protein	Meat, eggs, soya beans
Fat	Butter, cream
Water	
Vitamins	A, B_1, B_2, C, D and so on
Electrolytes	Na, K, Mg, chloride, phosphate and so on
Trace Elements	Zinc, copper, manganese and so on

NUTRIENTS IN DETAIL

CARBOHYDRATES

In the process of metabolising or transforming food into usable chemical units, some energy is generated and absorbed. Energy is now measured in ***Joules***, where formerly the ***Calorie*** was employed; 1,000 Joules are equivalent to 239 calories, so 1,000 kiloJoules are equivalent to 239 Calories (kilocalories).

Carbohydrates such as starch and the sugars are our principal sources of energy. They yield approximately 17 kiloJoules per gram.

FATS

The main function of fats is to supply energy, to form energy reserves and insulation, and to provide essential fatty acids. Even though they are of secondary importance to carbohydrates as an energy source, they nevertheless constitute a more efficient energy source, yielding 38 kiloJoules per gram.

PROTEINS

Proteins are important as structural components of all body cells and tissues as well as of enzymes. They are composed of subunits called peptides which are further subdivided into amino acids (methionine, lysine, histidine and so on). The 15 amino acids required for life are divided into two groups: essential and non-essential. The 10 essential amino acids cannot be synthesised by the body, while the five non-essential amino acids are manufactured by the body in amounts proportional to its requirements. Proteins are sometimes referred to as the "building blocks" of tissues. They yield approximately the same energy per gram as do the carbohydrates.

WATER

About 70% of the body mass is present as water. It is essential for all life processes and is the principal component of all body fluids.

ELECTROLYTES

Acid-base balance, fluid volume and other essential functions are regulated by the electrolytes: sodium, potassium, magnesium, calcium, acetate, chloride, sulphate and phosphate.

VITAMINS

These are not sources of energy but are essential components for the normal functioning of the body. They are required in small quantities and are sometimes referred to as "biological catalysts"—agents which have to be present for a particular reaction or process to occur.

TRACE ELEMENTS

Like vitamins, trace elements influence the structure of particular proteins or act as integral parts of enzymes. The roles played by zinc, copper, manganese, chromium and iodine are fairly well understood. Much remains to be understood about the body's requirements for less common trace elements such as molybdenum, selenium and vanadium. However, it has recently been reported that long-term selenium deficiencies may precipitate cardiomyopathy in adults and infants.

ENTERAL NUTRITION

While parenteral nutrition represents a commonly employed method of correcting nutritional deficiencies, it is not the only method. For patients whose alimentary tract is functional, the administration of appropriately formulated diets by normal oral feeding, sip feeding or feeding via fine-bore silastic nasogastric tubes, gastrostomies or jejunostomies may offer satisfactory but less potentially hazardous alternatives to parenteral feeding. The previous chapter discussed the technique in detail.

A useful reference on the subject is *Developments in Clinical Nutrition*, proceedings of a symposium held at the Royal College of Physicians, London, 20 Oct 1978, edited by I. D. A. Johnston and H.A. Lee. The publication is available from Roussel Laboratories ltd.

FIGURE 12: CRITERIA FOR SELECTION OF NUTRITIONAL THERAPY

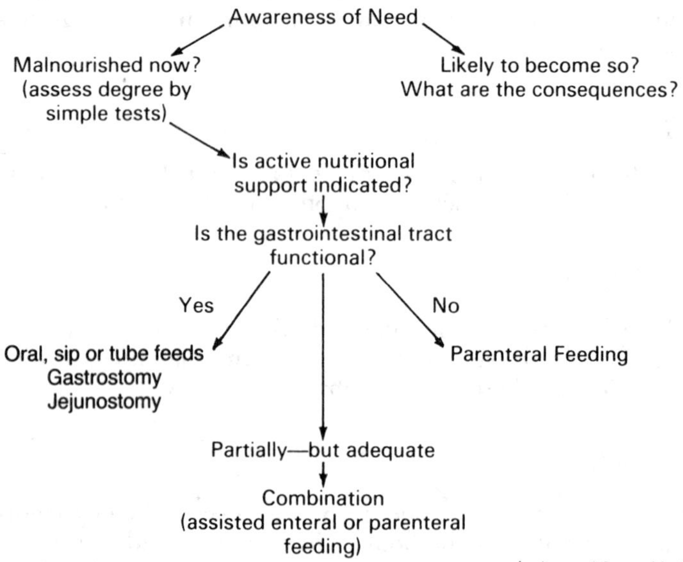

(adapted from H. A. Lee)

INDICATIONS FOR PARENTERAL NUTRITION

The indications for PN are numerous and increasing as our understanding of the nutritional needs of patients continues to grow. Table 118 includes most of the generally accepted indications for this therapy. Although not exhaustive, this does provide a guide to the large number of medical conditions in which impairment of normal nutritional processes has a significant effect upon the outcome of the disease state.

An example is the recent realisation that the nutritional status of patients is often indicative of the status of their immunity from infection. For patients facing major surgery, this is of particular importance since the extent of immune competence may ultimately determine their ability to survive the procedure.

Table 118
Indications for Parenteral Nutrition

1. Postsurgical patients, not expected to receive oral intake for seven days.
2. Debilitated patients prior to elective surgery.
3. Patients with impaired immune competence, prior to elective surgery.
4. Gastrointestinal fistulae.
5. Chronic intestinal obstruction.
6. Short bowel syndrome.
7. Inflammatory bowel disease.
8. Crohn's disease.
9. Massive burns.
10. Severe trauma.
11. As an adjunct in patients receiving cancer chemotherapy or radiotherapy.
12. Cancer of the oesophagus.
13. Cancer of the gastrointestinal tract.
14. Anorexia nervosa.
15. Acute hypercatabolic renal failure.
16. Infants with idiopathic diarrhoea or malabsorption syndrome.

METHODS OF DELIVERY OF PARENTERAL NUTRITION

Parenteral nutrition may be delivered in several different ways. There are two basic methods from which a number of variations have evolved. First, there is the administration of ***sequential*** bottles of near-isosmolar solutions into a peripheral vein; 3.5% amino acid solution and 10% dextrose may be administered in parallel with fat emulsions. Second is the ***single bottle/bag technique*** in which a strongly hyperosmolar dextrose amino-acid solution is infused via a central-venous catheter into a major vessel, usually the superior vena cava.

MULTIPLE BOTTLE TECHNIQUES

Traditionally the ***multiple-bottle peripheral approach*** has enjoyed much popularity in Europe and the United Kingdom. The need for multiple bottles has come about because the major solution components (dextrose, amino acids or fat emulsions) are unstable when mixed together prior to heat sterilisation. European workers have relied largely on fat emulsions (for example *Intralipid*) as their primary energy source. There are certain advantages in this method, the principal of these being that fat emulsions exert little osmotic effect and can be administered safely by the peripheral route. (The validity of this method has been challenged on the basis that fat emulsions are claimed by some to be irritating to the vein even though the effect is unrelated to osmolarity.) Another advantage is the high energy content of fat emulsions; 500 mL of a 20% solution yields 4.2 megaJoules. When administered through a Y-connector in conjunction with hyperosmolar 10% dextrose injection and solutions of amino acids, the lipid dilutes the other solutions, so reducing their osmolarity to a level tolerated by a peripheral vein. Fat emulsions are freely available in Europe and the UK at moderate cost; this has much to do with the popularity of the method.

"3-in-1" FORMULATIONS

Many workers in this field now believe that the best-tolerated regimes employ both ***fat*** and ***carbohydrate*** to satisfy daily energy needs. Up to 25% of these requirements may be provided by a fat emulsion while the balance can be delivered from high-concentration glucose solutions. A recent trend is to provide the total day's nutrient requirements in a single container. These "3-in-1" formulations require the mixing of the ***fat emulsion*** with the ***glucose*** and ***amino-acid solutions*** just before use, since combining them in this manner reduces the stability of the fat emulsion quite dramatically. Further, fat emulsions are particularly sensitive to the amount of calcium and magnesium salts added to them, and these factors combine to limit the usefulness of the "3-in-1" technique.

The potential hazards associated with central-venous catheterisation required for the single bottle/bag method in the US makes the multiple bottle/peripheral method seem quite attractive, particularly in view of the fact that it carries with it a comparatively lessened risk of systemic infection. However, it does have drawbacks; outside the UK and Europe, fat emulsions may cost in the vicinity of twelve times the equivalent amount of dextrose (glucose) upon which the American method is based. Also it has been argued that the protein-sparing effects of fat are considerably less than those of amino acids and dextrose.

DEXTROSE BASED METHODS

In the United States and Australia, the ***single bottle/bag dextrose-based methods*** (as originally described by Dudrick and Wilmore) are in wide use. In the US this is understandable since fat emulsions have only recently been introduced to the market in the late 1970s. The technique involves the administration of aseptically combined admixtures of commercially prepared dextrose and amino acid solutions with the addition of electrolytes, vitamins, trace elements and other components to tailor the solutions to the patient's individual needs. These may change daily or even more frequently. Because these solutions are rich sources of nutrients, it is not surprising to find that they can support profuse growth of microorganisms, particularly yeasts and fungi. In 1971 Deeb and Natsios reported contamination rates of up to 38% in solutions prepared "at the bedside" by medical and nursing staff.

Preparation of PN Solutions

The amount of manipulation required to prepare each solution is considerable, and it is imperative that the strictest standards of asepsis be employed throughout the procedure. These conditions may be met when the solutions are prepared by pharmacists skilled in this work and employing laminar air flow equipment in which a sterile controlled environment may be maintained. Rigorous standards of cleanliness must apply. No justification exists for preparing and manipulating PN solutions anywhere but in a laminar flow cabinet.

Formula Components

Table 119 lists the basic components of a PN solution intended for adult use. Table 120 gives a typical adult formulation. The average daily requirement of the solution given in Table 120 will be three litres. The solution is strongly hyperosmolar and can only be administered through a central venous catheter. (Portal catheters and arteriovenous shunts are alternative routes, but their use is rare.) Regions of rapid blood flow are essential to dilute the solution as quickly as possible after it enters the vein. In this example, the osmolarity will be in the vicinity of 1900 mOsm/L. (Remember that plasma osmolarity is 282 mOsm/L.) One litre of this formula will yield about 3900 kiloJoules, 6.5 grams of nitrogen (6.5 × 6.25 or 40.6 grams of protein), and one litre of water.

Calculating Daily Requirements

The aim of parenteral nutrition is to supply energy in excess of the patient's basal energy expenditure rate (BEE), which can be simply calculated. In the average 70-kg male, it may be to the order of 6700 kJ which represents the minimum energy requirement to maintain metabolic processes. It does not take into account any additional energy required for exercise or exertion of any kind, nor does it allow for the elevated energy requirements associated with stress or trauma.

The required energy input under stress is to the order of 1.7 to 2.1 times the BEE (1.7 in mild to moderate stress, above 2 in severe stress), which allows an excess of energy over the minimum metabolic requirement to take part in protein synthesis. Three litres of the formula given in Table 120 will provide 11 700 kJ (3900 × 3 kJ), which is approximately 1.76 times a BEE of 6700 kiloJoules suitable for a mildly stressed patient.

Three litres of the solution will also have provided 19.5 g of nitrogen in the form of amino acids. This is equivalent to 19.5 × 6.25 or 122 g of protein. The ratio between energy and grams of nitrogen available from the solution is important for balanced nutrition and proper utilisation of the amino acids. Current opinion favours the use of solutions containing approximately 630 kJ per gram of nitrogen; the above solution closely approximates this with a ratio of 11 700 kJ to 19.5 grams of nitrogen or 600 : 1.

Electrolyte content may require adjustment from day to day in response to the patient's measured levels. Thus patients who are receiving PN must be monitored closely and constantly (see the monitoring schedule in the Appendix).

Table 119
Components of Parenteral Nutrition Solutions

1. Dextrose — as an energy source
2. Amino acid solution — as a protein source
3. Water — essential for all biochemical processes
4. Electrolytes
5. Vitamins — both water soluble and oil soluble
6. Trace elements — at least zinc (Zn) and copper (Cu)
7. Heparin — to maintain catheter patency
8. Insulin — optional; when used, promotes glucose uptake and acts as an anabolic agent apart from its effect on glucose metabolism.

Table 120
A Typical Adult Formulation

Dextrose 50% in water	500 mL
8% amino acid solution*	500 mL
Potassium	30 mmol
Sodium	35 mmol
Magnesium	2.5 mmol
Calcium	3 mmol
Chloride	37 mmol
Phosphate	15 mmol
Acetate	65 mmol
Zinc	30 micromoles
Copper	8 micromoles
Dayamin or MVI multiple vitamin injection	0.3 mL
Heparin sodium	300 Units
Soluble insulin	(optional) as indicated by the patient's blood glucose
Approximate final volume	1000 mL

* Brands of amino acid solutions in common use are *Synthamin, Aminoplex, Aminofusin* and *Vamin.*

PARENTERAL NUTRITION IN PAEDIATRICS

PN finds an increasing role in paediatric practice. Patients with surgical disease of the gastrointestinal tract, especially newborn infants, form one important group. Other patients in whom total parenteral nutrition is used are those with chronic intestinal obstruction resulting from adhesion or peritoneal sepsis, bowel fistulas, chronic severe diarrhoea, extensive body burns and abdominal tumours treated by surgery, irradiation and chemotherapy. Low birth-weight infants have also been treated with TPN and, among others, the Melbourne group headed by Professor McMahon has achieved internationally-acknowledged success since the mid-1970s. The nutritional requirements of the paediatric patient are similar in many respects to those of the adult patient, which are detailed above. However the proportions of protein and calorie intake may vary, as Tables 119 and 122 indicate. Paediatric electrolyte and mineral requirements also differ in amounts from those of adults (Table 123).

Table 121
Paediatric and Adult Protein Requirements

Condition	Infants, young children	Adults
Normal, healthy	2.4 g/kg/day	1.0-1.5 g/kg/day
After surgery	2.5-3.0 g/kg/day	1.3-1.5 g/kg/day
Infection	2.5-3.5 g/kg/day	1.5-1.8 g/kg/day
Severe sepsis	3.0-3.5 g/kg/day	1.7-2.2 g/kg/day
Burns (30% to 100% body surface area)	3.5-4.0 g/kg/day	1.8-2.7 g/kg/day

Table 122
Paediatric Energy Requirements

Age	kiloJoules/day
0-6 months	500 kJ/kg/day
6-12 months	418 kJ/kg/day
over 12 months	4180 + (418 × age in years) kJ

Table 123
Paediatric and Adult Electrolyte and Mineral Requirements

Element	Infants, young children	Adults
Sodium	3-5 mmol/kg/day	60 mmol/day or more
Potassium	3-5 mmol/kg/day	60 mmol/day or more
Chloride	same as for sodium	same as for sodium
Calcium	0.5-1 mmol/kg/day	5-10 mmol/day
Phosphorus	0.65-1.3 mmol/day	10-15 mmol/day
Magnesium	0.15-0.25 mmol/day	5-15 mmol/day

Trace element requirements are more critical in paediatric TPN than in the treatment of adults, and these differ in amounts from one group to the other. Fluid volume requirements are critical in paediatric patients and particularly so in the newborn. Fat emulsions (10% to 20%) are widely employed as energy sources because of their high yield (38 kJ/g) and their low osmolarity.

TPN in paediatrics demands a high degree of vigilance on the part of nursing and medical staff. Extensive and continuous biochemical and haematological monitoring is particularly important in the newborn and infants. The consequences of metabolic complications or a septic episode may easily be fatal in these patients; by comparison, an adult is usually more resilient and less prone to exhibit the symptoms of these events.

VENOUS ACCESS AND COMPLICATIONS

Hyperosmolar PN solutions may be delivered by two routes: ***peripheral catheters and cannulae,*** and ***central venous catheters.*** Peripheral administration requires solutions to be rendered essentially isosmolar at the point of delivery; the Y adapter method with fat emulsions makes this possible.

The administration of PN solutions containing 50% or 70% dextrose necessitates delivery through a large vessel with a high rate of blood flow. The subclavian and jugular veins have classically been utilised for this purpose. In the adult, the subclavian route is preferred. Access may be gained in two ways: direct catheterisation of the subclavian or jugular vein, or peripheral (antecubital) placement of a long central catheter. In either case, the aim is to place the catheter tip in the superior vena cava. This necessitates radiological control and for this reason, all catheter materials must be radio-opaque.

CATHETER MATERIALS

Three types of catheter are available: PVC (polvinyl chloride), PTFE (Teflon) and silicone rubber (Silastic). The silicone-rubber type is gaining in popularity because of its inert nature, its softness and flexibility, and its surface characteristics tend to impede blood clotting on the tip and formation of a fibrin sheath around the catheter, a common occurrence with the other materials.

The actual process of catheter insertion, and a description of the vital role played by the nurse during this procedure, is too detailed for this brief overview of PN. The reader is directed to an excellent account of these techniques in Ada Lawrence Plumers' book, *Principles and Practice of Intravenous Therapy,* second edition, 1975, published by Little, Brown and Company, Boston.

TECHNICAL COMPLICATIONS OF CENTRAL VENOUS CATHETERISATION

The act of gaining access to the superior vena cava is a hazardous one. Many complications can occur, including pneumothorax, hydrothorax, haemothorax and inadvertent arterial puncture. Fortunately their occurrence is infrequent. Clotting of the catheter tip is an occasional complication which may necessitate its removal.

CARE OF THE CATHETER

One of the most potent causes of complications in PN is catheter sepsis. The catheter tip presents an ideal foreign body for colonisation and once infected, must be removed ***without delay.*** There is little point in administering antibiotics to sterilise the catheter *in situ*—almost invariably this is unsuccessful.

Use of the central venous line for other than delivery of parenteral nutrition solutions (for example, administering other drugs, central venous pressure monitoring, drawing blood, and so on) should be a contraindication because it increases the probability of infection.

It took a number of years for it to be recognised that an alarmingly high incidence of catheter sepsis associated with the development of parenteral nutrition mostly had as its source the patient's own skin flora. Migration of microorganisms from the patient's skin down the outer wall of the catheter may easily occur unless a well-planned and clearly-defined programme of regular catheter entry-site dressing is maintained in a highly disciplined manner. It is no exaggeration to suggest that the nurse may hold in her hands the success or failure of TPN depending upon her attitude to this vitally important procedure.

The organism most commonly found to infect catheter tips and to be associated with PN-related fungaemias is *Candida albicans.* It is typical of the yeasts, moulds and fungi which are resistant to inhibition by these hyperosmolar solutions. Bacteria display variable ability to survive and multiply in PN fluids. Iodine is an effective agent against both fungi and bacteria and (particularly in the form of povidone-iodine) is widely and successfully used in catheter insertion and routine exitsite dressings. The dressing procedure employed by Dudrick has been found to be effective, and a method based upon this is described in detail in Plumer's *Principles and Practice of Intravenous Therapy.*

A team approach to PN has been advocated; a paper published by Freeman *et al* in 1972 claimed a reduction in catheter related sepsis from 21.2% to 2.3% following the introduction of a "TPN Team" in which a small number of team nurses dressed catheters and nursed patients according to a strict protocol. It cannot be over-emphasised that an almost obsessive approach to catheter care by the nurse is a major contribution to the PN patient's progress.

CYCLIC PARENTERAL NUTRITION

Traditionally, PN was delivered on a round-the-clock basis and, in the case of patients who are moderately to severely ill, this is generally still the case. However, another method which is gaining support is to administer PN on an intermittent or "cyclic" basis, perhaps feeding the patient over 10 to 12 sleeping hours, then disconnecting, heparinising and capping the catheter to allow the patient total mobility throughout the day. The psychological advantages to the patient of this method are obvious. Other advantages claimed are that the metabolic demands placed upon the liver by PN are significantly reduced and that the often-observed elevation of liver enzymes in PN patients will be minimised accordingly.

HOME PARENTERAL NUTRITION

Cyclic PN gives the opportunity for many patients who (apart from an inoperative gut) are fit and healthy enough to return home and be treated by home parenteral nutrition (HPN). Usually these patients receive their total nutritional requirements by the parenteral route; hence the term Home TPN is applicable.

INFUSION DEVICES

Although much of the PN administered in the UK is by gravity, the use of positive pressure volumetric infusion pumps makes the technique demonstrably safer and simpler. (These devices should not be confused with the more usual drip controllers of the type, which are not well suited for this application.) The need for accuracy in infusion rate is paramount; glycosuria is a common occurrence when drip rate variations take place. Maintaining accurate administration rates in the absence of pumps can render PN particularly time consuming for nursing staff. An infusion pump or some other automatic regulating device is essential for HPN.

REQUIREMENTS FOR SAFE ADMINISTRATION OF PARENTERAL NUTRITION

An important rule in PN is that if the infusion falls behind schedule, ***do not attempt to catch up!*** Metabolic complications are likely to occur, and glycosuria will almost certainly result. Never cease a PN infusion abruptly. Because the pancreas has adjusted its insulin output to meet the high dextrose load, a tailing off period of some hours is usually necessary to avoid risk of hypoglycaemia. If a PN infusion has to be ceased because of some unforeseen circumstance, a container of 10% dextrose should be hung in its place. (This is less of a problem now than in the former years of hyperalimentation in which energy intakes of 16 000 kiloJoules and above (per day) were not uncommon.)

COMPLICATIONS

The principal complication is ***sepsis***. In former years, sepsis rates in excess of 25% were reported. Today, in well-run programmes, the average sepsis rate is 3%. In the majority of cases, sepsis is related directly to the catheter. It has become unusual for a contaminated solution to be the primary source of infection.

Osmotic diuresis may be a complication when large volumes of hyperosmolar dextrose are administered too rapidly. Glycosuria is likely to be observed under these circumstances. Deficiency states may develop unless comprehensive monitoring is maintained. Respiratory failure may occur in critically ill patients whose respiration is impaired and who are administered excessive levels of dextrose.

Other metabolic complications include hyperosmolar non-ketotic coma, hypoglycaemia, hypophosphataemia, acid-base imbalance, electrolyte imbalance, calorie-to-nitrogen ratio imbalance, prerenal azotaemia and hyperammonaemia.

NURSING IMPLICATIONS

Many institutions have developed policies and protocols for the administration of parenteral nutrition. Nurses must be familiar with local policy, and be involved with its formulation and review. Aspects usually covered include: changing of solutions and lines, care of catheter insertion sites and dressing techniques, patient monitoring and personnel involved.

Assessment

Accurate fluid balance records must be maintained during parenteral nutrition. Other signs of fluid and electrolyte imbalances, especially fluid overload, should be carefully and frequently monitored. Urinalysis for glucose content needs to be frequent. Serum electrolytes will be measured regularly. Patient observation should be related to the complications of parenteral nutrition listed above.

Infusion pumps or regulators often will be used to maintain flow rates. Their functions and alarm signals should be checked regularly. Patency of the infusion lines is essential, so all tubing should be checked regularly for kinks, leaks, obstruction and integrity.

Since sepsis is such a potential danger, the nurse must be alert for any signs of infection that might relate to the parenteral nutrition. These include: sudden rises in core temperature; inflammation or pain at the catheter insertion site, arm or shoulder; and changes in cardiovascular, respiratory or neurological status suggestive of septic shock.

Patients receiving parenteral nutrition are often critically and/or chronically ill. The addition of multiple bottles and tubes and frequent monitoring could add significantly to the anxiety the patient and his family already feel about his or her condition. Their need and ability to understand the reasons for methods of treatment should be assessed.

Administration

Frequent checks and accurate calculation of flow rates are essential. If the infusion falls behind schedule, it must ***not*** be "caught up", but the discrepancy should be reported and documented clearly. Metabolic complications are likely to occur if the infusion is too rapid, and glycosuria will almost certainly result. Allowance should be made for changes in the patient's position, in maintaining flow rates.

Infusions should never be ceased abruptly. Because the pancreas has adjusted its output to meet the high load of kiloJoules from the dextrose, a tailing-off period of some hours is advisable to avoid the risk of hypoglycaemia. If a TPN infusion has to be ceased because of some unforeseen circumstance, a container of 10% dextrose should be hung in its place.

Lines should be changed in the same way as other central venous lines, preventing entry of air into the line. Aseptic technique must be scrupulous with regard to: handling of solution containers, giving sets and connections; changing lines and containers; and dressing catheter sites. Dressings must be kept dry. Use of transparent dressings, such as *"Opsite"*, allows for observation without disturbing the dressing.

Parenteral nutrition lines should not be used for: administration of other medications; administration of blood products; blood sampling or central venous-pressure monitoring.

Obstruction of the catheter or known or suspected contamination of the catheter necessitates its removal and insertion of a new catheter. The medical officer must be informed immediately if the site needs to be changed or if any abnormality occurs.

Total parenteral nutrition solutions should be refrigerated until needed. The pharmacy should be notified immediately if there is any change or discontinuation of an order. Due to the high cost of these solutions, waste should be minimised.

As full an explanation as is appropriate (of the reasons for and expected results of the therapy) should be provided to the patient and his or her family. Reference to parenteral nutrition as a method of "feeding", the frequency with which it is currently used, and current success rates will help to reduce anxiety about an obviously complicated form of treatment. The patient will be encouraged by information about weight gains and stability of blood chemistry.

Evaluation

Maintenance of prescribed schedules, prevention of complications, weight gain, stabilisation of blood chemistry, and anxiety reduction indicate successful therapy. Any discrepancies between goals and achievements must be thoroughly documented.

The basic rule of parenteral nutrition is:

PN is DDD — *Different* from routine IV therapy.
Demanding of nursing and medical staff.
Deadly if not managed in a responsible and skilful manner

SELF-EVALUATION TEST

1. All of the following are nutritional requirements for patients receiving PN, except:
   (a) amino acids
   (b) starches
   (c) electrolytes and minerals
   (d) vitamins
2. Select the true statement.
   (a) One gram of glucose yields approximately 17 kiloJoules.
   (b) One mL of dextrose 50% yields approximately 8.36 megaJoules.
   (c) One gram of fat yields 38 kiloJoules.
   (d) All of the above are true.
3. All of the following trace elements may become deficient after several weeks of TPN except:
   (a) zinc
   (b) copper
   (c) manganese
   (d) platinum
4. Select the false statement.
   (a) 630 non-protein kiloJoules should be administered with each gram of nitrogen.
   (b) There is one gram of nitrogen in each 6.25 grams of protein.
   (c) 42 to 64 non-protein kiloJoules per gram of protein are considered optimal for anabolism.
5. Gluconeogenesis is a natural process for conversion of fat to glucose in the pancreas.
   (a) True. (b) False.
6. Which of the following substrates produces the highest energy yield?
   (a) Protein
   (b) Fat
   (c) Glucose
7. BEE is an abbreviation for ....
8. Septic complications may be expected in . . . per cent of patients managed by a PN team.
   (a) 0%
   (b) 3%
   (c) 13%
   (d) 21.3%
9. A 19-year-old male with a 60% body surface-area burn would be expected to require approximately .... parenterally administered kiloJoules to maintain nutritional balance.
   (a) 4000 kiloJoules
   (b) 12 000 kiloJoules
   (c) 21 000 kiloJoules
   (d) 33 000 kiloJoules
10. Heparin is included in PN solutions for its anabolic effect as well as its anticoagulant properties.
    (a) True. (b) False.

Table 124
Summary — Parenteral Nutrition

Drug Group	Drug Name	Use	Action	Adverse Reactions	Nursing Implications
Total parenteral nutrition solutions	Composed of essential nutrients, e.g. dextrose, amino acids, electrolytes, trace elements, vitamins, fat	Metabolic support for patients who cannot eat, are suffering from starvation, who require "gut rest"	Nutrition	Catheter complications, sepsis, osmotic, diuresis, metabolic complications	***Assess:*** fluid balance, weight, observe for fluid overload, urinalysis for glucose, frequent serum electrolytes, signs of sepsis — temperature, inflammation, pain; cardiovascular, respiratory, neurological status; anxiety. ***Administer:*** infusion regulator; do not "catch up" slow infusions; document all discrepancies between orders and flow rates achieved; taper off, rather than cease abruptly; strict aseptic technique and care of catheter, handling solutions and lines; do not administer other medications, blood products through line, or take blood samples, or monitor central-venous pressure; inform medical officer immediately if catheter obstructs, or is contaminated; refrigerate all solutions. ***Evaluate:*** achievement of prescribed schedules, weight gain, blood chemistry, anxiety reduction. ***Teach:*** purpose and expected results of therapy to patient and family.

34
INTRAVENOUS THERAPY

Virginia E. Richardson

OBJECTIVES

At the conclusion of this chapter, the reader should be able to:

1. list the principles involved in maintenance of body fluid, electrolyte and pH balance;
2. describe the principles involved in the replacement of nutritional deficits by IV therapy;
3. appreciate the effects of surgical intervention and the disease process on fluid, electrolyte and pH balance;
4. list the hazards associated with administration of IV fluids;
5. understand the principles and problems associated with the addition of drugs to IV fluids.

PREREQUISITE KNOWLEDGE

1. An understanding of the distribution of body fluids, electrolytes and nutrients.
2. An understanding of the chemistry of acids, bases and buffer systems.
3. A knowledge of the diseases and procedures likely to cause imbalances in fluids and electrolyte levels and acid/base balance.
4. A knowledge of aseptic procedures used in administering large-volume parenteral fluids to patients.
5. A knowledge of aseptic procedures involved in addition of drugs to large-volume parenteral fluids.

INTRODUCTION

At least 50% of normal body weight is composed of body fluid (water). Body fluids are either extracellular or intracellular. Extracellular fluid may be interstitial or intravascular.

Normal homeostatic controls maintain fluid balance in the healthy individual. Certain diseases and procedures upset this balance. The balance then must be rectified. Surgical intervention, trauma, burns and fever will upset normal fluid balance as will certain diseases, for example cardiovascular disease, renal disease and certain endocrine conditions.

Under normal conditions, fluid intake and output are in dynamic balance, but any change in normal intake and output can easily upset this balance. Vomiting, diarrhoea, excessive perspiration, exudation from denuded surfaces, gastric suction and enterocutaneous fistulae can rapidly deplete body fluid. In disorders such as congestive heart disease or renal disease, fluid may be retained rather than lost, and oedema will ensue. Excessive depletion or retention of body water leads to concomitant loss or retention of electrolytes.

The major body cations are sodium, postassium, calcium and magnesium. Major anions are chloride, bicarbonate, phosphate and sulphate. Losses must be replaced and excesses depleted appropriately.

FLUID VOLUME, ACID/BASE AND ELECTROLYTE CHANGES

At first it would appear that the treatment of fluid and electrolyte imbalances might be relatively simple. Sometimes this is true, and replacement of a deficit may be easily accomplished by oral administration of water containing suitable quantities of electrolytes. More often, however, deficits must be replaced intravenously, a more complex situation sometimes further complicated by the presence of disease.

In this chapter we will examine some of the major fluid and electrolyte and acid/base imbalances which can occur and appropriate treatments will be discussed.

CHANGES IN FLUID VOLUME

Fluid volume deficit

Deficit of body fluid is caused by lack of intake, excessive losses or a combination of both. Volume deficits may occur slowly or rapidly depending on circumstances, and the resultant condition is known as dehydration or hypovolaemia.

The patient will have dry skin and mucous membranes, a wrinkled tongue, oliguria, lowered body temperature, fatigue, increased pulse and respiration rate, lowered BP and central venous pressure (CVP) and over 5% weight loss. Haemoglobin and packed cell volume may be raised.

Treatment of fluid-volume deficit is by oral or parenteral replacement of water. It must be appreciated that water alone is never lost from the body. Water loss will always be accompanied by electrolyte losses, most commonly sodium and potassium. Lost electrolytes must be replaced along with lost fluid.

Fluid volume excess

Excessive fluid volume may be caused by overload of oral or parenteral fluids, or may be the result of diseases such as congestive cardiac failure, renal failure or portal hypertension.

The patient's BP, central venous pressure (CVP) and body weight will be increased, pulmonary oedema and pleural effusion may occur and ascites may occur in the presence of liver disease. The blood urea will be elevated in cases of congestive cardiac failure or renal disease but lowered in the presence of hepatic disease. The plasma will be diluted leading to an apparent decrease in formed elements. Imbalances in electrolyte and plasma-protein levels will occur depending on the underlying cause of the fluid volume excess.

Treatment is usually accomplished by restriction of fluid intake and concomitant use of diuretic therapy.

CHANGES IN ACID/BASE BALANCE

Any change in normal blood pH is serious. Acidosis is regarded as being present when the pH of body fluids is less than 7.35. Alkalosis is regarded as being present when the pH of body fluids is above 7.45.

There are a number of buffer systems in the body which aid in maintaining normal pH. Buffer systems operate by "mopping up" excess amounts of acid or base (alkali) in the body. In the blood the most important buffer systems are the bicarbonate buffer, the haemoglobin buffer and plasma-protein buffers. There are also several urinary buffer systems, namely the bicarbonate buffer, the phosphate buffer and the ammonium buffer, which work in the same manner as the blood buffer systems.

So what is a buffer, and how does it work? A buffer is a system of weak acid, base and hydrogen ion (H^+) which acts to resist pH changes in the following way.

1. When hydrogen ions (acids) are introduced, not all these ions are allowed to remain in free form to make more acid (or lower the pH) of the solution to which they are added. Some of the added hydrogen ions will combine with (or be "mopped up" by) the base of the buffer system and so be inactivated.
2. When hydrogen ions are removed from a solution it will become more basic (alkaline) and the pH will rise. Buffers will limit the extent of pH increase because the weak acid of the buffer system dissociates and gives off hydrogen ions to replace those which have been lost.

The major blood buffer is the bicarbonate buffer system which is the body's main mechanism for adding or removing hydrogen ions from the blood. When the acid load or base load is too much for the buffer systems to handle, then acidosis or alkalosis will develop.

There are two types of acidosis and alkalosis: metabolic acidosis or metabolic alkalosis and respiratory acidosis or respiratory alkalosis. Metabolic acidosis and alkalosis are caused by metabolic disturbances, while respiratory acidosis and alkalosis are caused by respiratory dysfunction.

FIGURE 13: BLOOD BUFFER SYSTEMS

Bicarbonate	H_2CO_3 weak acid (carbonic acid)	$\rightleftharpoons$	H^+	$+ HCO_3^-$ base (bicarbonate ion)
Haemoglobin	Hb–H weak acid	$\rightleftharpoons$	H^+	$+ Hb^-$ base
Protein Buffers	Pr–COOH weak acid (carboxylic acid from protein)	$\rightleftharpoons$	H^+	$+$ Pr–COO$^-$ base (carboxylate ion)
	Pr–NH_3^+ weak acid (amino group from protein)	$\rightleftharpoons$	H^+	$+$ Pr-NH_2 base

FIGURE 14: URINE BUFFER SYSTEMS

Bicarbonate	H_2CO_3 weak acid	$\rightleftharpoons$	H^+	$+ HCO_3^-$ base
Phosphate	$H_2PO_4^-$	$\rightleftharpoons$	H^+	$+ HPO_4^{=}$
Ammonium	NH_4^+	$\rightleftharpoons$	H^+	$+ NH_3$

Metabolic Acidosis

Metabolic acidosis may be caused by renal disease (acute and chronic renal failure and renal tubular acidosis), ketoacidosis (induced by diabetes, alcoholism or starvation), lactic acidosis (secondary to circulatory and respiratory failure or from drugs and toxins), severe vomiting and diarrhoea, thyrotoxicosis and overload of intravenous saline solutions.

The characteristics of metabolic acidosis are fatigue, confusion, stupor and coma. Hyperventilation may be evident, and shock and vascular collapse can occur. Reduction of plasma bicarbonate levels, lowering of blood pH (with compensatory PCO_2 reduction) and hyperkalaemia may occur.

Treatment depends on the cause and severity of the acidosis. In cases of chronic renal failure and renal tubular acidosis, the metabolic acidosis should be corrected with bicarbonate infusions. Patients suffering from acidosis due to acute renal failure are usually adequately treated by dialysis. Diabetic ketoacidosis normally responds to insulin therapy, and only in extreme cases can the use of bicarbonate infusions be justified. Ketoacidosis secondary to alcoholism responds to infusions of dextrose and saline. Lactic acidosis requires treatment of the underlying cause.

Acidosis associated with severe vomiting and diarrhoea is usually associated with electrolyte abnormalities such as hypokalaemia and with fluid-volume depletion. Treatment is by administration of suitable intravenous fluids containing the required electrolytes.

Metabolic alkalosis

Metabolic alkalosis results from increased plasma levels of base bicarbonate. Chloride-ion depletion from vomiting, gastrointestinal suction or diuretic therapy, severe potassium depletion and excessive oral or IV alkali intake will cause a metabolic alkalosis. Alkalosis may result from hyperadrenocorticism, for example, primary aldosteronism and Cushing's syndrome.

Characteristics include apathy, confusion and stupor, slow shallow respiration, irregular pulse, cardiac dilation or decompensation and finally muscle tetany and convulsions. Plasma bicarbonate and PCO_2 are elevated. Urinary and plasma pH are elevated. Plasma potassium and sodium levels may be low and ECG abnormalities may ensue due to hypokalaemia.

The first aim of treatment is to remove the underlying cause of the alkalosis. Infusions of sodium chloride will replace lost water, sodium ions and chloride ions; administration of potassium chloride is usually required as well. In rare instances following prolonged and severe gastrointestinal losses, intravenous therapy with acidifying agents such as ammonium chloride and arginine hydrochloride may be required.

Respiratory acidosis

The basic cause is respiratory dysfunction which leads to inadequate excretion of carbon dioxide by the lungs. Respiratory dysfunction may result from pneumonia, emphysema, drug intoxication, congestive cardiac failure, bronchiectasis, pulmonary oedema, cerebral disease, neuromuscular disorders, chest trauma or airway obstruction.

Characteristics are respiratory distress, tachycardia, cyanosis, weakness and coma. Urinary and plasma pH levels are low. Plasma bicarbonate and sodium are elevated, PCO_2 is elevated and plasma chloride is low.

The mainstay of treatment is to remove the underlying cause of the acidosis. Administration of bicarbonate or lactate infusions may also be required.

Respiratory alkalosis

The basic cause of respiratory alkalosis is an increase in the rate and depth of respiration leading to excessive loss of carbon dioxide. This is known as hyperventilation and is caused by hysteria, anxiety, fever, salicylate intoxication, CNS disease, trauma, high altitudes, acute bacteraemia, lung disease and heart disease, and may occur with mechanical ventilation.

Characteristics are light-headedness, paraesthesia, tetany and ultimately convulsions and loss of consciousness. Elevated plasma and urinary pH levels are found, along with low plasma sodium and bicarbonate levels. Plasma chloride may be normal or raised. PCO_2 is low.

The basis of treatment is to remove the underlying cause. Infusions of sodium chloride may be of use. In acute cases rebreathing into a bag may help.

CHANGES IN ELECTROLYTE BALANCE

Sodium deficit (hyponatraemia)

Sodium is the major extracellular electrolyte. Loss of sodium without corresponding water loss or increased water load without an increased sodium load may cause sodium deficit, as may prolonged vomiting or gastric suction, excessive sweating, adrenal insufficiency or excessive infusions of dextrose in water.

Characteristics are anxiety, weakness, stupor, abdominal cramps, muscle twitching, convulsions, oliguria or anuria and vasomotor collapse. Plasma sodium and chloride are low, and the specific gravity of the urine is low.

Treatment is by oral or parenteral replacement of sodium and chloride ions.

Sodium excess (hypernatraemia)

This can be caused by a decrease in water intake or increased water output or an increase in sodium intake or decrease in sodium output. Repeated saline infusions, tracheobronchitis, diarrhoea and inadequate water intake will cause hypernatraemia.

Characteristics are thirst, dry mucous membranes, firm tissue turgor, oliguria, agitation, convulsions and coma. Elevated plasma sodium and chloride levels, and elevated specific gravity of the urine are characteristic.

Treatment is by infusion of fluids with low sodium content.

Potassium deficit (hypokalaemia)

Potassium is the major intracellular electrolyte in the body. Prolonged inadequate potassium intake or excessive losses of potassium-rich secretions from diarrhoea may cause potassium deficit, as may ulcerative colitis, vomiting, burns, and the use of diuretics (especially thiazides). Recovery from diabetic acidosis, starvation or low potassium diet or prolonged use of adrenocorticosteroid therapy may induce hypokalaemia. Hypokalaemia is often associated with a metabolic alkalosis.

Characteristics are muscle weakness, anorexia, malaise, gastrointestinal tract distension, absence of bowel sounds, tremor, disorientation, paraesthesia and heart block. Plasma potassium and chloride levels are low. Plasma bicarbonate is elevated. ECG abnormalities may be found.

Treatment is by oral or parenteral replacement of potassium. Oral replacement may be by high potassium foods or by oral tablets or solutions containing potassium. Potassium may be replaced parenterally by administering intravenous infusions of solutions containing potassium chloride. The administration rate of these solutions should be adjusted so that no more than 20 millimoles of potassium per hour is administered, and the total daily dose should not normally exceed 80 mmol. No more than 43 mmol of potassium should be added to one litre of IV fluid unless exceptional circumstances prevail.

Potassium chloride must ***never*** be given by bolus intravenous injection.

Potassium excess (hyperkalaemia)

This may be caused by excessive potassium intake from too rapid infusion, inadequate potassium excretion in renal failure, the release of potassium from damaged cells after burns or crushing injury, or adrenal insufficiency and overuse of potassium-sparing diuretics.

Characteristics are oliguria followed by anuria, weakness, intestinal colic and diarrhoea, hypotension and bradycardia, cardiac arrhythmias leading to ventricular fibrillation and cardiac arrest. Serum-potassium levels are elevated and ECG abnormalities may be found.

The treatment is to cease potassium intake and to administer intravenous calcium gluconate, dextrose and insulin. Oral or rectal potassium-removing resins may be administered, and dialysis may be necessary in some cases.

Calcium deficit (hypocalcaemia)

Calcium deficit may be caused by: inadequate dietary intake of calcium, metabolic abnormalities such as malabsorption states, vitamin D deficiency or hypoparathyroidism, abnormal calcium losses from diarrhoea or wound exudates, diseases such as sprue or pancreatitis and infections and excessive infusions of citrated blood.

Characteristics are muscle cramps, tingling of extremities and in severe cases, tetany and convulsions. Prolonged hypocalcaemia predisposes the patient to osteomalacia and osteoporosis. Low plasma calcium levels and ECG abnormalities are found.

Treatment is by oral or IV calcium replacement. If hypoparathyroidism is the cause, vitamin D replacements must be given along with calcium replacements.

Calcium excess (hypercalcaemia)

This may be caused by tumours, excessive vitamin D intake or hyperactivity of the parathyroid gland.

Characteristics are muscle relaxation, fractures, renal calculi. A hypercalcaemic crisis is typified by intractable vomiting leading to dehydration, stupor, azotaemia, coma and cardiac arrest. Elevated plasma calcium levels and ECG abnormalities are found.

Treatment is by control of underlying disease and promotion of calcium excretion. Excess calcium may be removed from the body by administering disodium edetate, which is a calcium chelating agent.

Magnesium deficit (hypomagnesaemia)

This is caused by chronic alcoholism, prolonged vomiting or gastric suction, diarrhoea, impaired intestinal absorption, enterostomy drainage or low dietary intake.

Characteristics are increased CNS irritability manifested by disorientation, confusion, visual hallucinations, convulsions and tachycardia. Patients will exhibit low plasma magnesium levels.

Treatment is by intravenous replacement of magnesium; 50 mmol of magnesium sulphate may be added to a solution such as 1 L of 5% glucose and given over 12–24 hours.

Magnesium excess (hypermagnesaemia)

Hypermagnesaemia is a result of excessive magnesium ingestion or failure to excrete, for example, in chronic renal insufficiency or untreated diabetic acidosis.

Characteristics are CNS depression, impaired conduction at the neuromuscular endplate, loss of deep tendon reflexes, respiratory paralysis and cardiac arrest. Elevated plasma magnesium levels and ECG abnormalities are evident.

Calcium will antagonise magnesium, so infusions rich in calcium will be helpful. In severe cases, haemodialysis may be necessary.

NUTRITIONAL DEFICIT

In addition to fluid and electrolyte losses and pH imbalance, carbohydrate and protein losses may occur. Should these eventuate, then carbohydrate and protein must be replaced either orally or by infusion.

Protein depletion

This may be caused by inadequate dietary intake, increased catabolism, stress response, wound healing, neoplastic disease, trauma, haemorrhage, burns, ulcers or debilitating disease.

Characteristics are anorexia, pallor, fatigue, breakdown of body tissue leading to weight loss, loss of muscle tone and mass and respiratory disease due to starvation. Haemoglobin and erythrocyte counts are low, along with total plasma protein and plasma albumin levels.

Oral protein replacement is desirable where possible. Intravenous infusion of essential and non-essential synthetic L-amino acids is possible where oral replacement is not feasible. In severe cases, infusions of protein solutions, hypertonic dextrose and fat may be required. These infusions must be given via a central vein, and the technique is known as total parenteral nutrition (see Chapter 33).

MAINTENANCE OF FLUID VOLUME, ACID/BASE BALANCE AND ELECTROLYTE REQUIREMENTS IN THE PATIENT

Maintenance of fluid, acid/base and electrolyte balance is important in all patients, especially in the patient undergoing surgery. Most patients undergoing routine surgery (particularly abdominal surgery) will require a period of intravenous replacement until their normal gastrointestinal function returns.

In the uncomplicated postoperative patient, routine fluid therapy is a two-phase procedure:

Phase 1 — therapy during the first 24 hours; this includes the time during which the patient undergoes surgery;

Phase 2 — maintenance therapy which is carried out during each subsequent 24-hour period of the postoperative phase.

Extracelluar fluid volume is reduced after surgery. It is postulated that during surgical procedures extracellular fluid is lost into a "third space" which is probably located around the operation site. The volume of fluid lost into the "third space" will vary according to the severity of the operation, and this volume of fluid must be replaced. Replacement of "third-space" losses is usually carried out during phase 1, using sodium and water infusions. Other losses during phase 1 are due to urinary and insensible (sweat and respiration) losses.

Phase 1 replacement of fluids and electrolytes should therefore be as follows: 2 litres to replace urine losses, 1 litre to replace insensible losses, and 1 litre (or up to 4 litres in certain circumstances) to replace losses into the "third space". The anaesthetist usually replaces "third-space" losses during the operation by administering the appropriate volume of a balanced salt solution (such as Hartmann's) at the rate of 10 to 15 mL/kg for the first hour then 10 mL/kg/hour for each subsequent hour up to four hours. Hartmann's solution contains 131 mmol sodium, 5 mmol potassium, 111 mmol chloride, 2 mmol calcium and 29 mmol lactate in each litre.

Phase 2 replacement is during subsequent twenty four-hour postoperative periods. Patients require approximately three litres of replacement fluid per day under normal circumstances (that is two litres to replace urinary losses and one litre to replace insensible losses).

In addition to sufficient fluid volume during phase 2, a 70 kg patient with no postoperative complications requires adequate daily intake of electrolytes and calories.

Table 125
Baseline Daily Requirements for a 70 kg Patient

Volume (mL)	Glucose (g)	KiloJoules	Na (mmol)	K (mmol)	Cl mmol)
3000	200	3430	150	80	230

The usual daily intake of sodium is about 100 mmol; however, post-surgical patients may develop hyponatraemia if only 100 mmol is given. Providing that renal and cardiovascular status are normal, then 150 mmol is more appropriate therapy. The normal daily loss of potassium is around 80 mmol. Provided renal function and urine output are normal, potassium replacement should be at the rate of 80 mmol daily. KiloJoules in the form of glucose (approximately 200g or 3430 kiloJoules daily) are required to prevent gluconeogenesis and subsequent development of negative nitrogen balance. KiloJoule intake may not be critically important in a previously well-nourished patient who will only be on IV therapy for a few days, but it is nevertheless good practice to administer sufficient kiloJoules in the form of glucose. In obese patients, adequate kiloJoule intake will reduce fat catabolism and prevent the release of excessive amounts of free fatty acid into the plasma.

It is common and desirable practice to administer Vitamin B complex and Vitamin C daily during IV replacement therapy to improve the patient's nutritional status and to promote tissue healing.

All surgical patients should be managed in a fashion which ensures as accurate a balance of fluids, kiloJoules and electrolytes as possible. Fluid balance charts should be maintained, and serum-electrolyte measurements should be used as a guide when ordering IV therapy. Table 126 lists the composition of some commonly used intravenous fluids.

Table 126
Composition of Some Commonly Used IV Fluids

Fluid	Volume (mL)	Glucose (g)	kJ	Na	K (millimoles)	Cl	Ca	Lactate
5% dextrose in 0.9% saline	1000	50	3430	154	—	154	—	—
Normal saline 0.9%	1000	—	—	150	—	150	—	—
Hartmann's solution (lactated Ringer's)	1000	—	—	131	5	111	2	29
0.18% sodium chloride and 4% dextrose	1000	40	686	30	—	30	—	—
0.18% sodium chloride and 4% dextrose 20 mmol KCl	1000	40	686	30	20	50	—	—
5% dextrose in water	1000	50	3430	—	—	—	—	—

As most patients will require administration of at least three litres of fluid daily in the postoperative phase, routine use of only one type of IV fluid (for example normal saline or dextrose 5% in water) will, in time, produce abnormalities in the patient's electrolyte balance. Consider the following examples.

(a) If a patient is administered three litres of normal saline per day during the postoperative phase, he or she actually receives 3000 mL fluid, 450 mmol sodium and 450 mmol chloride per day — no calories and no potassium.
(b) If a patient is given three litres of dextrose 5% in water per day, he or she will receive 3000 mL fluid, 150 g glucose, 10 290 kiloJoules, and no electrolytes.
(c) If a patient is given three litres of Hartmann's solution per day, the

result will be 3000 mL fluid, 393 mmol sodium, 15 mmol potassium, 333 mmol chloride, 6 mmol calcium and 87 mmol lactate. He or she receives no kiloJoules and an undesirable balance of electrolytes.

From these examples, it becomes obvious that no single commercially available intravenous fluid provides baseline postsurgical requirements over a three litre per day regime. Therefore we must use alternating fluids containing some additives to provide patients with adequate fluid, calories and electrolytes. A suitable regime is made up of dextrose 5% in water alternating with dextrose 5% in normal saline, as shown in Table 127.

Table 127
A Regime to Provide Daily Maintenance Therapy Using a Combination of Solutions

Fluid	Volume (mL)	Glucose (g)	kJ	Na	K (millimoles)	Cl	Ca	Lactate
5% dextrose in N/ saline + 20 mmol KCl	1000	50	858	154	20	174	—	—
5% dextrose in water + 30 mmol KCl	1000	50	858	—	30	30	—	—
5% dextrose in water + 30 mmol KCl + vitamin B complex + vitamin C	1000	50	858	—	30	30	—	—
Total in 24 hours	3000	150	2574	154	80	234	—	—
Average normal daily requirements	3000	200	3430	150	80	230	—	—

Not all patients follow an uncomplicated postoperative course. Many patients will require adjustments to the standard Phase 1 and Phase 2 replacement-therapy regimens. Some of these circumstances are listed as follows:

(a) **In renal disease,** potassium replacements should not normally be administered to patients. The amount of fluid and sodium given to these patients may have to be significantly reduced.

(b) **If the patient is dehydrated** (that is, has low tissue turgor and is hypotensive) then more than the baseline three litres in 24 hours must be given. The extra fluid volume should be administered evenly over 24 hours, and central venous pressure should be monitored.

(c) **Variations in body mass and age** – adjustments in fluid volume may be necessary in the very young or elderly and in patients who are overweight or underweight. A useful method of calculating baseline fluid volume according to age and body weight is:

- first 10-kg body weight — 150 mL/kg/day of IV fluid
- second 10-kg body weight — 50 mL/kg/day of IV fluid

- all weight above 20 kg — 20 mL/kg/day IV fluid (if younger than 50 years); 15 mL/kg/day IV fluid (if older than 50 years)

(d) **In congestive cardiac disease,** a reduction in fluid volume and quantity of sodium administered will be necessary. The CVP should be monitored to prevent fluid overload, and adequate potassium supplements should be given, especially if the patient is receiving digoxin therapy.

(e) **After abnormal losses of fluid from the gastrointestinal tract** – These losses may result from nasogastric suction, vomiting, diarrhoea, ileostomy or colostomy loss, fistulae, T-tube or jejunostomy loss. As well as replacing lost fluid, attention must be given to replacement of lost electrolytes and albumin.

(f) **In pyloric stenosis,** fluid and potassium losses result from vomiting. Care must be taken to ensure adequate fluid and potassium replacement in patients with pyloric stenosis.

HAZARDS ASSOCIATED WITH ADDING DRUGS TO INTRAVENOUS FLUID CONTAINERS

Surveys have shown that between 40% and 60% of IV fluids administered to patients have drugs added to them. The practice of adding drugs to IV fluid packs is fraught with problems, many of which are not well recognised. Broaching the container of an IV fluid may alter the identity, strength, purity, sterility and toxicity of the final product. Some of the potential hazards are listed below.

BREAKDOWN OF STERILITY

Broaching the container of IV fluid may lead to contamination of the fluid with microorganisms. Sources of microorganisms may be the environment (airborne); exposed surfaces of stoppers on IV bottles or additive vials; the skin, nasal passages or clothing of the operator. The risk of microbiological contamination is minimised by using correct aseptic technique in a controlled environment such as a laminar air flow cabinet.

PARTICULATE CONTAMINATION

Introduction of microscopic particles into an IV fluid may lead to microbiological contamination of the fluid, vein damage, thrombophlebitis or thrombus formation. Sources of particles may be: airborne dust; skin or hair shed by the operator; lint; particles of glass from ampoules; particles of rubber from IV bottles or vials or organic matter from reconstituted powdered drugs.

Good operating techniques and the use of controlled environmental conditions (laminar air flow cabinets and membrane filters) will minimise the risk of particulate contamination.

THROMBOPHLEBITIS

This may be caused by particulate contamination of the IV fluid, or more often is caused by low pH of the infusion fluid. Needle irritation and the length of time cannulae are left *in situ* may also be contributing factors. Addition of even small amounts of drugs to IV fluids may be sufficient to lower the pH of the IV fluid and hence cause thrombophlebitis.

ALTERATIONS IN DRUG AVAILABILITY

An IV fluid may be considered to be a sustained release preparation. Depending on the infusion rate, it is likely that drugs with short plasma half-lives may not reach therapeutic blood concentrations if only the usual injection dose is added to a large volume of fluid to be administered over a prolonged period. In addition, some drugs when added to infusion containers may adsorb onto the glass or plastic of the container and not be available to reach the patient's circulation and the site of action.

MEDICATION ERRORS

The procedure of adding drugs to IV fluid containers must be carefully supervised with regard to dosage calculations and labelling the final container.

DRUG INCOMPATIBILITY

There are many factors which influence the compatibility of drugs with each other and with IV fluids. Differences in buffers, preservatives, vehicles, temperatures, concentrations and even in the order of mixing may all have an effect on compatibility. Lack of visual alteration in an IV fluid after addition of a drug is insufficient proof that the drug is compatible with the IV fluid.

Incompatibilities may be broadly classified as visual or chemical.

Visual (or sometimes called physical) incompatibilities are the result of poor solubility of drugs in solution or of acid/base reactions between oppositely charged ionic species in solution. They may be typified by formation of an obvious precipitate, evidence of turbidity or cloudiness, a colour change or evolution of gas (bubbles). Some examples are diazepam injection which will form a precipitate when mixed with solutions of dextrose 5% in water, and phenytoin sodium which (in sufficient concentration) will precipitate when added to aqueous solutions.

Chemical incompatibility involves the irreversible degradation of drugs in solution to form therapeutically inactive or, occasionally, toxic compounds. These incompatibilities may or may not be visually apparent. An example is the degradation of ampicillin sodium when mixed with dextrose 5% in water and stored at room temperature for more than four hours. Many of these degradation reactions are time and temperature dependent. As in the case of many antibiotics, degradation may be slowed down by storing the reconstituted product under refrigeration.

In clinical practice, it is acceptable to administer parenteral drugs provided less than 10% inactivation has occurred.

If contemplating multiple drug products for IV fluids, consult the pharmacy *first.*

It is not within the scope of this chapter to list the known drug/drug and drug/IV-fluid incompatibilities. This would require a complete book in itself. There are a variety of texts and reference books available on this topic, and the reader is directed to these for more detailed information.

NURSING IMPLICATIONS

Assessment

The clinical features of specific fluid and electrolyte disturbances and potential causes of disturbance (such as vomiting or wound drainage) must be documented so that the patient's response to therapy can be evaluated. Patients undergoing surgery will be assessed before surgery to establish a baseline of physiological parameters. Assessment should include weight, cardiovascular and respiratory parameters, temperature and neurological status. The condition of the skin, mucous membranes and tissue turgor are useful guides to hydration.

If an arm vein or hand vein is to be cannulated, the patient will be less restricted if the non-dominant side is chosen, wherever possible.

Nurses must be familiar with local policy directing the management of intravenous therapy, with regard to: prescriptions and documentation of administration; addition of medications to infusions; checking of solutions to be administered; selection and changing of giving sets; management of cannulation sites; and nursing observations and records.

Administration

Cannulae must be secured, but the site should be able to be inspected easily. Safety and patient comfort are appropriate criteria in the selection of a method for dressing the cannula site and securing tubing.

Flow rates must be maintained according to the prescription, so frequent and regular checking is essential. Giving sets delivering small or large drops, with or without burettes, should be selected according to the patient's needs and local policy. Giving sets with burettes (delivering small drops) enable greater control of flow rate, and reduce the potential for over-infusion. Infusion pumps are used where greater control is needed. Nurses must be familiar with the operation and limitations of pump devices. The cannulation site must be inspected frequently, since pumps can deliver fluid into tissues if cannulae dislodge. The appropriate giving set must be selected for use with the pump. However, no giving set or pump makes skilled nursing management unnecessary. A "timing tape", attached to the container and showing the expected fluid level at regular intervals, is a useful aid to monitoring flow over long periods.

As general rule, infusions that are running well behind schedule should not be "caught up" quickly, because of the dangers of fluid overload. Solutions containing potassium should never be infused faster than the prescribed rate. Discrepancies between the prescribed regime and the actual delivery over a period of hours must be reported to the prescriber, so that the schedule can be adjusted if necessary.

Adjustments to flow rates may be necessary if medications are added to burettes intermittently. These medications must be delivered at the rate prescribed for them, and the primary infusion adjusted after delivery of the medication. Great care should be taken with labelling, and to avoid infusing medications too rapidly.

Flow may be reduced or stopped by a change in limb position, restrictive clothing, the cannular tip being occluded by the vessel wall, or by the cannula piercing the vessel wall, allowing fluid to leak into the tissues. Thrombus formation at the tip of the cannula or in the lumen can occlude flow. Thrombus may be aspirated from the cannula, using aseptic technique, but must *never* be irrigated into the vein, because of the danger of embolus. Air bubbles must be removed from the giving set for the same reason.

If doubt exists about the position or patency of the cannula, the fluid container can be momentarily lowered below the level of the cannula — backflow of blood into the tubing indicates that the cannula is properly positioned.

When arterial pressures are recorded with a sphygmomanometer, the cuff should not be applied to the cannulated limb, if possible. The vein will be temporarily occluded as the cuff is inflated to systolic pressure, flow will be interrupted, and the cannula may have to be replaced if it becomes dislodged.

Accurate fluid balance records must be maintained during intravenous therapy. The record usually acts as both an intake and output record, and the documentation of the administration of prescribed substances. Often the prescription is written also on the fluid balance record, and it must then be treated and filed as a legal document. Daily weight records are a reliable adjunct to the fluid balance chart.

Evaluation

The patient's response to intravenous therapy is evaluated by his clinical state, and by monitoring blood chemistry and haematological parameters. Cardiovascular and respiratory signs should be observed regularly. The urine output and specific gravity should be monitored with regard to the patient's original condition, and the volume and nature of the fluid infused. Changes in thirst, capillary filling, condition of the mucous membranes and skin turgor should be evaluated in comparison with the initial assessment.

A rise in temperature, even with no other signs of infection, may indicate catheter sepsis. Pyrogenic reactions can occur if the infusion fluid is contaminated with bacterial endotoxins. Symptoms usually occur within 30 to 60 minutes of commencing the infusion, and include a sudden rise in temperature, headache, malaise, nausea and rigors. The medical officer must be notified, and the infusion will be stopped, and the cannula removed. Infusion fluids and cannulae may be sent for microbiological examination. Pyrogenic symptoms may be treated by administration of an antipyretic drug, for example, aspirin.

The cannula site must be inspected regularly, so that the appropriate action can be taken if tissue infiltration or thrombophlebitis occur. Local infiltration is signified by a sluggish flow rate, pain and swelling around the vein. Hypertonic, acidic or basic solutions and some medications can cause tissue necrosis. Thrombophlebitis and inflammation around the cannula site result from chemical, mechanical or microbiological irritation to the vein. The signs are pain, redness and swelling. The infusion should be discontinued and the cannula resited if either of these problems occur.

Cardiovascular and respiratory status must be evaluated for signs of circulatory overload or air embolus. Circulatory overload results from infusion of excessive volumes of fluid. Symptoms are elevated venous pressure (and sometimes arterial pressure), venous distension, dyspnoea and production of frothy sputum, indicating pulmonary oedema. The medical officer must be notified, and the infusion slowed down to a rate sufficient only to maintain patency of the cannula. The cannula should not be removed, since intravenous drug treatment might be necessary.

Air embolus results from air being infused through the giving set, and a large bubble or bubbles lodging in the pulmonary circulation. Symptoms are dyspnoea, cyanosis, hypotension, tachycardia and loss of consciousness. The infusion must be stopped. Oxygen should be administered, with the patient lying on his left side, with his head down. The vital signs should be recorded, and the medical officer notified immediately.

Teaching

The reasons for the intravenous therapy, its expected duration, and the limitations it will impose on his movement and activities should be explained to the patient. He should know to report any pain at the cannula site or breathlessness. If the initial disturbance was caused by a fluid or dietary-intake problem, advice about avoiding the problem in the future will be appropriate.

SELF-EVALUATION TEST

1. All of the following are characteristics of fluid volume depletion except:
   (a) oliguria
   (b) hypotension
   (c) increased pulse rate
   (d) increased CVP
2. All of the following are components of buffer systems except:
   (a) base
   (b) strong acid
   (c) hydrogen ions
3. One of the following is an important cause of metabolic acidosis.
   (a) fever
   (b) acute renal failure

(c) diuretic therapy
(d) primary aldosteronism

4. In the condition of metabolic alkalosis, one of the following statements is true.
   (a) Hyperkalaemia is common.
   (b) ECG abnormalities may occur.
   (c) Plasma sodium levels are elevated.
   (d) Infusion of sodium bicarbonate will reverse the alkalosis.
5. Adrenal insufficiency and massive crushing injuries are both potential causes of hyperkalaemia.
   (a) True
   (b) False
6. A 29-year-old man, weighting approximately 72 kg, undergoes a routine abdominal surgical procedure with no complications. During the surgical phase and for the first 24 hours after surgery, a suitable IV fluid replacement regime would be: first 8-hour period — 1 litre Hartmann's solution; second 8-hour period — 1 litre Hartmann's solution; third 8-hour period — 1 litre normal saline containing 10 mmol potassium chloride.
   (a) True
   (b) False
7. Patients who require postsurgical IV fluid replacement therapy and who are also receiving digoxin therapy for CCF require the following adjustments to their postoperative fluid replacement regimes: less fluid volume intake than normal patients and no potassium or sodium supplements. This statement is:
   (a) True
   (b) False
8. Thrombophlebitis is likely to be caused by which (if any) of the following factors?
   (a) Contamination of an IV fluid by microscopic glass particles.
   (b) Leaving the IV cannula *in situ* for prolonged periods of time.
   (c) An infusion fluid with a low pH.
9. A patient develops malaise, nausea and a temperature of 39.5°C about 40 minutes after the commencement of an infusion of normal saline containing 25 mmol per litre of potassium chloride. The symptoms indicate one of the following.
   (a) thrombophlebitis
   (b) air embolus
   (c) hyperkalaemia
   (d) contamination of the IV fluid by bacterial endotoxin
   (e) circulatory overload
10. A drug is compatible with an intravenous fluid if upon addition of the drug to the IV fluid there is no visible change in the fluid.
    (a) True
    (b) False

SECTION 10

35

WARD DIAGNOSTIC REAGENTS

A. Paul Harding

OBJECTIVES

At the conclusion of this chapter the reader should be able to:

1. list the reasons for examination of urine and the clinical significance of results;
2. correctly perform a urine test using either a reagent strip or tablet;
3. describe the differences between qualitative and quantitative test procedures;
4. correctly handle and store reagent strips and tablets;
5. name the most common substances which may interfere with reagent tests;
6. measure specific gravity and correctly describe the appearance of normal and abnormal urines.

EXAMINATION OF URINE

THE SPECIMEN

No matter how accurate the test, the result is only as good as the specimen. The best results are obtained on freshly voided specimens. Testing should take place within one hour of voiding. Specimens should be well mixed, not centrifuged. If urine cannot be tested immediately, the specimen should be refrigerated to avoid deterioration. Before testing, refrigerated specimens must be allowed to return to room temperature as some tests (for example, enzymatic tests for glucose or blood) are temperature dependent.

URINE COLLECTION

The container should be clean, well rinsed and clear of contaminants such as hypochlorites, which will give false results with some tests, such as protein.

APPEARANCE

Urine specimens should initially be observed for colour, odour and turbidity as the appearance of urine will provide useful clues as to the presence of many substances in the specimen.

The odour of urine is affected by many components, such as urine concentration, food pigments, dyes, blood and drugs. The intensity of colour of normal urine is dependent on the concentrations. The colour of urine should therefore be noted from the normal amber through the lighter straw colours and darker yellows, and including any other colour which appears abnormal.

Normal, fresh urine has a characteristic odour. Urine that stands for any length of time develops an ammoniacal odour due to the decomposition of urea. Urine may vary from a fruity odour (in diabetes) to a foul odour (possibly urinary-tract infection).

Normal, fresh urine is usually clear or transparent but may have a cloudy or turbid appearance. The character of the urine should therefore be noted, in addition to a description of any sediment, for example, mucus, crystals or pus.

SPECIFIC GRAVITY

The specific gravity of urine indicates the relative proportions of dissolved solid components to the total volume of the specimen. It reflects the relative degree of concentration of dilution of the specimen. Under appropriate and standardised conditions of fluid restriction or increased intake, specific gravity measures the concentrating and diluting abilities of the kidney.

The specific gravity of urine can be determined with a urinometer, which is floated in a cylinder containing the urine. The urinometer measures directly the relative density of urine on a scale calibrated to read 1.000 in distilled water at a specific temperature (usually 15.6°C). The depth to which the urinometer sinks in the urine indicates the specific gravity, which is read on the urinometer scale at the junction of the urine with air.

It is important to remember that, for accurate results, certain corrections must be made on readings obtained with a urinometer. Correction for temperature is accomplished by adding (or subtracting) 0.001 for each 3°C above (or below) the calibration temperature. Corrections are also recommended when glucose or protein are present — 0.003 should be subtracted from the urinometer reading for each 1000 mg/dL (10 mg/mL) of glucose and protein. The urinometer requires large urine volume and is cumbersome to perform.

Alternative methods of direct and indirect determination are available of which the most common (and newest) is a reagent strip method utilising *Multistix-SG* or *N-Multistix-SG*. This recent development enables specific gravity to be read by colour change in conjunction with normal screening procedures (refer Chemical Test Procedures) thus providing greater convenience compared to the classical methods. No corrections for temperature, glucose or protein are required, whilst for increased accuracy, 0.005 may be added to readings from urines with a pH equal or greater than 6.5.

CHEMICAL TEST PROCEDURES

Chemically impregnated reagent strips are available for rapid determinations of urine specific gravity, pH, protein, glucose, ketones, bilirubin, haemoglobin, nitrite, urobilinogen and ascorbic acid. These strips are used in basic urinalysis and have replaced the older, more cumbersome methods. In addition, other reagent strips and chemical tablets are available for special determinations. Instrumentation is available which can process reacted reagent strips to allow standardisation of results.

The reactions employed in reagent strips are kinetic in nature and such results are time-dependent. The manufacturers' directions should be followed closely and, where additional equipment is required to perform the test, the recommended equipment should be used. For example, the *Clinitest* copper-reduction test utilises test tubes and droppers designed to give optimum results. The *Clinitest* droppers will dispense a standard volume, and the test tubes are of a specific diameter and length to give best results.

When using reagent strips, two methods can be employed.

Qualitative: this method is generally used for screening where multiple urine tests such as *N-Multistix-SG* or *Combur 9* are used. After dipping the reagent strip in urine, the results are read in 30 to 60 seconds. Any colour changes occurring within this time are to be considered a positive result.

Quantitative: where it is important to know how much of a substance is present, it is necessary to follow the timings specified by the manufacturer. All enzymatic tests need to be timed accurately if quantitative results are to be obtained.

SENSITIVITY

The level of sensitivity of urine reagent strips and tablets varies from one manufacturer to another, and this must be kept in mind when testing patients' urine specimens. It is important to know if the sensitivity of the test is sufficient for the task, and how the sensitivity relates to normal physiological concentrations of the substance in urine.

SPECIFICITY

Some urine reagent tests are specific for the substance being tested, but others are non-specific and will react with a range of substances in urine. An example is *Clinitest*, which will detect a range of reducing sugars in urine including glucose. By comparison, the enzymatic glucose strip tests *(Diastix, BM Test Glucose)* are specific for glucose only.

CLINICAL SIGNIFICANCE

The results obtained from testing urine provide valuable clinical information and assist the physician in arriving at a diagnosis.

Table 128 provides a concise summary of the results expected from urinalysis when various disease states are examined.

INTERFERING FACTORS

Many substances that may be present in urine can interfere with urine tests. The number and combination of drugs administered to patients may also cause misleading results. Table 129 presents a summary of the more common substances that may affect urine test results.

EXAMINATION OF BLOOD

REAGENT STRIP PROCEDURE

Several reagent strips are available for the determination of blood glucose levels – the only substance for which blood is tested in wards. The manufacturers' instructions should be followed exactly when utilising these products. All products utilise whole blood obtained from a finger prick.

The major differences between reagent strips relate to details of technique, the time taken to perform the test and the ability of the strip to be read in a blood-glucose meter or by visual interpretation of colour change.

Blood-glucose meters have been especially developed to enable accurate quantitation of the blood-glucose result. More precise results can thus be obtained, as the meter objectively determines the extent of any reagent colour change by measuring the amount of light reflected off the reagent area.

Most of these meters are portable and can be used at the patient's bedside or in the home, in addition to their widely accepted use in hospital wards. The manufacturers' operating manuals should be studied prior to using any of these instruments.

QUALITY CONTROLS

Quality-control solutions enable operators to ensure that their technique is correct when using reagent strips. Quality-control solutions for blood-glucose reagent strips are used in place of the patient's blood and will give a known result providing that the correct technique is utilised. These solutions are therefore invaluable for ensuring accuracy of results.

STORAGE OF REAGENTS

Urine and blood reagents are stable when stored and handled properly, but by virtue of their composition, are hygroscopic in nature. Prolonged exposure to moisture will lead to altered reagent activity. The desiccant packs or tablets supplied with reagents should not be removed. In general, reagents should be stored in a cool, dry area away from heat, sunlight, strong vapours and moisture. Reagents should not be refrigerated.

NURSING IMPLICATIONS

Assessment

Due consideration should be given to the need for a test and the clinical significance of results. Unnecessary testing constitutes a waste of health-care resources.

Implementation

Specific collection procedures need to be observed, particularly the double-void procedure for diabetic patients. If the desired time for testing is 11am, the patient is asked to void at 10.30am, then again at 11am, the second specimen being used for testing. This ensures that the urine-glucose level reflects the blood level as nearly as possible. Observe the following standard precautions for urine testing.

Use fresh, well-mixed, uncentrifuged urine.

Always replace the reagent bottle cap immediately.

Protect all reagent products against ambient moisture, light and heat.

Store reagents at temperatures under 30°C (86°F).

Accurate timing of reagent strip tests is essential for quantitative results.

Do not touch reagent test areas or excessively handle reagent tablets.

Remove excess urine from reagent strips by drawing the strip across the rim of the container.

Compare reagent colour development with colour charts in good, natural light whenever possible.

Record results of tests according to institutional policy.

Evaluation

Monitor reagents for expiry date. Check at each use for damage from moisture, light and heat. Monitor testing procedures to ensure optimum use of equipment.

Patient education

Many patients need to perform their own tests, particularly blood-glucose monitoring and urine testing for glucose and ketones. Teaching of these skills will need to occupy several sessions, with ample time allowed for the patient to perform the test under supervision and have questions answered. Thus teaching will need to begin well before discharge for an inpatient, or to occupy several sessions as an outpatient. The outpatient will need to know how to ensure a constant source of supplies and where to contact a resource person in case of future enquiries.

SELF-EVALUATION TEST

1. A normal fresh urine would best be described as which of the following?
   (a) colour – straw, amber or yellow
   (b) turbidity – clear, translucent or cloudy
   (c) odour – fruity, ammoniacal or aromatic
2. (a) What is the difference between a qualitative and quantitative procedure?
   (b) For general screening purposes, which procedure would be adequate?
3. How would you explain a positive result with *Clinitest* tablets and a negative result with *Diastix* on the same urine specimen?
4. What are the most important points to remember with regard to storage of reagent strips and tablets?
5. Why is it necessary to replace the cap immediately after removing reagent strips or tablets from the bottle?
6. What correction factors should be made when utilising a urinometer to measure specific gravity of urine?
7. Which of the following substances would you expect to find in the urine of a patient suspected of having diabetes?
   (a) blood
   (b) protein
   (c) glucose
   (d) ketones
   (e) all of the above
8. Why are quality controls important?
9. Which of the following substances may be detected in urine using currently available reagent strips?
   (a) protein
   (b) glucose
   (c) ketones
   (d) specific gravity
   (e) blood
   (f) potassium
   (g) bilirubin
   (h) vitamin A
   (i) urobilinogen
10. Where would you obtain technical information on urine or blood reagents if you did not have ready access to the manufacturer?

Table 128
Urine Chemistry Tests

	Renal	**Hepatic**	**Pancreatic**
Specific Gravity	Acute renal failure ▼ Renal tubular defects ▼ Polyuria ▼ Oliguria ▲	Hepatic disease ▲	Diabetes mellitus ▲ Diabetes insipidus ▼
pH	Renal tubular acidosis ▲ Bacterial infections ▲ Chronic renal failure ▲		Diabetic acidosis ▼
Protein	Nephrotic syndrome ▲ Pyelonephritis ▲ Glomerulonephritis ▲ Kimmelstiel-Wilson syndrome ▲ Malignant hypertension ▲		
Glucose	Lowered renal threshold ▲ Renal tubular disease ▲		Pancreatitis ▲ Diabetes mellitus ▲
Ketones		von Gierke's disease (glycogen storage disease) ▲	Diabetic acidosis
Bilirubin		Complete and partial obstructive jaundice ▲ Viral and drug-induced hepatitis ▲ Cirrhosis ▲	Carcinoma of the head of the pancreas ▲
Blood	**Haematuria in:** Acute nephritis Passive congestion of the kidneys Calculi Malignant papilloma Renal carcinoma Nephrotic syndrome Polycystic kidneys	**Haematuria in:** Cirrhosis (impaired prothrombin function)	**Haemoglobinuria in:** Kimmelstiel-Wilson syndrome
Nitrite	Significant Bacteriuria ▲ ($\geqslant 10^5$)		
Urobilinogen		Obstruction of the bile duct ▼ Liver cell damage ▲ Cirrhosis ▲	Carcinoma of the head of the pancreas ▼

The above findings are characteristic of the conditions listed but are not necessarily found consistently in all cases. Definitive diagnosis must rely upon clinical acumen and the results of other indicated procedures.

Gastrointestinal	Cardiovascular	Other	
		High fluid intake ▼ Dehydration ▲ Adrenal insufficiency ▲	
Diarrhoea ▼ Pyloric obstruction ▲ Malabsorption-**N** or ▲	Congestive heart failure-**N**	Dehydration ▼ Starvation ▼ Low-carbohydrate diets ▲	Acetazolamide therapy ▲ Metabolic acidosis ▼ Metabolic alkalosis ▲ Emphysema ▼
	Benign hypertension ▲ Congestive heart failure ▲ Subacute bacterial endocarditis ▲	Toxaemia of pregnancy ▲ Gout ▲ Acute febrile state ▲ Eclampsia ▲	Carbon Tetrachloride poisoning ▲ Electric-current injury ▲ Potassium depletion ▲ Orthostatic proteinuria ▲
Alimentary glycosuria ▲	Coronary thrombosis ▲	Phaeochromocytoma ▲ Hyperthyroidism ▲ Acromegaly ▲	Shock ▲ Pain ▲ Excitement ▲
Vomiting ▲		Starvation ▲ Low-carbohydrate diets ▲ Eclampsia ▲ Hyperthyroidism ▲	Trauma ▲ Chloroform or ether anaesthesia ▲
Choledocholithiasis ▲	Congestive heart failure in the presence of jaundice ▲	Recurrent idiopathic jaundice of pregnancy ▲	Noxious fumes ▲ Chlorpromazine hepatitis ▲
Haematuria in: Diverticulosis of the colon	**Haemoglobinuria in:** Bacterial endocarditis Intravascular haemolysis Hypertension with renal involvement	**Haemoglobinuria in:** Chronic infections Chronic phenacetin ingestion Sulfonamide therapy Sickle-cell disease **Myoglobinuria in:** Severe burns	Haemolytic anaemias Transfusion reaction Sudden cold Eclampsia Allergic reactions Multiple myeloma Alkaloids-poisonous mushrooms
Suppression of the gut flora ▼ (antibiotic therapy)	Congestive heart failure ▲ Extravascular haemolysis ▲	Noxious fumes ▲ Hepatitis associated with infectious mononucleosis ▲ Thalassaemia ▲ Pernicious anaemia ▲ Haemolytic anaemias ▲ Chlorpromazine hepatitis ▼	

N = Normal, ▲ = Increased ▼ = Decreased

Table 129
Factors Affecting Urine Chemistry Tests

Test	Urine constituents affecting results	The specific gravity test area on N-MULTISTIX® and other Ames reagent strip tests	T.S. Meter (refractometer)	Urinometer (hydrometer)
Specific gravity	Protein	Moderate concentrations may cause elevated results	Subtract 0.003 for every 1 g/dL protein	Subtract 0.003 for every 1 g/dL protein
	1% or more glucose	No effect	Subtract 0.004 for every 1 g/dL glucose	Subtract 0.004 for every 1 g/dL glucose
	pH	Add 0.005 for urine pH≥6.5	No effect	No effect
	X-ray contrast media	No effect	Elevated results	Elevated results
	Temperature	No effect	Most refractometers are temperature compensated between 60-100°F	A correction of 0.001 should be made for each 3°C above the calibration temperature indicated on the urinometer (usually 15.6°C or 60°F)

Test		Enzyme Strip Tests		Copper Reduction Tests	
Glycosuria	**Urine constituents causing false positive or negative reactions**	**Glucose test area KETO*DIASTIX® DIASTIX® N-MULTISTIX® and other Ames Multiple Reagent Strips**	**CLINISTIX®**	**Benedict's Solution**	**CLINITEST®**

	Sugars other than glucose				
	Galactose	No effect	No effect	Reacts positively	Reacts positively
	Lactose	No effect	No effect	Reacts positively	Reacts positively
	Levulose (fructose)	No effect	No effect	Reacts positively	Reacts positively
	Maltose	No effect	No effect	Reacts positively	Reacts positively
	Pentose	No effect	No effect	Reacts positively	Reacts positively
	Urine Constituents				
	Creatinine	No effect	No effect	May cause false +	No effect
	Uric acid	No effect	No effect	May cause false +	No effect
	Ketone bodies (Acetoacetic acid)	40 mg/dL AAA may cause false negative at glucose concentration of 100 mg/dL	No effect	No effect	No effect
If the enzyme test for glucose is positive and CLINITEST® is	High Specific Gravity	No effect	Depresses colour development	No effect	No effect
negative on the same specimen, it may be due to a concentration of glucose below the sensitivity range for which CLINITEST® is designed.	Low Specific Gravity	No effect	Intensifies colour development	No effect	No effect
A positive CLINITEST and negative enzyme test on the same	Drug Metabolities or Contaminants in Urine				
specimen is usually due to the presence of non-glucose reducing substances, i.e., lactose, galactose, etc.	Salicylates (aspirin)	No effect	Large concentrations may depress colour development	May cause false +	No effect
False positives can occur with	Penicillin (massive doses)	No effect	No effect	May cause false +	No effect
Benedict's more frequently than	Chloral hydrate	No effect	No effect	May cause false +	No effect
with CLINITEST because of	Glucosamine	No effect	No effect	May cause false +	No effect
differences in sensitivities of the	Streptomycin	No effect	No effect	May cause false +	No effect
two tests. By design, CLINITEST	Isoniazid	No effect	No effect	May cause false +	No effect

will detect approximately 0.25% levels of reducing substances. In contrast, Benedict's Solution has a sensitivity range from .07% to 0.15% and may react with those interfering substances listed.	Para-aminosalicylic acid	No effect	No effect	May cause false +	No effect
	Ascorbic Acid (AA)	50 mg/dL AA may cause false negative results by one colour block at glucose concentration of 100 mg/dL	May cause false negative reaction	May cause false + with large quantities	May cause false + with 250 mg/dL in urine
	Hypochlorite or Chlorine	May cause false+	May cause false+	No effect	No effect
	Peroxide	May cause false+	May cause false+	No effect	No effect
	L-Dopa	Large concentrations may depress colour development	Large concentrations may depress colour development	No effect	No effect
	Nalidixic acid (NegGram®)	No effect	No effect	May cause false +	May cause false +
	Cephalosporins (Keflin® Keflex®)	No effect	No effect	May cause false +	May cause false + or atypical reaction
	Probenecid (Benemid®)	No effect	No effect	May cause false +	May cause false +
	X-ray Contrast Media (Hypaque® Meglumine)	No effect	No effect		May cause false negative reaction

Proteinuria	**Urine constituents causing false positive or negative reactions**	**The protein test area on N-MULTISTIX® and other Ames reagent strip tests**	**Sulfosalicylic acid or Exton's Reagent**	**Heat and acetic acid or nitric acid ring test**
	Urine turbidity	No effect	May confuse reading	May confuse reading
	X-ray contrast media	No effect	May cause false +	May cause false +
	Tolbutamide (Rastinon)	No effect	May cause false +	May cause false +
	Penicillin (massive doses)	No effect	May cause false +	May cause false +
	Sulphafurazole (Gantrisin®)	No effect	May cause false +	No effect

	Para-aminosalicylic acid in urines containing certain preservative agents	No effect		
	Highly buffered alkaline urine	May cause false +	May cause false −	May cause false −
	Quaternary Ammonium Salts	May cause false +	No effect	No effect
	Tolmetin Sodium (Tolectin®)	No effect	May cause false +	May cause false +
Ketonuria	**Urine constituents causing false positive or negative reactions**	**The improved ketone test area on N-MULTISTIX® and other Ames reagent strip tests**	**ACETEST® Reagent Tablets, Rothera or liquid nitroprusside**	**Gerhardt or liquid ferric chloride**
	L-Dopa	False Positive (trace or less)	False Positive (atypical colour)	False Positive
	PKU (large quantities of phenylketones)	No effect	False Positive	No effect
	BSP	No effect	False Positive	No effect
	Salicylate or metabolities of aspirin	No effect	False Positive	False Positive
	Highly pigmented urines	May produce positive (trace or less) results		
Bilirubinuria	**Urine constituents causing false positive or negative reactions**	**The bilirubin test area on N-MULTISTIX® and other Ames reagent strip tests**	**ICTOTEST® Reagent Tablets**	**Watson or liquid ferric ion test**
	Salicylate	No effect	No effect	Interfering colour may give false positive
	Pyridium® and other highly coloured compounds	Could mask small reaction	Could mask small reaction	No effect if blank is used
	Rifadin®	Could mask or mimic positive reaction	Could mask small reaction	No effect if blank is used.

	Ascorbic Acid	25 mg/dL AA may cause False Negative Reaction	Very large quantities may cause False Negative Reaction	Very large quantities may cause False Negative Reaction
	Chlorpromazine (e.g. Largactil®) metabolites	False Positive with large quantities	False Positive with large quantities	No effect
	Not freshly voided urine specimen	May give false negative	May give false negative	
Occult Blood	**Urine constituents causing false positive or negative reactions with tests for hematuria and hemoglobinuria**	**The occult blood test area on N-MULTISTIX® and other Ames reagent strip tests**	**Microscopic examination of urine sediment**	
	High specific gravity urines	May reduce reactivity	No effect	
	Elevated protein levels in urines	May reduce reactivity	No effect	
	Oxidizing contaminants, i.e. hypochlorite	May produce false positives	No effect	
	Microbial peroxidase from urinary tract infection	May produce false positives	No effect	
	Ascorbic acid (5 mg/dL or greater) in urines	May cause false negatives at trace level	No effect	
	Myoglobin	Reacts positively	Will not be detected	
	Erythrocytes settled out in container (not a well-mixed urine)	May cause false negative reaction	May not be detected	
	Lysed erythrocytes	Reacts postively	May not be detected	
Nitrite	**Urine constituents causing false positive or negative reactions**	**The nitrite test area on N-MULTISTIX® reagent strip**		
	Azo Dye Metabolites (Pyridium®)	Could Mask or Mimic Positive Reaction	**Note: Consult latest product insert for complete information on any of the Ames Tests.**	
	Pink spots or pink edges	Do not interpret as a positive result		
	Any degree of uniform pink colour development	Interpret as a postive result suggesting presence of 10^5 or more organisms per ml; colour		

		development is not proportional to number of bacteria		
	Urinary tract infections caused by organisms not containing reductase to convert nitrate to nitrite	Negative results		
	When urine has not been retained in bladder long enough (4 hours +) to reduce nitrate to nitrite	May yield negative results		
	Lack of dietary nitrate in presence of organisms	Negative results		
	High specific gravity urines	Sensitivity is reduced		
	Ascorbic acid (25 mg/dL. or greater) in urines.	May cause false negative results if urine contains nitrite ion in concentrations of 0.03 mg/dL or less		
Urobilinogenuria	**Urine constituents causing false positive or negative reactions with tests for urobilinogenuria**	**The urobilinogen test area on N-MULTISTIX®**	**Wallace and Diamond dilution**	**Watson semi-quantiative**
	Bilirubin	No effect	Masks colour	Masks colour
	Blood	No effect	May obscure result	No effect if blank is used
	Interfering substances i.e. para-amino salicylic acid, known to react with Ehrlich's reagent	Will react with test area	Atypical	No effect if blank is used
	Drugs containing azo dyes (i.e. Azo Gantrisin)	May give a masking golden colour	Atypical	No effect if blank is used
	Detection of Porphobilinogen	Not reliable by this method		
	Absence of Urobilinogen	Cannot be determined with this test		

Reproduced by permission of Ames Division, Miles Laboratories Limited, Stoke Poges, Slough, Berks.

Table 130
Urine Chemistry Tests

Reproduced with kind permission of BCL (Boehringer Corporation (London) Limited)

Rapid Diagnostics

○ qualitative

◐ semiquantitative

	Urine									Blood	Faeces	
	Leucocytes	Nitrite	pH	Protein	Glucose	Ketones	Uribilinogen	Bilirubin	Blood	Glucose	Albumin	
BM Test 8®		○	◐	◐	◐	○	◐	○	◐			Routine screening
BM Test 7®			◐	◐	◐	○	◐	○	◐			
BM Test 5L®			◐	◐	◐	○			◐			
BM Test 4®		○	◐	◐	◐							
BM Test 3®			◐	◐	◐							
BM Test Meconium®											○	
Keto-Diabur-Test 5000®					◐	○						Diabetes mellitus
Diabur-Test 5000®					◐							
Ketur-Test®						○						*Semiquantitative visually; qualitative with meter
BM-Test-Glycemie 1-44®										*		
Nephur Test + Leucocytes®	◐	○	◐	◐	◐				◐			Kidneys and urinary tract
Albym Test®				◐								
Sangur Test®									◐			
Bilugen Test®							◐	○				Liver

APPENDIX A

INTERPRETATION OF MEDICAL PRESCRIPTION ABBREVIATIONS

1. Relating to weight, measure or strength

mL, ml, cc	millilitre
L, l	litre
mcg, microg, μg	microgram
mg	milligram
g	gram
kg	kilogram
mEq	milliequivalent
i.u.,IU	international units
mmol	millimole
micromol, μmol	micromole

2. Relating to dose form

cap, caps	capsules
elix	elixir
gtt, guttae	eyedrops
inj	injection
lin	liniment
linct	linctus
mist, mixt	mixture
neb	spray for inhalation
oc	eye ointment
pess	pessary
pulv	powder
sol, soln	solution
supp	suppositories
susp	suspension
tab, tabs	tablets
tinct, tr	tincture

3. Relating to route of administration

p.o.	by mouth
p.r.	by rectum
p.v.	by vagina
HI	hypodermic injection
IM	intramuscular
IV	intravenous
SC, s.c.	subcutaneous
LE	left eye
RE	right eye

4. Relating to time of administration

a.c.	before meals
c.c, c̄.c	with meals
p.c.	after meals
m, mane	morning
n, nocte	night
h.s.	bedtime
b.d., bid	twice a day
tds, tid	three times a day
qds, qid	four times a day
q4h, qqh	every four hours
q6h	every six hours
stat	immediately, at once
sos	if necessary
prn	when necessary

5. Miscellaneous

p.d.	for pain
et	and
aq	water
ex aq	with water
c̄	with
K	potassium
KCl	potassium chloride
NaCl	sodium chloride
Fe	iron
$FeSO_4$	ferrous sulphate

APPENDIX B

MEDICAL ABBREVIATIONS USED IN THE TEXT

ADR	Adverse Drug Reaction
ADT	Adsorbed Diphtheria and Tetanus
ALG	Antilymphocyte Globulin
ANS	Autonomic Nervous System
AV	Atrioventricular
BEE	Basal Energy Expenditure
BP	British Pharmacopoeia
BPC	British Pharmaceutical Codex
BUN	Blood Urea Nitrogen
Cal	Calorie (N.B. often used to mean *kilo*calories)
CCF	Congestive Cardiac Failure
CDT	Combined Diphtheria and Tetanus
CML	Chronic Myelocytic Leukaemia
CNS	Central Nervous System
CPR	Cardiopulmonary Resuscitation
CSF	Cerebrospinal Fluid
CVP	Central Venous Pressure
DES	Diethylstilboestrol
DNA	Deoxyribose Nucleic Acid
DVT	Deep Venous Thrombosis
ECG	Electrocardiogram
EDTA	Ethylene Diamine Tetra-acetic Acid
ENT	Ears Nose and Throat
ESR	Erythrocyte Sedimentation Rate
GABA	Gamma-amino Butyric Acid
GIT	Gastrointestinal Tract
HCG	Human Chorionic Gonadotrophin
5-HT	5-Hydroxytryptamine
IPPR	Intermittent Positive Pressure Respiration
IPPV	Intermittent Positive Pressure Ventilation
kJ	kiloJoules
MAO	Monoamine Oxidase
MAOI	Monoamine Oxidase Inhibitor

MCT	Medium Chain Triglyceride
MRSA	Methicillin-resistant *Staphylococcus aureus*
NS	Normal Saline
NSAID	Non-steroidal Anti-inflammatory Drug
PET	Pre-eclamptic Toxaemia
PN	Parenteral Nutrition
QAC	Quaternary Ammonium Compound
REM	Rapid Eyeball Movement
RDS	Respiratory Distress Syndrome
RNA	Ribonucleic Acid
SLE	Systemic Lupus Erythematosus
TDB	Tripotassium Dicitrato Bismuthate
TPN	Total Parenteral Nutrition
USP	United States Pharmacopeia
UV	Ultraviolet
WHO	World Health Organization

APPENDIX C

GUIDELINES FOR THE INTRAVENOUS ADMINISTRATION OF ANTI-INFECTIVE AGENTS

Note: the information contained in these tables should serve as a guide only. Reference should be made to other sources (manufacturers and the literature) to obtain more complete information.

Anti-infective Agent	Compatible IV Fluids	Some Important Incompatibilities	Preparation and Administration
Amikacin sulphate	Sodium chloride 0.9% Dextrose 5%	Heparin	Add 500 mg/2 mL to 200 mL of fluid and administer over 30 to 60 min
Ampicillin sodium	Sodium chloride 0.9% Dextrose 5% Dextrose/saline Water for injections Normosol/plasmalyte	Aminophylline Chloramphenicol Clindamycin Lincomycin Gentamicin Heparin Sulphadiazine Vitamins B and C	Reconstitute with sodium chloride or water for injections, diluting 1 g to 20 mL and administer over 10 to 15 min; 30 to 40 min for doses less than 500mg/5mL
Amoxycillin sodium	Sodium chloride 0.9% Water for injections Stable at room temp for 2 to 3 hours in Dextrose 5%	Blood products Proteinaceous fluids Lipid emulsions	Reconstitute with sodium chloride or water for injections, diluting 1 g to 20 mL and administer IV at least over 3 to 4 min, preferably 15 min; may be given by IV infusion over 30 to 60 min; a transient pink discolouration or slight opalescence may appear during reconstitution; use solutions within 30 min of reconstitution, potency may decrease after this period
Amphotericin	Water for injections—to reconstitute, Dextrose 5% preservative free to infuse	Sodium chloride Calcium salts Potassium chloride Benzylpenicillin Carbenicillin Gentamicin Hydrocortisone	Reconstitute with water for injections then add to dextrose to produce a concentration of 0.1 mg/1 mL and administer immediately over a period of six hours. Do not include a membrane filter in the line.
Benzylpenicillin	Sodium chloride 0.9% Dextrose 5% Dextrose/saline Water for injections Normosol/plasmalyte	Aminophylline Gentamicin Heparin Lincomycin Sulphadiazine Vitamins B and C	Reconstitute with sodium chloride or water for injections, 600 mg to 10 mL and administer over 2 min; do not exceed an infusion rate of 300 mg per min

Carbenicillin sodium	Sodium chloride 0.9% Dextrose 5% Dextrose/saline	Chloramphenicol Erythromycin Gentamicin Heparin Lincomycin Vitamins B and C	Reconstitute with water for injections, diluting 1 g to 5 to 10 mL and administer over 3 to 5 min; may be given at an infusion over 30 to 40 min.
Cefotaxime	Sodium chloride 0.9% Dextrose 5% Dextrose/saline Water for injections Lactated Ringer's	Aminoglycosides — do not admix (e.g. amikacin, gentamicin, tobramycin) Sodium bicarbonate	Reconstitute with water for injections, diluting 1 g to at least 4 mL and administer over 3 to 5 min For intermittent IV infusion, dilute 2 g to 40 mL of water for injections or compatible IV fluid and infuse over 20 to 30 min For continuous IV infusion, dissolve 2 g in 100 mL of sodium chloride 0.9% or dextrose 5% and infuse over 4 h
Cefoxitin sodium	Sodium chloride 0.9% Dextrose 5%, 10% Dextrose/saline Water for injections Lactated Ringer's	Do not admix in same syringe or infusion container with any other antibiotic as precipitation may occur; manufacturer claims cefoxitin is stable with aminoglycosides when admixed in 200 mL of sodium chloride 0.9% or dextrose 5%	Reconstitute with water for injections, diluting 1 g or 2 g to 10 mL and administer over 3 to 5 min May be given by IV infusion
Cephaloridine	Sodium chloride 0.9% Dextrose 5% Dextrose/saline Water for injections		Reconstitute 500 mg with 2 mL of water for injections then dilute to 10 mL or 1 g with 2.5 mL and dilute to 20 ml; inject over 3 to 5 min
Cephamandole nafate	Sodium chloride 0.9% Dextrose 5%, 10% Dextrose/saline Water for injections Normosol M in D5W	Amikacin Calcium chloride; Gentamicin Lignocaine HCl (greater than 0.5%) Tobramycin Calcium gluconate Precipitation may occur with solutions containing magnesium salts	Reconstitute with water for injections, dextrose 5% or sodium chloride 0.9%, diluting 1 g to 10 mL and administer over 3 to 5 min; for an intermittent infusion, if water for injections is used to reconstitute, dilute 1 g with 20 mL to avoid a hypotonic solution; for continuous IV infusion, reconstitute 1 g with 10 mL water for injections and add to compatible IV fluid

continued

Cephalothin sodium	Sodium chloride 0.9% Dextrose 5% Dextrose/saline Water for injections Normosol/plasmalyte	Aminophylline Benzylpenicillin Calcium salts Erythromycin Gentamicin	Reconstitute 2 g with 10 mL of water for injections and inject over 3 to 5 min; may be administered in a larger volume over 15 to 20 min
Cephazolin sodium	Sodium chloride 0.9% Dextrose 5% Dextrose/saline Water for injections	Aminophylline Calcium salts Erythromycin Gentamicin Heparin	Reconstitute with water for injections or sodium chloride and dilute 1 g to at least 10 mL; Inject over 3 to 5 min; may be administered in a larger volume over 30 to 60 min
Cephradine	Sodium chloride 0.9% Dextrose 5% Water for injections	Calcium salts Lignocaine	Reconstitute 1 g with 10 mL of water for injections and inject slowly over 3 to 5 min
Chloramphenicol sodium succinate	Sodium chloride 0.9% Dextrose 5% Dextrose/saline Water for injections Normosol/plasmalyte	Aminophylline Ampicillin Benzylpenicillin Carbenicillin Sulphadiazine Vitamins B and C	Reconstitute with 11 mL of water for injections to produce a solution containing 100 mg/mL (10%); inject over 1 min
Clindamycin phosphate	Sodium chloride 0.9% Dextrose 5% Dextrose/saline Normosol/plasmalyte	Aminophylline Ampicillin Vitamins B and C	Must be diluted prior to intravenous administration to a concentration of 600 mg/100 mL (6 mg/mL) at least; infuse over 20 min or longer. Not to be given by IV bolus
Cloxacillin sodium	Sodium chloride 0.9% dextrose 5% Dextrose/saline Water for injections	Gentamicin Lincomycin	Reconstitute 500 mg with 2 mL of water for injections or sodium chloride and inject slowly over 3 to 4 min. Doses of 1 g should be diluted to at least 20 mL
Colistin	Sodium chloride 0.9% Dextrose 5% Dextrose/saline Water for injections	Cephalothin Erythromycin Sodium Hydrocortisone	Reconstitute 150 mg with 2 mL of water for injections to produce a solution containing 75 mg/mL; Inject slowly over 3 to 5 min

Erythromycin lactobionate	Sodium chloride 0.9% Dextrose 5%	Carbenicillin Cephalothin Chloramphenicol Heparin Lincomycin Vitamins B and C	Reconstitute with 10 mL of water for injections. Further dilute to 1 g per 100 mL or more with infusion solution. Infuse 100 mL of solution over 30 to 45 min
Flucloxacillin sodium	Sodium chloride 0.9% Dextrose 5% Dextrose/saline Water for injections	Avoid mixing with proteinaceous materials	Reconstitute with 10 mL of water for injections (1 g to 20 mL) and inject slowly over 3 to 4 min
Gentamicin	Sodium chloride 0.9% Dextrose 5% Dextrose/saline Normosol/plasmalyte	Amphotericin Cephalothin Chloramphenicol Heparin Penicillins Sulphadiazine	Dilute 80 mg to 10 mL with fluid and inject over 3 to 5 min; or for infusion, add gentamicin to fluid to produce a solution containing 1 mg/mL and infuse at a rate of 100 mL over 30 to 45 min
Latamoxef disodium	Sodium chloride 0.9% Dextrose 5% Dextrose/saline Water for injections Normosol-M/Plasmalyte in D5W Lactated Ringer's Ringer's	Aminoglycosides — do not admix Avoid alcohol-containing solutions	Reconstitute with water for injections, sodium chloride 0.9% or dextrose 5%, diluting 1 g to 10 mL and administer over 3 to 5 min; for intermittent IV infusions, if water for injections is used to reconstitute, dilute 1 g to 20 mL to avoid a hypotonic solution; for continuous IV infusion, reconstitute 1 g with 10 mL water for injections and add to compatible IV fluid
Lincomycin	Sodium chloride 0.9% Dextrose 5% Dextrose/saline Normosol/plasmalyte	Carbenicillin Cloxacillin Heparin Sulphadiazine	Must be diluted prior to intravenous administration to a concentration of 600 mg/60 mL (10 mg/mL) and infused over 1 hour
Methicillin	Sodium chloride 0.9% Dextrose 5% Dextrose/saline Water for injections Normosol/plasmalyte	Hydrocortisone Sulphadiazine	Reconstitute with 5 mL of water for injections and inject over 5 to 10 min
Metronidazole	Sodium chloride 0.9% Dextrose 5% Dextrose/saline	Do not admix with other anti-infective agents	Infuse at a rate of 5 mL per minute (solution contains 5 mg/mL)

continued

Miconazole	Sodium chloride 0.9% Dextrose 5%		Must be diluted prior to intravenous administration with at least 200 mL of fluid and infused over 30 to 60 min
Netilmicin	Sodium chloride 0.9% Dextrose 5%, 10% Water for injections Lactated Ringer's Ringer's	Manufacturer recommends to avoid admixing with other drugs	Dilute to 10 mL with water for injections and inject slowly over 3 to 5 min; or for infusion, dilute in 50 mL to 200 mL of sodium chloride or dextrose 5% and infuse over 30 min to 2 hours
Piperacillin sodium	Sodium chloride 0.9% Dextrose 5% Dextrose/saline Water for injections Lactated Ringer's Dextran in sodium chloride; the above IV fluids containing potassium chloride	Amikacin Cephalosporins Sodium bicarbonate Tobramycin Whenever piperacillin is administered concurrently with another antibiotic, the two drugs should be administered separately. Do not mix in the same solution.	Reconstitute with water for injections, diluting 1 g to 5 mL and administer IV over 3 to 5 min; solution may be further diluted prior to injection; for IV infusion, add the reconstituted solution to at least 50 mL of compatible IV fluid and infuse over 20 to 40 min
Sodium fusidate (fusidic acid)	Sodium chloride 0.9%		Reconstitute in 50 mL of buffer solution, then must be diluted prior to intravenous administration with 250 to 500 mL of fluid and infused over 2 to 4 hours

Sulphadiazine sodium	Sodium chloride 0.9%	Aminophylline Cephalothin Chloramphenicol Gentamicin Heparin Hydrocortisone Lincomycin Penicillins	Administer as an infusion or as a solution containing no more than 1 g per 20 mL over 20 min Do not admix with other drugs.
Ticarcillin	Sodium chloride 0.9% Dextrose 5% Dextrose/saline Water for injections Normosol/plasmalyte	Gentamicin Tobramycin	Reconstitute 1 g with 4 mL of water for injections, then dilute further to produce a solution containing 1 g per 20 mL; Inject slowly over 5 to 10 min or administer as an IV infusion
Tobramycin	Sodium chloride 0.9% Dextrose 5% Dextrose/saline	Calcium salts Cephalosporins Heparin Penicillins	Add to 50 or 100 mL of infusion solution and administer over 20 to 45 min
Trimethoprim-Sulphamethoxazole	Sodium chloride 0.9% Dextrose 5% Dextrose/saline	Avoid admixing with other drugs	Dilute one ampoule, 5 mL (80 mg:400 mg) to 125 mL with infusion solution and administer over 60 to 90 min
Vancomycin	Sodium chloride 0.9% Dextrose 5% Dextrose/saline Water for injections	Chloramphenicol Benzylpenicillin	Reconstitute 500 mg with 10 mL of water for injections; dilute further to 100 to 200 mL and infuse over 20 to 30 min
Vidarabine	Sodium chloride 0.9% Dextrose 5% Dextrose/saline Normosol/plasmalyte	Avoid admixing with other drugs	Shake the vial well prior to use; pre-warm the intravenous fluid to 37°C, then add the suspension slowly, swirling the IV container. Do not add more than 500 mg to 1 litre of fluid. Infuse slowly over 12 or more hours. Include an in-line filter in the line.

APPENDIX D

PARENTERAL NUTRITION PROTOCOL
TOTAL PARENTERAL NUTRITION TEAM — WODEN VALLEY HOSPITAL (AUSTRALIA)

Parenteral nutrition is of increasing importance to medicine, but this expensive therapy must be used correctly to ensure maximum benefit and minimal morbidity. The following are guidelines.

1. *Costs*

When contemplating initiation of parenteral nutrition, consideration should be given to the potential benefit to the patient opposed to the cost of therapy.

2. *Indications for Parenteral Nutrition*

Providing there is no preceding nutritional impairment, 5% dextrose suffices to provide the calories required to prevent ketosis for the usual three to four days' post-operative starvation period, or in acute medical conditions where normal oral intake of food is interrupted for this time.

Parenteral nutrition should not be undertaken lightly but should be part of a general plan of management of patients who are extremely debilitated and who would be benefited by (and are not able to take) oral nourishment. Enteral feeding with prepared formulations such as *Ensure* or *Isocal* through fine-bore nasogastric tubes should be considered as the preferable alternative to parenteral nutrition when possible.

Broad indications for intravenous nutrition are:

1 *Medical Conditions*
- (a) Severe ulcerative colitis
- (b) Severe Crohn's disease
- (c) Acute hypercatabolic renal failure
- (d) Severe malabsorption syndromes
- (e) Malignant disease of the alimentary tract with cachexia
- (f) Starvation states
- (g) Loss of body protein due to excessive vomiting or diarrhoea
- (h) Dysphagia

2 *Surgical Conditions*
- (a) Starvation longer than five days
- (b) High intestinal fistulae
- (c) Breakdown of intestinal anastamosis
- (d) Peritonitis
- (e) Severe trauma
- (f) Renal failure of traumatic or surgical origin
- (g) Short bowel syndrome
- (h) Severe burns
- (i) Impaired immune competence prior to surgery

3. *Contraindications to Parenteral Nutrition*

1 Fat solutions should be used with caution in severe blood dyscrasias, gross hepatic insufficiency and hyperlipaemias.
2 Diabetes mellitus, unless meticulously supervised.
3 Fluid overload conditions, e.g. cardiac failure, cerebral oedema.
4 Hepatic failure, which precludes amino acid and fat solutions.

4. *Requirements*

A standard formulation of Total Parenteral Nutrition solution is available. This is referred to as "TPN-1". Additional requirements are supplied on a daily basis, according to each patient's fluid, electrolyte, lipid and calorie requirements. Broadly speaking, parenteral nutrition is based on daily requirements of:

Water	35 mL/kg
Calories	30 kcal/kg (125 kiloJoules)
Carbohydrates	2 g/kg
Protein (as amino acids)	1 g/kg

5. *Formulation of Solutions*

The solution in use has been formulated on the following basis:

The ratio between available non-nitrogen calories and the nitrogen content of the solution (in grams) should be between 145:1 and 215:1 for complete utilisation of the nitrogen.

1 Dextrose is the calorie source of choice; it is both safe and cheap. It yields approximately 4 kilocalories (about 17 kJ) per gram.
2 Costly lipid emulsions such as *Intralipid* are not employed as primary calorie sources, but rather on an intermittent basis to avoid essential fatty acid deficiency. However, circumstances sometimes dictate their use as an energy course in a non-routine manner.
3 Small doses of insulin may be added as needed to assist the patient to utilise the carbohydrate load and for their anabolic effect.

6. *Solution Available*

Parenteral nutrition at Woden Valley Hospital is administered from a standard formula detailed below. This is prepared in bulk and can only be modified after manufacture by addition of compatible substances. The solution is strongly hypertonic and is administered only through a central venous catheter.

It is intended that a therapeutic goal be determined and the appropriate daily volume of solution be chosen upon which to base the regimen.

TPN–1

1 litre of TPN–1 yields 6.5 g of nitrogen (equivalent to 42 g of protein) and 940 kcal (3929 kJ).

At the usual administration rate of 3 litres per day, TPN–1 provides approximately 20 g of nitrogen and 2820 kcal.

The therapeutic goal largely indicates the volume to be administered daily.

In 1 Litre

Synthamin 13 (8% 1-amino acids)	500 mL
Dextrose 50%	500 mL

Electrolytes

Sodium	35 mmol (35 mEq)
Potassium	30 mmol (30 mEq)
Magnesium	2.5 mmol (5 mEq)
Acetate	65 mmol (65 mEq)
Chloride	37 mmol (37 mEq)
Phosphate	15 mmol (45 mEq)
Calcium	3 mmol (6 mEq)

Trace Elements

Trace Elements Formula (WVH)	0.5 mL
Heparin Sodium	1000 units
Insulin BP	(as needed)

Calorie-To-Nitrogen Ratio

The formula listed contains baseline electrolytes and the regime is tailored to the patient's needs by the administration of additional electrolytes, vitamins, insulin, etc., immediately before the solution is released from the pharmacy.

Compatibility of Ingredients

Note: Some components of TPN therapy such as calcium and folic acid may be unstable or incompatible in TPN solutions under certain circumstances. Formulation and routes of administration may require adjustment in these cases.

Vitamins

Vitamin requirements are supplied by daily 1 mL doses of *Dayamin* to the first TPN bag of the day.

Dayamin contains in 1 mL:

Thiamine HCl	10 mg	Vitamin A —4000 IU
Riboflavin	2.5 mg	Vitamin D — 500 IU
Niacinamide	37.5 mg	Vitamin E — 1 IU
Sodium pantothenate	5 mg	
Pyridoxine	2.5 mg	
Vitamin C	50 mg	
Cyanocobalamin	2 micrograms	

Trace Elements

Woden Valley Hospital has adopted a standard Trace Element Formulation for use in parenteral nutrition based upon recommendations of the (US) AMA Expert Panel on Essential Trace Element Preparations for Parenteral Use, 1979.

Contained in 0.5 mL		*Recommended Daily Intake (1.5 mL)*
Copper	0.5 mg	1.5 mg
Manganese	0.16 mg	0.48 mg
Zinc	2.0 mg	6.0 mg
Chromium	5 micrograms	15 micrograms

Suggested Dosage: 0.5 mL per litre of PN solution

Additional Zinc Requirements

In addition to the zinc provided by this formulation, doses of 15 mg or more per day may be considered in patients for whom there is the need to promote wound healing. In this case, zinc chloride to make up the total dose is added to the TPN solution during preparation.

7. *Additional Requirements in Long-Term TPN*

In long-term parenteral nutrition, certain deficiencies occur and need to be replenished from the third week. These are:

1 Essential fatty acids, available in *Intralipid*. Give 500 mL of 10% emulsion by the peripheral route each week.
2 Trace elements, zinc, copper, manganese and chromium. Give up to 1.5 mL of WVH formula daily.
3 Folic acid, 7.5 mg IV weekly.
4 Vitamin K, 10 mg IV weekly.
5 Calcium, depleted from bone stores. Give 10 mmol (20 mEq) per day.

Blood and Human Serum Albumin are given when indicated.

Adjust daily requirements according to daily serum electrolytes and 24-hour urine losses. Additional losses of protein, electrolytes and bicarbonate from nasogastric tube and wound drains must also be accounted for.

Whenever adequate nutrition can be accomplished by oral or nasogastric tube feeding, parenteral nutrition should be ceased.

8. *Commencing And Ceasing Therapy*

Since a standard formulation is employed, the strength of solutions remain unchanged. The therapy is gradually introduced to the patient according to the following plan:

Litres of PN-Solution	*Hours*	*mL / hour*
1	24	42
2	24	84
3 (full regime)	24	125

The need for addition of insulin to the PN-solution is assessed during this period. Doses to the order of 40 units per litre are added after day 3 if *Clinitest* urinalysis shows a result in excess of 1% sugar.

Therapy should be ceased gradually to avoid the possibility of rebound hypoglycaemia. In the event of sudden cessation becoming necessary, dextrose 5% should replace the TPN solution.

9. *Monitoring The Patient*

1 *Dextrostix* test of blood sugar level using the Ames Reflectance meter should be performed four-hourly initially, then daily after regime is stabilised.
Clinitest urinalysis should take place four-hourly.
Maintain a blood sugar level of 70 mg/100 mL (4 mmol/L) to 200 mg/100 mL (11 mmol/L). The renal threshold for glucose is normally exceeded and some glycosuria is to be expected, but 2% glycosuria is unacceptable. Hence increase or decrease the added soluble insulin accordingly.
2 The fluid balance chart must be carefully kept.
3 Weigh patient daily if possible.
4 *Biochemical And Haematological Monitoring Plan*
4a Initial Work-Up for New Patients:
SMAC
24-hour urinary urea
Serum Mg
Serum Zn
Serum Fe and Total Iron-binding Capacity
Serum Trace Elements (copper, manganese, chromium)
Serum Vit. D
Serum Vit. B_{12}
Full Blood Count
Serum Folate
Prothrombine Time
4b During Introduction of Full Regime:
Monday–6/60
Tuesday–6/60
Wednesday–SMAC, FBC, Zn, Mg
Thursday–6/60, 24-hour urinary urea
Friday–6/60
Saturday–6/60
Sunday–6/60
4c Patient Stable on Full Regime:
Monday–6/60
Wednesday–SMAC, FBC, Zn, Mg
Thursday–24-hour urinary urea
Friday–6/60
4d Patient at home:
Wednesday–SMAC, FBC, Zn, Mg

10. *Intravenous Techniques*

1 The preferred sites of IV catheterisation are the subclavian and internal jugular veins. The catheter is inserted under aseptic conditions (gown, gloves, mask, cap, drapes) and sutured in place. Currently, silastic catheters are favoured. A chest X-ray examination must be carried out immediately after IV cannulation to check the position of the tip of the catheter and to exclude the possibility of pneumothorax.

2 This catheter is for parenteral nutrition only. Three-way taps must not be inserted in the line, and the line is not to be used for blood sampling. CVP measurements or antibiotics. These measures are essential to prevent infection.
3 Antibacterial terminal filters (e.g. *Ivex-2*) are used routinely on both central and peripheral lines. (They must be removed if blood or *Intralipid* are infused). They should be replaced every 72 hours.
4 All catheters removed will have the tips aseptically severed and sent for culture, both for bacteria and fungi.
5 The catheter is changed only if it blocks or kinks, the patient shows unexplained fever, or there is obvious insertion site infection.

11. *Catheter Dressings*

1 These dressings will be carried out by trained nursing staff each Monday, Wednesday and Friday.
2 With usual aseptic precautions, the skin will be defatted using acetone or isopropanol swabs. The site is disinfected for five minutes with *Betadine* solution applied by swabsticks.
3 *Betadine* ointment will then be applied at the catheter insertion site.
4 An *Op-Site* occlusive dressing will then be applied.
5 Any evidence of infection, catheter kink, leak or malfunction should be reported to a member of the TPN team.
6 A new giving set is supplied already fitted to each bag of TPN solution.

Suggested References for Further Reading

Avery, G. S., *Drug Treatment*. Sydney: Adis Press.
Aviado, D. M., *Pharmacological Principles of Medical Practice*. Baltimore: Williams and Wilkins.
Ball, A. P., Gray, J. A. and Murdoch, J. McC., *Antibacterial Drugs Today*. Sydney: Adis Press.
British National Formulary. London: British Medical Association and The Pharmaceutical Society of Great Britain.
Goodman, L. S. and Gilman, A., *The Pharmacological Basis of Therapeutics*. London: Macmillan.
Martin, E. W., *Hazards of Medication*. Philadelphia: Lippincott.
Martindale, *The Extra Pharmacopoeia*. London: The Pharmaceutical Press.

INDEX

Trade names are in *italics*.

Remember — drug names marked with a dagger (†) in the text are not currently available at NHS expense.

It has always been the duty of the nurse to administer drugs to patients, but this often simple act of drug administration carries with it a broader responsibility. The nurse must carry out this duty with accuracy and care, and with an understanding of what benefits and hazards the drug may bring to the patient. The nurse will be required to give a degree of informed and responsible information when patients enquire about their drugs. In addition to defining drug groups, drug action, uses, adverse reactions and precautions, this text has the following unique features: the information has been directed towards the needs of the practising nurse; a section on nursing implications of drug use is included in all chapters; learning objectives and self evaluation questions are included. The original Australian book was written by a team of hospital pharmacists and other health professionals with clinical experience at ward level and involvement in nurse education.

This British edition has been thoroughly adapted for use in the United Kingdom and the Republic of Ireland by a team from the Westminster Hospital, London.

F. Mary Wellington SRN, RNT
Senior Nurse: Education
The Wolfson School of Nursing of Westminster

Denise Victoria Hoare BSc(Hons), MPS
Staff Pharmacist
The Westminster Hospital

Jeremy Hyde PhD, BPharm(Hons), MPS
Assistant General Manager
Charing Cross Hospital, London
Formerly Principal Pharmacist, The Westminster Hospital

Brigid Mary Knight SRN, OND, DN (Lond), DipNEd (Lond)
Tutor, The Wolfson School of Nursing of Westminster

Dee Montague-Johnstone RGN, RCNT, DipNEd (Lond)
Tutor, The Wolfson School of Nursing of Westminster

Diane Roberts SRN, RSCN, RCNT
Clinical Teacher
The Wolfson School of Nursing of Westminster

ISBN 0-7020-1169-X

Baillière Tindall
33 The Avenue, Eastbourne
East Sussex BN21 3UN

9 780702 011696